NUTRITION
and ALCOHOL

Linking Nutrient Interactions and Dietary Intake

NUTRITION
and ALCOHOL

Linking Nutrient Interactions
and Dietary Intake

Edited by
Ronald Ross Watson
Victor R. Preedy

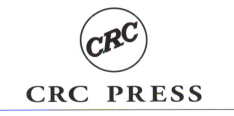

CRC PRESS

Boca Raton   London   New York   Washington, D.C.

Library of Congress Cataloging-in-Publication Data

Nutrition and alcohol : linking nutrient interactions and dietary intake
/ edited by Ronald R. Watson and Victor R. Preedy
    p. ; cm.
  Includes bibliographical references and index.
  ISBN 0-8493-1680-4 (alk. paper)
  1. Alcohol — Nutritional aspects. 2. Alchoholism — Pathophysiology. 3.
  Drug–nutrient interactions
[DNLM: 1. Ethanol — metabolism. 2. Ethanol — pharmacology. 3.
Alcohol-Induced disorders — physiopathology. 4. Alcoholic
Beverages — adverse effects. 5. Food–Drug Interactions. 6.
Nutrition — physiology. QV 84 N976 2003] I. Watson, Ronald R. (Ronald
Ross) II. Preedy, Victor R. III. Title.
RC565.N874 2003
616.86′1—dc22
                                                      2003060241

Visit the CRC Press Web site at www.crcpress.com

© 2004 by CRC Press LLC

No claim to original U.S. Government works
International Standard Book Number 0-8493-1680-4
Library of Congress Card Number 2003060241
Printed in the United States of America 1 2 3 4 5 6 7 8 9 0
Printed on acid-free paper

Preface

Humankind has had a complex relationship with alcohol from the beginning of recorded history. In most societies, some level of alcohol consumption is acceptable. In the United States, about 60% of high school students use alcohol. Alcohol-altered nutrition directly affects 10 million alcohol-abusing adults. It costs people in the United States more than $250 billion in health care, lost work, etc. Alcohol research is in a golden era. With more powerful tools for data collection and analysis and increased funding, the epidemiology of alcohol consumption, dietary consequences, role of nutrition in treatment of alcohol's pathology, and alcohol-related health issues are being better elucidated.

Chronic alcohol use is associated with heart, liver, brain, and other organ pathology. Alcohol is a drug of abuse and a caloric food. It causes poorer intake and absorption of nutrients, thus playing a major role in many aspects of clinical consequences. Alcohol use lowers consumption of fruit and vegetables, lowers tissue nutrients, and, in some cases, requires nutritional therapy by clinicians.

Nutrition and Alcohol: Linking Nutrient Interactions and Dietary Intake helps to define the causes and types of nutritional changes due to alcohol use and how nutrition can be used to ameliorate its consequences. Chapters deal with application of current nutritional knowledge by physicians and dietitians. An intimate, detailed knowledge of the effects of alcohol on the biochemical reactions and nutritional changes is critical in preventing or treating biomedical consequences.

Specific areas involving alcohol-related damage due to nutritional changes are reviewed. These include heart disease, obesity, digestive tract cancers, lactation, brain function, and liver disease. In addition, alcohol's effects on absorption of minerals and nutrients, a key role in causing damage, are treated. Diet is an important factor in modifying alcohol and its metabolite damage, or sometimes in enhancing them. Finally, efforts to explain alcohol's damage in addition to nutrient absorption and utilization include its role in peroxidation, methyl transfer, and production of acetaldehyde.

The book will become a desk reference for alcohol therapists and researchers as well as primary care physicians and dietitians. These professionals frequently need information on the nutritional effects of alcohol as well as the role of nutritional supplementation and diet in the therapy of alcohol pathology. The research progress over the past decade since the first book, *Nutrition and Alcohol*, edited by Dr. Ronald Watson in 1992, encourages us to summarize and evaluate in detail advances in understanding changes in nutritional biochemistry and physiology caused by ethanol (alcoholic beverages). It will assist the clinician, student, and dietitian to comprehend the complex changes caused by direct and indirect effects of ethanol at the cellular level via its nutritional modification. This book will stimulate research while educating health-oriented laypersons as well as scientists and health-care professionals.

About the Editors

Ronald Ross Watson, Ph.D., has edited 54 biomedical books. He directs several NIH-funded biomedical grants relating to the causes of heart disease and has studied the importance of fats in the diet for 20 years. His model studies have used both deficiency and excess. He is an internationally recognized nutritionist and immunologist, and recently edited two books on heart disease: *Alcohol and Heart Disease* (2002) and *AIDS and Heart Disease* (2002). He has contributed several chapters to this book, using research from his four NIH grants given by the National Heart, Lung, and Blood Institute to study cardiovascular disease. He also initiated and directed the National Institute of Alcohol Abuse and Alcoholism (NIAAA) Alcohol Research Center at the University of Arizona College of Medicine where the main goal was to understand the role of ethanol-induced immunosuppression on immune function and disease resistance in animals. Dr. Watson attended the University of Idaho but graduated from Brigham Young University in Provo, Utah, with a degree in chemistry in 1966. He completed his Ph.D. degree in 1971 in biochemistry from Michigan State University. His postdoctoral schooling was completed at the Harvard School of Public Health in Nutrition and Microbiology, which included 2 years of postdoctoral research experience in immunology. Dr. Watson is a member of several national and international nutrition, immunology, and cancer societies and research societies on alcoholism.

Victor R. Preedy, Ph.D., D.Sc., F.R.C. Path., is a professor in the Department of Nutrition and Dietetics, King's College, London. He directs studies regarding protein turnover, cardiology, nutrition, and, in particular, the biochemical aspects of alcoholism. Dr. Preedy graduated in 1974 from the University of Aston with a combined honors degree in biology and physiology with pharmacology. He received his Ph.D. in 1981 in the field of nutrition and metabolism, specializing in protein turnover. In 1992, he received his membership in the Royal College of Pathologists, based on his published works, and in 1993 a D.Sc. degree for his outstanding contribution to the study of proteins and metabolism. At the time, he was one of Aston University's youngest recipients of this distinguished award. Dr. Preedy was elected a fellow of the Royal College of Pathologists in 2000. He has published more than 450 articles, which include more than 135 peer-reviewed manuscripts based on original research, and 70 reviews. His current major research interests include the role of alcohol in enteral nutrition, and the molecular mechanisms responsible for alcoholic muscle damage.

List of Contributors

Junko Adachi
Department of Legal Medicine
Kobe University Graduate School of
  Medicine
Kobe, Japan

David J. Baer
Diet and Human Performance Lab
Beltsville Human Nutrition Research
  Center
Beltsville, Maryland

Giorgio Bedogni
University of Modena and Reggio
  Emilia
Modena, Italy

Stefano Bellentani
Centro Studi Fegato
Modena and Trieste, Italy

Adrian B. Bonner
Director of the Addictive Behaviour
  Group
Division of Psychiatry
Kent Institute of Medicine and Health
  Sciences
University of Kent
United Kingdom

Beverly A. Clevidence
Diet and Human Performance Lab
Beltsville Human Nutrition Research
  Center
Beltsville, Maryland

Christopher C. H. Cook
Psychiatry of Alcohol Misuse
Division of Psychiatry
Kent Institute of Medicine and Health
  Science
University of Kent
United Kingdom

David Crabb
Department of Medicine
Indiana University School of Medicine
  and
Richard L. Roudebush Veteran's Affairs
  Medical Center
Indianapolis, Indiana

Kevin D. Croft
Royal Perth Hospital Unit
School of Medicine and Pharmacology
University of Western Australia
Perth, Australia

Samuel W. French
Harbor UCLA Medical Center
Torrance, California

J. Michael Gaziano
Department of Medicine
Brigham and Women's Hospital,
  VA Boston Healthcare System, and
  Harvard Medical School
Boston, Massachusetts

Emilio González-Reimers
Servicio de Medicina Interna
Hospital Universitario de Canarias
Facultad de Medicina
Universidad de La Laguna
Tenerife, Spain

Armin Imhof
Department of Internal Medicine II –
  Cardiology
University of Ulm
Ulm, Germany

Fumiyasu Ishikawa
Yakult Central Institute for
  Microbiological Research
Tokyo, Japan

Mitsuyoshi Kano
Yakult Central Institute for
  Microbiological Research
Tokyo, Japan

Dawn Warner Kershner
Department of Medicine
Brigham and Women's Hospital and
  Harvard Medical School
Boston, Massachusetts

Hugo Kesteloot
Department of Epidemiology
School of Public Health
Catholic University of Leuven
Leuven, Belgium

Wolfgang Koenig
Department of Internal Medicine II –
  Cardiology
University of Ulm
Ulm, Germany

Michael Koll
Department of Nutrition and Dietetics
King's College London
London, England

David Mantle
Department of Agricultural and
  Environmental Science
Newcastle University
Newcastle upon Tyne
United Kingdom

Julie A. Mennella
Member and Director of Education
  Outreach
Monell Chemical Senses Center
Philadelphia, Pennsylvania

Robert R. Miller, Jr.
Department of Biology
Hillsdale College
Hillsdale, Michigan

Misako Okita
Department of Nutritional Services
Faculty of Health and Welfare Sciences
Okayama Prefectural University
Okayama, Japan

Vinood B. Patel
Clinical Biochemistry
King's College London
London, England

Timothy J. Peters
Clinical Biochemistry
King's College London
London, England

Victor R. Preedy
Department of Nutrition and Dietetics
King's College London
London, England

Ian B. Puddey
Professor of Medicine
Royal Perth Hospital Unit
School of Medicine and Pharmacology
University of Western Australia
Perth, Australia

Vijay A. Ramchandani
Laboratory of Clinical Studies
National Institute on Alcohol Abuse and
  Alcoholism
National Institutes of Health
Bethesda, Maryland

William V. Rumpler
Diet and Human Performance Lab
Beltsville Human Nutrition Research
  Center
Beltsville, Maryland

Ragnar Rylander
Department of Environmental Medicine
Göteborg University
Gothenburg, Sweden

Mikko P. Salaspuro
Research Unit of Substance Abuse
  Medicine
Biomedicum Helsinki
University of Helsinki
Finland

Francisco Santolaria
Servicio de Medicina Interna
Hospital Universitario de Canarias
Facultad de Medicina
Universidad de La Laguna
Tenerife, Spain

Takayo Sasagawa
Department of Nutritional Services
Faculty of Health and Welfare Sciences
Okayama Prefectural University
Okayama, Japan

Helmut K. Seitz
Laboratory of Alcohol Disease, Liver
  Disease, and Nutrition
Department of Medicine
Salem Medical Center
University of Heidelberg
Heidelberg, Germany

A. G. Shaper
Professor Emeritus of Clinical
  Epidemiology
Department of Primary Care and
  Population Sciences
Royal Free and University College
  Medical School
London, England

Patrick J. Skerrett
Department of Medicine
Brigham and Women's Hospital and
  Harvard Medical School
Boston, Massachusetts

Felix Stickel
Department of Medicine I
University of Erlangen-Nuremberg
Erlangen, Germany

Andrew Sumner
Division of Cardiology
Department of Medicine
Pennsylvania State University College
  of Medicine
Hershey, Pennsylvania

Allan D. Thomson
Kent Institute of Medicine and Health
  Sciences
University of Kent
United Kingdom

Claudio Tiribelli
Centro Studi Fegato, Modena and
  Trieste, Italy and
University of Trieste, Italy

Thomas C. Vary
Department of Cellular and Molecular
  Physiology
Pennsylvania State University College
  of Medicine
Hershey, Pennsylvania

Y.-J.Y. Wan
Department of Pharmacology,
  Toxicology, and Therapeutics
University of Kansas Medical Center
Kansas City, Kansas

Xiang-Dong Wang
Nutrition and Cancer Biology
  Laboratory
Jean Mayer USDA Human Nutrition
  Research Center on Aging
Tufts University
Boston, Massachusetts

S. Goya Wannamethee
Department of Primary Care and
  Population Sciences
Royal Free and University College
  Medical School
London, England

Simon Worrall
Department of Biochemistry and
  Molecular Biology
Alcohol Research Unit
School of Microbial and Molecular
  Sciences
The University of Queensland
Australia

Junko Yokoyama
Department of Nutritional Services
Faculty of Health and Welfare Sciences
Okayama Prefectural University
Okayama, Japan

Min You
Department of Medicine
Indiana University School of Medicine
  and Richard L. Roudebush Veteran's
  Affairs Medical Center
Indianapolis, Indiana

Jianjou Zhang
Hipple Cancer Research Center and
  Department of Community Health
Wright State University
School of Medicine
Dayton, Ohio

Renate R. Zilkens
Royal Perth Hospital Unit
School of Medicine and Pharmacology
University of Western Australia
Perth, Australia

Table of Contents

SECTION IV   Alcohol: Metabolism and Metabolites

SECTION V Alcohol and Nutrients

Section I

Overview of Nutrition and Alcohol

1 Alcohol and Nutrition: an Integrated Perspective

Francisco Santolaria and Emilio González-Reimers

CONTENTS

1.1 INTRODUCTION

Alcohol abuse is common in Western countries. Nutritional disorders remain among the most relevant medical problems of alcoholic patients since they are related to advanced alcoholism and to survival.

Ethanol is a highly energetic (7.1 kcal/g), readily oxidizable compound often present in the Western diet. It accounts for 5.6% of the total energy intake of the average American diet, despite the fact that about one third of the population is teetotaller.[1] Ethanol accounts for up to 10% of the total energy intake among social drinkers, this proportion reaching more than 50% in heavy alcoholics. Because of ethanol's high caloric content, ethanol consumption has been considered a risk factor for weight gain and obesity. However, weight loss is common among heavy drinkers, and there is controversy regarding changes in body weight and moderate alcohol consumption.[2]

0-8493-1680-4/04/$0.00+$1.50

From a nutritional point of view, ethanol is an energetic compound, but lacks any other nutritional value. On the other hand, it is also the most frequently abused psychoactive drug, the consumption of which leads to behavioral alterations, family and social problems, and dependence. Moreover, it is a toxic substance, which may potentially affect every organ or system, either directly or via acetaldehyde, its main metabolite. The ways in which these three properties may affect nutritional status are discussed below and constitute the main focus of this review.

1.2 PRIMARY MALNUTRITION

1.2.1 SHIFT OF NUTRIENTS

Moderate ethanol consumption increases rather than decreases dietary intake. Indeed, Westerterp-Plantenga and Verwegen (1999) showed that 24-h energy intake was higher on days in which a drink was consumed as an aperitif.[3] In contrast, heavy alcoholism leads to a substantial reduction of dietary intake, so consumption of other nutrients progressively decreases as ethanol intake increases.[4,5] Moreover, since heavy alcoholics underreport the amount of ethanol consumed, but overreport their nonalcoholic energy intake, this effect is probably even more important.[6,7]

Despite the fact that alcoholic beverages may account for up to 5% of the total energy intake, they should not be considered a food or, in the best of cases, only as a poor-quality food since they provide only one nutrient, lacking proteins, essential lipids, minerals, and the majority of trace elements and vitamins. Therefore, although the diet of a heavy drinker matches or even surpasses the caloric requirements, it may be inadequate in terms of protein, essential lipid, and other nutrient consumption.

In addition, ethanol may cause satiety because it delays gastric emptying.[8] There is controversy about the effect of ethanol on leptin (an anorexigenic protein) secretion. Whereas acute ethanol intake in healthy volunteers reduces serum leptin levels, these are increased in heavy alcoholics with dependence and decreased in alcoholics admitted for organic complications.[9–11]

1.2.2 ETHANOL-MEDIATED CALORIC WASTAGE

Pirola and Lieber (1972) in classic studies found a weight loss of about 1 kg after consumption for 14 d of a diet in which 50% of calories were substituted by ethanol. Moreover, no significant weight gain was observed when 2000 kcal (in the form of ethanol) were added to the diet, whereas subjects experienced a weight gain of nearly 3 kg when the same amount of calories was consumed in the form of chocolate. These findings were attributed to the metabolism of ethanol by energy-wasting pathways in chronic alcoholics.[12,13]

Ethanol is a xenobiotic product, which cannot be stored in the body, but becomes rapidly oxidized, displacing other fuels. Two main mechanisms are involved in ethanol metabolism: the alcohol dehydrogenase (ADH) pathway and the microsomal ethanol oxidizing system (MEOS). The ADH pathway requires reduction of NAD to NADH + H, but MEOS requires oxidation of NADPH to NADP, a process that consumes ATP and dissipates heat. Therefore, the ADH pathway yields 16 mol

ATP/mol of ethanol oxidized, whereas MEOS yields only 10. The MEOS pathway scarcely works in occasional ethanol consumers but is induced in chronic alcoholics.[14,15] Moreover, the existence of a futile metabolic cycle involving both systems has been proposed: ethanol would be transformed into acetaldehyde by MEOS and acetaldehyde, again to ethanol by ADH, a process which would consume six ATP molecules.[16,17]

1.2.3 INCREASED ENERGY EXPENDITURE

The effect of ethanol on energy expenditure, oxygen consumption, and thermogenesis has been studied by indirect calorimetry. In healthy volunteers, short-term ethanol administered as 25% of the total energy requirements, either added to the diet or given instead of other food, increases 24-h energy expenditure.[18,19] Since this experiment was carried out in healthy nondrinkers, ethanol should have been mainly metabolized by the ADH system and not by the MEOS. Therefore, mechanisms other than MEOS must be involved in the alcohol-mediated increase in energy expenditure, such as acetaldehyde-induced catecholamine secretion. When moderate amounts of ethanol, 5 to 10% of total daily calories, were added to the diet (as occurs with social drinkers), no change was observed in resting energy expenditure (REE).[20,21] However, Addolorato et al. (1998) report an increase in REE in long-term heavy drinkers (mean consumption of 195 g ethanol/d) when compared with social drinkers; chronic alcoholics show a significantly lower weight due to lower fat mass and increased fat oxidation.[22,23] Levine et al. (2000) also showed an increased fat oxidation and an increased REE, which is related to ethanol ingestion since both decrease 4 d after withdrawal.[24] Thus, it seems that ethanol increases REE, not only due to an enhanced MEOS metabolism, but also due to increased catecholamine secretion and uncoupled oxidative phosphorylation due to mitochondrial damage.[25,26]

1.2.4 EFFECT OF ETHANOL ON FAT OXIDATION

Ethanol may inhibit fat mobilization due to the antilipolytic effect of acetate.[27] In addition, an increased NADH/NAD ratio may enhance liver fatty acid and triglyceride synthesis. Suter et al. (1992) have shown in healthy nonalcoholic individuals that consumption of 96 g ethanol (about 25% of the daily caloric requirement) reduces the lipid oxidation rate by about 30%, an effect which was only observed during the period of the day in which ethanol was consumed and metabolized.[18] No significant effect was observed on protein and carbohydrate metabolism. Moreover, Siler et al. (1999) report that the intake of 24 g of ethanol by eight healthy volunteers led to an increase in hepatic *de novo* lipogenesis (from 2 to 30%), while 77% of the amount of ethanol was cleared and converted to acetate, which entered systemic circulation. Release of nonsterified fatty acids by adipose tissue decreased by 53%, and whole lipid oxidation by 73%. Therefore, the liver metabolizes ethanol into acetate, and this major end product of ethanol inhibits lipolysis.[28]

These changes would theoretically favor lipid accumulation and weight gain. However, epidemiologic studies support the conclusion that moderate ethanol consumers (less than 50 g/d), despite an increase in the total energy intake, show weight loss.[29,30] This apparent paradox — the loss of weight in moderate drinkers — has been interpreted by an ethanol-induced increased muscle sensitivity to insulin and a downregulation of insulin effect on adipose tissue, decreasing fat mass.[31]

Studies dealing with changes in body composition in chronic heavy drinkers describe fat loss. Addolorato et al. (1998), in chronic heavy drinkers (195 g/d) without liver cirrhosis or malabsorption, found a lower body weight due to fat mass reduction (the triceps skinfold was reduced but not the midarm muscle circumference), and a preferential use of lipids as fuel when compared with social drinkers. Fat distribution was also different in heavy drinkers than in social drinkers. Heavy drinkers showed a raised waist-to-hip ratio (both in men and women), a pattern which has been related to visceral fat deposition and liver steatosis, even in non-alcoholic subjects.[22,23] These metabolic changes improved 1 month after withdrawal, and totally reversed 3 months after alcohol cessation. A normalization of BMI and fat mass, and a decrease of fat oxidation with a parallel increase in carbohydrate oxidation, were recorded, and remained unchanged 6 months later (provided alcohol abstinence).[32]

1.2.5 EFFECTS OF ETHANOL ON PROTEIN METABOLISM

Ethanol increases urinary nitrogen excretion.[33,34] Reinus et al. (1989) studied eight alcoholic patients continuously fed by nasogastric tube. When ethanol accounted for 30% of the total caloric intake (about 100 g/d, an amount which does not surpass hepatic clearance rate), negligible ethanol concentrations were detected in blood, and no increase in urea nitrogen excretion was observed. However, when the amount of ethanol was increased to 40 to 60% of the total calories (about 180 g), blood ethanol concentration ranged from 250 to 300 mg/dl, urinary urea nitrogen and 3-methyl histidine increased (pointing to muscle wastage), and weight loss ensued.[35]

Ethanol administered to rats leads to reduced protein synthesis and type II muscle fiber atrophy, an effect probably dependent more on acetaldehyde than on ethanol itself. Type IIb fiber atrophy is more intense when a low-protein diet is added to ethanol.[36] The association of ethanol, malnutrition, and muscle atrophy is complex. It has been clearly shown that ethanol leads to muscle atrophy and cardiomyopathy in the absence of any kind of nutritional impairment.[37] However, malnutrition is frequently associated with alcoholic myopathy.[38] Histologically assessed muscle atrophy was found in one third of 64 heavy alcoholic drinkers of 217 g ethanol/d. Patients with muscle atrophy showed an impaired nutritional status, affecting not only muscle mass, but also subcutaneous fat.[39] Fernandez-Sola et al. (1995) reported that protein-calorie malnutrition is an independent predictive factor of type II fiber atrophy.[40] However, muscle atrophy implies a reduction in total body protein burden and is thus, in itself, a criterion of malnutrition. In any case, as Fernandez-Sola et al. (2000) show, alcoholic myopathy only appears with heavy ethanol consumption, at levels at which malnutrition is frequent. Interestingly, it may recover without total abstinence, only lowering the dose of ethanol consumption.[41]

In addition to muscle protein, ethanol and acetaldehyde may alter protein synthesis in every body tissue. It decreases protein synthesis in the majority of the tissues, such as bone, decreasing collagen, liver, decreasing albumin, prealbumin, IGF-1, its binding protein IGF1BP3, and osteocalcin, and whole-body nitrogen balance, but it also increases liver collagen synthesis.[42]

1.2.6 SOCIOECONOMIC STATUS, SOCIAL AND FAMILY PROBLEMS, AND IRREGULAR FEEDING

Malnutrition has been more frequently reported among skid-row and lower-class alcoholics than in middle-class ones.[43,44] In this sense, Goldsmith et al. (1983) found that only 8% of alcoholics of middle and high socioeconomic status were malnourished, in contrast with 32% of those belonging to a low social class.[45] Alcoholics frequently have social and family problems which disrupt social links and lead to an irregular lifestyle. Meals of lonely male alcoholics are often irregular. As alcoholics increase ethanol intake, they change their feeding habits, some meals are missed, and the quality of the diet consumed is poor.[5]

In a study performed on drug addicts — mainly heroin consumers — admitted for detoxification, we found that disruption of social and family links was related to anorexia and poor food intake and also to a more intense drug addiction.[46] In our culture, regular meals and adequate food intake are related to family life, family rupture leading to progressive marginalization and poverty. These factors, together with the anorexigenic effect of alcohol and the lack of interest in everything except ethanol consumption, may lead to progressive malnutrition. In this line, we studied 181 alcoholic patients, consumers of about 180 g ethanol daily. The heaviest drinkers showed the most irregular feeding habits and were severely underweight. The worst situation was suffered by the skid-row alcoholics, all of them unemployed, homeless, and without family support. Most of these patients (73%) showed a BMI below 20 kg/m^2, a finding which was observed only in 11% of nonskid-row alcoholics and in none of the controls. Skid-row alcoholics also showed an intensely decreased lean and fat mass assessed by midarm anthropometry and double energy x-ray absorptiometry (DEXA), and, subsequently, decreased hand grip strength. However, skid-row alcoholics did not show more somatic complications.[47]

Alcoholics eat frequently in bars or taverns instead of at home. They miss meals, meals are scanty, and portions are small and deficient in protein. Alcoholics who confessed irregular feeding habits had more social and family problems, drank more ethanol, and suffered a more intense malnutrition with decreased fat, lean and bone mass (pointing to a possible relationship between malnutrition and osteopenia); they showed low serum albumin, prealbumin and transferrin, cholesterol and triglyceride, and also serum folate and magnesium, and had a decreased hand-grip strength when compared with the remaining alcoholics. Thus, irregular feeding and loneliness may be the link between social and family problems and malnutrition.[47,48]

Alcohol abuse in teenagers may impair growth. The height of alcoholic patients was 4 cm less than that of the controls. Height of the alcoholics was related to age at the onset of drinking, which was before 15 years in nearly half the cases. Alcoholics who drank before 15 years of age were 3 cm shorter than the remaining alcoholics who did not drink at this age, and also showed a higher current ethanol intake.[47] Alcohol intake was related to decreased serum IGF-1 and osteocalcin levels, even among those alcoholics without liver disease.[47–49] A study performed on Harris lines, which may be related to growth arrest due to metabolic stress, showed a relation with ethanol intake during growth.[50]

Serum folate levels are reduced in alcoholics.[47,49,51–53] In a study on 103 male alcoholics (drinkers of a mean of 205 g/d) we found decreased serum folate and B_6 levels but increased B_{12} ones. Thirty percent of our alcoholics showed serum folate levels below 3 ng/l. The decrease in serum folate was not related to liver function impairment or to ethanol intake, despite the well-known interference of ethanol with folate metabolism and the ethanol-mediated enhancement of folate urinary excretion;[54,55] instead, it was related with nutritional data, especially with irregular feeding habits (only one meal per day, and one dish per meal) and poor consumption of one or more of the main food groups. Decreased B_6 levels were also related to malnutrition. Serum folate and B_6 levels were inversely related to homocysteinaemia.[56] Ethanol abuse may lead to hyperhomocysteinaemia,[52] which is more frequent (84%) in alcoholics with the TT polymorphism of methylentetrahydrofolate reductase.[56] Stroke is highly prevalent among heavy alcoholics. Indeed, heavy alcohol consumption — in contrast with light or moderate consumption — is a risk factor for stroke, despite high HDL levels. This increased risk could be attributed to hypertension, arrhythmia, or altered coagulation, three factors frequently observed in alcoholics, but which also could be related to hyperhomocysteinaemia.

1.3 SECONDARY MALNUTRITION

Many alcohol-related diseases may lead to malnutrition, mainly by interfering with intake or absorption of nutrients. Chronic gastritis, with anorexia and vomiting, and diarrhea, are common complications of alcohol consumption. However, chronic pancreatitis and liver disease are the two main causes of secondary malnutrition in alcoholics. Moreover, alcoholics frequently suffer episodes of infections and injuries, leading to superimposed stress malnutrition. Nicolás et al. (1993), in a study performed on 250 male chronic alcoholics, who drank a mean of 235 g ethanol per day, with stable social status and familial support, and who entered a treatment program for alcoholism, found that impaired nutritional status was mainly due to organic complications but not to alcohol itself. Indeed, nutritional status of alcoholics without organic complications was similar to that of the controls.[57] On the other hand, alcohol dependence does not seem to play an important role in alcoholic malnutrition. Alcoholics with major withdrawal symptoms, either at admission or during hospital stay, showed a nutritional status similar to those without withdrawal symptoms.[47]

1.3.1 CHRONIC ALCOHOLIC PANCREATITIS

Chronic alcoholic pancreatitis severely impairs nutritional status when exocrine pancreatic failure and diabetes mellitus with hypoinsulinemia (another cause of malnutrition) are present. Morillas et al. (1997) found malnutrition in 72% of patients with chronic alcoholic pancreatitis.[58] However, subtle pancreatic dysfunction leading to malnutrition may exist even in asymptomatic heavy drinkers. Aparisi et al. (2000)

found exocrine pancreatic dysfunction in 26% of 105 heavy drinkers (mean of 195 g/d) without any signs or symptoms of pancreatic alteration 30 d after withdrawal. One third of the affected cases had steatorrhea. All these alterations were related to an impaired nutritional status.[59]

1.3.2 LIVER CIRRHOSIS

Compensated liver cirrhosis may be associated with a normal or only slightly impaired nutritional status. In cirrhotics, interpretation of decreased serum albumin, transferrin, and prealbumin levels may be difficult since they may be secondary to liver failure rather than to malnutrition, or may even be related to infection or injury.[60] Serum IGF-1 and IGFBP3 levels show a better correlation with liver function than with nutritional status.[49,61]

Alcoholics with liver disease show some metabolic disturbances which may clearly influence nutritional status. A hypermetabolic state with increased thermogenesis has been observed in these patients, especially in those with superimposed alcoholic hepatitis.[62–65] However, these changes are not specific to alcoholic liver disease, since they are also observed in other forms of liver disease such as postviral cirrhosis.[66,67] Furthermore, not all cirrhotics are hypermetabolic. In fact, Muller et al. (1992) report hypermetabolism in 18% and hypometabolism in 31% of their cirrhotics. Those who were hypermetabolic showed a reduced muscle mass, whereas those who were hypometabolic, an increased fat mass.[68] Hypermetabolism has been related to increased serum levels of pro- and antiinflammatory cytokines.[69]

The substrate oxidation pattern becomes altered in the majority of cirrhotic patients. Cirrhotics cannot store glycogen and show resistance to insulin, so glucose oxidation decreases and lipid oxidation increases in nearly all the patients.[62,66,68,70] Leptin, an anorexigenic protein which also enhances the metabolic rate, is increased in cirrhotics studied by Campillo et al. (2001), Nicolás et al. (2001), and Lyn et al. (2002), but not in those reported by Onodera et al. (2001), who presented normal values. We also found normal leptin values in compensated cirrhosis but decreased ones in cirrhotics with ascites.[10,11,70–72]

In contrast to cirrhotics with ascites, compensated cirrhotics show a better nutritional status, even with 52% being overweight (BMI above 25 kg/m²). This overweight is related to an excess of fat, as lean mass was shown to be reduced both by creatinine excretion and by absorptiometry. Indeed, arm lean mass and hand-grip strength were both decreased to a similar degree in compensated cirrhotics and noncirrhotic alcoholics.[11,47–49] Other studies have also shown an excess of fat in cirrhosis. Overweight was reported in 18% of the 883 male cirrhotics who entered the Italian Multicentre Study (1994), and Bunout et al. (1983) found higher values of body weight (110% of ideal weight) and midarm fat area (113% of the standard) in alcoholics with cirrhosis or alcoholic hepatitis.[73,74] Therefore, obesity is not an uncommon finding in cirrhotics. However, the increased fat mass often coexists with a decreased lean mass, which is a criterion of malnutrition. In this sense Lautz et al. (1992), in a series of cirrhotic patients selected for liver transplantation, report that in about the half of those who were malnourished, total weight was normal in the face of a reduced lean mass and an increased fat mass, i.e., they suffered an obese type malnutrition.[75]

Nutritional status of decompensated cirrhotics (mainly by ascites or alcoholic hepatitis) is worse than that of noncirrhotic alcoholics.[11,47,49,76,77] Cirrhotics with ascites showed reduced lean and fat mass. Ascites causes anorexia and early satiety due to gastric compression and abdominal distension but not to altered gastric emptying: large volume paracentesis improves satiety and dietary intake but has no effect on gastric emptying.[78] Ascites drainage by peritoneovenous shunting improves fat and muscle mass, serum albumin and transferrin, and lymphocyte count.[79,80] Transjugular intrahepatic porto-systemic shunt (TIPS), the current therapeutic approach for refractory ascites, decreases portal hypertension and improves intestinal absorption. Allard et al. (2001) studied 10 cirrhotics with refractory ascites who underwent TIPS, before the procedure and during a follow-up period of 12 months. Total body nitrogen, total body fat, REE, caloric intake, and muscle strength were all reduced at baseline, but showed a marked improvement 12 months later, although no change was observed in serum albumin and the increase in caloric intake was not significant. Body weight did not change, despite recovery, but dry weight increased by 7 kg. Therefore, a recovery in fat and lean mass matched with a loss of retained water results in unchanged body weight.[81]

Thus, body weight is a misleading method to detect nutritional changes in cirrhotics. Both fluid retention and obese-type malnutrition (decreased lean mass with increased fat mass) are common in cirrhotics, emphasizing the importance of nutritional assessment by compartments. Moreover, decreased albumin, prealbumin, transferrin, and IGF-1 are unreliable nutritional markers, since they may depend more on liver function than on nutritional impairment.

Nutritional assessment by body compartments may be performed either by anthropometry, bioelectrical impedance, or absorptiometry. DEXA is the most accurate of these procedures, and allows a separate evaluation of fat, lean, and bone mass, although it has the drawback that retained water as ascites or edema is counted as lean mass.[82] However, since fluid retention is habitually less pronounced or absent in arms, compartmental analysis of the upper limbs allows an accurate assessment of lean mass.[47]

1.4 ALCOHOL ABUSE, MALNUTRITION, AND SURVIVAL

Malnutrition, irrespective of its etiology, is related to a poor prognosis since it depresses immunity and favors infection. Therefore, mortality of malnourished alcoholic inpatients is increased to a similar degree as that of similarly undernourished nonalcoholics.[83]

The prognostic value of malnutrition in alcoholics has been extensively analyzed in those affected by liver disease: acute alcoholic hepatitis and liver cirrhosis. The prognosis of decompensated liver cirrhosis is very poor, with a 2- to 5-year mortality of 50%.[84,85] The Child system is a widely used prognostic score of liver disease. Subjective nutritional assessment was included in the first version of the Child and Turcotte classification (1964), although this parameter was later substituted by prothrombin in the Child–Pugh score (1973).[86,87] Therefore, in the current version of the Child–Pugh score, no nutritional parameter is included, with the possible exception of serum albumin, the levels of which, as commented before, are more closely dependent on liver function or on acute phase reaction than on malnutrition. Similarly, low serum IGF-1 levels, in relation to liver failure, have a prognostic value in cirrhotics.[88,89]

The question is, therefore, whether nutritional data — other than liver synthesized proteins and BMI in cases of fluid retention — may improve the prognostic value of the Child–Pugh score regarding survival. In this line, Abad et al. (1993) showed that midarm circumference (MAC) improves the prognostic capacity of the Child–Pugh score, a result also obtained by Alberino et al. (2001) with midarm muscle circumference (MAMC) and triceps skinfold (TSF), MAMC yielding a closer prognostic value than TSF.[84,90] Merli et al. (1996) found that a MAMA below the 5th percentile is associated with an increased mortality in Child class A and B patients, but not in class C ones, whereas a decrease in adipose tissue did not worsen the prognosis in any of the Child groups.[85] Mendenhall et al. (1995) report that in patients with acute alcoholic hepatitis, creatinine excretion and hand grip strength — both related to muscle mass — are better indicators of survival than other nutritional parameters.[91] Diverse studies in patients subjected to orthotopic liver transplantation (OLT) have shown that preoperative malnutrition is related to shorter long-term survival.[92] Selberg et al. (1997) report that hypermetabolic subjects (REE > 20%) and patients with reduced body cell mass (<35% of body weight) have reduced survival between 1 and 5 years after OLT.[93] Taken together, these observations suggest that the protein compartment, — especially muscle protein — is clinically more important than body fat stores in patients with liver disease.

1.5 PREVALENCE OF MALNUTRITION IN ALCOHOLISM

Reports on the prevalence of malnutrition among alcoholics yield variable results, ranging from 5% found by Koehn et al. (1993) in hospitalized patients to 100% reported by Mendenhall et al. (1984) in decompensated cirrhotics.[77,94] These differences probably reflect the heterogeneity of these patients and the lack of uniformity in the criteria used to define malnutrition. Malnutrition has been defined on the basis of defective caloric and/or protein intake; as reduced weight (either as BMI or in relation to ideal weight) or altered anthropometric parameters; as altered visceral proteins or creatinine excretion, using bioimpedance or whole-body DEXA; or as functional impairment such as reduced grip strength, lymphocyte count, or anergy. In addition, some authors define malnutrition using only one parameter, whereas others require the alteration of any of the aforementioned data or a combination of them.

However, most studies report a prevalence of malnutrition of about 30%. Nicolás et al., defining malnutrition as weight below 80% of ideal weight or a 10% reduction in lean mass, found malnutrition in 33% of patients; the Italian Multicentre Study reported a 30% prevalence. Thulavauth and Triger, using a MAMA below the 5th percentile as a defining criterion, reported 35%; Caregaro et al., using either MAMA or TSF below the 5th percentile reported a 34% prevalence, and our group, using a MAMA below the 5th percentile, reported a 33% prevalence, 29% showed a DEXA arm lean mass below the control 5th percentile. As shown, the most frequently used criterion is muscle mass assessed by anthropometry.[47,49,57,73,95,96]

1.6 MALNUTRITION IN ALCOHOLICS IS MULTIFACTORIAL

As mentioned, many factors predispose to malnutrition in alcoholics, such as the amount of ethanol intake, the disruption of social and family links, irregularity of meals, and the development of organic complications. All these factors may be related to each other. Therefore, in order to discern which of them yield an independent value in the development of malnutrition, as well as their hierarchical importance, we performed a multivariate analysis, defining malnutrition as a DEXA assessed reduction in lean mass in the upper limbs. Irregularity of food habits was the parameter most closely related to malnutrition, and liver cirrhosis with ascites also showed a predictive value. In turn, the irregularity of feeding habits was dependent on disruption of social and family links, and on the amount of ethanol intake.[47]

The clinical relevance of malnutrition in alcoholics resides in its relation with a poor prognosis and enhanced risk of infection. Malnutrition in alcoholics is a chronic process which ensues over years and is related to heavy and prolonged consumption. In most studies dealing with this problem, alcohol intake was higher than 200 g/d and lasted for 20 years or more. As we have shown, malnutrition in alcoholics is related to irregular feeding; family, social, and work-related problems; and heavy drinking. Probably, all these factors are in play for a long time before malnutrition becomes a clinical problem. Finally, superimposed organic complications — such as chronic pancreatitis, decompensated liver cirrhosis, acute alcoholic hepatitis, acute or chronic infections, and injury — may further impair nutritional status, making recovery unlikely.

References

1. Block G, Dresser CM, Hartman AM, and Carroll MD. Nutrient sources in the American diet: quantitative data from the NHANES II survey. II. Macronutrients and fats. *Am. J. Epidemiol.*, 1985; 122: 27–40.
2. Hellerstedt WL, Jeffery RW, and Murray DM. The association between alcohol intake and adiposity in the general population. *Am. J. Epidemiol.*, 1990; 132: 594–611.
3. Westerterp-Plantenga MS and Verwegen CR. The appetizing effect of an aperitif in overweight and normal-weight humans. *Am. J. Clin. Nutr.*, 1999; 69: 205–212.
4. Gruchow HW, Sobocinski KA, Barboriak JJ, and Scheller JG. Alcohol consumption, nutrient intake, and relative body weight among US adults. *Am. J. Clin. Nutr.*, 1985; 42: 289–295.
5. Hillers VN and Massey LK. Interrelationships of moderate and high alcohol consumption with diet and health status. *Am. J. Clin. Nutr.*, 1985; 41: 356–362.
6. Orrego H, Blake JE, Blendis LM, Kapur BM, and Israel Y. Reliability of assessment of alcohol intake based on personal interviews in a liver clinic. *Lancet*, 1979; 2: 1354–1356.
7. Zhang J, Temme EH, and Kesteloot H. Alcohol drinkers overreport their energy intake in the BIRNH study: evaluation by 24-hour urinary excretion of cations. Belgian Interuniversity Research on Nutrition and Health. *J. Am. Coll. Nutr.*, 2001; 20: 510–519.
8. Mushambi MC, Bailey SM, Trotter TN, Chadd GD, and Rowbotham DJ. Effect of alcohol on gastric emptying in volunteers. *Br. J. Anaesth.*, 1993; 71: 674–676.

9. Röjdmark S, Calissendorff J, and Brismar K. Alcohol ingestion decreases both diurnal and nocturnal secretion of leptin in healthy individuals. *Clin. Endocrinol.*, 2001; 55: 639–647.

10. Nicolás JM, Fernandez-Sola J, Fatjo F, Casamitjana R, Bataller R, Sacanella E, Tobias E, Badia E, and Estruch R. Increased circulating leptin levels in chronic alcoholism. *Alc. Clin. Exp. Res.*, 2001; 25: 83–8.

11. Santolaria F, Perez-Cejas A, Aleman MR, Gonzalez-Reimers E, Milena A, De La Vega MJ, Martinez-Riera A, and Gomez-Rodriguez MA. Low serum leptin levels and malnutrition in chronic alcohol misusers hospitalized by somatic complications. *Alcohol Alcohol.*, 2003; 38: 60–66.

12. Pirola RC and Lieber CS. The energy cost of the metabolism of drugs, including alcohol. *Pharmacology*, 1972; 7: 185–196.

13. Pirola RC and Lieber CS. Hypothesis: energy wastage in alcoholism and drug abuse: possible role of hepatic microsomal enzymes. *Am. J. Clin. Nutr.*, 1976; 29: 90–93.

14. Lieber CS and DeCarli LM. Ethanol oxidation by hepatic microsomes: adaptive increase after ethanol feeding. *Science*, 1968; 162: 917–918.

15. Oneta CM, Lieber CS, Li J, Ruttimann S, Schmid B, Lattmann J, Rosman AS, and Seitz HK. Dynamics of cytochrome P4502E1 activity in man: induction by ethanol and disappearance during withdrawal phase. *J. Hepatol.*, 2002; 36: 47–52.

16. Cronholm T, Jones AW, and Skagerberg S. Mechanism and regulation of ethanol elimination in humans: intermolecular hydrogen transfer and oxidoreduction *in vivo*. *Alc. Clin. Exp. Res.*, 1988; 12: 683–6.

17. Lands WEM and Zakhari S. The case of missing calories. *Am. J. Clin. Nutr.*, 1991; 54: 47–48.

18. Suter PM, Schutz Y, and Jequier E. The effect of ethanol on fat storage in healthy subjects. *N. Engl. J. Med.*, 1992; 326: 983–987.

19. Suter PM, Jequier E, and Schutz Y. Effect of ethanol on energy expenditure. *Am. J. Physiol.*, 1994; 266: 1204–1212.

20. Rumpler WV, Rhodes DG, Baer DJ, Conway JM, and Seale JL. Energy value of moderate alcohol consumption by humans. *Am. J. Clin. Nutr.*, 1996; 64: 108–114.

21. Cordain L, Bryan ED, Melby CL, and Smith MJ. Influence of moderate daily wine consumption on body weight regulation and metabolism in healthy free-living males. *J. Am. Coll. Nutr.*, 1997; 16: 134–139.

22. Addolorato G, Capristo E, Greco AV, Stefanini GF, and Gasbarrini G. Influence of chronic alcohol abuse on body weight and energy metabolism: is excess ethanol consumption a risk factor for obesity or malnutrition? *J. Intern. Med.*, 1998; 244: 387–395.

23. Addolorato G, Capristo E, Marini M, Santini P, Scognamiglio U, Attilia ML, Messineo D, Sasso GF, Gasbarrini G, and Ceccanti M. Body composition changes induced by chronic ethanol abuse: evaluation by dual energy x-ray absorptiometry. *Am. J. Gastroenterol.*, 2000; 95: 2323–2327.

24. Levine JA, Harris MM, and Morgan MY. Energy expenditure in chronic alcohol abuse. *Eur. J. Clin. Invest.*, 2000; 30: 779–786.

25. Lieber CS. Perspectives: do alcohol calories count? *Am. J. Clin. Nutr.*, 1991; 54: 976–982.

26. Cederbaum AI, Lieber CS, and Rubin E. Effects of chronic ethanol treatment of mitochondrial functions damage to coupling site I. *Arch. Biochem. Biophys.*, 1974; 165: 560–569.

27. Crouse JR, Gerson CD, DeCarli LM, and Lieber CS. Role of acetate in the reduction of plasma free fatty acids produced by ethanol in man. *J. Lipid Res.*, 1968; 9: 509–512.

28. Siler SQ, Neese RA, and Hellerstein MK. *De novo* lipogenesis, lipid kinetics, and whole-body lipid balances in humans after acute alcohol consumption. *Am. J. Clin. Nutr.*, 1999; 70: 928–936.

29. Colditz GA, Giovannucci E, Rimm EB, Stampfer MJ, Rosner B, Speizer FE, Gordis E, and Willett WC. Alcohol intake in relation to diet and obesity in women and men. *Am. J. Clin. Nutr.*, 1991; 54: 49–55.

30. Mannisto S, Uusitalo K, Roos E, Fogelholm M, and Pietinen P. Alcohol beverage drinking, diet and body mass index in a cross-sectional survey. *Eur. J. Clin. Nutr.*, 1997; 51: 326–332.

31. McCarty MF. The alcohol paradox. *Am. J. Clin. Nutr.*, 1999; 70: 940–942.

32. Addolorato G, Capristo E, Greco AV, Caputo F, Stefanini GF, and Gasbarrini G. Three months of abstinence from alcohol normalizes energy expenditure and substrate oxidation in alcoholics: a longitudinal study. *Am. J. Gastroenterol.*, 1998; 93: 2476–2481.

33. McDonald JT and Margen S. Wine versus ethanol in human nutrition. I. Nitrogen and calorie balance. *Am. J. Clin. Nutr.*, 1976; 29: 1093–1103.

34. Bunout D, Petermann M, Ugarte G, Barrera G, and Iturriaga H. Nitrogen economy in alcoholic patients without liver disease. *Metabolism*, 1987; 36: 651–653.

35. Reinus JF, Heymsfield SB, Wiskind R, Casper K, and Galambos JT. Ethanol: relative fuel value and metabolic effects *in vivo*. *Metabolism*, 1989; 38: 125–135.

36. Conde A, Gonzalez-Reimers E, Gonzalez-Hernandez T, Santolaria F, Martinez-Riera A, Romero-Perez JC, and Rodriguez-Moreno F. Relative and combined roles of ethanol and protein malnutrition on skeletal muscle. *Alcohol Alcohol.*, 1992; 27: 159–163.

37. Urbano-Marquez A, Estruch R, Navarro-Lopez F, Grau JM, Mont L, and Rubin E. The effects of alcoholism on skeletal and cardiac muscle. *N. Engl. J. Med.*, 1989; 320: 409–415.

38. Duane P and Peters TJ. Nutritional status in alcoholics with and without chronic skeletal muscle myopathy. *Alcohol Alcohol.*, 1988; 23: 271–277.

39. Romero JC, Santolaria F, A Conde, Díaz Flores L, and González-Reimers E. Chronic alcoholic myopathy and nutritional status. *Alcohol*, 1994; 11: 549–555.

40. Fernández Sola J, Sacanella E, Estruch R, Nicolás JM, Grau JM, and Urbano A. Significance of type II fiber atrophy in chronic alcoholic myopathy. *J. Neurol. Sci.*, 1995; 130: 69–76.

41. Fernandez Sola J, Nicolás JM, Sacanella E, Robert J, Cofan M, Estruch R, and Urbano A. Low-dose ethanol consumption allows strength recovery in chronic alcoholic myopathy. *Q. J. Med.*, 2000; 93: 35–40.

42. Preedy VR, Reilly ME, Patel VB, Richardson PJ, and Peters TJ. Protein metabolism in alcoholism: effects on specific tissues and the whole body. *Nutrition*, 1999; 15: 604–608.

43. Salaspuro M. Nutrient intake and nutritional status in alcoholics. *Alcohol Alcohol.*, 1993; 28: 85–88.

44. Gelberg L, Stein JA, and Neumann CG. Determinants of undernutrition among homeless adults. Public Health Rep. 1995; 110: 448–454.

45. Goldsmith RH, Iber FL, and Miller PA. Nutritional Status of alcoholics of different social class. *J. Am. Coll. Nutr.*, 1983; 2: 215–220.

46. Santolaria F, Gómez Sirvent JL, González-Reimers E, Batista N, Jorge JA, Rodríguez Moreno F, Martínez Riera A, and Hernández García MT. Nutritional assessment of drug addicts. *Drug Alcohol Depend.*, 1995; 38,11–18.

47. Santolaria F, Pérez Manzano JL, González-Reimers E, Milena A, Alemán MR, Martínez Riera A, and de la Vega MJ. Nutritional assessment in alcoholic patients. Its relationship with alcoholic intake, feeding habits, organic complications and social problems. *Drug Alcohol Depend.*, 2000; 59: 295–304.

48. Santolaria F, Gonzalez-Reimers E, Perez-Manzano JL, Milena A, Gomez-Rodriguez MA, Gonzalez-Diaz A, de la Vega MJ, and Martinez-Riera A. Osteopenia assessed by body composition analysis is related to malnutrition in alcoholic patients. *Alcohol*, 2000; 22: 147–157.

49. Santolaria F, González G, González-Reimers E, Martínez-Riera A, Milena A, Rodríguez-Moreno F, and González-García C. Effects of alcohol and liver cirrhosis on the GH-IGF-I axis. *Alcohol Alcohol.*,1995; 30: 703–708.

50. González-Reimers E, Santolaria F, Moreno A, Batista N, and Rodríguez-Moreno F. Harris lines: a marker of alcohol consumption during growth period? *Int. J. Anthropology*, 1993; 8: 21–25.

51. Gloria L, Cravo M, Camilo ME, Resende M, Cardoso JN, Oliveira AG, Leitao CN, and Mira FC. Nutritional deficiencies in chronic alcoholics: relation to dietary intake and alcohol consumption. *Am. J. Gastroenterol.*, 1997; 92: 485–489.

52. Cravo ML, Gloria LM, Selhub J, Nadeau MR, Camilo ME, Resende MP, Cardoso JN, Leitao CN, and Mira FC. Hyperhomocysteinemia in chronic alcoholism: correlation with folate, vitamin B-12, and vitamin B-6 status. *Am. J. Clin. Nutr.*, 1996; 63: 220–224.

53. Fernando OV and Grimsley EW. Prevalence of folate deficiency and macrocytosis in patients with and without alcohol-related illness. *South. Med. J.*, 1998; 91: 721–725.

54. Halsted CH, Villanueva JA, Devlin AM, and Chandler CJ. Metabolic interactions of alcohol and folate. *J. Nutr.*, 2002; 132: 2367S-2372S.

55. McMartin KE, Collins TD, Shiao CQ, Vidrine L, and Redetzki HM. Study of dose dependence and urinary folate excretion produced by ethanol in humans and rats. *Alc. Clin. Exp. Res.*, 1986; 10: 419–424.

56. de la Vega MJ, Santolaria F, Gonzalez-Reimers E, Aleman MR, Milena A, Martinez-Riera A, and Gonzalez-Garcia C. High prevalence of hyperhomocysteinemia in chronic alcoholism: the importance of the thermolabile form of the enzyme methylenetetrahydrofolate reductase (MTHFR). *Alcohol*, 2001; 25: 59–67.

57. Nicolás JM, Estruch R, Antúnez E, Sacanella E, and Urbano Marquez A. Nutritional status in chronically alcoholic men from the middle socio-economic class and its relation to ethanol intake. *Alcohol Alcohol.*, 1993; 28: 551–558.

58. Morillas C, Hernandez Mijares A, Morillas MJ, Aparisi L, Lluch I, Ascaso JF, and Carmena R. Nutritional status assessment in diabetes mellitus secondary to chronic alcoholic pancreatitis. *Med. Clin. (Barc.)*, 1997; 108: 373–376.

59. Aparisi L, Navarro S, Perez Mateo M, and Bautista D. Prevalence of malnutrition and morphofunctional alterations of the pancreas in asymptomatic chronic alcoholic patients. *Med. Clin. (Barc.)*, 2000; 114: 444–448.

60. Simko V, Connell AM, and Banks B. Nutritional status in alcoholics with and without liver disease. *Am. J. Clin. Nutr.*, 1982; 35: 197–203.

61. Caregaro L, Alberino F, Amodio P, Merkel C, Angeli P, Plebani M, Bolognesi M, and Gatta A. Nutritional and prognostic significance of insulin-like growth factor 1 in patients with liver cirrhosis. *Nutrition*, 1997; 13: 185–190.

62. Schneeweiss B, Graninger W, Ferenci P, Eichinger S, Grimm G, Schneider B, Laggner AN, Lenz K, and Kleinberger G. Energy metabolism in patients with acute and chronic liver disease. *Hepatology*, 1990; 11: 387–93.

63. Muller MJ, Fenk A, Lautz HU, Selberg O, Canzler H, Balks HJ, von zur Muhlen A, Schmidt E, and Schmidt FW. Energy expenditure and substrate metabolism in ethanol-induced liver cirrhosis. *Am. J. Physiol.*, 1991; 260 E338–344.

64. Campillo B, Bories P, Pornin B, Devanlay M, Linsker S, Guillemin A, Wirquin E, and Fouet P. Energy expenditure and the use of nutriments in cirrhotic patients fasting and at rest. Influence of alcoholic hepatitis and the severity score of the disease. *Gastroenterol. Clin. Biol.*, 1989; 13: 544–550.

65. John WJ, Phillips R, Ott L, Adams LJ, and McClain CJ. Resting energy expenditure in patients with alcoholic hepatitis. *J. Parenter. Enteral Nutr.*, 1989; 13: 124–127.

66. Greco AV, Mingrone G, Benedetti G, Capristo E, Tataranni PA, and Gasbarrini G. Daily energy and substrate metabolism in patients with cirrhosis. *Hepatology*, 1998; 27: 346–350.

67. Tajika M, Kato M, Mohri H, Miwa Y, Kato T, Ohnishi H, and Moriwaki H. Prognostic value of energy metabolism in patients with viral liver cirrhosis. *Nutrition*, 2002; 18: 229–234.

68. Muller MJ, Lautz HU, Plogmann B, Burger M, Korber J, and Schmidt FW. Energy expenditure and substrate oxidation in patients with cirrhosis: the impact of cause, clinical staging and nutritional state. *Hepatology*, 1992; 15: 782–794.

69. Plauth M and Schutz ET. Cachexia in liver cirrhosis. *Int. J. Cardiol.*, 2002; 85: 83–87.

70. Campillo B, Sherman E, Richardet JP, and Bories PN. Serum leptin levels in alcoholic liver cirrhosis: relationship with gender, nutritional status, liver function and energy metabolism. *Eur. J. Clin. Nutr.*, 2001; 55: 980–988.

71. Lin SY, Wang YY, and Sheu WH. Increased serum leptin concentrations correlate with soluble tumour necrosis factor receptor levels in patients with cirrhosis. *Clin. Endocrinol.*, 2002; 57: 805–811.

72. Onodera K, Kato A, and Suzuki K. Serum leptin concentrations in liver cirrhosis: relationship to the severity of liver dysfunction and their characteristic diurnal profiles. *Hepatol. Res.*, 2001; 21: 205–212.

73. Italian Multicentre Cooperative Project on Nutrition in Liver Cirrhosis, Nutritional status in cirrhosis. *J. Hepatol.*, 1994; 21, 317–325.

74. Bunout D, Gattas V, Iturriaga H, Pérez C, Pereda T, and Ugarte G. Nutritional status in alcoholic patients: its possible relationship to alcoholic liver damage. *Am. J. Clin. Nutr.*, 1983; 38, 469–473.

75. Lautz HU, Selberg O, Korber J, Burger M, and Muller MJ. Protein-calorie malnutrition in liver cirrhosis. *Clin. Invest.*, 1992; 70: 478–486.

76. Sarin SK, Dhingra N, Bansal A, Malhotra S, and Guptan RC. Dietary and nutritional abnormalities in alcoholic liver disease: a comparison with chronic alcoholics without liver disease. *Am. J. Gastroenterol.*, 1997; 92: 777–783.

77. Mendenhall CL, Anderson S, Weesner RE, Goldberg SJ, and Crolic KA. Protein-calorie malnutrition associated with alcoholic hepatitis. Veterans Administration Cooperative Study Group on Alcoholic Hepatitis. *Am. J. Med.*, 1984; 76: 211–222.

78. Scolapio JS, Ukleja A, McGreevy K, Burnett OL, and O'Brien PC. Nutritional problems in end-stage liver disease: contribution of impaired gastric emptying and ascites. *J. Clin. Gastroenterol.*, 2002; 34: 89–93.

79. Franco D, Charra M, Jeambrun P, Belghiti J, Cortesse A, Sossler C, and Bismuth H. Nutrition and immunity after peritoneovenous drainage of intractable ascites in cirrhotic patients. *Am. J. Surg.*, 1983; 146: 652–657.

80. Blendis LM, Harrison JE, Russell DM, Miller C, Taylor BR, Greig PD, and Langer B. Effects of peritoneovenous shunting on body composition. *Gastroenterology*, 1986; 90: 127–134.

81. Allard JP, Chau J, Sandokji K, Blendis LM, and Wong F. Effects of ascites resolution after successful TIPS on nutrition in cirrhotic patients with refractory ascites. *Am. J. Gastroenterol.*, 2001; 96: 2442–2447.

82. Woodrow G, Oldroyd B, Turney JH, and Smith MA. Influence of changes in peritoneal fluid on body-composition measurements by dual-energy x-ray absorptiometry in patients receiving continuous ambulatory peritoneal dialysis. *Am. J. Clin. Nutr.*, 1996; 64: 237–241.

83. Bienia R, Ratcliff S, Barbour GL, and Kummer M. Malnutrition and hospital prognosis in the alcoholic patient. *J. Parenter. Enteral Nutr.*, 1982; 6: 301–303.

84. Abad-Lacruz A, Cabre E, Gonzalez-Huix F, Fernandez-Banares F, Estevez M, Planas R, Llovet JM, Quer JC, and Gassull MA. Routine tests of renal function, alcoholism, and nutrition improve the prognostic accuracy of Child-Pugh score in nonbleeding advanced cirrhotics. *Am. J. Gastroenterol.*, 1993; 88: 382–387.

85. Merli M, Riggio O, and Dally L. Does malnutrition affect survival in cirrhosis? PINC (Policentrica Italiana Nutrizione Cirrosi). *Hepatology*, 1996; 23: 1041–1046.

86. Child CG and Turcotte JG. The surgery and portal hypertension. In: *The Liver and Portal Hypertension*. Child CG (Ed.), WB Saunders, Philadelphia, (1964). pp. 50–51.

87. Pugh RN, Murray-Lyon IM, Dawson JL, Pietroni MC, and Williams R. Transection of the oesophagus for bleeding oesophageal varices. *Br. J. Surg.*, 1973; 60: 646–649.

88. Caregaro L, Alberino F, Amodio P, Merkel C, Angeli P, Plebani M, Bolognesi M, and Gatta A. Nutritional and prognostic significance of insulin-like growth factor 1 in patients with liver cirrhosis. *Nutrition*, 1997;13: 185–190.

89. Moller S, Becker PU, Juul A, Skakkebaek NE, and Christensen E. Prognostic value of insulin-like growth factor I-IGF-I — and its binding protein IGFBP-3 in alcoholic liver disease. *Ugeskr. Laeger.*, 1997; 159: 4636–4640.

90. Alberino F, Gatta A, Amodio P, Merkel C, Di Pascoli L, Boffo G, and Caregaro L. Nutrition and survival in patients with liver cirrhosis. *Nutrition*, 2001; 17: 445–450.

91. Mendenhall CL, Moritz TE, Roselle GA, Morgan TR, Nemchausky BA, Tamburro CH, Schiff ER, McClain CJ, Marsano LS, Allen JI, et al. The VA Cooperative Study Group #275. Protein energy malnutrition in severe alcoholic hepatitis: diagnosis and response to treatment. *J. Parenter. Enteral Nutr.*, 1995; 19: 258–265.

92. Merli M, Nicolini G, Angeloni S, and Riggio O. Malnutrition is a risk factor in cirrhotic patients undergoing surgery. *Nutrition*, 2002; 18: 978–986.

93. Selberg O, Bottcher J, Tusch G, Pichlmayr R, Henkel E, and Muller MJ. Identification of high- and low-risk patients before liver transplantation: a prospective cohort study of nutritional and metabolic parameters in 150 patients. *Hepatology*, 1997; 25: 652–657.

94. Koehn V, Burnand B, Niquille M, Paccaud F, Magnenat P, and Yersin B. Prevalence of malnutrition in alcoholic and nonalcoholic medical inpatients: a comparative anthropometric study *J. Parenter. Enteral Nutr.*, 1993; 17: 35–40.

95. Thuluvath PJ and Triger DR. Evaluation of nutritional status by using anthropometry in adults with alcoholic and nonalcoholic liver disease. *Am. J. Clin. Nutr.*, 1994; 60: 269–273.

96. Caregaro L, Alberino F, Amodio P, Merkel C, Bolognesi M, Angeli P, and Gatta A. Malnutrition in alcoholic and virus-related cirrhosis. *Am. J. Clin. Nutr.*, 1996; 63: 602–609.

2 Antioxidant and Pro-Oxidant Effects of Alcoholic Beverages: Relevance to Cardiovascular Disease

Ian B. Puddey, Renate R. Zilkens, and Kevin D. Croft

CONTENTS

2.1 INTRODUCTION

Atherosclerotic vascular disease, with its major manifestations of heart attack and stroke, is still by far the leading cause of death in Western communities. Together with the corresponding very high morbidity from both coronary artery disease and cerebrovascular disease, this has been a major impetus to better definition of those

0-8493-1680-4/04/$0.00+$1.50
© 2004 by CRC Press LLC

processes integral to the initial development of an atherosclerotic plaque, together with identification of the genetic and environmental risk factors which may modify its subsequent course and consequences. In this regard, the relatively recent appreciation of lipid peroxidation as an essential element in the pathogenesis of atheroma[1] has meant that there has been a major focus on nutritional and lifestyle factors which may influence redox state, now understood as a critical element in the initial development of fatty streaks in a blood vessel wall. Understanding the potential, therefore, for antioxidant and pro-oxidant effects from regular ingestion of alcoholic beverages to modify the course of atherosclerotic vascular disease has major public health implications.

Antioxidant effects are postulated on the basis of a variety of antioxidant phytochemicals that have been identified in alcoholic beverages. These largely comprise polyphenolic compounds and may include flavonoids, procyanidins, phenolic acids, hydroxystilbenes, and isoflavones. Given their plant source, these compounds not surprisingly are identified in most alcoholic beverages, although the profile and amount will vary considerably from one beverage to another. This variability has led to speculation that if such antioxidant substances are physiologically active, then those beverages with the highest concentrations (e.g., red wine) will have unique properties that may account, at least in part, for the already well-documented protection against the development of atheroma of regular light-to-moderate drinking. Such speculation, however, needs to be weighed against the equally well-documented antiatherosclerotic actions of alcohol *per se*. Alcohol has been shown to increase high-density lipoprotein cholesterol (HDL), a lipoprotein which promotes reverse cholesterol transport from the arterial wall and which therefore is associated with reduced incidence of atherosclerotic vascular disease. Alcohol may also have anticoagulant effects, resulting in lower levels of fibrinogen, decreased platelet adhesiveness and enhanced fibrinolysis, all of which may make a further contribution to the diminished likelihood of atherosclerosis in regular drinkers. Finally, alcohol has increasingly recognized antiinflammatory and immunomodulatory effects which may influence the inflammatory processes that also characterize development of atheroma. Speculation about any preventive role against atherosclerosis from antioxidant polyphenolic compounds in alcoholic beverages also needs to encompass the fact that the metabolism of alcohol itself, especially when consumed in excess, results in a cascade of events which may be pro-oxidant in nature. At the same time, high levels of alcohol intake will result in higher blood pressure, cardiac arrhythmias, higher risk for diabetes mellitus, and disadvantageous changes in the lipid profile with an increase in triacylglycerol. It is therefore important to recognize, as outlined below, that any protection against atherosclerotic events from light-to-moderate regular alcohol consumption may well be attenuated or reversed at higher levels of consumption and with binge drinking.

2.2 ALCOHOL AND CARDIOVASCULAR DISEASE

Differential effects of light-to-heavy intakes of alcohol on the major risk factors modifying atherogenesis mean that the interrelationships of alcohol with cardiovascular disease are complex. In the first ever meta-analysis of the relationship between alcohol and coronary artery disease,[2] an L-shaped relationship was reported. In that analysis of 42 carefully selected prospective population studies carried out up until 1993, most of the protective effect of alcohol against cardiovascular disease was established at one standard drink per day or every second day (5 to 10 g alcohol) and no further decrease in risk was seen at higher levels of consumption. A more recent meta-analysis[3] attempted to examine the nature of the relationship more carefully by only including the 28 cohort studies assessed as being of the highest quality. That analysis overall identified the relationship as a J-shaped curve. The nadir of the curve was at 20 g ethanol per day where the mean decrease in relative risk was approximately 20%.[3] Any protective effect of alcohol was lost, however, at the level of 72 g/d and at intakes greater than 89 g/d there was a mean 5% increase in relative coronary risk.

The relationships of alcohol consumption with cerebrovascular disease are even more complex than those seen with coronary artery disease. Much of this complexity is a consequence of the multifaceted nature of stroke. Stroke may first be ischemic in nature, arising from occlusive vascular disease of the intracranial or extracranial vasculature. In such a setting, similar pathophysiological processes to atherosclerotic coronary artery disease may be operative and a similar favorable effect of alcohol to protect against stroke might therefore be anticipated. In prospective cohort studies[4,5] as well as case-control comparisons,[6,7] such a protective relationship has been identified mainly in middle-aged and older subjects. However, in binge and heavy drinkers, there is often an increased risk of ischemic stroke.[8] Second, stroke may be secondary to intracerebral hemorrhage, and in both case-control comparisons and longitudinal studies, there is compelling evidence that intracerebral hemorrhage is increased in heavy drinkers.[9] A comprehensive systematic review of the association between alcohol and stroke has recently been published and included 41 studies where careful categorization had been performed of the type of stroke and amount of alcohol consumed.[10] For ischemic stroke, the authors observed a similar J-shaped relationship to that reported for coronary heart disease events. However, the evidence linking light-to-moderate consumption with a reduction in risk was thought to be inconsistent, while that linking increased consumption, especially recent consumption and binge drinking,[8] to increased risk of both ischemic and hemorrhagic stroke was considered strong.

2.3   FLAVONOIDS AND CARDIOVASCULAR DISEASE

If the polyphenolic flavonoids in alcoholic beverages, especially red wine, are having an influence on atherogenesis, their widespread use in the community should, at least to some extent, be contributing to a measurable link between dietary flavonoid intake and cardiovascular disease outcomes. This remains to be firmly established. In one of the first reports in this area, Hertog and colleagues[11] identified a relationship between average flavonoid intake across populations and coronary artery disease mortality in the Seven Countries Study, a relationship which was independent of differences in alcohol intake. However, there was no analysis of the potential associations with predominant alcoholic beverage preference across the 16 cohorts involved. In the Finnish Mobile Clinic Health Examination Survey of more than 10,000 men and women, persons with the highest quercetin intakes had a 21% lower relative risk of mortality from coronary artery disease,[12] while intakes of the major flavonoids, kaempferol, naringenin, and hesperetin, were associated with a significantly reduced risk of cerebrovascular disease.[12] The food sources predominantly responsible for these associations were identified as apples, onions, oranges, and grapefruit. Four other studies have shown similar findings.[13–16] Three of these were from Holland where the major dietary flavonoid source was black tea.[13–15] The fourth was carried out in a cohort of American women and flavonoid intake was reported to reduce the incidence of coronary artery disease death but not stroke mortality, with the major flavonoid food source identified as broccoli.[16] Two other large studies, one in American males and the other in Welsh men, have not identified such associations.[17,18] Resolution of the issue as to whether dietary flavonoid intake independently reduces cardiovascular outcomes therefore awaits further population-based studies and may only be fully resolved through a large-scale intervention trial. The question as to whether alcoholic beverages that are rich in flavonoids can further influence any associations between flavonoid intake and CVD is not yet supported by epidemiological evidence.

2.4 ALCOHOLIC BEVERAGE PREFERENCE AND CARDIOVASCULAR DISEASE

If the polyphenolic flavonoids in alcoholic beverages are having a significant influence on atherogenesis, we would also expect consistent differences in cardiovascular outcomes according to alcoholic beverage preference given the substantially higher levels of polyphenolic compounds seen in red wine. Several reports from ecological studies have demonstrated that in France, despite a relatively high intake of saturated fat, there is a relatively low mortality from CHD.[19–21] This has nurtured the concept of a "French paradox" which has been ascribed, at least in part, to a corresponding relatively high wine consumption, especially red wine. However, Rimm and colleagues[22] in a systematic review of studies that have attempted to define cardiovascular outcomes according to predominant beverage preference came to the conclusion that a substantial proportion of the lower risk of coronary heart disease is from alcohol rather than from any components of each type of alcoholic drink. A further recent meta-analysis[23] suggests that the currently accepted potential mechanisms for a protective effect of regular light-to-moderate drinking relate largely to direct effects of alcohol on cardiovascular risk factors rather than to any specific beverage constituents. In that analysis, the pooled results from 42 intervention studies[23] confirmed dose-dependent effects of alcohol to raise high-density lipoprotein cholesterol (HDL-C) by approximately 0.1 mmol/l for every 30 g/d of pure ethanol, whether consumed as beer, wine, or spirits. In a smaller number of studies, dose-dependent effects of alcohol to reduce fibrinogen levels were also seen[23,24] and as previously discussed, alcohol has also been associated with an increase in fibrinolysis[25] and a decrease in platelet activation.[26] These combined effects of moderate regular alcohol use on lipids and hemostatic factors are sufficient to account for at least a 25% decrease in coronary artery disease mortality[23] with the predominant influence being that of alcohol to raise HDL-C.[27] This represents the majority of the anticipated decrease in coronary risk from regular alcohol consumption. Hence, antioxidant flavonoids in red wine, or any other putative protective components in alcoholic beverages apart from alcohol, are only likely to be making a very small further contribution, if at all.

Therefore, the observation, that in some studies red wine drinkers have beneficial outcomes for total mortality[28] and stroke,[29] with neutral or adverse effects for those whose preference is for beer or spirits, is more likely to relate to a residual confounding influence of important unmeasured variables.[30,31] For example, wine preferrers compared to beer preferrers eat more fresh fruit and vegetables, eat less red meat, take fewer salty snacks, use more olive oil and are more likely to trim fat from meat and use less fatty spreads.[32] They often have a higher socioeconomic status and hence better access to health care.[33,34] Other correlates of predominant beverage preference include aspects of personality, smoking habits, and different volumes and patterns of drinking,[35,36] each of which constitutes further alternative and plausible explanations for the more favorable profile for cardiovascular outcomes reported in wine vs. beer or spirits drinkers. These caveats aside, the intriguing possibility remains that the high concentrations of flavonoids and other polyphenols in red wine may contribute, at least in part, to lower cardiovascular disease risk. The antioxidant effects of such compounds, together with strong evidence for a link between oxidative stress and cardiovascular disease and demonstrated effects of polyphenolics on platelet function,[37] inflammatory processes,[38,39] and endothelial[40,41] and vascular smooth muscle function[42] continue to fuel research in this area.

2.5 RED WINE POLYPHENOLS

The type and amount of phenolic constituents can vary greatly from one wine to another,[43] with the total polyphenol content of red wines as high as 2000 mg/l. Red wine contains the flavonoids catechin, epicatechin, and quercetin in addition to polymeric phenols and tannins as major components. The anthocyanins give red wine its characteristic color (for examples of these structures, see Figure 2.1). Red wine also contains significant quantities of phenolic acids such as gallic acid, caffeic acid, and coumaric acid (Figure 2.1). The hydroxystilbenes, *cis* and *trans* resveratrol, are present in low concentrations (approximately 1 mg/l) but are of interest because of their biological activity.[44]

2.6 ABSORPTION AND BIOAVAILABILITY OF POLYPHENOLS

The bioavailability of dietary polyphenols has been reviewed in detail.[45] Research in this area has increased over the last decade with improved methods for analysis of specific polyphenols and their metabolites. While intestinal absorption can be high for some polyphenols, plasma concentrations of specific compounds rarely

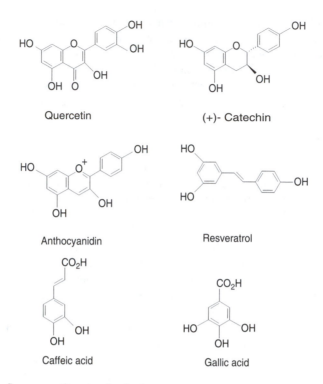

FIGURE 2.1 Some constituents of red wine.

exceed 1 μM even after consumption of between 10 to 100 mg of that substance.[45] However, many unknown or unidentified compounds or metabolites may be present which could contribute to the overall bioactivity. Bioavailability is influenced by the structure of polyphenols but there is as yet little understanding of the relationship between structure and absorption. There is also large individual variation in absorption between subjects, which may be related to the composition of colonic microflora which plays a role in transformation of polyphenols prior to intestinal absorption. Metabolic transformations include methylation and conjugation. Donovan et al.[46] studied the absorption and metabolism of catechin, the major flavonoid in red wine, using gas chromatography–mass spectrometry (GC–MS). Volunteers consumed 120 ml of red wine containing 35 mg of catechin, and plasma catechin concentration peaked after 1 h at 0.09 μM, regardless of whether it was normal or de-alcoholized wine. Catechin was present in plasma either as the 3-O-methylcatechin or conjugated metabolites. If flavonoids are protective nutrients then it is likely that the active forms are metabolites rather than the initial form which exists in a food or beverage. This is also highlighted in the study by Caccetta et al.[47] in which phenolic acid absorption was studied by GC–MS following ingestion of red wine. The major phenolic acids, caffeic and gallic acid, peaked after 2 h, and all the gallic acid was in the form of the 4-O-methylgallic acid. In the same study, it was noted that the antioxidant activity of the methylated form of gallic acid was significantly less than the unmethylated form.[47]

Some investigators have suggested that red wine is a poor source of bioavailable flavonoids.[48] These investigators, using the flavonoid quercetin as a marker compound, found that flavonoids from red wine are absorbed relatively less than those from onions or tea. While many aspects of flavonoid and phenolic acid absorption and metabolism remain unknown, there is enough overall evidence to suggest that some of these compounds will be absorbed in sufficiently high concentration to have physiological effects. Improvements in methodologies for measuring phenolic compounds or their metabolites in plasma and urine are essential in this area if useful information in relation to potential physiological effects of polyphenolics in alcoholic beverages is to be provided.

2.7 ANTIOXIDANT ACTIVITY OF WINE POLYPHENOLS

Dietary polyphenols may have physiological antioxidant properties, quenching reactive oxygen and nitrogen species and hence potentially modifying pathogenic mechanisms relevant to cardiovascular disease. The antioxidant activity of phenolic compounds is due to the ease with which they can donate a hydrogen atom from an aromatic hydroxyl (OH) group to a free radical.[49] The phenolic radical so formed is relatively stable due to delocalization around the aromatic ring. Different substituents on the aromatic structure can affect antioxidant activity, and structure activity relationships for the flavonoids have been studied in detail.[50–53]

Numerous studies have confirmed that polyphenolic compounds from red wine in particular have antioxidant activity in a range of *in vitro* chemical oxidation systems using low-density lipoprotein (LDL) or plasma as a substrate.[54–57] However, it has been less clear whether such antioxidant effects occur *in vivo*. Of the *in vivo* studies conducted to date, most have used indirect measures of lipid and lipoprotein damage or nonspecific measures of plasma antioxidant capacity.[58] In general, red wine or grape phenolics appear to increase the antioxidant capacity of plasma, and while mechanisms have not been specifically investigated in these studies, it is presumed that the beverage phenolics are absorbed sufficiently to contribute to the radical trapping capacity of the plasma. Effects on *ex vivo* LDL oxidation have been variable and largely inconclusive, partly due to differences in study design and methodology of LDL isolation and oxidation conditions.[47,59–67] Using F_2-isoprostanes, a specific biomarker of *in vivo* lipid peroxidation, it was shown in a randomized trial in smoking subjects that 2 weeks' consumption of de-alcoholized red wine significantly reduced *in vivo* oxidative stress.[68] Normal red wine containing 13% alcohol had no effect on oxidative stress in the same study, perhaps suggesting a counter balance between the antioxidant effects of polyphenols and the pro-oxidant action of alcohol metabolism. In support of this concept, alcohol consumption alone has been shown to increase isoprostane production in humans.[69]

It should also be pointed out that redox active phenolic compounds can also act as pro-oxidants under some conditions. This is particularly the case in metal ion catalyzed systems as demonstrated with flavonoids.[70] Caffeic acid can also have pro-oxidant activity on Cu^{++}-induced oxidation of LDL.[71,72] In the healthy body, metal ions appear to be largely sequestered in forms unable to catalyze free radical reactions,[72] whereas injury to tissues may release iron or copper[73] and in this context catalytic metal ions have been measured in atherosclerotic lesions.[74] If metal ions do play a role in lipoprotein oxidation *in vivo,* then possible pro-oxidant effects of phenolic compounds should not be ignored.

2.8 ANTIATHEROSCLEROTIC EFFECTS OF RED WINE — INSIGHTS FROM ANIMAL STUDIES

The apolipoprotein E deficient (apoE -/-) mouse develops human-like atherosclerotic plaques as early as 5 weeks of age.[75] When placed on a normal chow diet, these animals have been observed to develop complex lesions within 6 months, similar to plaques observed in late-stage human atherosclerosis. This model has been considered particularly useful for the study of the oxidation hypothesis of atherosclerosis. However, the results of studies involving red wine interventions in animal models of atherosclerosis have been inconsistent.

Hayek et al.[76] found reduced progression of atherosclerosis in apoE-deficient mice following consumption of red wine, or its polyphenols quercetin or catechin, and this was associated with reduced susceptibility of LDL to oxidation. However, red wine did not reduce mature atherosclerosis in apoE-deficient mice.[77] We have found that red wine polyphenols reduce atherosclerosis development in apoE deficient mice independent of effects on lipid peroxidation (unpublished data). A recent study by Stocker and O'Halloran (personal communication) also shows that red wine polyphenols decrease atherosclerosis in this model without inhibiting lipoprotein oxidation in the vessel wall. In another recent report, plasma and heart F_2-isoprostanes were measured in Sprague-Dawley rats after dietary flavonoid supplementation and failed to reveal any suppression of lipid peroxidation beyond that seen with simultaneous α-tocopherol supplementation.[78] These authors again questioned whether such compounds can suppress lipid peroxidation *in vivo*.[78] In the fat-fed hamster model of atherosclerosis, red wine, de-alcoholized red wine, and grape juice all inhibited atherosclerosis over a 10-week period.[79] Although largely based on animal studies, the above data suggest overall that there is a potential for polyphenolic compounds to have beneficial effects in preventing atherosclerosis, but probably independent of any antioxidant effect.

2.9 OTHER BIOACTIVITY OF WINE POLYPHENOLS RELEVANT TO ATHEROSCLEROSIS

Polyphenolic compounds derived from red wine, grape juice, and grape skin have been shown to induce endothelium-dependent vasorelaxation of the precontracted rat aorta,[42] an effect that appears to be mediated by the nitric oxide cyclic GMP pathway. Wine polyphenols fed to stroke-prone hypertensive rats for 8 weeks attenuated the elevation in blood pressure and improved aortic biomechanical properties compared to control animals.[80] Grape polyphenols administered to rats reduced thrombin-induced platelet aggregation,[37] and grape juice inhibited platelet activity and thrombosis in stenosed canine coronary arteries.[81] Phenolic acids such as caffeic acid have been shown to protect cultured endothelial cells against the cytotoxic effects of oxidized LDL, possibly by blocking the intracellular signalling triggered by oxLDL.[82] Some phenolic acids are potent and specific inhibitors of nuclear transcription factor NF-κB,[83] and since activation of NF-κB is induced by a number of inflammatory agents, its inhibition by these compounds may explain some of their antiinflammatory properties.

Three recent reports suggest that red wine polyphenols may alter the expression and activity of endothelial nitric oxide synthase.[40,84,85] Resveratrol, when incubated with cultured endothelial cells, was able to upregulate the expression of eNOS mRNA in a time- and dose-dependent manner as well as increasing NO production.[84] Red wine polyphenol extract was also shown to increase eNOS expression[40,85] and subsequent NO release from cultured human endothelial cells.[85] Although based on *in vitro* studies, this work does raise the possibility that effects on endothelial NO with a subsequent improvement in endothelial function may explain the beneficial effects of red wine polyphenols on the development of atherosclerosis, at least in animal models discussed earlier, and possibly also in humans. Endothelial dysfunction is generally considered to be an important pathogenic mechanism for atherosclerosis and may be one of the earliest manifestations of this disease.[86]

2.10 WINE POLYPHENOLS, ALCOHOL, AND ENDOTHELIAL FUNCTION IN HUMANS

The antiatherosclerotic potential of any effect of beverage phenolics to improve endothelial function is highlighted by the fact that the human endothelium has been estimated to cover an approximate area of 1000 m^2 and weigh 1.5 kg, making it similar in size to the liver. The endothelium is an important endocrine and paracrine organ which responds to a variety of physical and chemical stimuli by synthesis and release of a variety of vasoactive and thromboregulatory molecules and growth factors. In particular, the synthesis and release of endothelium-derived nitric oxide (NO) is a pivotal molecule in the regulation of vascular homeostasis. NO activates vascular smooth muscle soluble guanylate cyclase, increasing cyclic GMP that in turn stimulates vascular smooth muscle cell relaxation. NO is not only a potent vasodilator but also inhibits smooth muscle cell proliferation and migration, platelet aggregation and adhesion, leukocyte–endothelial interactions, and expression of adhesion molecules by endothelial cells.[87]

Central to the development of endothelial dysfunction is a loss of bioactive endothelial NO. The loss of NO bioactivity can result not only from reduced synthesis and release of NO by endothelial cells but also increased oxidative inactivation of subendothelial NO by reactive oxygen intermediates such as superoxide. The noninvasive measurement of flow-mediated dilatation of the brachial artery (FMD) following forearm occlusion is a functional assay in humans that allows quantification of the degree of endothelial dysfunction. This method utilizes the shear stress response of endothelial cells to release NO and monitors by ultrasound the subsequent dilatation of the brachial artery. The *in vivo* improvement in FMD following the acute or chronic administration of antioxidant vitamins to humans in conditions associated with increased levels of oxidative stress[88,89] supports the *in vitro* evidence that oxidative stress is one of the pathogenic mechanisms causing endothelial dysfunction. It also has been the catalyst for a large number of studies utilizing red wine or grape juice to ascertain whether the antioxidant polyphenolics in such beverages can improve endothelial function in humans.

However, any effects of alcoholic beverage polyphenolics on endothelial function need to be understood in the context of possible effects of alcohol to also modulate endothelial function. Such potential effects have previously been reviewed[90] and to date there have been three studies that have further explored the possible relationships between alcohol use and endothelial function as measured by FMD.[91–93] In the first study, 20 men with a history of heavy drinking, defined as more than 75 g of alcohol per day in the past 8 years, and who were in an abstinence phase for 3 months were compared with 20 controls who reported no alcohol consumption.[91] After 3 months of abstinence, however, the ex-drinkers had significantly impaired endothelial function when compared to the control group despite being nonsmokers, normotensive, normocholesterolemic, and free of cardiovascular disease. The second was a cross-sectional study of 108 male subjects with newly diagnosed coronary artery disease.[92] Of the 54 subjects who drank alcohol, none drank wine, 24 drank beer, 14 drank sake, 4 drank Japanese vodka, and 4 drank whisky. FMD was higher in drinkers, especially the subgroups who consumed light (1 to 20 g/d) and moderate (21 to 50 g/d) amounts of alcohol. The third study[93] was an intervention trial to determine whether reducing alcohol intake in 16 men who were moderate-to-heavy drinkers (40 to 110 g/d) would improve conduit artery endothelial function as assessed by FMD and the endothelial biomarkers, E-selectin, endothelin-1, and von Willebrand factor. Despite a substantial reduction in alcohol intake, there was no improvement in either FMD or the biomarkers over a 4-week intervention period.

Similar carefully controlled intervention studies with red wine or grape juice polyphenolics are yet to be reported, with most of the inferences in this area having been drawn from studies of their acute effects on endothelial function[94–96] or from uncontrolled interventions.[97,98] In the first acute study,[94] red wine was administered together with a high-fat meal and found to have no effect on postprandial FMD. It remains possible, however, that the ingestion of the fat meal may have interfered with the absorption of any polyphenol compounds. In the second acute study, conducted in New Zealand,[95] both red wine and de-alcoholized red wine were administered to healthy subjects immediately prior to measurement of endothelial function. While the de-alcoholized red wine elicited an improved endothelial response as reflected by an increase in FMD, the red wine which contained alcohol had no such effect. The explanation for a lack of detectable improvement after the red wine was that the baseline resting vessel diameter, blood flow, and heart rate were all increased by stimulation by the alcohol component of the red wine. In the third study, conducted in Japan, the beverages examined included Japanese vodka, red wine, de-alcoholized red wine, and water.[96] Again the baseline vessel diameter was increased by the beverages that contained alcohol (i.e., Japanese vodka and red wine); however, on this occasion the red wine led to an acute improvement in endothelial function, while the vodka led to impairment. The de-alcoholized red wine in this study led to an improvement in endothelial function just as it had in the New Zealand study.[95] These studies suggest that endothelium-dependent vasodilation may improve after the acute ingestion of either red wine or de-alcoholized red wine in humans and that it is the nonalcohol constituents of red wine and not the alcohol that are responsible

Two intervention studies have reported that short-term ingestion of purple grape juice improves FMD in adults with coronary artery disease.[97,98] Unfortunately these studies were neither randomized nor did they have a control beverage group with a low flavonoid content for comparison. In both studies, the grape juice was consumed on the morning of the assessment of endothelial function, making it difficult to ascertain whether the improvement was a result of "acute" or "short-term" intake. Although the authors of both studies suggested that the polyphenols in purple grape juice may be beneficial for endothelial function, identification of longer-term effects of red wine and/or grape juice to improve FMD and endothelial function await the results of further, more rigorous intervention studies.

2.11 ALCOHOL AS A PRO-OXIDANT

As appealing as the concept might be that an alcoholic beverage such as red wine may be beneficial for health because of its antioxidant content, it needs to be tempered by the knowledge that the metabolism of alcohol itself has pro-oxidant effects. Such pro-oxidant effects may lead to enhanced lipid peroxidation and hence contribute to the increased risk of cardiovascular disease evident at high levels of alcohol intake. Alcohol consumption has already been demonstrated in a human intervention study to increase the oxidizability of LDL[99] and, as mentioned previously, the levels of urinary F_2-isoprostanes, which are a group of prostaglandin-like products of nonenzymatic lipid peroxidation,[100] are acutely increased by alcohol in healthy volunteers.[101] Increased F_2-isoprostane levels have been identified in human atherosclerotic plaque and in one study the levels in plaque were higher in drinkers compared to nondrinkers.[102] Chronic alcohol administration to rhesus monkeys (as 2.6 g artificially flavored ethanol/kg/d over 3 years — the equivalent of about 14 standard drinks per day in a 70-kg man) caused an 80% increase in plasma F_2-isoprostanes with concomitant alcohol-induced liver damage.[103] Chronic alcohol exposure in patients with alcoholic liver disease was also associated with increased urinary F_2-isoprostanes which decreased with abstinence.[104]

The mechanism for such pro-oxidant effects of alcohol is the subject of continuing investigation. Direct measurement of free radical production through the use of free radical trapping agents suggests that hepatic metabolism of alcohol leads to local free radical generation.[105] It is also highly likely that ethanol or its major metabolic product, acetaldehyde, can lead to the production of free radical species in other sites[106] with such pro-oxidant effects responsible for a variety of alcohol-related tissue toxicity and injury. The production of free radical species can occur during several stages of the metabolism of alcohol. It is oxidized to acetaldehyde by alcohol dehydrogenase, the microsomal ethanol oxidizing system, and by catalase, with each representing possible points at which excess free radical generation may result. Alcohol may alter the activities of the antioxidant enzymes superoxide dismutase and glutathione peroxidase,[107] while acetaldehyde can bind with cysteine or glutathione,[108] both potentially important pathways for scavenging free radicals and prevention of lipid peroxidation.

2.12 BLOOD PRESSURE

The presence of pro-oxidants and antioxidants in alcoholic beverages may be relevant to the well-established relationship between alcohol and blood pressure. A recent meta-analysis of 15 randomized controlled alcohol intervention trials confirmed a dose–response relationship,[109] with the estimation that a reduction in daily alcohol intake by two thirds in a population drinking three to six drinks/d, could lower average systolic and diastolic BP by 3.3 and 2 mm Hg, respectively.[109] Changes of this magnitude are considerable when one notes that a 2 mm Hg population-based reduction in diastolic BP would result in a 17% decrease in the prevalence of hypertension, a 6% reduction in the risk of coronary heart disease, and a 15% reduction in the risk of stroke.[110]

Hypertension is increasingly recognized as a state of heightened oxidative stress[111] and pro-oxidant effects of alcohol may be a component in mediating the blood pressure raising effect of alcohol. Evidence supportive of this concept comes from the well-documented direct association of plasma levels of gamma-glutamyl-transpeptidase (γGT) with levels of blood pressure in cross-sectional[112] and longitudinal population studies.[113] A membrane-bound ectopeptidase, γGT cleaves the glutamyl group from glutathione, the first step in the uptake of extracellular glutathione. The vasodilator nitric oxide also increases intracellular glutathione levels in aortic endothelial cells through a pathway that is γGT–dependent, and both nitric oxide and the glutathione cycle appear to be co-ordinately regulated.[114] Maintenance of intracellular glutathione levels is integral to redox homeostasis and an increase in γGT with chronic alcohol ingestion may be a marker for those subjects who develop increased oxidative stress and/or nitric oxide depletion with alcohol and therefore exhibit a greater sensitivity to development of alcohol-related hypertension. This hypothesis garners further support from the results of Japanese and Korean studies[115,116] in which, after drinking and nondrinking subjects were categorized on the basis of high or low levels of γGT, only drinkers with a high γGT demonstrated increasing levels of blood pressure and increased risk of hypertension with increasing alcohol intake. Moreover, in both normotensive and hypertensive Japanese drinkers, following a 4-week period of moderating their alcohol intake, blood pressure levels decreased more markedly in those who initially had the highest γGT levels.[117]

The polyphenolics in red wine have been characterized in *in vitro* experiments as having potent vasodilator activity[42,118,119] which, as discussed earlier, may be a result of effects to enhance vascular NO synthesis or release. This has led to speculation that red wine will have less of an effect to elevate blood pressure compared to other alcoholic beverages. The Kaiser Permanente study reported similar effects on blood pressure in North Americans who drank beer, wine, or spirits.[120] Furthermore, studies from countries in which the population drinks predominantly sake[121] or wine[122,123] or beer[124,125] have all shown relationships between alcohol and blood pressure of similar magnitude. However, there is other epidemiological evidence that wine drinking is associated with smaller effects on blood pressure. In the

Lipid Clinics Prevalence Study[126] regression data from subjects who reported drinking only one type of alcoholic beverage showed significant positive regression coefficients for beer and spirits and blood pressure but no significant relationships for wine drinkers. The PRIME study also found a weaker association for wine and blood pressure compared with beer.[127] These studies need to be interpreted in the knowledge of the previously invoked differences in diet and other behaviors between groups drinking predominantly wine, beer, or spirits.[32] They should also be considered against results from a recent 4×4 week, cross-over trial from our group comparing effects of wine, de-alcoholized red wine, beer, and water on 24-h ambulatory blood pressure in 26 men, where similar increases in blood pressure were observed with the two alcohol-containing beverages (Zilkens et al., personal communication) with an increase in awake systolic blood pressure of 2.9 mm Hg for red wine and 1.9 mm Hg for beer compared with the water control. In addition no fall in ambulatory BP was recorded during the period when only the de-alcoholized wine was consumed.

2.13 ALCOHOLIC BEVERAGES AND HOMOCYSTEINE LEVELS

Alcoholic beverages and their antioxidant and pro-oxidant constituents may also have implications for atherosclerotic vascular disease through an impact on another increasingly recognized independent risk factor for cardiovascular disease — plasma homocysteine levels. Homocysteine is an intermediate generated in almost all human tissues during the metabolism of methionine with normal fasting plasma levels ranging from 5 to 15 μmol/l. Folate and vitamin B_{12} are essential for the reconversion of homocysteine to methionine via the remethylation cycle. Vitamin B_6 is essential for the transulfuration pathway that converts homocysteine to cysteine. Cysteine may, in turn, be incorporated into glutathione, a major intracellular regulator of redox status, or be further metabolized to sulfate and excreted in the urine.

A meta-analysis of available data has estimated that a 5 μmol/l increment in homocysteine is associated with an increase in CVD risk to the same extent as a 0.5 mmol/l increase in cholesterol.[128] Potent reactive oxygen species (including superoxide, hydrogen peroxide, and the hydroxyl radical) are produced during the auto-oxidation of homocysteine and have been implicated in the vascular effects of hyperhomocysteinemia.[129] The generation of reactive oxygen species may lead to oxidative damage to vascular endothelial cells, increased proliferation of vascular smooth muscle cells, and oxidative modification of low-density lipoprotein.

The general consensus is that moderate-to-heavy alcohol consumption can elevate homocysteine levels[130–133] and hence may be relevant to the increased risk of atherosclerotic vascular disease in heavy drinkers. However, Koehler et al.[134] have described a J-shaped relation between homocysteine and alcohol consumption where moderate alcohol consumption of <2 drinks/d was associated with lower homocysteine, while heavier alcohol consumption was associated with increased homocysteine, consistent with the J-shaped relationship between alcohol and CVD.

Alcoholic beverage type may also be a confounding determinant of the ultimate relationship between alcohol and homocysteine. The metabolic removal of homocysteine requires folate as a cofactor, so it has been suggested that a negative association between beer intake and homocysteine levels reported in a number of studies[131,132,135,136] could have resulted from the relatively high content of folate in beer (6 to 9 µg/100 ml). In alcoholics consuming on average 2.78 g alcohol/kg/d, those who drank beer had significantly lower homocysteine levels than those drinking wine or spirits.[132] However, the extremely heavy beer intake was still associated with a higher homocysteine level than in the 30 g alcohol/d control group. In the Caerphilly Cohort follow-up study in South Wales where the predominant alcoholic beverage was beer, alcohol intake was a significant negative determinant of homocysteine[135] supporting the finding of a cross-sectional study conducted in the predominantly beer-drinking Czechoslovakian population where the heavier drinkers also had lower homocysteine levels.[136] In the Framingham Offspring Cohort,[131] consumption of spirits was strongly associated with higher homocysteine, weakly related to consumption of red wine, and not related to consumption of white wine or beer. The notion that components in beer benefit homocysteine levels has also been supported by a 3-week cross-over study involving 11 healthy middle-aged men which found that a daily intake of 40 g alcohol sourced from either red wine or spirits raised homocysteine, while an identical intake of beer had no effect.[137]

This finding contrasts with those of a 4-treatment parallel intervention study involving 60 healthy males who abstained from alcohol use for 3 months prior to study entry.[138] In that study the consumption of 30 g alcohol/d for 6 weeks in the form of either beer, red wine, or spirits all raised homocysteine levels, with no increase found in the mineral water control group.[138] In a more recent randomized cross-over intervention study involving 16 healthy men, an increase in beer consumption from an average of 8 g alcohol/d/4 weeks to 72 g alcohol/d/4 weeks led to a 9% increase in plasma homocysteine levels.[93] Thus, although the epidemiological data suggest a negative association between beer drinking and plasma homocysteine levels in some populations, most of the recent intervention studies suggest that regardless of which type of alcohol is consumed, drinking more than 30 g alcohol/d is likely to raise plasma homocysteine levels.

Chlorogenic acid, a polyphenol that occurs in large amounts in coffee and black tea polyphenols, has been shown to raise plasma homocysteine concentrations,[139] so there is also theoretical speculation that the polyphenols found in red wine might also increase homocysteine levels. It is proposed that during the metabolism of dietary polyphenols from tea and coffee, the polyphenols accept a methyl group that has been released during the metabolism of methionine to homocysteine.[139,140] Thus, consumption of a high dose of polyphenols might increase homocysteine production through increased methylation reactions. Although such a mechanism offers an explanation for any elevation of homocysteine with red wine, it does not explain the homocysteine-raising effects of beer or spirits. Further research is required to elucidate the mechanism behind the homocysteine-raising effect of all types of alcoholic beverages.

2.14 CONCLUSION

The overall interrelationships of alcohol to atherosclerotic vascular disease and the major cardiovascular endpoints of myocardial infarction and stroke are complex. This complexity is also reflected in the inter-relationships of alcohol with the major risk factors for cardiovascular disease. Understanding these complex relationships and seeking to gain insights into their etiology and pathogenesis are essential if balanced and appropriate advice is to be promulgated on either the safe levels of alcohol consumption for cardiovascular disease or the potential advantages and disadvantages of one alcoholic beverage over another. The antioxidant and pro-oxidant effects of alcoholic beverages are likely to be highly relevant in advancing such an understanding. What is well established at the present time is that the regular consumption of 1 to 2 glasses of alcohol per day (10 to 20 g) confers a measurable cardiovascular advantage with an estimated 20% reduction in incidence of coronary artery disease. Similar effects for the incidence of ischemic stroke are also highly probable on available evidence. These effects, however, appear independent of the predominant alcoholic beverage choice. Claims for a potential advantage of red wine compared to beer or spirits have a feasible basis because of its high levels of antioxidant flavonoids and hence greater anticipated benefits for atherosclerosis prevention. However, such anticipated benefits remain to be convincingly demonstrated either for cardiovascular risk factor modification in intervention trials or for hard cardiovascular endpoints in population-based epidemiological studies. Any claims for unique cardiovascular benefits from the ingestion of red wine also need to be counterbalanced by the knowledge that excessive alcohol consumption, no matter what alcoholic beverage, will have adverse consequences for cardiovascular and other diseases which may in part be mediated by pro-oxidant effects of alcohol metabolism.

References

1. Esterbauer, H., Wag, G., and Puhl, H., Lipid peroxidation and its role in atherosclerosis, *Brit. Med. Bull.*, 49, 566–576, 1993.
2. Maclure, M., Demonstration of deductive meta-analysis: ethanol intake and risk of myocardial infarction, *Epidemiol. Rev.*, 15, 328–351, 1993.
3. Corrao, G. et al., Alcohol and coronary heart disease: a meta-analysis, *Addiction*, 95, 1505–1523, 2000.
4. Stampfer, M.J. et al., A prospective study of moderate alcohol consumption and the risk of coronary disease and stroke in women, *N. Engl. J. Med.*, 319, 267–273, 1988.
5. Klatsky, A.L., Armstrong, M.A., and Friedman, G.D., Alcohol use and subsequent cerebrovascular disease hospitalizations, *Stroke*, 20, 741–746, 1989.
6. Jamrozik, K. et al., The role of lifestyle factors in the etiology of stroke. A population-based case-control study in Perth, Western Australia, *Stroke*, 25, 51–59, 1994.
7. Sacco, R.L. et al., The protective effect of moderate alcohol consumption on ischemic stroke, *JAMA*, 281, 53–60, 1999.
8. Hansagi, H. et al., Alcohol consumption and stroke mortality. 20-year follow-up of 15,077 men and women, *Stroke*, 26, 1768–1773, 1995.

9. Monforte, R. et al., High ethanol consumption as risk factor for intracerebral hemorrhage in young and middle-aged people, *Stroke*, 21, 1529–1532, 1990.

10. Mazzaglia, G. et al., Exploring the relationship between alcohol consumption and non-fatal or fatal stroke: a systematic review, *Addiction*, 96, 1743–1756, 2001.

11. Hertog, M.G. et al., Flavonoid intake and long-term risk of coronary heart disease and cancer in the Seven Countries Study, *Arch. Int. Med.*, 155, 381–386, 1995.

12. Knekt, P. et al., Flavonoid intake and risk of chronic diseases, *Am. J. Clin. Nutr.*, 76, 560–568, 2002.

13. Hertog, M.G., Feskens, E.J., and Kromhout, D., Antioxidant flavonols and coronary heart disease risk, *Lancet*, 349, 699, 1997.

14. Keli, S.O. et al., Dietary flavonoids, antioxidant vitamins, and incidence of stroke. The Zutphen Study, *Arch. Int. Med.*, 156, 637–642, 1996.

15. Geleijnse, J.M. et al., Inverse association of tea and flavonoid intakes with incident myocardial infarction: the Rotterdam Study, *Am. J. Clin. Nutr.*, 75, 880–886, 2002.

16. Yochum, L. et al., Dietary flavonoid intake and risk of cardiovascular disease in postmenopausal women, *Am. J. Epidemiol.*, 149, 943–949, 1999.

17. Rimm, E.B. et al., Relation between intake of flavonoids and risk for coronary heart disease in male health professionals, *Ann. Int. Med.*, 125, 384–389, 1996.

18. Hertog, M.L. et al., Antioxidant flavonols and ischemic heart disease in a Welsh population of men — the Caerphilly Study, *Am. J. Clin. Nutr.*, 65, 1489–1494, 1997.

19. Renaud, S. and de Lorgeril, M., Wine, alcohol, platelets, and the French paradox for coronary heart disease, *Lancet*, 339, 1523–1526, 1992.

20. Renaud, S.C. et al., Alcohol and mortality in middle-aged men from Eastern France, *Epidemiology*, 9, 184–188, 1998.

21. Criqui, M.H. and Ringel, B.L., Does diet or alcohol explain the French paradox?, *Lancet*, 344, 1719–1723, 1994.

22. Rimm, E.B. et al., Review of moderate alcohol consumption and reduced risk of coronary heart disease: is the effect due to beer, wine, or spirits? *Br. Med. J.*, 312, 731–736, 1996.

23. Rimm, E.B. et al., Moderate alcohol intake and lower risk of coronary heart disease: meta-analysis of effects on lipids and haemostatic factors, *Br. Med. J.*, 319, 1523–1528, 1999.

24. Dimmitt, S.B. et al., The effects of alcohol on coagulation and fibrinolytic factors — a controlled trial, *Blood Coag. Fibrinol.*, 9, 39–45, 1998.

25. Hendriks, H.F.J. et al., Effect of moderate dose of alcohol with evening meal on fibrinolytic factors, *Br. Med. J.*, 308, 1003–1006, 1994.

26. Renaud, S.C. et al., Alcohol and platelet aggregation: the Caerphilly Prospective Heart Disease Study, *Am. J. Clin. Nutr.*, 55, 1012–1017, 1992.

27. Langer, R.D., Criqui, M.H., and Reed, D.M., Lipoproteins and blood pressure as biological pathways for effect of moderate alcohol consumption on coronary heart disease, *Circulation*, 85, 910–915, 1992.

28. Gronbaek, M. et al., Mortality associated with moderate intakes of wine, beer, or spirits, *Br. Med. J.*, 310, 1165–1169, 1995.

29. Truelsen, T. et al., Intake of beer, wine, and spirits and risk of stroke. The Copenhagen City Heart Study, *Stroke*, 29, 2467–2472, 1998.

30. Rimm, E.B., Invited commentary — alcohol consumption and coronary heart disease: good habits may be more important than just good wine, *Am. J. Epidemiol.*, 143, 1094–1098, 1996.

31. Klatsky, A.L., Is it the drink or the drinker? Circumstantial evidence only raises a probability, *Am. J. Clin. Nutr.*, 69, 2–3, 1999.

32. Tjonneland, A. et al., Wine intake and diet in a random sample of 48763 Danish men and women, *Am. J. Clin. Nutr.*, 69, 49–54, 1999.

33. Mortensen, E.L. et al., Better psychological functioning and higher social status may largely explain the apparent health benefits of wine: a study of wine and beer drinking in young Danish adults, *Arch. Intern. Med*, 161, 1844–1848, 2001.

34. Klatsky, A.L., Diet, alcohol, and health: a story of connections, confounders, and cofactors, *Am. J. Clin. Nutr.*, 74, 279–280, 2001.

35. Klatsky, A.L., Armstrong, M.A., and Kipp, H., Correlates of alcoholic beverage preference: traits of persons who choose wine, liquor or beer, *Brit. J. Addict.*, 85, 1279–1289, 1990.

36. Burke, V., Puddey, I.B., and Beilin, L.J., Mortality associated with wines, beers, and spirits — Australian data suggest that choice of beverage relates to lifestyle and personality, *Br. Med. J.*, 311, 1166, 1995.

37. Xia, J.M., Allenbrand, B., and Sun, G.Y., Dietary supplementation of grape polyphenols and chronic ethanol administration on LDL oxidation and platelet function in rats, *Life Sci.*, 63, 383–390, 1998.

38. Blanco-Colio, L.M. et al., Red wine intake prevents nuclear factor-kappa B activation in peripheral blood mononuclear cells of healthy volunteers during postprandial lipemia, *Circulation*, 102, 1020–1026, 2000.

39. Lin, Y.L. et al., Theaflavin-3,3'-digallate from black tea blocks the nitric oxide synthase by down-regulating the activation of NF-kappaB in macrophages, *Eur. J. Pharmacol.*, 367, 379–388, 1999.

40. Wallerath, T. et al., Red wine increases the expression of human endothelial nitric oxide synthase: a mechanism that may contribute to its beneficial cardiovascular effects, *J. Am. Coll. Cardiol.*, 41, 471–478, 2003.

41. Andriambeloson, E. et al., Natural dietary polyphenolic compounds cause endothelium-dependent vasorelaxation in rat thoracic aorta, *J. Nutr.*, 128, 2324–2333, 1998.

42. Fitzpatrick, D.F., Hirschfield, S.L., and Coffey, R.G., Endothelium-dependent vasorelaxing activity of wine and other grape products, *Am. J. Physiol.*, 265, H774–H778, 1993.

43. Soleas, G.J. et al., Toward the fingerprinting of wines: cultivar-related patterns of polyphenolic constituents in Ontario wines, *J. Agric. Food Chem.*, 45, 3871–3880, 1997.

44. Pendurthi, U.R., Williams, J.T., and Rao, L.V.M., Resveratrol, a polyphenolic compound found in wine, inhibits tissue factor expression in vascular cells. A possible mechanism for the cardiovascular benefits associated with moderate consumption of wine, *Arterioscler. Thromb. Vasc. Biol.*, 19, 419–426, 1999.

45. Scalbert, A. and Williamson, G., Dietary intake and bioavailability of polyphenols, *J. Nutr.*, 130, 2073S–2085S, 2000.

46. Donovan, J.L. et al., Catechin is present as metabolites in human plasma after consumption of red wine, *J. Nutr.*, 129, 1662–1668, 1999.

47. Caccetta, R.A. et al., Ingestion of red wine significantly increases plasma phenolic acid concentrations but does not acutely affect *ex vivo* lipoprotein oxidizability, *Am. J. Clin. Nutr.*, 71, 67–74, 2000.

48. De Vries, J.H.M. et al., Red wine is a poor source of bioavailable flavonols in men, *J. Nutr.*, 131, 745–748, 2000.

49. Croft, K.D., The chemistry and biological effects of flavonoids and phenolic acids, *Ann. NY Acad. Sci.*, 854, 435–442, 1998.

50. Rice-Evans, C.A., Miller, N.J., and Paganga, G., Structure-antioxidant activity relationships of flavonoids and phenolic acids, *Free Radic. Biol. Med.*, 20, 933–956, 1996.

51. van Acker, S.A.B.E. et al., Flavonoids as scavengers of nitric oxide radical, *Biochem. Biophys. Res. Comm.*, 214, 755–759, 1995.
52. Lien, E.J. et al., Quantitative structure-activity relationship analysis of phenolic antioxidants, *Free Radic. Biol. Med*, 26, 285–294, 1999.
53. van Acker, S.A. et al., Structural aspects of antioxidant activity of flavonoids, *Free Radic. Biol. Med*, 20, 331–342, 1996.
54. Abu-Amsha, R. et al., Phenolic content of various beverages determines the extent of inhibition of human serum and low-density lipoprotein oxidation *in vitro* — identification and mechanism of action of some cinnamic acid derivatives from red wine, *Clin. Sci.*, 91, 449–458, 1996.
55. Frankel, E.N. et al., Inhibition of oxidation of human low-density lipoprotein by phenolic substances in red wine, *Lancet*, 341, 454–457, 1993.
56. Kanner, J. et al., Natural antioxidants in grapes and wines, *J. Agric. Food Chem.*, 42, 64–69, 1994.
57. Deckert, V. et al., Prevention of LDL alpha-tocopherol consumption, cholesterol oxidation, and vascular endothelium dysfunction by polyphenolic compounds from red wine, *Atherosclerosis*, 165, 41, 2002.
58. Morton, L.W. et al., Chemistry and biological effects of dietary phenolic compounds: relevance to cardiovascular disease, *Clin. Exp. Pharmacol. Physiol.*, 27, 152–159, 2000.
59. Carbonneau, M.A. et al., Supplementation with wine phenolic compounds increases the antioxidant capacity of plasma and vitamin E of low-density lipoprotein without changing the lipoprotein Cu_2^+-oxidizability — possible explanation by phenolic location, *Eur. J. Clin. Nutr.*, 51, 682–690, 1997.
60. de Rijke, Y.B. et al., Red wine consumption does not affect oxidizability of low-density lipoproteins in volunteers, *Am. J. Clin. Nutr.*, 63, 329–334, 1996.
61. Fuhrman, B., Lavy, A., and Aviram, M., Consumption of red wine with meals reduces the susceptibility of human plasma and low-density lipoprotein to lipid peroxidation, *Am. J. Clin. Nutr.*, 61, 549–554, 1995.
62. Kondo, K. et al., Inhibition of oxidation of low-density lipoprotein with red wine, *Lancet*, 344, 1152, 1994.
63. Maxwell, S., Cruickshank, A., and Thorpe, G., Red wine and antioxidant activity in serum, *Lancet*, 344, 193–194, 1994.
64. Miyagi, Y., Miwa, K., and Inoue, H., Inhibition of human low-density lipoprotein oxidation by flavonoids in red wine and grape juice, *Am. J. Cardiol.*, 80, 1627, 1997.
65. Nigdikar, S.V. et al., Consumption of red wine polyphenols reduces the susceptibility of low-density lipoproteins to oxidation *in vivo*, *Am. J. Clin. Nutr.*, 68, 258–265, 1998.
66. Serafini, M., Maiani, G., and Ferroluzzi, A., Alcohol-free red wine enhances plasma antioxidant capacity in humans, *J. Nutr.*, 128, 1003–1007, 1998.
67. Whitehead, T.P. et al., Effect of red wine ingestion on the antioxidant capacity of serum, *Clin. Chem.*, 41, 32–35, 1995.
68. Caccetta, R.A.A. et al., Red wine polyphenols, in the absence of alcohol, reduce lipid peroxidative stress in smoking subjects, *Free Radic. Biol. Med.*, 30, 636–642, 2001.
69. Meagher, E.A. et al., Alcohol-induced generation of lipid peroxidation products in humans, *J. Clin. Invest.*, 104, 805–813, 1999.
70. Cao, G., Sofic, E., and Prior, R.L., Antioxidant and prooxidant behavior of flavonoids: structure-activity relationships, *Free Radic. Biol. Med.*, 22, 749–760, 1997.
71. Yamanaka, N., Oda, O., and Nagao, S., Prooxidant activity of caffeic acid, dietary non-flavonoid phenolic acid, on Cu^{2+}-induced low density lipoprotein oxidation, *FEBS Lett.*, 405, 186–190, 1997.

72. Halliwell, B. and Gutteridge, J.M., The antioxidants of human extracellular fluids, *Arch. Biochem. Biophys.*, 280, 1–8, 1990.
73. Halliwell, B., Gutteridge, J.M., and Cross, C.E., Free radicals, antioxidants, and human disease: where are we now? *J. Lab. Clin. Med.*, 119, 598–620, 1992.
74. Smith, C. et al., Stimulation of lipid peroxidation and hydroxyl-radical generation by the contents of human atherosclerotic lesions, *Biochem. J.*, 286, 901–905, 1992.
75. Tamminen, M. et al., Ultrastructure of early lipid accumulation in ApoE-deficient mice, *Arterioscler. Thromb. Vasc. Biol.*, 19, 847–853, 1999.
76. Hayek, T. et al., Reduced progression of atherosclerosis in apolipoprotein E-deficient mice following consumption of red wine, or its polyphenols quercetin or catechin, is associated with reduced susceptibility of LDL to oxidation and aggregation, *Arterioscler. Thromb. Vasc. Biol.*, 17, 2744–2752, 1997.
77. Bentzon, J.F. et al., Red wine does not reduce mature atherosclerosis in apolipoprotein E-deficient mice, *Circulation*, 103, 1681–1687, 2001.
78. Willcox, J.K., Catignani, G.L., and Roberts, L.J., Dietary flavonoids fail to suppress F_2-isoprostane formation *in vivo*, *Free Radic. Biol. Med.*, 34, 795–799, 2003.
79. Vinson, J.A., Teufel, K., and Wu, N., Red wine, dealcoholized red wine, and especially grape juice, inhibit atherosclerosis in a hamster model, *Atherosclerosis*, 156, 67–72, 1999.
80. Mizutani, K. et al., Extract of wine phenolics improves aortic biomechanical properties in stroke-prone spontaneously hypertensive rats (SHRSP), *J. Nutr. Sci. Vitaminol.*, 45, 95–106, 1999.
81. Demrow, H.S., Slane, P.R., and Folts, J.D., Administration of wine and grape juice inhibits *in vivo* platelet activity and thrombosis in stenosed canine coronary arteries, *Circulation*, 91, 1182–1188, 1995.
82. Vieira, O. et al., Effect of dietary phenolic compounds on apoptosis of human cultured endothelial cells induced by oxidized LDL, *Brit. J. Pharmacol.*, 123, 565–573, 1998.
83. Natarajan, R. et al., Signaling mechanisms of nuclear factor-kappab-mediated activation of inflammatory genes by 13-hydroperoxyoctadecadienoic acid in cultured vascular smooth muscle cells, *Arterioscler. Thromb. Vasc. Biol.*, 21, 1408–1413, 2001.
84. Wallerath, T. et al., Resveratrol, a polyphenolic phytoalexin present in red wine, enhances expression and activity of endothelial nitric oxide synthase, *Circulation*, 106, 1652–1658, 2002.
85. Leikert, J.F. et al., Red wine polyphenols enhance endothelial nitric oxide synthase expression and subsequent nitric oxide release from endothelial cells, *Circulation*, 106, 1614–1617, 2002.
86. Mano, T. et al., Endothelial dysfunction in the early stage of atherosclerosis precedes appearance of intimal lesions assessable with intravascular ultrasound, *Am. Heart J.*, 131, 231–238, 1996.
87. Loscalzo, J., Nitric oxide and vascular disease, *N. Engl. J. Med.*, 333, 251–253, 1995.
88. Title, L.M. et al., Oral glucose loading acutely attenuates endothelium-dependent vasodilation in healthy adults without diabetes: an effect prevented by vitamins C and E, *J. Am. Coll. Cardiol.*, 36, 2185–2191, 2000.
89. Hirai, N. et al., Insulin resistance and endothelial dysfunction in smokers: effects of vitamin C, *Am. J. Physiol.*, 279, H1172–H1178, 2000.
90. Puddey, I.B. et al., Alcohol and endothelial function: a brief review, *Clin. Exp. Pharmacol. Physiol.*, 28, 1020–1024, 2001.
91. Maiorano, G. et al., Noninvasive detection of vascular dysfunction in alcoholic patients, *Am. J. Hypertens.*, 12, 137–144, 1999.

92. Teragawa, H. et al., Effect of alcohol consumption on endothelial function in men with coronary artery disease, *Atherosclerosis*, 165, 145–152, 2002.
93. Zilkens, R.R. et al., Effects of alcohol intake on endothelial function in men: a randomized controlled trial, *J. Hypertens.*, 21, 97–103, 2003.
94. Djousse, L. et al., Acute effects of a high-fat meal with and without red wine on endothelial function in healthy subjects, *Am. J. Cardiol.*, 84, 660–664, 1999.
95. Agewall, S. et al., Does a glass of red wine improve endothelial function? *Eur. Heart J.*, 21, 74–78, 2000.
96. Hashimoto, M. et al., Effect of acute intake of red wine on flow-mediated vasodilatation of the brachial artery, *Am. J. Cardiol.*, 88, 1457–60, A9, 2001.
97. Stein, J.H. et al., Purple grape juice improves endothelial function and reduces the susceptibility of LDL cholesterol to oxidation in patients with coronary artery disease, *Circulation*, 100, 1050–1055, 1999.
98. Chou, E.J. et al., Effect of ingestion of purple grape juice on endothelial function in patients with coronary heart disease, *Am. J. Cardiol.*, 88, 553–555, 2001.
99. Croft, K.D. et al., Oxidative susceptibility of low-density lipoproteins — influence of regular alcohol use, *Alcohol Clin. Exp. Res.*, 20, 980–984, 1996.
100. Morrow, J.D. et al., A series of prostaglandin F_2-like compounds are produced *in vivo* in humans by a non-cyclooxygenase, free radical-catalyzed mechanism, *Proc. Natl. Acad. Sci. U.S.A*, 87, 9383–9387, 1990.
101. Meagher, E.A. et al., Alcohol-induced generation of lipid peroxidation products in humans, *J. Clin. Invest.*, 104, 805–813, 1999.
102. Waddington, E.I. et al., Fatty acid oxidation products in human atherosclerotic plaque: an analysis of clinical and histopathological correlates, *Atherosclerosis*, 167, 111–120, 2003.
103. Pawlosky, R.J., Flynn, B.M., and Salem, N., Jr., The effects of low dietary levels of polyunsaturates on alcohol-induced liver disease in rhesus monkeys, *Hepatology*, 26, 1386–1392, 1997.
104. Hill, D.B. and Awad, J.A., Increased urinary F_2-isoprostane excretion in alcoholic liver disease, *Free Radic.*, 26, 656–660, 1999.
105. Kukielka, E., Dicker, E., and Cederbaum, A.I., Increased production of reactive oxygen species by rat liver mitochondria after chronic ethanol treatment, *Arch. Biochem. Biophys.*, 309, 377–386, 1994.
106. Nordmann, R., Ribiere, C., and Rouach, H., Ethanol-induced lipid peroxidation and oxidative stress in extrahepatic tissues, *Alcohol Alcohol.*, 25, 231–237, 1990.
107. Zidenberg-Cherr, S. et al., Ethanol-induced changes in hepatic free radical defense mechanisms and fatty-acid composition in the miniature pig, *Hepatology*, 13, 1185–1192, 1991.
108. Speisky, H. et al., Increased loss and decreased synthesis of hepatic glutathione after acute ethanol administration, *Biochem. J.*, 225, 565, 1985.
109. Xin, X. et al., Effects of alcohol reduction on blood pressure: a meta-analysis of randomized controlled trials, *Hypertension*, 38, 1112–1117, 2001.
110. Cook, N.R. et al., Implications of small reductions in diastolic blood pressure for primary prevention, *Arch. Int. Med.*, 155, 701–709, 1995.
111. Romero, J.C. and Reckelhoff, J.F., State-of-the-art lecture. Role of angiotensin and oxidative stress in essential hypertension, *Hypertension*, 34, 943–949, 1999.
112. Henningsen, N.C., Janzon, L., and Trell, E., Influence of carboxyhemoglobin, gamma-glutamyl-transferase, body weight, and heart rate on blood pressure in middle-aged men, *Hypertension*, 5, 560–563, 1983.

113. Nilssen, O. and Forde, O.H., Seven-year longitudinal population study of change in gamma-glutamyltransferase: the Tromso Study, *Am. J. Epidemiol.*, 139, 787–792, 1994.

114. Moellering, D. et al., The induction of GSH synthesis by nanomolar concentrations of NO in endothelial cells: a role for gamma-glutamylcysteine synthetase and gamma-glutamyl transpeptidase, *FEBS Lett.*, 448, 292–296, 1999.

115. Yamada, Y. et al., Alcohol, high blood pressure and serum gamma-glutamyl transpeptidase level, *Hypertension*, 18, 819–826, 1991.

116. Lee, D.H. et al., Gamma-glutamyltransferase, alcohol, and blood pressure. A four year follow-up study, *Ann. Epidemiol.*, 12, 90–96, 2002.

117. Yamada, Y. et al., Serum gamma-glutamyl transferase levels and blood pressure falls after alcohol moderation, *Clin. Exp. Hypertens.*, 19, 249–268, 1997.

118. Chen, C.K. and Pace-Asciak, C.R., Vasorelaxing activity of resveratrol and quercetin in isolated rat aorta, *Gen. Pharmacol.*, 27, 363–366, 1996.

119. Flesch, M., Schwarz, A., and Bohm, M., Effects of red and white wine on endothelium-dependent vasorelaxation of rat aorta and human coronary arteries, *Am. J. Physiol.*, 275, H1183-H1190, 1998.

120. Klatsky, A. et al., Alcohol consumption and blood pressure — Kaiser-Permanente Multiphasic Health Examination Data, *N. Engl. J. Med.*, 296, 1194–1200, 1977.

121. Ueshima, H. et al., Alcohol intake and hypertension among urban and rural Japanese populations, *J. Chron. Dis.*, 37, 585–592, 1984.

122. Lang, T. et al., Relationship between alcohol consumption and hypertension prevalence and control in a French population, *J. Chron. Dis.*, 40, 713–720, 1987.

123. Trevisan, M. et al., Alcohol consumption, drinking pattern and blood pressure: analysis of data from the Italian National Research Council Study, *Int. J. Epidemiol.*, 16, 520–527, 1987.

124. Keil, U., Chambless, L., and Remmers, A., Alcohol and blood pressure: results from the Luebeck blood pressure study, *Prev. Med.*, 18, 1–10, 1989.

125. Arkwright, P.D. et al., Effects of alcohol use and other aspects of lifestyle on blood pressure levels and prevalence of hypertension in a working population, *Circulation*, 66, 60–66, 1982.

126. Criqui, M.H. et al., Alcohol consumption and blood pressure. The Lipid Research Clinics Prevalence Study, *Hypertension*, 3, 557–565, 1981.

127. Marques-Vidal, P. et al., Relationships between alcoholic beverages and cardiovascular risk factor levels in middle-aged men, the PRIME study, *Atherosclerosis*, 157, 431–440, 2001.

128. Boushey, C.J. et al., A quantitative assessment of plasma homocysteine as a risk factor for vascular disease. Probable benefits of increasing folic acid intakes, *JAMA*, 274, 1049–1057, 1995.

129. Welch, G.N. and Loscalzo, J., Homocysteine and atherothrombosis, *N. Engl. J. Med.*, 338, 1042–1050, 1998.

130. Halsted, C.H., Lifestyle effects on homocysteine and an alcohol paradox, *Am. J. Clin. Nutr.*, 73, 501–502, 2001.

131. Jacques, P.F. et al., Determinants of plasma total homocysteine concentration in the Framingham Offspring cohort, *Am. J. Clin. Nutr.*, 73, 613–621, 2001.

132. Cravo, M.L. et al., Hyperhomocysteinemia in chronic alcoholism: correlation with folate, vitamin B-12, and vitamin B-6 status, *Am. J. Clin. Nutr.*, 63, 220–224, 1996.

133. Hultberg, B. et al., Elevated plasma homocysteine in alcoholics, *Alcohol Clin. Exp. Res.*, 17, 687–689, 1993.

134. Koehler, K.M. et al., Association of folate intake and serum homocysteine in elderly persons according to vitamin supplementation and alcohol use, *Am. J. Clin. Nutr.*, 73, 628–637, 2001.
135. Ubbink, J.B. et al., Homocysteine and ischaemic heart disease in the Caerphilly cohort, *Atherosclerosis*, 140, 349–356, 1998.
136. Mayer, O., Jr., Simon, J., and Rosolova, H., A population study of the influence of beer consumption on folate and homocysteine concentrations, *Eur. J. Clin. Nutr.*, 55, 605–609, 2001.
137. van der Gaag, M.S. et al., Effect of consumption of red wine, spirits, and beer on serum homocysteine, *Lancet*, 355, 1522, 2000.
138. Bleich, S. et al., Moderate alcohol consumption in social drinkers raises plasma homocysteine levels: a contradiction in the "French Paradox"? *Alcohol Alcohol.*, 36, 189–192, 2001.
139. Olthof, M.R. et al., Consumption of high doses of chlorogenic acid, present in coffee, or black tea increases plasma total homocysteine concentrations in humans, *Am. J. Clin. Nutr.*, 73, 532–538, 2001.
140. Hodgson, J.M. et al., Can black tea influence plasma total homocysteine concentrations? *Am. J. Clin. Nutr.*, 77, 907–911, 2003.

Section II

Alcohol and Liver Disease

3 Nutritional Factors in the Pathogenesis of Alcoholic Liver Disease: An Update

Samuel W. French and Y.-J.Y. Wan

CONTENTS

3.1   INTRODUCTION

There is little doubt that alcoholic liver disease (ALD) is a nutritional disease. It has been argued that ethanol is a direct liver toxin because of the formation of its metabolite, acetaldehyde, which forms adducts with proteins. However, the importance of acetaldehyde adducts in ALD pathogenesis is still at the theoretical level.

In fact, increasing the levels of blood acetaldehyde by giving acetaldehyde dehydrogenase inhibitors actually prevented liver injury in rats fed ethanol.[1] On the other hand, it has been clearly shown that a number of nutritional factors are involved in ALD pathogenesis, which is the subject of this review. Each of these factors will be discussed as follows: (1) alcohol changes the requirements of proteins, carbohydrates, and lipids by altering liver metabolism, (2) high blood ethanol levels decrease the NAD/NADH ratio and O_2 consumption rate, which changes the energy available for the metabolism of nutrients, (3) ethanol alters the enzymes involved in the methyl-donor-dependent pathways such as methyltransferases in the metabolism of *S*-adenosyl-methionine, in phosphatidyl choline synthesis, and the methylation of DNA, and (4) alcohol increases the requirement of antioxidants to reduce lipid peroxidation, i.e., manganese, copper, and zinc.

3.2 ALCOHOL INCREASES THE REQUIREMENTS OF PROTEINS, CARBOHYDRATES, AND LIPIDS BY ALTERING LIVER METABOLISM, AND DIETARY IRON INCREASES OXIDATIVE STRESS INJURY

3.2.1 CARBOHYDRATES

It has become clear that the amount of carbohydrate in the diet is critical because it influences the blood alcohol levels (BAL), the degree of liver pathology, and the level of CYP2E1 induction in experimental ALD. Originally, it was thought that the enhancement of ethanol-induced CYP2E1 was due to a high-fat diet[2–4] which was further enhanced by adding linoleate to the diet.[5] However, it now appears that it is the amount of carbohydrate-derived calories displaced by the high-fat diet which causes the increased induction of CYP2E1 and alters the rate of alcohol elimination. Sato et al. showed that the induction of CYP450 by ethanol was prevented by a high-carbohydrate diet.[6] In the absence of carbohydrate in the diet, CYP2E1 (MEOS) was maximally induced by alcohol, and the addition of a high-protein or high-fat diet did not affect the increase in CYP2E1 caused by the absence of carbohydrate in the diet.[7] This effect of reduced dietary carbohydrate is associated with an increase in liver pathology and is associated with higher blood alcohol levels when fed to rats *ad libitum*.[8,9] Using a low-carbohydrate diet, but otherwise a different diet composition, failed to cause a more severe liver pathology. It was confirmed, however, that the blood alcohol levels were higher compared with a diet rich in carbohydrate.[10] The blood alcohol levels varied from day to day but were generally higher, which could be important in ALD pathogenesis.

There is a problem in equating the results of the various dietary studies on the effect of carbohydrate when rats are fed *ad lib*. The problem is that the other dietary ingredients differ and those differences are unknown because the dietary compositions are not given. Specifically, the level of methyl donors such as choline and methionine is only stated in two studies.[9–12] This is an important aspect to consider because methyl donor deficiency leads to cirrhosis and potentiates the liver damage caused by ethanol feeding in rats.[13] Additionally, the vitamin and mineral content, especially those vitamins and minerals that are related to methyl donor metabolism and antioxidant activity, need to be equated in the diet to allow meaningful comparisons to be made between the results of the various studies reported. The vitamins and minerals in this category include vitamin B_6, vitamin B_{12}, and folic acid. The minerals involved include copper, zinc, and manganese. The role of dietary choline, vitamins, and minerals in protecting the liver from ethanol-induced liver damage was discussed in depth in a previous review.[14]

Antioxidant metabolites such as glutathione and antioxidant vitamins such as vitamins C and E are also important in protecting the liver from ethanol-induced oxidative stress and, therefore, also need to be equated for the purpose of comparing the results of the different dietary regimens used in the low carbohydrate studies.

Also important is the degree of carbohydrate deficiency. For instance, in one report the calories of carbohydrate fed was 11%,[9] in another study it was 5%,[10] in another study it was 2%,[8] and in another 0%.[15] None of these study diets is similar to the diets consumed by human alcoholics.[16]

3.2.2 PROTEINS

Both the quality and the quantity of protein may influence the degree of liver pathology induced by ethanol. In alcoholic liver disease in man, protein–calorie malnutrition may involve 100% of the patients in the alcoholic hepatitis stage of ALD.[17] In fact, dietary protein supplement and calories proved to be critical for survival in the treatment of ALD.[17]

In rats fed ethanol, the percent of calories derived from protein influences the degree of liver damage and fibrosis.[18,19] Young rats require that the dietary protein composition be 18% of calories for optimum growth. Growing rates are usually used to establish that the diet is adequate in studies on experimental alcohol disease in rats. When a diet deficient in protein was fed, liver enlargement was greater and fatty change and fibrosis were greater compared with rats fed ethanol and adequate protein.[19]

The quality of protein may also be important in ALD pathogenesis. For instance, casein contains more methionine than does soybean protein. In the case of alcoholic patients, the source of dietary protein in the form of meat or fish influences the incidence of alcoholic hepatitis and cirrhosis.[16] For instance, alcoholic hepatitis and cirrhosis were found to be more prevalent in alcoholic abusers who ate pork and pig products compared with those who eat beef or fish.[16] This is supported by the epidemiologic evidence that indicates that *per capita* pork consumption with or without alcohol consumption correlates positively with the incidence of cirrhosis.[20] In that study a detailed dietary history and one or more liver biopsies were available for each patient. Another variable in that study was the type of alcoholic beverage consumed. Those patients who drank wine had fatty liver or alcoholic hepatitis but had a lower incidence of cirrhosis than those patients who drank beer. The type of meat and beverage consumed were independent variables.[16]

3.2.3 DIETARY FAT

In a previous review, the type and amount of fat consumed by rats fed ethanol and the amount of fat consumed by alcoholic patients were shown to correlate with more advanced stages of ALD including fibrosis in rats and cirrhosis in man.[14] The type of dietary fatty acids consumed by alcoholics with ALD did not influence the stage of ALD in liver biopsied patients, however.[16] In rats fed ethanol, the type of fat plays a role in the pathogenesis of ALD as summarized in a previous review.[18] Medium-chain triglycerides and tallow both totally prevented ALD in the rat fed intragastrically, despite a high blood alcohol level being maintained and a high-fat diet. However, lard, sunflower oil, olive oil, safflower oil, corn oil, tallow + 18:2, and fish oil all support the development of ALD.[18] Only a small amount of linoleic acid (2.5%) is required to support the development of ALD. The pathology of ALD is less with olive oil, lard, and palm oil, and worse with fish oil except that fatty liver is found less often with fish oil (menhaden oil).[18,21] Fish oil is rich in eicosapentaenoic acid (20:5n-3) and docosahexaenoic acid (22:6n-3). Both are omega-3 polyunsaturated fatty acids which are antagonistic to omega-6 polyunsaturated fatty acids (i.e., 18:2, 20:4) and inhibit cytokine formation such as LTB_4 and thromboxane A_2 formation. Both types of fat support the inflammatory changes in the liver when ethanol is fed. However, the inflammation is greater in the rats fed ethanol and fish oil.[22] This increase may be related to a greater induction of CYP2E1 and increased lipid peroxidation.[22]

There is evidence that fatty acid metabolism shifts from β oxidation in the mitochondria and peroxisomes to the endoplasmic cytochrome P450 (CYP) enzymes which peroxidate, hydroxylate, and epoxidate long-chain polyunsaturated fatty acids to form bioactive intermediates such as hydroxy-eicosatetraenoic acids and epoxy-licosatrienoic acids[23] and enzymes that metabolize arachidonic acid to bioactive prostaglandins and thromboxanes.[24] The intermediates that form from fatty acid hydroxylation result from ethanol-induced CYP 4A1, 3A1, 2B1, and 1B1.[25–28]

3.3 HIGH BLOOD ALCOHOL LEVELS DECREASE THE NAD/NADH RATIO, O_2 CONSUMPTION RATE, AND ETHANOL ELIMINATION RATE, WHICH CHANGES THE TYPE OF ENERGY AVAILABLE FOR THE METABOLISM OF NUTRIENTS

When the intragastric tube continuous feeding model of ALD was first developed, a cyclic change in the rate of ethanol elimination was noted.[29] When blood alcohol levels were falling in this model, the rate of ethanol elimination was rising and, conversely, when the blood alcohol levels were rising, the rate of ethanol elimination was falling. Thus the cyclic rise and fall in the blood alcohol levels during continuous ethanol ingestion was due to the change in the rate of oxidation of alcohol by alcohol dehydrogenase activity.

Thus, the level of blood ethanol as a nutrient was somehow governing the rate of its own oxidation. This cycling of the rate of ethanol elimination depended on a cyclic change in body temperature and a change in the rate of O_2 consumption which were inversely proportional to the urine ethanol levels (equivalent to blood alcohol levels in this model).[30] When thyroid secretion of thyroxin (T4) was blocked by propylthiouracil, the cycle was eliminated.[30] When the pituitary stalk was cut, the cycle was also eliminated.[30,31] It was concluded that the cycle was dependent on an intact hypothalamic–pituitary–thyroid axis initiated by a fall in body temperature caused by the effect on the brain when high blood alcohol levels are achieved.

The main metabolic consequence of the cyclic changes in the blood alcohol levels was the decrease in O_2 consumption when the blood alcohol levels reached 300 to 400 mg%. ATP levels fell because of the reduced oxidative phosphorylation by the mitochondrial electron transport chain due to hypoxia at high BALs. The NAD/NADH ratio also falls due to liver hypoxia.[32] The drop in the NAD/NADH ratio reduces the rate of elimination of ethanol by alcohol dehydrogenase.

The hypoxia also reduces β-fatty acid oxidation by the mitochondria, and increases triglyceride storage by the liver. The steatohepatitis lesion of ALD is worse at the peaks.[30] Hypoxia was documented at the peaks using the hypoxia indicator pimonidazole. The activation of the hypoxic responsive element HIFα induces the expression of the VEGF gene. VEGF protein is increased at the peaks. Erythropoietin gene expression, which is upregulated by hypoxia, also increased.[33] Other changes in gene expression also differed at the peaks and troughs of the cycle.

Microarray analysis emphasized these differences[34] (Figure 3.1). JNK was increased at the troughs compared to the peaks (Figure 3.1). MAP kinase 3, DNA-damage-inducible protein 45, D-aminoacid oxidase, and catechol-*O*-methyl transferase were increased at the peaks (Figure 3.1). Cytochrome P450 isozymes and reductases were upregulated at the peaks (Figure 3.1), indicating rather profound differences in gene expression of proteins involved in the metabolism of macro- and micronutrients and ethanol as well as antioxidant requirements at the peak of the cycle which is rate-limited by the availability of NAD. The levels of ADH in the liver did not change significantly.[32] Hypoxia at the peaks was documented immunohistochemically, where an increased adduct formation of pimonidazole was observed *in vivo*.[32] Glycogen stores did not change at the peaks and troughs of the cycle, probably because glucose was continually infused with diet and ethanol.

Thus it appears that ethanol as a central nervous system depressant alters basic biochemical pathways of energy-dependent (ATP and O_2) and NAD-dependent enzyme activities such as alcohol dehydrogenase.

3.4 ETHANOL ALTERS THE ENZYMES INVOLVED IN THE METHYL DONOR-DEPENDENT PATHWAYS SUCH AS METHYL TRANSFERASES IN THE METABOLISM OF *S*-ADENOSYLMETHIONINE AND PHOSPHATIDYL CHOLINE SYNTHESIS, AND IN THE METHYLATION OF DNA

There is renewed interest in the effect of ethanol on the methionine-*S*-adenosyl-methionine-glutathione pathway of metabolism because of the depletion of glutathione (GSH) in the mitochondria[33] which responds to *S*-adenosylmethionine (SAMe) oral therapy[34] in the intragastric feeding model of rat ALD. With alcoholic patients, serum levels of methionine increase,[35] further suggesting a deficit in this pathway (Figure 3.2). The components of this pathway are numerous and involve numerous enzymes, transcription factors, nutrients, and vitamins (Figure 3.2). The

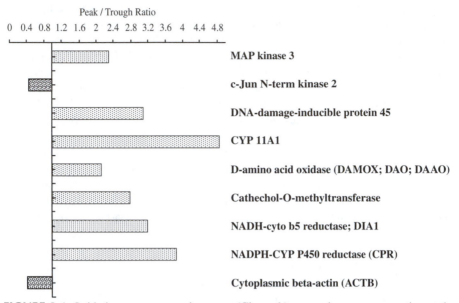

FIGURE 3.1 Oxidative stress gene microarray (Clontech) comparing gene expression at the peaks and troughs of the UAL cycle (peak/trough ratio). The values were normalized against the average values. The scale is fold increase or decrease. The data are derived from pooled samples from five pairs of rats. Only 2+ fold changed genes are listed.

transcription factors which are involved in the expression of most of these enzymes have been identified using hepatocyte RXRα-deficient mice.[36] When RXRα is deficient, it downregulates the expression of upregulate cystathionine β-synthase (CBS), γ-glutamyl cysteine ligase catalytic subunit (GLCLC), glycine-*N* methyl transferase (GNMT), methionine synthetase (MS) and 5, 10-methylenetetrahydro-folate reductase (MTHER), cysteine choline kinase (CK), and choline/ethanolamine-phospho-transferase (CEPT) genes. However, the expression of phosphatidylcholine transfer protein (PCTP) and adenosylhomocysteinase (AHCY) is upregulated in hepatocyte RXRα-deficient mice. Vitamins involved in the pathway include retinoic acid, folic acid, B_2, B_6, and B_{12}. Folate is involved in the activity of MTHFR, and B_6 is involved in the activity of CBS, THF, and betaine-homocysteine/*S*-methyl transferase (BHMT). B_2 is involved in MTHFR and B_{12} is involved in MS activity. One heavy metal, zinc, is involved in BHMT and CBS activity. Hence the pathway is very complex with numerous nutritional variables which are affected by ethanol ingestion and dietary composition.

Chronic ethanol ingestion affects the methionine-*S*-adenosylmethionine pathway adversely at several different sites of the pathway. First, ethanol causes a shift in predominance of methionine adenosyltransferase (MAT) with a decrease in the MATIA/MAT2A ratio expression, which leads to decreased SAMe, GSH, and DNA methylation levels, decreased homocysteine metabolism, and hyperhomocysteine-mia.[37] Possible pathologic consequences include decreased antioxidant defense, fibrogenesis, induction of TNFα, increased DNA strand breaks, and upregulation of c-*myc* expression.[37]

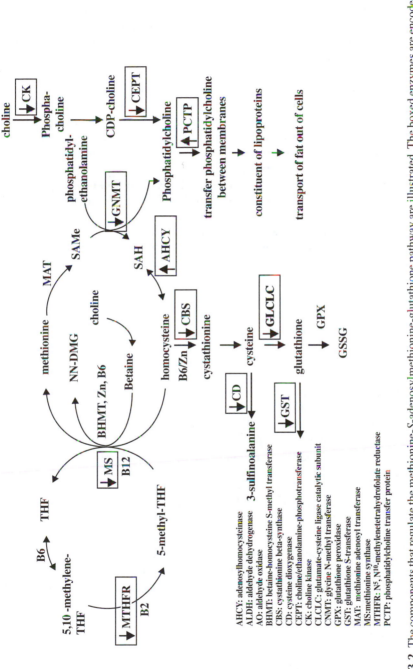

FIGURE 3.2 The components that regulate the methionine–S-adenosylmethionine-glutathione pathway are illustrated. The boxed enzymes are encoded genes regulated by RXRα deficiency. The arrows indicate up or down regulation.

AHCY: adenosylhomocysteinase
ALDH: aldehyde dehydrogenase
AO: aldehyde oxidase
BHMT: betaine-homocysteine S-methyl transferase
CBS: cystathionine beta-synthase
CD: cysteine dioxygenase
CEPT: choline/ethanolamine-phosphotransferase
CK: choline kinase
CLCLC: glutamate-cysteine ligase catalytic subunit
CNMT: glycine N-methyl transferase
GPX: glutathione peroxidase
GST: glutathione S-transferase
MAT: methionine adenosyl transferase
MS: methionine synthase
MTHFR: N^5, N^{10}-methylenetetrahydrofolate reductase
PCTP: phosphatidylcholine transfer protein

There are other sites of the pathway affected by chronic ethanol feeding with the net effect of a reduction of methionine and an increase in homocysteine where MS and CBS activity are reduced and betaine-homocysteine methyltransferase (BHMT) is increased.[37] Folate and B_{12} deficiency seen in alcoholics may play an important role in the ethanol-induced decrease in MS activity observed.[38] For instance, ethanol ingestion impairs folate absorption.[39] An increase in the homocysteine/SAMe ratio is observed.[38] Betaine is preempted in the synthesis of SAMe to compensate for reduced methionine resynthesis from homocysteine[40] but increases the requirement for folate and *vice versa*.[41] Both SAMe and betaine supplements may have a potential therapeutic value in the treatment of ALD for this reason.[37,40] Since humans lack choline oxidase which converts choline to betaine, the BHMT alternate pathway to convert homocysteine to methionine cannot compensate so that betaine supplements would be necessary for this pathway to become activated.[42] Ethanol ingestion in the rat enhances the fatty liver caused by either choline deficiency or B_6 deficiency.[43] Choline deficiency acts by reducing methionine and SAMe synthesis from homocysteine and export from the liver. B_6 deficiency acts by reducing conversion of homocysteine to cystathionine due to decreased CBS activity.

Treatment of ALD with SAMe supplements improves blood levels of SAMe and glutathionine (GSH).[44] SAMe blood levels are reduced in both human and experimental ALD. SAMe therapy also corrects abnormalities of Kupffer cell cytokine production in response to LPS.[45] Although SAMe supplements improve survival of patients with less severe ALD, the mechanisms involved in this treatment effect have not been determined.[37,46]

Both RXRα- and PPARα-regulated genes involved in liver metabolism are affected by chronic ethanol ingestion. For instance, in rats fed ethanol intragastrically, PPARα mRNA was downregulated, probably because of a reduction in the 20:4 levels in the livers of rats fed ethanol.[47] PPARα is directly regulated by the level of unsaturated fatty acid.[48,49] Ethanol inhibited PPARα activation of a reporter gene *in vitro* in a hepatoma cell line that expresses alcohol metabolizing enzymes. The inhibition was abolished by 4-methyl pyrazole and was increased by cyanamide, suggesting that acetaldehyde was the mediator. Acetaldehyde inhibited the binding of PPARα/RXR to PPAR response elements.[50] Fatty liver develops in PPAR-deficient mice,[51] suggesting that fatty liver may develop in ethanol-fed animals, in part, due to the failure of the regulation of fat metabolism because of the inhibition of the PPAR expression.

Ethanol feeding intragastrically did not affect the levels of RXR or RAR in rats fed intragastrically[47] but retinoic acid was markedly reduced in the liver (fivefold reduced) in this model.[52] This decrease in liver retinoic acid is associated with Ito cell activation,[47] *c-jun* overexpression,[53] and decreased expression of JNK which caused a decrease in apoptosis[54] and increased liver cell proliferation.[53,54] Retinoic acid is reduced because of an increased metabolism by ethanol-induced CYP2E1 activity.[55] Thus the PPARα/RXRα dimers which are downregulated by chronic ethanol ingestion have profound consequences on methyl donor metabolism, cytokine production, liver cell proliferation, and apoptosis as well as fatty acid storage, all of which may play a role in ALD pathogenesis.

3.5 ALCOHOL INCREASES THE REQUIREMENT OF ANTIOXIDANTS TO REDUCE LIPID PEROXIDATION, I.E., MANGANESE, COPPER, ZINC, AND DIETARY IRON INCREASE OXIDATIVE STRESS INJURY

The antioxidants which have dietary derived prosthetic groups include manganese superoxidase dismutase (Mn SOD) in the liver mitochondria and copper-zinc superoxide dismutase (CuZn SOD) in the liver cytosol. Mn SOD is downregulated at peak blood alcohol levels in chronic ethanol-fed rats, whereas CuZn SOD expression is unchanged.[56]

Dietary iron overload (650 mg/kg/diet), on the other hand, enhances lipid peroxidation in livers of rats.[57] Even a small increase in dietary iron fed to rats with ethanol accentuated oxidative stress,[58] and in liver Kupffer-cells-increased iron storage enhances the expression of TNFα.[59] The latter is thought to be key in the pathogenesis of ethanol-induced liver disease.[44]

ACKNOWLEDGMENTS

The authors are grateful for the assistance of Adriana Flores and Dr. F. Bardag-Gorce in the preparation of the manuscript, which was also supported by grants CA53596, AA014147, and NIH NIAA08116.

References

1. Lindros, K.O., Jolelaninen, K., and Nanji, A.A. Acetaldehyde prevents nuclear factor kappa B activation and hepatic inflammation in ethanol-fed rats. *Lab. Invest.*, 79: 799–806, 1999.
2. Kanayama, R., Takase, S., Matsuda, Y., and Takada, A. Effect of dietary fat upon ethanol metabolism in rats. *Biochem. Pharmacol.*, 33: 3283, 1984.
3. Joly, J.-G. and Hetu, C. Effects of chronic ethanol administration in the rat relative dependence on dietary lipids. I. Induction of hepatic drug metabolizing enzymes *in vitro. Biochem. Pharmacol.*, 24: 1475, 1975.
4. Winston, G.W. and Narayan, S. Alteration of liver microsomal monooxygenases and substrate competition with amiline hydroxylase from rats chronically fed low-fat containing alcohol diets. *J. Biochem. Toxicol.*, 3: 181, 1988.
5. Joly, J.-G. and Hetu, C. Effects of chronic ethanol administration in the rat: relative dependency on dietary lipids. II. Paradoxical role of linoleate in the induction of hepatic drug-metabolizing enzymes *in vitro. Can. J. Physiol. Pharmacol.*, 55: 34, 1977.
6. Sato, A., Najakima, T., and Kayama, Y. Interaction between ethanol and carbohydrate on the metabolism in rat liver of aromatic and chlorinated hydrocarbons. *Toxicol. Appl. Pharmacol.*, 68: 242, 1983.
7. Yonekura, I., Nakano, M., Nakajima, T., and Sato, A. Dietary carbohydrate intake as a modifying factor for the development of alcohol fatty liver. *Biochem. Arch.*, 5: 41, 1980.

8. Lindros, K.O. and Jarvelainen, H.A. A new oral low-carbohydrate alcohol liquid diet producing liver lesions: a preliminary account. *Alcohol Alcohol.*, 33: 347–353, 1998.

9. Tsukada, H., Wang, P.-Y., Kanedo, T., Wang, Y., Nakano, M., and Sato, A. Dietary carbohydrate intake plays an important role in preventing alcoholic fatty liver in the rat. *J. Hepatol.*, 29: 715–724, 1998.

10. Li, J., French, B.A., Riley, N., Bardag-Gorce, F., Fu, P., and French, S.W. Oral low-carbohydrate alcohol liquid diet induces experimental steatohepatitis in the rat. *Exp. Molec. Pathol.*, 71: 132–136, 2001.

11. Bardag-Gorce, F., French, B.A., Li, J., Riley, N.B., Yuan Q.X., Valinluk, V., Fu, P., Ingelman-Sundberg, M., Yoon, S., and French, S.W. The importance of cycling of blood alcohol levels in the pathogenesis of experimental alcoholic liver disease. *Gastroenterology*, 123: 325–335, 2002.

12. Morimoto, M., Reitz, R.C., Morin, R.J., Nguyen, K., Ingelman-Sundberg, M., and French, S.W. Fatty acid composition of hepatic lipids in rats fed ethanol and high fat diet intragastrically. Effect of CYP2E1 inhibitors. *J. Nutr.*, 125: 2953–2964, 1995.

13. French, S.W. Effect of chronic ethanol ingestion on liver enzyme changes induced by thiamine, riboflavin, pyridoxine, or choline deficiency. *J. Nutr.*, 88: 291–302, 1966.

14. French, S.W. Nutritional factors in the pathogenesis of alcoholic liver disease. In: *Nutrition and Alcohol*. Watson, R.R. and Watzl, B. (Eds.), CRC Press, Boca Raton, FL. pp. 337–361, 1992, Chap. 15.

15. French, S.W., Zhang-Gouillon, Z.Q., and Ingelman-Sundberg, M. The role of CYP2E1 induction by ethanol in the pathogenesis of alcoholic liver disease as determined by inhibitors of CYP2E1 transcription and posttransplantation modulating factors. *Alc. Clin. Exp. Res.*, 22: 738–739, 1998.

16. Bode, C., Bode, J.C., Erhardt, J.G., French, B.A., and French, S.W. Effect of the type of beverage and meat consumed by alcoholics with alcoholic liver disease. *Alc. Clin. Exp. Res.*, 22: 1803–1805, 1998.

17. Mendenhall, C.L., Moritz, T.E., Roselle, G.A., Morgan, T.R., Nemchansky, B.A., Tamburro, C.H., Schiff, E.R., McClain, C.J., Marsano, L.S., Allen, J.I., Samanta, A., Weesner, R.E., Henderson, W., Chen, T.S., French, S.W., Chedid, A., and the VA Cooperative Study Group #275. Protein energy malnutrition in severe alcoholic hepatitis. Diagnosis and response to treatment. *J. Parenteral Enteral Nutr.*, 19: 258–265, 1995.

18. French, S.W. Nutrition in the pathogenesis of alcoholic liver disease. *Alcohol Alcohol.*, 28: 97–109, 1993.

19. French, S.W., Miyamoto, K., Wong, K., Jui, L., and Briere, L. Role of the Ito cell in liver parenchymal fibrosis in rats fed alcohol and a high fat–low protein diet. *Am. J. Pathol.*, 132: 73–85, 1988.

20. Nanji, A.A. and French, S.W. Relationship between degree of histologic abnormality and serum alanine aminotransferase activity in experimental alcoholic liver disease. *Res. Commun. Subst. Abuse*, 9: 125–128, 1988.

21. Nanji, A.A, Zakim, D., Rahemtulla, A., Daly, T., Miao, L., Zhao, S., Khwaja, S., Tahan, S.R., and Dannenberg, A.J. Dietary saturated fatty acids down-regulate cyclooxygenase-2 and tumor necrosis factor alfa and reverse fibrosis in alcoholic-induced liver disease in the rat. *Hepatology*, 26: 1538–45, 1997.

22. Morimoto, M., Zern, M.A., Hagbjork, A.-L., Ingelman-Sundberg, M., and French, S.W. Fish oil, alcohol and liver pathology: role of cytochrome P450 2E1. *Proc. Soc. Exp. Biol. Med.*, 207: 197–205, 1994.

23. French, S.W., Morimoto, M., Reitz, R., Koop, D., Klopfenstein, B., Estes, K., Clot, P., Ingelman-Sundberg, M., and Albano, E. Lipid peroxidation, CYP2E1, and fatty acid metabolism in alcoholic liver disease. *J. Nutr.*, 127: 9075–9115, 1997.

24. Nanji, A.A., Miao, L, Thomas, P. et al. Enhanced cyclooxygenase-z gene expression in alcoholic liver disease in the rat. *Gastroenterology*, 112: 943–951, 1997.

25. Amet, Y., Lucas, D., Zhang-Gouillon, Z.Q., and French, S.W. P450-dependent metabolism of lauric acids in alcoholic liver disease: comparison between rat liver and kidney microsomes. *Alc. Clin. Exp. Res.*, 22: 455–462, 1998.

26. Amet, Y., Berthoum, F., and French, S.W. Alcohol-inducible P450 in rat liver and kidney microsomes. Fatty acid metabolism. *Alc. Clin. Exp. Res.*, 22: 744–746, 1998.

27. Amet, Y., Plee-Gautier, E., Berthou, F., Adas, F., and French, S.W. Adaption to chronic ethanol administration emphasized by fatty acid hydroxylations in rat liver and kidney microsomes. *Eur. J. Nutr.*, 39: 270–276, 2000.

28. Lytton, S.D., Helander, A., Zhang-Gouillon, Z.Q., Stokklan, K., Bordone, R., Arico, S., Albano, E., French, S.W., and Ingelman-Sundberg, M. Autoantibodies against cytochromes P450 2E1 and P450 3A in alcoholics. *Molec. Pharmacol.*, 55: 223–233, 1999.

29. Tsukamoto, H., French, S.W., Reidelberger, R.D., and Largeman, C. Cyclic pattern of blood alcohol levels during continuous intragastric ethanol infusion in rats. *Alc. Clin. Exp. Res.*, 9: 31–37, 1985.

30. Li, J., Nguyen, V., French, B.A., Parlow, A.F., Su, G.L., Fu, P., Yuan, Q.X., and French, S.W. Mechanism of the alcohol cyclic pattern: role of the hypothalamic-pituitary-thyroid axis. *Am. J. Physiol. Gast. Liver Physiol.*, 279: G118–G125, 2000.

31. French, S.W. Intragastric ethanol infusion model for cellular and molecular studies of alcoholic liver disease. *J. Biochem. Sci.*, 8: 20–27, 2001.

32. Bardag-Gorce, F., French, B.A., Li, J., Riley, N.E., Yuan, Q.X., Valinluck, V., Fu, P., Ingelman-Sundberg, M., Yoon, S., and French S.W. The importance of cycling of blood alcohol levels in the pathogenesis of experimental alcoholic liver disease. *Gastroenterology*, 123: 325–335, 2002.

33. Nanji, A.A., Su, G.L., Laposata, M., and French, S.W. Pathogenesis of alcoholic liver disease-recent advances. *Alc.Clin. Exp. Res.*, 26: 731–736, 2002.

34. Garcia-Ruiz, C., Morales, A., Colell, A., Ballesta, A., Rodes, J., Kaplowitz, N., and Fernandez-Checa, J.C. Feeding S-adenosyl-L-methionine attenuates both ethanol-induced depletion of mitochondrial glutathione and mitochondrial dysfunction in periportal and perivenous rat hepatocytes. *Hepatology*, 21: 207–214, 1995.

35. Loguercio, C., Del Vecchio Blanco, F., DeGirolamo, V., Disalvo, D., Nadri, G., Parente, A., and Del Vecchio Blanco, C. Ethanol consumption amino acid and glutathione blood levels in patients with and without chronic liver disease. *Alc. Clin. Exp. Res.*, 23: 1780–1784, 1999.

36. Wan, Y-J Y, An, D., Cai, Y., Repa, J.J., Chen, TH.-P, Flores, M., Postic, C., Magnuson, M.A., Chen, J., Chien, K.R., French, S., Mangelsdorf, D.J., and Sucov, H.M. Hepatocyte-specific mutation establishes retinoid X-receptor α as a heterodimeric integrator of multiple physiological processes in the liver. *Molec. Cell Biol.*, 20: 4436–4444, 2000.

37. Lu, S.C., Tsukamoto, H., and Mato, J.M. Role of abnormal methionine metabolism in alcoholic liver injury. *Alcohol*, 27: 155–162, 2002.

38. Halsted, C.H., Villanueva, J.A., Devlin, A.M., Niemela, O., Pakkila, S., Garow, T.A., Wallock, L.M., Shigenaga, M.K., Melinyk, S., and James, S.J. Folate deficiency disturbs hepatic methionine metabolism and promotes liver injury in ethanol-fed micropig. *Proc. Natl. Acad. Sci. USA*, 99: 10072–10077, 2002.

39. Halsted, C.H., Villanueva, J.A., Devlin, A.M., and Chandler, C.J. Metabolic interactions of alcohol and folate. *J. Nutr.*, 132: 2367S–2374S, 2002.
40. Barak, A.J., Beckenhauer, H.C., Kharbanda, K.K., and Tuma, D.J. Chronic ethanol consumption increases monocystein accumulation in hepatocytes. *Alcohol*, 25: 71–81, 2001.
41. Niculescu, M.D. and Zeizel, S.H. Diet methyl donors and DNA methylation: interactions between dietary folate, methionine and choline. *J. Nutr.*, 132: 2333S–23335, 2002.
42. Barak, A.J., Beckonhauer, H.C., and Tuna, D.J. Methionine synthase: a possible prime site of the ethanolic lesion in liver. *Alcohol*, 26: 65–67, 2002.
43. French, S.W. Effect of chronic ethanol ingestion on liver enzyme changes induced by thiamine, riboflavin, pyridoxine or choline deficiency. *J. Nutr.*, 88: 291–302, 1966.
44. McClain, C.J., Hill, D.B., Song, Z., Chawla, R., Watson, W.H., Chen, T., and Barve, S. S-adenosyl-methionine, cytokines and alcoholic liver disease. *Alcohol*, 27: 185–192, 2002.
45. Mato, J.M., Camara, J., Fernandez de Paz, J., Caballera, L., Coll, S., Caballero, A., Garcia-Buey, L., Beltran, J., Benita, V., Martin-Duce, A., Correa, J.A., Pares, A., Barrao, E., Garcia-Magaz, I., Puerta, J.L., Moreno, J., Boissard, G., Ortiz, P., and Rodes, J. S-Adenosylmethionine in alcoholic liver cirrhosis: a randomized, placebo-controlled, double-blind, multicentric clinical trial. *J. Hepatol.*, 30: 1081–1089, 1999.
46. Wan, Y-JY, Morimoto, M., Thurman, R.G., Bojes, HK., and French, S.W. Expression of the peroxisome proliferator-activated receptor gene is decreased in experimental alcoholic liver disease. *Life Sci.*, 56: 307–317, 1995.
47. Kliewer, S.A., Sundseth, S.S., Jones, S.A., Brown, P.J., Wisely, G.B., Koble, C.S., Deuchand, P., Wahli, W.S., Wilson, T.M., Lenhard, J.M., and Lehmann, J.M. Fatty acids and eicosanoids regulate gene expression through direct interactions with peroxisome proliferator-activated receptors α and γ. *Proc. Natl. Acad. Sci. USA*, 94: 4318–4323, 1997.
48. Wan, Y-JY, Cai Y, Li, J., Yuan, Q.X., French, B., Gonzalez, F.J., and French, S.W. Regulation of peroxisome proliferator activated receptor α-mediated pathways in alcohol fed cytochrome P450 2E1 deficient mice. *Hepatol. Res.*, 19: 117–130, 2001.
49. Galli, A., Pinaire, J., Fischer, M., Dorris, R., and Crabb, D.W. The transcriptional and DNA binding activity of peroxisome proliferator-activated receptor α is inhibited by ethanol metabolism. *J. Biol. Chem.*, 276: 68–75, 2001.
50. Lee, S.S., Pineau, T., Drago, J., Lee, E.J., Owens, J.W., Kroetz, D.L., Fernandez-Salguero, P.M., Westphal, H., and Gonzalez, F.J. *Molec. Cell Biol.*, 15: 3012–3022, 1995.
51. Takahashi, H., Wong, K., Jui, L., Nanji, A., McKibbon, D., Mendenhall, C.S., and French, S.W. Effect of dietary fat on Ito cell activation by chronic ethanol intake: a long term serial morphometric study on ethanol-fed and control rats. *Alc. Clin. Exp. Res.*, 15: 1060–1066, 1991.
52. Chung, J., Liu, C., Smith, D.E., Seitz, H.K., Russell, R.M., and Wang, X-D. Restoration of retinoic acid concentration suppresses ethanol-enhanced c-jun expression and hepatocyte proliferation in rat liver. *Carcinogenesis*, 22: 1213–1219, 2001.
53. Chung, J., Chavez, R.G., Russell, R.M., and Wang, X-D. Retinoic acid inhibits hepatic Jun N-terminal kinase-dependent signaling pathway in ethanol-fed rats. *Oncogene*, 21: 1539–1547, 2002.
54. Chun, L., Russell, R.M., Seitz, H.K., and Wang, X-D. Ethanol enhances retinoic acid metabolism into polar metabolites in rat liver via induction of cytochrome P450 2E1. *Gastroenterology*, 120: 179–189, 2001.

55. Shahed, A.R., Li, J., Yuan, Q., and French, S.W. Effect of ethanol cycling on gene expression in intragastric ethanol feeding rat model of alcoholic liver disease. *FASEB J.*, 15: A609, 2001.
56. Fischer, J.G., Glauert, H.P., Yin, T., Sweeney-Reeves, M.L., Larmonier, N., and Black, M.C. Moderate iron overload enhances lipid peroxidation in livers of rats, but does not affect NF-KB activation induced by the peroxisome proliferator, Wy-14, 643. *J. Nutr.*, 132: 2525–2531, 2002.
57. Tsukamoto, H., Horne, W., Kamimura, S., Niemela, O., Parkkila, S., Yla-Herttuala, S., and Brittenham, G.M. Experimental liver cirrhosis induced by alcohol and iron. *J. Clin. Invest.*, 96: 620–630, 1995.
58. Tsukamoto, H., Lin, M., Ohata, M., Giuliui, C., French, S., and Bittenham, G. Iron promes hepatic macrophages for NF-KB activation in alcoholic liver injury. *Am. J. Physiol.*, 277: G1240–G1250, 1999.
59. Tsukamoto, H. and Lu, S.C. Current concepts in the pathogenesis of alcoholic liver injury. *FASEB J.*, 15: 1335–1349, 2001.

4 Ethanol and Methyl Transfer: Its Role in Liver Disease and Hepatocarcinogenesis

Felix Stickel and Helmut K. Seitz

CONTENTS

4.1 SUMMARY

Several mechanisms have been described by which chronic alcohol consumption may interact with one-carbon metabolism and thereby disturb methylation reactions. Interactions may occur with absorption, storage, biologic transformation, and excretion of compounds which are closely involved with methyl group transfer. Among the factors that may be affected are folate, vitamin B_6, and lipotropes, such as choline, betaine, and methionine. In particular, the production of *S*-adenosyl-L-methionine (SAMe), the universal methyl group donor in methylation reactions, is impaired due to various mechanisms, including the formation of methyl groups, their transport by tetrahydrofolate, and finally their transfer to methionine, the precursors of SAMe. Alcohol interacts with SAMe synthesis through the inhibition of crucial metabolic enzymes such as methionine synthase and methionine adenosyltransferase either by producing oxidative stress or by direct inhibition of vitamin B_6, a coenzyme in various transmethylation reactions. Thus, alcohol inhibits the production of glutathione by inhibiting cystathionine-β-synthase, a reaction in which glutathione is formed via the intermediates cystathionine and cysteine. Due to the inhibition of SAMe production, the integrity of cellular membranes may be compromised by inhibiting methylation of membrane phospholipids.

Several possibilities exist by which chronic alcohol consumption may interact with methylation of certain genes and thereby contribute to liver damage and tumor development. It is well established that dietary depletion of lipotropes may cause hypomethylation of oncogenes leading to their activation. The decrease in methylation capacity caused by chronic alcohol consumption may therefore contribute to epigenetic alterations of genes involved in carcinogenesis. Whether alcohol consumption is sufficient to produce genetic hypomethylation to directly cause tumor initiation is not yet known but could be an explanation for the cocarcinogenic effects of alcohol in hepatocarcinogenesis

4.2 TOXICITY OF ALCOHOL

Alcohol is hepatotoxic through a variety of mechanisms that are carefully addressed in other chapters of this book. Briefly summarized, alcohol-induced liver damage is primarily based on the toxicity of its first metabolite, acetaldehyde, and several disturbances related to alcohol metabolism. With regard to the latter, an important pathophysiological event is the enhanced formation of reactive oxygen species (ROS) mainly caused by the induction of the ethanol-metabolizing isoenzyme cytochrome P450 2E1, which constitutes the microsomal ethanol-oxidizing system (MEOS). The elevated generation of ROS produces cytotoxic oxidative stress and increased lipid peroxidation. Thereby, the capacity of CYP2E1 to oxidize ethanol is markedly increased as alcohol is continuously consumed in larger quantities.[1,2] As an additional pathogenic factor, primary and secondary malnutrition further contribute to the development of liver damage. In alcoholics, numerous metabolic events are profoundly altered, either through direct interference with alcohol or its metabolite acetaldehyde, or due to the insufficiency of the composition and the amount of food intake.[2]

4.3 INTERACTION WITH LIPOTROPES

Among the many macro- and micronutrients that are affected by chronic alcohol consumption, several so-called lipotropes are particularly important. To this group of micronutrients belong choline, betaine, and methionine which are all essential for the generation, transport, and transfer of one-carbon units to target molecules, such as phospholipids, neurotransmitters, SAMe, and DNA, and for the formation of polyamines.[3] A series of experimental and epidemiological studies have convincingly demonstrated that chronic alcohol consumption causes a depletion of all these lipotropes because of a poor dietary supply in addition to detrimental interaction with their metabolism.[4–6] Consequently, alcohol interacts profoundly at various sites of one carbon transfer (Figure 4.1).

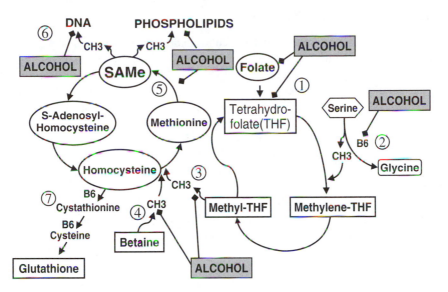

FIGURE 4.1 Acetaldehyde may interact with transmethylation at various sites: (1) inhibition of absorption and methylation of folate; (2) interaction with pyridoxal-5′-phosphate (vitamin B_6) and consequent generation of methyl groups; (3) inhibition of methionine synthase (MS); (4) betaine:homocysteine methyl transferase; (5) methionine adenosyltransferase (MATI/III); (6) DNA methyltransferase; (7) block of glutathione synthesis via inhibition of cystathionase and cystathionine-β-synthase.

4.3.1 INTERACTION WITH FOLATE

In addition to lipotrope depletion, a frequently encountered finding in chronic alcoholics is that of folate deficiency, which reaches a prevalence of more than 50%. In fact, in industrialized countries alcoholism is the most frequent cause of folate depletion, primarily due to poor dietary intake. For example, in a group of unselected alcoholics 37.5% showed a low serum folate level and 17.6% also had low red blood cell folate levels, commonly considered a more accurate measure of body folate stores than pure blood levels.[7] In a recent study from Portugal, Gloria and coworkers investigated the relationship between nutritional status and ethanol consumption in 33 chronic alcoholics devoid of clinical evidence for established liver disease.[8] One of the major findings in this study was that 51.5% of all alcoholics revealed significantly decreased red blood cell folate levels, while only 18.1% of the screened population were clinically malnourished. It is now agreed that folate deficiency in alcoholics is multifactorial and results from poor dietary intake, reduced absorption related to changes in the intestinal mucosal surface,[9] changes in hepatic folate retention capacity,[10] and increased urinary folate excretion.[11] Folate is an important participant in methyl group transfer since, after activation by the enzyme tetrahydrofolate reductase, tetrahydrofolate is the principal acceptor of methyl groups derived from the transformation of serine into glycine, in which carbon groups are generated through the action of the enzyme serine hydroxymethylase (Figure 4.1).

4.3.2 INTERACTION WITH VITAMIN B₆

Another possible interaction between alcohol and methyl group transfer may take place as methyl groups are transferred to homocysteine to form methionine, a cobalamin-dependent reaction mediated by the enzyme methionine synthase. Barak and associates have generated an extensive body of experimental data addressing this issue and have repeatedly shown that even short-term alcohol-feeding for 4 weeks decreases the activity of methionine synthase in rats.[4,12] In addition to the interaction with folate, alcohol also seems to interfere with pyridoxal-5′-phosphate (PLP, vitamin B₆). It was shown in experimental rats fed alcohol by using Lieber–DeCarli liquid diets as well as in alcoholics that in addition to serum folate levels, PLP levels were likewise suppressed, leading to impaired transmethylation as measured by decreased SAMe levels and increased S-adenosylhomocysteine (SAH) levels in the liver, probably through synergistic depletion of folate and vitamin B₆.[8,13,14] PLP deficiency in alcoholism is a common feature although its etiology is not yet fully understood. Possibly alcohol exerts its interaction with PLP again via acetaldehyde which displaces protein-bound PLP *in vivo* and thereby exposes the coenzyme to degrading phosphatases which are upregulated in alcoholics.[15]

4.3.3 INTERACTION WITH CHOLINE

For many years, choline deficiency has been incriminated as a primary etiologic cause of liver injury, especially in alcoholic liver disease. In experimental rats, choline deficiency produces fatty liver, a pathological finding frequently seen in alcoholic liver damage. The nutrient choline and its metabolites are important factors in numerous cellular processes, including the biosynthesis of phosphatidylcholine via the so-called Kennedy pathway and subsequently to sphingomyelin. Both compounds are essential for sustaining membrane integrity and fluidity for the transport of materials across membranes. Choline also serves as a methyl group donor through its conversion to betaine by the activity of choline oxidase. However, despite these observations, choline repletion was found to be ineffective to offset hepatic damage in alcoholics and, furthermore, high-dose supplementation with choline did not prevent alcohol-induced fatty liver in volunteers.[16] Moreover, even more severe liver damage including fibrosis and cirrhosis developed in nonhuman primates in spite of massive choline administration to the point of toxicity.[17] From experimental and clinical studies it became evident that rodents differ substantially from primates, including humans, with regard to choline requirements, a phenomenon which is related to differences in choline oxidase activity in the liver. Thus, rodents such as rats manage to replenish lipotrope stores by the conversion of choline to betaine, a reaction mediated by the action of choline oxidase. Accordingly, choline deficiency requiring supplementation has been documented only in patients receiving an extremely restricted diet.[18] Although choline is an important factor in the maintenance of hepatic integrity, at present the attention is rather drawn to betaine and methionine, which are in close relationship to choline.

4.3.4 INTERACTION WITH BETAINE

Because of the observed transformation of choline into betaine, it was assumed that betaine is a simple by-product of choline oxidation, but recent studies have convincingly shown that betaine is, in fact, an important methylating compound in the liver. Several lines of evidence indicate that betaine may be a significant compensatory source of methyl groups for the formation of methionine and, consequently, of SAMe. In methionine metabolism, the conversion of homocysteine to methionine is highly important in order to maintain hepatic methionine stores, to dispose of homocysteine, and for the production of SAMe. Two alternate metabolic pathways exist by which homocysteine is transformed into methionine: in the first reaction, which is mediated by the enzyme methionine synthase (MS; N^5-methyl-tetrahydrofolate:homocysteine methyl transferase), a one-carbon group is transferred from N^5-methyl-tetrahydrofolate to homocysteine to produce methionine. The second reaction involves a methyl group transfer from betaine to homocysteine catalyzed by the enzyme betaine:homocysteine methyl transferase (BHMT) to again produce methionine.[19] Experimental data from different laboratories have shown that chronic alcohol feeding leads to a marked decrease in hepatic betaine levels accompanied by an accumulation of N^5-methyl-tetrahydrofolate in the liver. An attractive explanation for this observation was findings demonstrating an alcohol-related inhibition of N^5-methyl-tetrahydrofolate:homocysteine methyl transferase (methionine synthase) leading to nonutilization of N^5-methyl-tetrahydrofolate, along with an adaptive increase of BHMT, thereby exhausting betaine stores. Indeed, it was further shown that this compensatory pathway is sufficient to maintain a coordinate production of methionine and SAMe in rodents.[20] In a long-term animal study, alcohol was fed to rats over a period of up to 4 months and parameters of transmethylation were investigated.[12] The data showed a continuous decrease of methionine synthase activity while BHMT activity increased, resulting in sustained hepatic SAMe levels. Although betaine levels eventually declined until cessation of the experiment, these results are suggestive of compensatory SAMe production via betaine in rodents when the classical way of remethylation via N^5-methyl-tetrahydrofolate is inhibited by alcohol. In a series of subsequent experiments, Barak's group aimed to test the hypothesis of betaine supplementation as being capable of inhibiting alcohol-related SAMe depletion and thereby preventing hepatic damage.[21–23] It was demonstrated that betaine supplementation at 0.5% not only restored hepatic SAMe stores to physiological levels but also prevented alcohol-induced liver damage including that of simple steatosis. Interestingly, hepatic steatosis was even prevented when alcohol feeding was continued. Considering these results, the relatively low cost of betaine and the lack of toxicity, as well as its ubiquitous availability, may render this compound a promising therapeutic agent in the treatment of liver disease.

4.3.5 ALCOHOL AND METHIONINE METABOLISM

With regard to transmethylation reactions, the influence alcohol has on methionine metabolism is pivotal, especially in alcoholic liver disease.

Considerable progress has been made in our understanding of certain nutritional factors in the pathogenesis of alcoholic liver disease and consecutive treatments. From the available data, it is evident that some nutrients are essential because they cannot be generated endogenously and, therefore, must be provided through the diet. Among these essential nutrients, methionine, a sulfur-containing amino acid, is very important, especially in the setting of alcoholic liver disease. Data from studies in humans show that methionine metabolism may be markedly hampered in alcoholics. While in some studies serum methionine levels were found to be normal,[24] other investigators reported elevated levels.[25,26] When methionine was administered to patients with advanced liver damage, both systemically and orally, a marked delay in methionine clearance from the circulation was detected.[27,28] This observation appears important since it has been shown by Mudd and Poole, as well as by Finkelstein et al., that normally 50% of the body's methionine metabolism and approximately 85% of all methylation reactions occur in the liver.[29,30] These disturbances in methionine homeostasis cannot simply be offset by the administration of methionine, and experimental data have shown that even a sevenfold increase in the normal dietary methionine content did not improve hepatic SAMe levels.[30] In fact, apart from its uselessness, methionine supplementation may even become toxic as a result of nonutilization.

Apart from its incorporation into proteins, methionine exerts several important key functions including the formation of nucleic acids, proteins, phospholipids, and biologic amines.[31] However, in order to participate in these biological processes, methionine requires activation in the liver or other organs, a process which is severely disturbed in chronic liver diseases.[32] The active metabolite of methionine in virtually all transmethylation reactions is SAMe. With regard to transmethylation reactions, the effects alcohol exerts on the metabolism of methionine and its bioactivation to SAMe are crucial since SAMe is the principal donor of methyl groups in virtually all biological methylation reactions. Several experimental studies in various animal species have equivocally shown that chronic ethanol administration markedly decreases hepatic SAMe concentrations while hepatic SAH concentrations are increased, leading to an impairment of the hepatic methylation capacity expressed as the SAMe/SAH ratio.[5,13,33]

SAMe is important, as mentioned above, because of its role as the most important methyl group donor and enzyme activator in hepatic transmethylation and transsulfuration. SAMe thereby contributes to homocysteine disposal and to establishing the antioxidative defense system.[3] Accordingly, a central role of SAMe in the regulation of homocysteine and methionine metabolism has been reported by Finkelstein et al., who demonstrated that SAMe is a potent activator of cystathionine-β-synthase, the major enzyme that converts homocysteine to cystathionine.[30] Cystathionine, in turn, is further hydrolyzed to form cysteine, which reacts with glutamate and glycine, resulting in the formation of glutathione, which forms the major antioxidative defense mechanism in humans.[34] As described above, oxidative stress plays an important role in alcohol-induced tissue damage, including hepatotoxicity and carcinogenicity. In this situation, glutathione, a tripeptide which contains the rate-limiting amino acid cysteine, plays an important part in antagonizing cytotoxic effects of ROS by providing sulfhydryl groups with reductive capacity.[35] Thus,

SAMe is important for the maintenance of the antioxidative defense capacity in the human body.

Furthermore, SAMe acts as the main provider of propylamine groups for the synthesis of polyamines by decarboxylation of SAMe and subsequent transfer of the aminopropyl group to putrescine and spermidine which finally results in the generation of polyamines. Due to this biological function, SAMe is essential, especially under conditions of increased polyamine synthesis such as liver regeneration.[36]

Another important function of SAMe is its potential to stabilize cellular membranes via enabling the formation of phosphatidylcholine (PPC) from phosphatidylethanolamine. PPC is a polyunsaturated phospholipid responsible for the integrity and fluidity of cellular membranes where it is integrated as an antioxidant against free radicals. Lieber and coworkers have demonstrated in numerous experimental studies that PPC may exert antioxidative, antiinflammatory, and antifibrotic effects in baboons chronically fed alcohol.[37] Recently, the results of a large randomized, controlled multicenter trial from the U.S. were presented in which the impressive number of 789 patients with biopsy-proven alcoholic liver damage were treated with 1.5 g of PPC daily or placebo for 4 to 6 years. While the overall comparison of the two groups failed to show a significant treatment effect by PPC, possibly due to their marked reduction of alcohol consumption, a subgroup of patients who continued to drink at least 6 drinks/d (n = 52 patients) showed a slight regression with PPC, whereas those on placebo progressed histologically.[38] This limited benefit as demonstrated in this trial seems somewhat disappointing considering the high expectations linked to PPC.

Possibly related to antioxidative and membrane-stabilizing properties are the antifibrotic effects of SAMe which have been described in different animal models of fibrosis in which SAMe decreased the accumulation of collagen together with a marked reduction of elevated liver enzyme levels.[39,40]

4.3.6 ALCOHOL AND SAMe FORMATION

SAMe is synthesized from L-methionine and adenosine triphosphate (ATP) in a two-step reaction catalyzed by an enzyme termed *methionine adenosyltransferase* (MAT; syn.: SAMe synthase), where the complete tripolyphosphate moiety is cleaved from ATP as SAMe is being formed.[41] In humans, MAT is the product of two different genes, namely *MAT1A* and *MAT2A*, which encode two different enzymes. *MAT1A* codes for the catalytic subunit α1 that organizes into dimers which form MAT III, and tetramers which generate MAT I, while *MAT2A* encodes a catalytic subunit α2 that forms MAT II.[41] The main differences between these two enzymes are related to their capacity to produce SAMe, and to their distribution in human organs. While MATI/III can maintain high intrahepatic SAMe levels, the capacity of MAT II to metabolize methionine is rather low.[41] *MAT1A*, coding for the enzymes MAT I and III, is almost exclusively expressed in adult liver, while *MAT2A* expression, encoding MAT II, in the liver is usually relatively low but high in nonhepatic tissues, fetal liver, and conditions with high hepatic cell turnover such as following partial hepatectomy and tumor growth. Functional transfection experiments have revealed that the *MAT1A* promotor is active not only in hepatocytes but also in hepatoma cells and in hamster ovary cells, indicating that the liver-restricted MAT I/III activity does not solely depend on tissue-specific factors.[42] An explanation for this phenomenon was the finding that the promotor of *MAT1A* is hypomethylated in adult hepatic tissue and therefore actively transcribed, whereas it is hypermethylated and therefore silenced in fetal and regenerating liver, as well as in hepatocellular carcinoma.[43] In conclusion, there is compelling evidence that SAMe levels are not only related to MAT I/III activity in the liver, but SAMe itself also actively takes part in the regulation of *MAT1A* expression, thereby influencing MAT I/III activity.

As mentioned above, oxidative stress is an important pathogenic feature in alcoholic liver damage, contributing to tissue damage and promoting tumor development. On the posttranscriptional level, it has been demonstrated that nitric oxide (NO) and reactive oxygen species (ROS), the latter being a by-product of microsomal alcohol oxidation, may inactivate both MAT I and MAT II through nitrosylation and oxidation.[44] On the other hand, hepatic MAT I and MAT III inactivation is effectively reversed by physiologic concentrations of glutathione.[45]

Recently, a knockout mouse which is deficient in hepatic MAT synthesis has been introduced with which it is possible to examine the consequences of a chronic reduction of SAMe levels in the liver.[46] These so-called *MAT0* mice reveal markedly elevated blood methionine levels and decreased hepatic SAMe concentrations when compared to wild-type mice. At the age of 3 months, *MAT0* mice show marked hepatic hyperplasia and fatty liver and, moreover, reveal an increased susceptibility toward toxic insults such as with carbon tetrachloride. After a mean of 8 months, *MAT0* mice develop steatohepatitis; ongoing experiments will unravel whether this particular mouse strain is more likely to develop fibrosis and cirrhosis, and possibly hepatoma, and whether this will be related to changes of methylation patterns in certain genes.

4.3.7 SAMe as a Treatment for Alcoholic Liver Disease

The therapeutic benefit of SAMe to treat certain liver diseases has been demonstrated. For example, SAMe was shown to relieve pruritus and to lower elevated liver enzymes in patients with cholestatic liver disease such as intrahepatic cholestasis, primary biliary cirrhosis (PBC), and chronic viral hepatitis.[47] So far, three clinical trials have suggested a favorable effect of SAMe treatment in ALD. Thus, oral administration of SAMe improved alcohol-induced glutathione deficiency in red blood cells and the liver,[48,49] while the most impressive data come from a randomized, placebo-controlled, double-blind multicenter trial in alcoholic cirrhotics.[50] In this trial, 123 patients with various stages of liver cirrhosis as assessed by the Child–Pugh index were treated with 1200 mg/d of oral SAMe for 2 years. Death from liver-related complications and liver transplantation were chosen as primary endpoints. The overall mortality at the end of the trial was 30% in the placebo group and 16% in the patients receiving SAMe. This result failed just short of reaching significance ($p = 0.077$), but after exclusion of Child C patients, the reduction of the rate of mortality or liver transplantation became significant (29% vs. 12%, $p = 0.025$). It should be further emphasized that patients' compliance was excellent and adverse treatment effects were equal to placebo level. Although these encouraging results require confirmation in other clinical trials, they suggest that SAMe represents an effective, relatively cheap, and nontoxic drug for the treatment of chronic ALD.

4.3.8 SAMe AND DNA METHYLATION

The term *DNA methylation* is used to describe a postreplicative modification in which a DNA residue receives a covalently bound methyl group. The attached methyl adduct can either be the result of an interaction with an alkylating chemical or it can be the normal consequence of an enzymatic transfer reaction, termed *biological methylation*. It is the latter which is referred to in this chapter. Alterations of genes may occur either due to genetic changes such as point mutations, chromosome deletions, or DNA strand breaks, or due to epigenetic variations of gene expression such as defects of DNA repair enzymes, changes in histone acetylation, or methylation patterns. DNA methylation is an important determinant in controlling gene expression, whereby hypermethylation has a silencing effect on genes, and hypomethylation may lead to increased gene expression which has important implications for carcinogenesis (Figure 4.2). Thus, DNA methylation is a powerful mechanism for the suppression of gene activity.[51] Methyl group transfer occurs via the transfer of methyl groups from SAMe due to the activity of enzymes termed *DNA methyl transferases* of which two distinct patterns of activity can be distinguished: *de novo* DNA methyl transferase and maintenance DNA methyl transferase. The former is responsible for the addition of methyl groups to a target sequence devoid of preexisting methylation, while the latter restores hemimethylated DNA substrates.[52] DNA methylation primarily occurs at the fifth carbon atom of the nucleotide cytosine within CpG dinucleotides, which leads to the formation of methylated CpG-islands that are often located nearby or within the promotor region of genes (Figure 4.3). Functionally, the gene-silencing effect of methylation is related to several mechanisms:

1. The strong effect of 5-methylcytosine in mammalian promotor regions indicates that DNA methylation inhibits transcription initiation by interference with DNA-protein interaction and by inhibiting the elongation of amino acid chains.
2. DNA methylation reduces the binding affinity of sequence-specific transcription factors.[53]
3. Transcriptional repression by DNA methylation may occur due to changes in chromatin structure and histone acetylation, which alters the accessibility of genes through a sequence-independent process.[54]

The biological functions of DNA methylation which have been suggested include the inactivation of viral invaders such as viruses and plasmides and the control of gene expression during development and differentiation. Another example represents the silencing of the second X chromosome in women. In this line fits the hypothesis by Bird that DNA methylation evolved as a mechanism to reduce transcriptional "background noise."[55]

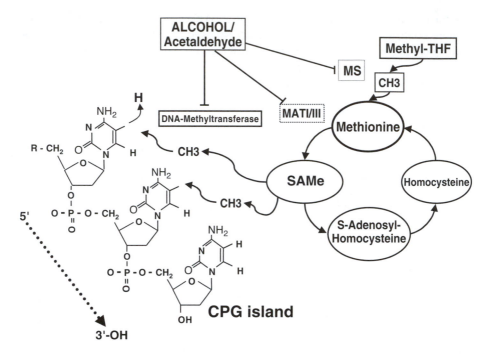

FIGURE 4.2 Alcohol/acetaldehyde inhibits the entire methyl group transfer cascade including the formation of methionine (MS, methionine synthase), SAMe (MATI/III, methionine adenosyltransferase), and methylation of dinucleotides (DNA methyl transferase). Hydrogen atoms are replaced by one-carbon units through enzymatic reaction and are attached to the fifth carbon atom of cytosine. Hypermethylated dinucleotides represent CpG islands located in the promotor region of genes.

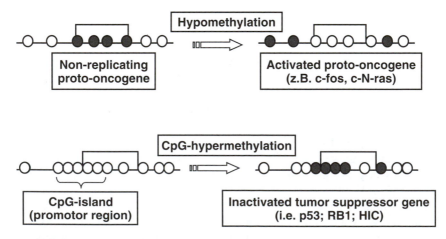

FIGURE 4.3 Methylation alters the expression of genes important in tumor development. Hypomethylation of proto-oncogenes leads to their activation (i.e., *c-fos, c-ras*), hypermethylation of actively transcribing tumor suppressor genes (i.e., *p53*) may cause its inactivation.

Numerous lines of evidence demonstrate that chronic alcohol consumption may enhance the risk of developing cancers of several organs including the oropharynx, esophagus, colorectum, and the liver.[56,57] With regard to human cancers, changes in the degree of global DNA and site-specific methylation of certain genes are frequently encountered. For example, in hepatocarcinogenesis, general hypomethylation may be coupled with areas of regional hypermethylation. Thus, hypermethylation of tumor suppressor genes can result in decreased gene transcription of *p53* and *HIC-1*,[58] and hypomethylation of certain oncogenes such as *c-myc* and *c-N-ras* may lead to dedifferentiation and proliferation.[59,60] Recently, it has been suggested that aberrant DNA hypermethylation may be associated with genetic instability as determined by loss of heterozygosity and microsatellite instability in human HCC due to chronic viral hepatitis.[61,62] Iwata et al. detected hypermethylation of the *14-3-3 sigma* gene which has been implicated as a key inducer of cell cycle arrest associated with *p53* in 89% of investigated human HCCs.[63] However, genetic alterations in animal models and human hepatocarcinogenesis differ substantially. Thus, it was shown that activation of *N-myc* and *c-myc* oncogenes is frequent in woodchuck hepatitis virus-associated HCC, although no *p53* can be found. This mutational pattern is reversed in humans where *p53* mutations are frequent, while oncogene activation seems to play a minor role.[64,65]

Importantly, modifications of the degree of hepatic DNA methylation have also been observed in experimental models of chronic alcoholism.[66,67] Hypomethylation is a plausible consequence of metabolic alterations in the setting of ethanol consumption. As mentioned above, alcohol has a marked impact on hepatic methylation capacity as reflected by decreased levels of *S*-adenosylmethionine (SAM), an important methyl group donor, increased levels of SAH, resulting in an up to 2.5-fold decrease of the SAM/SAH ratio.[13] Apart from lowering the hepatic methylation capacity, alcohol may furthermore inhibit the activity of DNA methylase which transfers methyl groups to DNA in rats,[66] a finding which could not be confirmed in humans.[68]

To date, it is well established that dietary depletion of lipotropes, including methionine, choline, betaine, SAM, and folate, leads to DNA hypomethylation, particularly hypomethylation of oncogenes (i.e., c-*Ha-ras*, c-*Ki-ras*, and c-*fos*) and to DNA strand breaks, all of which are associated with an increased incidence of hepatocellular carcinoma in rats.[69,70] It has been shown that DNA and site-specific hypomethylation are reversible, either spontaneously[71,72] or by therapeutic intervention.[64] With regard to the latter, data from animal studies using different models of tumor initiation with chemical carcinogens in rats demonstrate that both patterns of impaired methyl group metabolism and DNA methylation as well as tumor development can be effectively prevented by administering SAMe.[73-75] However, the effect of alcohol on methylation in the setting of chemically induced carcinogenesis in experimental animals has not yet been investigated. Likewise, a study investigating the chemopreventive effect of lipotropes, i.e., SAM, in humans with HCC has not been performed.

4.4 CONCLUSION

The interaction between alcohol and transmethylation is undisputed and several features of alcohol-related organ damage are certainly related to impaired methyl group transfer. Among these are pathological changes of cellular membranes and the antioxidative defense capacity leading to acute organ damage, especially in the liver. Moreover, chronic effects related to impaired methylation alterations may inhibit tissue regeneration and DNA methylation. Whether the alcohol-related hypomethylation of DNA and certain genes involved in hepatocarcinogenesis are sufficient to accelerate tumorigenesis requires further investigation. Future research will have to focus on this issue since the impact of alcohol on tumor development may be significant considering its widespread consumption.

References

1. Tsukamoto, H. and Lu, S.C., Current concepts in the pathogenesis of alcoholic liver disease, *FASEB J.*, 15, 1335, 2001.
2. Lieber, C.S., Alcohol and the liver: 1994 update, *Gastroenterology*, 106, 1085, 1994.
3. Lieber, C.S. and Packer, L., S-Adenosylmethionine: molecular, biological, and clinical aspects — an introduction, *Am. J. Clin. Nutr.*, 76 (suppl.), 1148S, 2002.
4. Barak, A.J. and Beckenhauer, H.C., The influence of ethanol on hepatic transmethylation, *Alcohol Alcohol.*, 23, 73–7, 1988.
5. Trimble, K.C. et al., The effect of ethanol on one-carbon metabolism: increased methionine catabolism and methyl-group wastage, *Hepatology*, 18, 984, 1993.
6. Martinez-Chantar, M.L. et al., Importance of a deficiency in S-adenosyl-L-methionine synthesis in the pathogenesis of liver injury, *Am. J. Clin. Nutr.*, 76(suppl), 1177S, 2002.
7. World, M.J. et al., Differential effect of chronic alcohol intake and poor nutrition on body weight and fat stores, *Alcohol*, 19, 281, 1984.
8. Gloria, L. et al., Nutritional deficiencies in chronic alcoholics: relation to dietary intake and alcohol consumption, *Am. J. Gastro.*, 92, 485, 1997.
9. Halsted, C.H., Chronic alcoholism, malnutrition, and folate deficiency, in *Alcohol: A Molecular Perspective*, Palmer, T.N. (Ed.), Plenum Press, New York, 1991, pp. 237–51.
10. Hidiroglu, N. et al., Effect of chronic ethanol ingestion on hepatic folate distribution in the rat, *Biochem. Pharm.* 47, 1561, 1994.
11. Russell, R.M. et al., Increased urinary excretion and prolonged turnover time of folic acid during ethanol ingestion, *Am. J. Clin. Nutr.*, 38, 64, 1983.
12. Barak, A.J. et al., Effects of prolonged ethanol feeding on methionine metabolism in rat liver, *Biochem. Cell Biol.*, 65, 230, 1986.
13. Stickel, F. et al., Effect of chronic alcohol consumption on total plasma homocysteine levels in rats, *Alcohol Clin. Exp. Res.* 24, 259, 2000.
14. Brussaard, J.H. et al., Dietary and other determinants of vitamin B6 parameters, *Eur. J. Clin. Nutr.*, 51(suppl.), S39, 1997.
15. Fonda, M.L. et al., Concentration of vitamin B6 and activity of enzymes of B6 metabolism in the blood of alcoholic and nonalcoholic men, *Alc. Clin. Exp. Res.*, 3, 804, 1989.

16. Rubin, E. and Lieber, C.S., Alcohol induced hepatic injury in nonalcoholic volunteers, *N. Engl. J. Med.*, 278, 869, 1968.

17. Lieber C.S. et al., Choline fails to prevent liver fibrosis in ethanol-fed baboons but causes toxicity, *Hepatology*, 5, 561, 1985.

18. Chawla, R.K. et al., Choline may be an essential nutrient in malnourished patients with cirrhosis, *Gastroenterology*, 97, 1514, 1989.

19. Barak, A.J., Beckenhauer, H.C., and Tuma, D.J., Betaine, ethanol, and the liver: a review, *Alcohol*, 13, 395, 1996.

20. Barak, A.J. et al., Adaptive increase in betaine:homocysteine methyltransferase activity maintains hepatic S-adenosylmethionine levels in ethanol-treated rats, *IRCS Med. Sci.*, 12, 866, 1984.

21. Barak, A.J. et al., Dietary betaine promotes generation of hepatic-S-adenosylmethionine and protects the liver from ethanol-induced fatty infiltration, *Alc. Clin. Exp. Res.*, 17, 552, 1993.

22. Barak, A.J., Beckenhauer, H.C., and Tuma, D.J., S-adenosylmethionine generation and prevention of alcoholic fatty liver by betaine, *Alcohol*, 11, 501, 1994.

23. Barak, A.J. et al., The effect of betaine in reversing alcoholic steatosis, *Alc. Clin. Exp. Res.*, 21, 1100, 1997.

24. Iob, V. et al., Free amino acids in liver, plasma and muscle of patients with cirrhosis of the liver, *J. Surg. Res.*,7, 41, 1967.

25. Fischer, J.E. et al., Plasma amino acids in patients with hepatic encephalopathy, *Am. J. Surg.*, 127, 40, 1974.

26. Montanari, A. et al., Free amino acids in plasma and skeletal muscle of patients with liver cirrhosis, *Hepatology*, 8, 1034, 1988.

27. Kinsell L., et al., Rate of disappearance from plasma of intravenously administered methionine in patients with liver damage, *Science*, 106, 589, 1947.

28. Horowitz, J.H. et al., Evidence for impairment of transsulfuration pathway in cirrhosis, *Gastroenterology*, 81, 668, 1981.

29. Mudd, S.H. and Poole, J.R., Labile methyl balances for normal humans on various dietary regimens, *Metabolism*, 24, 721, 1975.

30. Finkelstein, J.D., Methionine metabolism in mammals, *J. Nutr. Biochem.*, 1, 228, 1990.

31. Lu, S.C., S-adenosylmethionine, *Int. J. Biochem. Cell Biol.*, 32, 391, 2000.

32. Avila, M.A. et al., S-Adenosylmethionine revisited: its essential role in the regulation of liver function, *Alcohol*, 27, 163, 2002.

33. Halsted, C.H. et al., Ethanol feeding of micropigs alters methionine metabolism and increases hepatocellular apoptosis and proliferation, *Hepatology*, 23, 497, 1996.

34. Selhub, J., Homocysteine metabolism, *Ann. Rev. Nutr.*, 19, 217, 1999.

35. Valencia, E., Marin, A., and Hardy, G., Glutathione — nutritional and pharmacological viewpoints, *Nutrition*, 17, 485, 2001.

36. Mato, J.M. et al., S-adenosylmethionine synthesis: molecular mechanisms and clinical implications, *Pharmacol. Ther.*, 73, 265, 1997.

37. Lieber, C.S., Alcoholic liver disease: new insights in pathogenesis lead to new treatments, *J. Hepatol.*, 32(suppl 1), 113, 2000.

38. Lieber, C.S. et al., Effect of moderation of ethanol consumption combined with PPC administration on liver injury in alcoholics: prospective, randomized, placebo-controlled, multicenter VA trial (CSP 391) (Abstract), *Hepatology*, 36, 381A, 2002.

39. Muriel, P. and Castro, V., Effects of S-adenosyl-L-methionine and interferon-alpha2b on liver damage induced by bile duct ligation in rats, *J. Appl. Toxicol.*,18, 143, 1998.

40. Gasso, M. et al., Effects of S-adenosylmethionine on lipid peroxidation and liver fibrogenesis in carbon tetrachloride-induced cirrhosis, *J. Hepatol.*, 25, 200, 1997.

41. Kotb, M. et al., Consensus nomenclature for the mammalian methionine adenosyltransferase genes and gene products, *Trends Genet.*, 13, 51, 1997.

42. Alvarez, L. et al., Characterization of rat liver-specific methionine adenosyltransferase gene promotor. Role of distal upstream *cis*-acting elements in the regulation of the transcription activity, *J. Biol. Chem.*, 272, 22875, 1997.

43. Torres, L. et al., Liver-specific methionine adenosyltransferase *MAT1A* gene expression is associated with a specific pattern of promotor methylation and histone acetylation: implications for *MAT1A* silencing during transformation, *FASEB J.*, 14, 95, 2000.

44. Sanchez-Gongora, E. et al., Interaction of liver methionine adenosyltransferase with hydroxyl radical, *FASEB J.*, 11, 1013, 1997.

45. Corrales, F.J., Ruiz, F., and Mato, J.M., *In vivo* regulation by glutathione of methionine adenosyltransferase *S*-nitrosylation in rat liver, *J. Hepatol.*, 31, 887, 1999.

46. Lu, S.C. et al., Methionine adenosyltransferase 1A knockout mice are predisposed to liver injury and exhibit increased expression of genes involved in proliferation, *Proc. Natl. Acad. Sci. USA*, 98, 5560, 2001.

47. Frezza, M. et al., Oral *S*-adenosylmethionine in the symptomatic treatment of intrahepatic cholestasis, a double-blind, placebo-controlled study, *Gastroenterology*, 99, 211, 1990.

48. Vendemiale, G. et al., Effect of oral *S*-adenosyl-L-methionine on hepatic glutathione in patients with liver disease, *Scand. J. Gastroenterol.*, 24, 407, 1989.

49. Loguerico, C. et al., Effect of *S*-adenosyl-L-methionine administration on red blood cell cysteine and glutathione levels in alcoholic patients with and without liver disease, *Alcohol Alcohol.*, 29, 597, 1994.

50. Mato, J.M. et al., *S*-adenosylmethionine in alcoholic liver cirrhosis: a randomized, placebo-controlled, double-blind, multicentre clinical trial, *J. Hepatol.*, 30, 1081, 1999.

51. Kass, S., Pruss, D., and Wolffe, A.P., How does DNA methylation repress transcription? *Trends Genet.*, 13, 444, 1997.

52. Bestor, T.H. and Tycko, B., Creation of genomic methylation patterns, *Nat. Genet.*, 12, 363, 1996.

53. Prendergast, G.C. and Ziff, E.B., Methylation-sensitive sequence-specific DNA binding by the c-myc basic region, *Science*, 251, 186, 1991.

54. Bestor, T.H., Gene silencing. Methylation meets acetylation, *Nature*, 393, 311, 1998.

55. Bird, A.P., Gene number, noise reduction and biological complexity, *Trends Genet.*, 11, 94, 1995.

56. Seitz, H.K., Poeschl, G., and Simanowski, U.A., in *Alcohol and Cancer*, Galanter, M. (Ed.), Recent developments in alcoholism, Plenum Press, New York, 1998, pp. 67–95.

57. Stickel, F. et al., Cocarcinogenic effects of alcohol in hepatocarcinogenesis, *Gut*, 51, 132, 2002.

58. Kanai, Y. et al., DNA hypermethylation at the D17S5 locus and reduced HIC-1 mRNA expression are associated with hepatocarcinogenesis, *Hepatology*, 29, 703, 1999.

59. Wainfan, E. et al., Rapid appearance of hypomethylated DNA in livers of rats fed cancer-promoting methyl-deficient diets, *Cancer Res.*, 49, 4094, 1989.

60. Shen, L. et al., Correlation between DNA methylation and pathological changes in human hepatocellular carcinoma, *Hepato-Gastroenterol.*, 45, 1753, 1998.

61. Kondo, Y. et al., Genetic instability and aberrant DNA methylation in chronic hepatitis and cirrhosis — a comprehensive study of loss of heterozygosity and microsatellite instability at 39 loci and DNA hypermethylation on CpG islands in microdissected specimens from patients with HCC, *Hepatology*, 32, 970, 2000.

62. Kanai, Y. et al., Aberrant methylation precedes loss of heterozygosity on chromosome 16 in chronic hepatitis and liver cirrhosis, *Cancer Lett.*, 148, 73, 2000.

63. Iwata, N. et al., Frequent hypermethylation of CpG islands and loss of expression of the 14-3-3 sigma gene in human hepatocellular carcinoma, *Oncogene*, 19, 5298, 2000.

64. Pascale, R.M., Simile, M.M., and Feo, F, Genomic abnormalities in hepatocarcinogenesis. Implications for a chemopreventive strategy, *Anticancer Res.*, 13, 1341, 1993.

65. Hui, A.M. and Makuuchi, M., Molecular basis of multistep hepatocarcinogenesis: genetic and epigenetic events, *Scan. J. Gastroenterol.*, 8, 737, 1999.

66. Garro, A.J. et al., Ethanol consumption inhibits fetal DNA methylation in mice: implications for the fetal alcohol syndrome, *Alcohol Clin. Exp. Res.*, 15, 395, 1991.

67. Choi, S.W. et al., Chronic alcohol consumption induces genomic but not p53-specific DNA hypomethylation in rat colon, *J. Nutr.* 129, 1945, 1999.

68. Miyakawa, H. et al., Effect of alcohol drinking on gene expression of hepatic O6-methylguanine DNA methyltransferase in chronic liver diseases, *Alcohol Clin. Exp. Res.*, 20(suppl), 297, 1996.

69. Zapisek, W.F. et al., The onset of oncogene hypomethylation in the livers of rats fed methyl-deficient, amino acid-defined diets, *Carcinogenesis*, 13, 169, 1992.

70. Pogribny, I.P. et al., Breaks in genomic DNA and within the *p53* gene are associated with hypomethylation in livers of folate/methyl-deficient rats, *Cancer Res.*, 55, 1894, 1995.

71. Ramchandani, S. et al., DNA methylation is a reversible biological signal, *Proc. Natl. Acad. Sci. USA*, 96, 6107, 1999.

72. Christman, J.K. et al., Reversibility of changes in nucleic acid methylation and gene expression induced in rat liver by severe dietary methyl deficiency, *Carcinogenesis*, 14, 551, 1993.

73. Pascale, R.M. et al., Chemoprevention of rat liver carcinogenesis by S-adenosyl-L-methionine: a long-term study, *Cancer Res.*, 52, 4979, 1992.

74. Pascale, R.M. et al., Chemoprevention by S-adenosyl-L-methionine of rat liver carcinogenesis initiated by 1,2-dimethylhydrazine and promoted by orotic acid, *Carcinogenesis*, 16, 427, 1995.

75. Simile, M.M. et al., Persistent chemopreventive effect of S-adenosyl-L-methionine on the development of liver putative preneoplastic lesions induced by thiobenzamide in diethylnitrosamine-initiated rats, *Carcinogenesis*, 17, 1533, 1996.

5 Alcohol and Nutrition as Risk Factors for Chronic Liver Disease

Stefano Bellentani, Claudio Tiribelli, and Giorgio Bedogni

CONTENTS

5.1 INTRODUCTION

The liver is the major gland in the body involved in the intermediate metabolism of nutrients absorbed from the intestine. For this reason, it is intuitive to think that this

organ could be vulnerable to metabolic stress. However, the definition, the pathogenesis, the natural history, and the clinical features of metabolic-induced liver
damage have been identified only in the past 10 years. For example, liver steatosis
or fatty liver (FL), an infiltration of fat inside the hepatocyte, has been traditionally
considered a benign and reversible condition, usually the expression of a nonspecific
response of the liver to metabolic stress of different origin. In the light of new
knowledge, steatosis, especially macrosteatosis, is increasingly recognized as a
condition that could evolve to cirrhosis and HCC, and its etiology is correlated not
just to alcohol abuse. As shown in Figure 5.1, FL may progress to fibrosis and
cirrhosis both in alcoholic liver disease (left panel) and in nonalcoholic liver disease
(right panel), with possible shunting that could rapidly worsen the disease when
acute hepatitis occurs.

Fibrosis leading to cirrhosis can accompany virtually any chronic liver disease
(CLD) that is characterized by the presence of hepatobiliary distortion and/or inflammation.[1] The main causes worldwide of progression from fibrosis to cirrhosis and
HCC are chronic viral hepatitis (HBV- or HCV-induced) and steatohepatitis associated with either alcohol abuse (ASH in Figure 5.1) or obesity (NASH in Figure 5.1).
Other causes include metabolic disorders (such as diabetes, hyperlipidemia, and
parenteral nutrition), autoimmune disease, neonatal and congenital rare disease,
storage disease, drug toxicity, and vascular derangement.

In this chapter, we shall overview the prevalence, natural history, and risk factors
of CLD induced by alcohol abuse (ASH) and obesity (NASH), and try to give
updated information on the causes of progression of steatohepatitis to cirrhosis in
both cases.

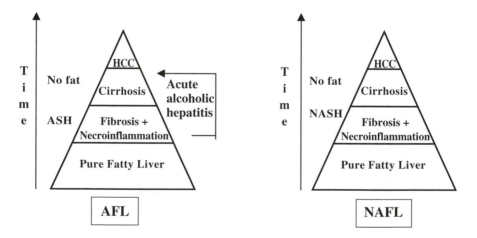

FIGURE 5.1 Common natural history pathway of alcoholic fatty liver (AFL: left panel) and
nonalcoholic fatty liver (NAFL: right panel). Liver steatosis (= Pure Fatty Liver) induced
either by alcohol or other nutritional and metabolic causes may progress to alcoholic or nonalcoholic steatohepatitis (ASH and NASH), then to cirrhosis and hepatocellular carcinoma
(HCC).

5.2 ALCOHOL AS RISK FACTOR FOR CLD

5.2.1 MECHANISMS INVOLVED IN THE PROGRESSION OF FL TO FIBROSIS AND CIRRHOSIS

The mechanisms that may contribute to steatosis-related fibrogenesis are addressed in another chapter. It is well recognized that both ASH and NASH can lead to hepatic fibrosis and cirrhosis through at least four different pathways[1]:

1. Oxidant stress due to *Cyp2E1* and *Cyp4A*. This pathway is specific to steatohepatitis induced by alcohol (ASH). In alcoholic liver disease (ALD), saturation of alcohol dehydrogenase pathways leads to induction of cytochrome P450, which can also metabolize alcohol, in particular cytochrome P450 2E1 (*Cyp2E1*); oxidation of alcohol by *Cyp2E1* or *Cyp4A* generates reactive oxygen species (ROS) that can damage hepatic cells and stimulate the fibrogenesis by stellate cells.
2. Inflammation with release of fibrogenic cytokines by infiltrating lympho-cytes and neutrophils as well as paracrine and autocrine secretion of mediators, such as chemokines, interleukins, and growth factors that stimulate hepatic stellate cells. Recently, Paradis et al.[2] demonstrated that hyperglycemia and hyperinsulinemia induce the secretion of the fibro-genic cytokine connective tissue growth factor (CTGF) in cultured stellate cells, providing direct potential evidence of progression to fibrosis involved in NASH.
3. Downregulation and deregulation of the activity of peroxisome prolifer-ator activated receptor (PPAR) signaling, involved in the pathogenesis of NASH.
4. Dysregulation of leptin expression and signaling, a pathogenetic mecha-nism that may explain the clinical link between obesity and NASH.

5.2.2 THE SAFE DOSE OF ALCOHOL FOR THE LIVER

The major and best-known determinant of fibrosis and CLD progression is continued alcohol abuse, and there is no doubt that excessive alcohol consumption leads to liver disease, from simple FL to cirrhosis in certain individuals. Patients with fibrosis who continue to drink are virtually certain of the progression of liver damage, but only a proportion of the general population, ranging from 6 to 30%, develop CLD.[3–6] Thus, one is forced to postulate that the relation between alcohol consumption and cirrhosis is a multifactorial phenomenon, also involving the interplay of other factors. The search for other potential factors has been extensive but inconclusive, probably because only one factor (usually gender) has been studied at any one time. Moreover, it has been impossible to determine if more than one factor acting simultaneously predisposes the heavy drinker to the various forms of ALD (steatosis, steatohepatitis, cirrhosis).[7–17] Multivariate analyses have not been performed until very recently. Furthermore, in spite of the axiom "No alcohol, no ALD," the epidemiological data correlating alcohol consumption and risk of ALD suggest that alcohol consumption might not be the only determinant of this disease (nor of this group of diseases).

Clinical observations commonly suggest a wide individual susceptibility to ALD.[18–22] On the other hand, the dose-threshold, that is, the amount of alcohol ingested which separates the populations with near zero risk of liver damage from those where the risk is greater than zero, varies from series to series, that is, it varies with differences in the characteristics of the population studied as well as with study design (retrospective, prospective, case-control, or cohort).[18] Dose–response curves between lifetime alcohol ingested and the relative risk of cirrhosis have been reported in the last 20 years,[19–27] and all the data available clearly demonstrate that the risk of developing cirrhosis increases exponentially with the amount of alcohol ingested throughout the subject's lifetime. But the "real" main question each apparently healthy subject asks his doctor and that often remains unanswered is, "How much alcohol is too much for me?"

When, some years ago, we tried to determine the safe daily or lifetime dose for alcohol intake in a normal subject, we found different recommendations in the data of the literature, ranging from 20 to 80 g of alcohol per day consumed for at least 10 to 12 years. This is surely in part due to the fact that the design of the other studies was different and the majority of them have been retrospective, performed in selected series and not in the general population. Furthermore, the major limits of these studies is that the measurement of alcohol intake is uncontrolled and that reliable controls are lacking.[3–5,18–26] Almost 10 years ago, our group started the Dionysos Study,[6,17,28] with the aim of defining the real prevalence of CLD in the general adult population, its etiology, and possibly, following this population for at least 10 years, its natural history. The Dionysos Study was designed in two parts: the first part, aiming to know the prevalence of CLD, was performed in 1991–1993, when almost 7000 people were enrolled and their livers were studied; the second part, which started in 2001 and is ongoing was designed to learn the 10-year incidence and the natural history of CLD in the same population. The Dionysos population is composed of the residents of two towns in northern Italy: Campogalliano and Cormons. About 70% of the population was followed-up for 10 years. The two towns were chosen because they were comparable for economic and demographic features, but they differ for drinking and dietary habits. As far as alcohol-induced liver disease is concerned, other causes of chronic liver disease, such as viral-induced hepatitis and drug-induced liver damage were excluded. Particular care was taken to use a reliable method of measurement of alcohol consumption: a semiquantitative color-illustrated food questionnaire was employed and submitted to each subject by trained personnel. The questionnaire has been validated and the alcohol intake was also crosschecked with the family members and with the total amount of alcohol consumed in the drug stores and pubs during the 2 years' duration of the study, with a 90% correlation. Presence of alcoholic liver disease (ALD) was defined on the basis of the persistent alteration of the common biochemical blood tests used as markers for alcohol abuse and hepatocyte necrosis (alanine aminotransferase, aspartate aminotransferase, γ-glutamyl-transpeptidase, mean corpuscular volume, and platelet count); patients with any clinical sign of liver disease or an abnormal blood test underwent liver ultrasonography, and, when necessary, liver biopsy was performed in order to reach the final diagnosis. In the Dionysos population, we were able to demonstrate that the risk threshold of alcohol consumption for ALD in both sexes is 30 g/d.[17] No significant risk for noncirrhotic liver disease or cirrhosis was present up to this level of intake, but above that level the risk of having either noncirrhotic CLD or cirrhosis increased proportionally with the amount of daily alcohol intake. Alcohol abusers, i.e., people who drank more than 120 g of alcohol per day, had a risk of cirrhosis 62 times higher than alcohol abstainers.[6] According to these data, the safe dose one can drink every day in order to preserve the liver from damage is 30 g; that is the equivalent of almost three standard drinks per day or 21 drinks per week. This value is very similar to that calculated by Becker et al.[24] in 13,285 subjects participating in the prospective Copenhagen City Heart Study. In this study, the threshold dose for alcohol-induced liver disease was above 7 to 13 drinks per week for women and 14 to 27 drinks per week for men. The Dionysos Study also showed that CLD does not develop below a lifetime alcohol ingestion of 100 kg, and that the effects of alcohol intake on the liver are independent of such variables as body mass index (BMI) or type of alcoholic beverage (wine, beer, and spirits).

5.2.3 EPIDEMIOLOGICAL FEATURES OF ALCOHOL-INDUCED LIVER DAMAGE

The true picture of the prevalence, incidence, and natural history of CLD induced by alcohol in the general population is not fully understood, and the majority of the available data belongs to retrospective studies on mortality or on hospitalized patients, which provides only a glimpse into the entire phenomenon, that is, the tip of the so-called "iceberg phenomenon," well-known to epidemiologists. By studying ALD in the general population of the Dionysos Study, the overall prevalence of cirrhosis in the general population of this cohort was found to be 1.1%, that is, more than three times the one commonly reported in northern Italy on the basis of mortality rate and hospital discharge. The majority of the people with cirrhosis were asymptomatic: almost 40% of the cases of cirrhosis were alcohol related, meaning that the prevalence of alcoholic cirrhosis in the general population, at least in northern Italy, is 0.42%. After exclusion of the subjects infected by either HBV or HCV virus, the prevalence of population at risk for liver damage (according to the level of risk of 30 g of alcohol per day, as indicated above) was 17.8%. The prevalence of alcohol-induced liver damage was 1.1%, while the prevalence of "pure" alcoholic cirrhosis (after excluding the other types of cirrhosis, such as primary biliary cirrhosis or hereditary hemochromatosis) was 0.5%; not surprisingly only 10% were symptomatic. The Dionysos Study allowed to better define the iceberg phenomenon (see Figure 5.2). Starting from a prevalence of alcoholic cirrhosis in the general apparently healthy population of 0.50%, that is, 500 over 100,000 apparently healthy cirrhotic subjects, 50 over 100,000 of them are symptomatic and need medical support; only 11 over 100,000 of them die every year. In other words, the prevalence of symptomatic alcoholic cirrhosis in the general population is probably 45 times higher than the one estimated by the annual mortality rate.

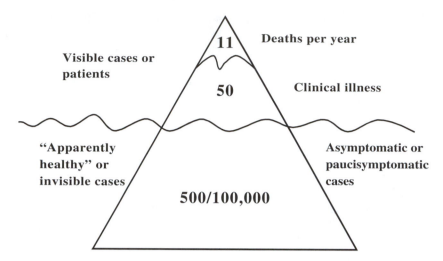

FIGURE 5.2 The "iceberg" phenomenon. Prevalence and natural history of alcoholic cirrhosis in the general population of two towns in northern Italy (Dionysos Study[6,23,38]) from healthy subjects to bedside.

5.2.4 DRINKING HABITS AND PATTERN OF DRINKING: DO THEY INFLUENCE THE RISK OF CLD?

Other questions patients frequently ask the doctor are: "what is the safest time of the day to drink?" and "what kind of beverages should I choose?" Previously, studies have shown that a sustained alcohol intake induces ALD with greater frequency than binge drinking.[19] This has been attributed to the possibility that alcohol binging might give liver cells a chance to recover at least in part. Furthermore, a sustained alcohol intake is more likely to produce inadequate food intake and malnutrition than binging or social drinking. Malnutrition clearly aggravates ALD. A number of studies, derived in part from alcohol abuse treatment programs, suggest that heavy drinkers with cirrhosis have a less severe pattern of alcohol dependency and perhaps less psychosocial difficulties than heavy drinkers without cirrhosis.[29,30] An interesting observation was made by Gronbaek et al.[31] who, in confirming the known association between total alcohol intake and the risk of upper gastrointestinal tract malignancies, noted that there was a carcinogenic effect for beer and liquor but not for wine. This may be partly due to the protective effect of resveratrol, present in wine but not in beer and liquor.[32,33] Two recent studies confirmed these findings. Roizen et al.[34] explored the mortality for alcoholic cirrhosis in the U.S. during the last 50 years and showed a significant association with the consumption of liquor, but not with the consumption of other alcoholic beverages. Another study by Becker et al.[35] showed a lower risk of developing cirrhosis in wine drinkers in comparison to both liquor and beer drinkers. However, these studies are contradicted by others. For instance, Guallar-Castillón et al.[36] recently showed that moderate drinking of beer or spirits may be just as "healthy" as wine drinking and that it is the overall quantity of alcohol consumed rather than the type of alcoholic beverage that has the greatest impact on health. More work is needed to reconcile, if possible, these discrepancies.

The Dionysos Study[6,17] showed that, in addition to the total amount of alcohol ingested, the pattern of drinking is a determinant of the development of ALD. For equal amounts of alcohol, individuals who ingested at mealtime and outside mealtime had an incidence of ALD and cirrhosis from three to five times higher than that of the individuals ingesting it only at mealtime. This increased risk began to be significant in heavy drinkers from age 50 on. Furthermore, while the type of alcoholic beverage *per se* had no demonstrable effect on the incidence of ALD, the use of multiple types (wine, beer, and liquor) was associated — within the same range of total alcohol consumption — with a significantly higher incidence of ALD and cirrhosis.

5.2.5 GENETIC FACTORS: ARE THEY INVOLVED IN THE PROGRESSION OF ALD?

Several studies link ALD with different genes, such as those encoding for alcohol dehydrogenase (*ADH2, ADH3*) and aldehyde dehydrogenase (*ALDH2*), as well as those encoding for the microsomal ethanol oxidation system known as Cytochrome P4502E1 (*CYP2E1*).[9–16] However, results are often conflicting for various reasons such as selected or few patients, or the difficulty of a precise definition of the disease. The Dionysos Study also helped in shedding some light on this complicated issue. The distributions of nine different polymorphisms in three genes involved in alcohol metabolism (*ADH2, ADH3,* and *CYP2E1*) were investigated among the drinkers reporting comparably high amounts of ethanol intake (more than 120 g/d for more than 10 years) but differing for the presence or absence of clinical and biochemical signs of liver damage. In the inhabitants of Campogalliano, the C2 allele in the promoter region of the *CYP2E1* gene had a frequency significantly higher in heavy drinkers with cirrhosis as compared with healthy, heavy drinkers. In Cormons, whose inhabitants have a different genetic derivation, a prominent association between ALD and homozygosity for allele *ADH3*2* of *ADH3* was observed, with a prevalence in heavy drinkers with or without ALD of 31 and 7%, respectively.[37] These results indicate that the presence of either at least one allele C2 of cytochrome P4502E1 or of the homozygosity for the *ADH3*2* allele are predisposing factors for the development of ALD in this population. The identification of two genetic polymorphisms predisposing to ALD reinforces the notion that ALD is a multigenic disorder.

5.2.6 GENDER DIFFERENCES: ARE WOMEN AT GREATER RISK FOR ALD?

Previous studies showed that the relative risk of alcoholic cirrhosis rises in females much more steeply with increasing levels of alcohol intake than in males.[37,38] It had been reported that in women, clinical liver disease occurs after a shorter period of alcohol intake.[39] Pharmacokinetic studies had indicated that blood levels in women after the ingestion of a standard dose of alcohol are significantly higher than in males, due either to a smaller distribution volume or to a lower gastric alcohol dehydrogenase activity (ADH).[40,41] These gender-related differences, however, were found only in selected populations. In large, open-population cohort studies like the Dionysos Study, no gender-related difference was found in either the minimum quantity of alcohol necessary to increase the risk or the susceptibility to ALD.[6] Therefore, the suggested greater susceptibility of women to ALD remains unproven and further research is warranted.

5.2.7 CHRONIC VIRAL INFECTION AS FACTOR OF RISK FOR ALD PROGRESSION

Chronic alcoholism appears to cause, in patients already suffering from chronic hepatitis B and C, more severe ALD, which more rapidly and more frequently progresses to cirrhosis and to hepatocellular carcinoma (HCC).[42,43] Recent data have demonstrated that, among patients with alcoholic cirrhosis, the risk of developing HCC is 8.3 times higher in HCV-positive than in HCV-negative subjects,[44] and in a large European cooperative study on HCV-related chronic hepatitis, an alcohol intake greater than 50 g/d significantly increases the percentage of fibrosis within the liver.[45] We also showed in the Dionysos Study that the percentage of either cirrhosis or HCC in people who abuse alcohol and are infected with either virus B or virus C is significantly higher than in people who are excessive drinkers but who did not get any viral infection. The consensus of opinion on this matter seems to indicate the virus — especially HCV — as the main factor responsible for the progression of chronic liver disease in patients who have viral hepatitis and are also heavy drinkers, independent of which factor started first. Because of these considerations, the so-called healthy HBV and HCV carriers should either abstain from alcohol completely or at least reduce its intake to levels below the risk threshold of 30 g/d.

5.3 NUTRITION AS RISK FACTOR FOR CLD

5.3.1 ALCOHOL ABUSE AND OBESITY AS RISK FACTORS FOR THE PROGRESSION OF CLD

Although the roles of alcohol abuse and obesity in inducing FL have been reported, their relative roles are still undefined, and the real prevalence of FL in the general population has long been controversial. Previous studies[46] reported a prevalence of steatosis from 3 to 22%, which is probably explained by the different types of populations studied. In spite of this variability in prevalence, there is an overall agreement to consider that fatty liver occurs more frequently in men and that obesity, alcohol abuse, and hyperinsulinemia may be important in determining this. The Dionysos Study allowed understanding the "real" prevalence of FL and defining the subjects at risk for the hepatic fat accumulation. After exclusion of HBV- and HCV-positive subjects, and those who consumed any type of drugs during the previous 6 months, an intracohort case control study[28] was performed. The risk ratio of steatosis significantly increased in heavy drinkers (2.8), obese (4.6), and obese and heavy drinkers (5.8). Obesity increased 2.0 times the risk of steatosis in heavy drinkers while heavy drinking was associated with only a 1.0-fold risk in obese subjects. Collectively, this study allowed us to conclude that steatosis is frequently encountered in healthy subjects (16%) and it is almost always present in obese subjects drinking more than 60 g alcohol per day (95%). Most important was the demonstration that steatosis is more strongly associated with obesity (76%) than heavy drinking (46%), suggesting a greater role for overweight than for inappropriate alcohol consumption in inducing fat accumulation in the liver, and in the pathogenesis of NASH, as other authors in Spanish and Japanese populations also reported recently.[38,47] Alcoholic patients often show a severe distortion of their diets, but no association between low intake of specific nutrients and chronic liver disease is usually detected.[4] There is compelling evidence that ALD is more frequent in obese patients, who may be subjected to CLD 2.5 to 3 times more frequently than the general population.[48]

5.3.2   NONALCOHOLIC FATTY LIVER DISEASE (NAFLD)

5.3.2.1   Definition, Prevalence, and Natural History of NAFLD

NAFLD is a condition characterized by a significant accumulation of lipids inside the hepatocytes without a history of excessive alcohol consumption.[49] NAFLD encompasses a wide spectrum of liver injury, ranging from steatosis to steatohepatitis, fibrosis, and cirrhosis.[50] Nonalcoholic steatohepatitis (NASH) is a stage of NAFLD characterized by histological lesions similar to those of alcoholic steatohepatitis (ASH).[50] While simple steatosis has a benign clinical course, NASH may evolve into fibrosis, cirrhosis, and, possibly, hepatocarcinoma.[49] Because NASH cannot be distinguished from ASH on histological grounds, its diagnosis relies heavily on the determination of the quantity of alcohol consumed by the patient.[51] However, there is lack of consensus on what represents excessive alcohol consumption. Studies on NAFLD published before 1990 allowed no alcohol consumption, while those published subsequently allowed up to 210 g per week, i.e., 30 g/d.[51] Hepatic steatosis can, however, be induced by a quantity of alcohol of 20 g/d and this is the upper limit employed by recent studies on NAFLD.[51] The worldwide prevalence of NAFLD is unknown. According to imaging and autopsy studies,[49] about 20 to 30% of adults in the U.S. and other Western countries are estimated to have NAFLD and 2 to 3% to have NASH. NASH is becoming increasingly recognized in children and may lead to cirrhosis during childhood.[49]

5.3.2.2   Nutrition as a Risk Factor for NAFLD

Obesity, type 2 diabetes, and hyperlipidemia are risk factors for NAFLD. As reviewed by Angulo,[52] the prevalence of obesity in patients with NAFLD varies between 30 and 100%, that of type 2 diabetes between 10 and 75%, and that of hyperlipidemia between 20 and 92%. In the Dionysos study, the prevalence of NAFL was 4.6 times higher in obese than in nonobese individuals.[28] Insulin resistance is common in obesity and hyperlipidemia and is the hallmark of type 2 diabetes.[53] Moreover, it is frequently detected in patients with NAFLD[54–57] and also in those without obesity and diabetes. Thus, insulin resistance may be the minimum common denominator of most cases of NAFLD.[52,58] Insulin resistance, impaired glucose tolerance, obesity, and hyperlipidemia are all elements of the metabolic syndrome[53] that causes NAFLD to be considered as another "disease of affluence."[58] In a recent study,[54] Marchesini et al. have assessed the prevalence of the metabolic syndrome in 304 consecutive NAFLD patients without diabetes. A total of 18% of normal-weight and 67% of obese subjects had the metabolic syndrome. Of the patients with NASH, 88% had the metabolic syndrome as compared to 53% of those with simple steatosis. Interestingly, the metabolic syndrome was a predictor of fibrosis. All these data point to the conclusion that insulin resistance *per se* may be a risk factor for the progression of simple steatosis to NASH, even if a cause–effect relationship can be disclosed only by prospective studies. Insulin is hypothesized to play a central role in the pathogenesis of NASH by the so-called two-hit theory.[58-60] The "first hit" consists in the development of hepatic steatosis owing to insulin resistance. The "second hit" would be oxidative stress, mainly in the form of an excessive production of reactive oxygen species from the mitochondria of lipid-laden hepatocytes. In light of recent studies showing that insulin resistance is a risk factor for NASH,[54,56,57] insulin itself may possibly act as a "second hit."[58] Obesity, type 2 diabetes, hyperlipidemia, and insulin resistance can be considered nutritional risk factors in view of their association with nutritional status. However, contrary to cardiovascular and metabolic disease,[53] there is at present no evidence that dietary intake is associated with NAFLD or its progression to NASH. Musso et al.[61] have recently described a higher intake of saturated fatty acids and cholesterol and a lower intake of polyunsaturated fatty acids, fiber, ascorbic acid, and tocopherol in 25 patients with NASH as compared to 25 healthy controls. Although obtained in a selected sample, these findings are of interest because they are similar to those obtained for cardiovascular and metabolic disease, at least as far as fats and fiber are concerned.[53] Clearly, further prospective and larger studies are necessary to provide this important and practical information.

5.4 CONCLUSION

From what has been indicated above, it is clear that several dark aspects are still present in the long-known, though poorly defined, correlation linking liver damage with what we drink and eat. What we ought to understand is whether the *amount* of alcohol is the most important side of the coin or the mere *consumption* of alcohol. The same applies to food quality and quantity. But most important, it seems to us, is to understand whether what will be derived from studies performed in one population (Caucasian, for example) can be extrapolated to other races, thus making what is discovered applicable worldwide. In reviewing previous data, this seems not to be the case, leading researchers to the role of genes in the production of or protection from liver damage. Certainly, investigators in this field will be kept rather busy in the future.

ACKNOWLEDGMENTS

Many of the results described in this chapter and obtained through the Dionysos Study were possible thanks to the grants offered by: Fondo per lo Studio delle Malatie del Fegato– ONLUS; Assessorato Sanità Regione Friuli Venezia Giulia and Regione Emilia Romagna; Fondazioni Cassa di Risparmio di Trieste, Gorizia, and Modena.

References

1. Friedman S.L. Liver fibrosis — from bench to bedside. *J. Hepatol.*, 38 Suppl 1, S38, 2003.
2. Paradis V. et al. High glucose and hyperinsulinemia stimulate connective tissue growth factor expression: a potential mechanism involved in progression to fibrosis in non-alcoholic steatohepatitis. *Hepatology*, 34, 738, 2001.
3. Diehl A.M. Alcoholic liver disease. *Med. Clin. North. Am.*, 73, 815, 1989.
4. Bunout D. Nutritional and metabolic effects of alcoholism: their relationship with alcoholic liver disease. *Nutrition*, 15, 583, 1999.
5. Derr R.F. et al. Is ethanol per se hepatotoxic? *J. Hepatol.*, 10, 381, 1990.
6. Bellentani S. et al. Drinking habits as cofactors of risk for alcohol induced liver damage: the Dionysos Study Group. *Gut*, 41, 845, 1997.
7. Devor E.J. et al. Genetics of alcoholism and related end-organ damage. *Semin. Liver Dis.*, 8, 1, 1988.
8. Davis M. Alcoholic liver injury. *Proc. Nutr. Soc.*, 47, 115, 1988.
9. Day C.P. et al. Investigation of the role of polymorphisms at the alcohol and aldehyde dehydrogenase loci in genetic predisposition to alcohol-related end-organ damage. *Hepatology*, 14, 798, 1991.
10. Chao Y.C. et al. Alcoholism and alcoholic organ damage and genetic polymorphisms of alcohol metabolizing enzymes in Chinese patients. *Hepatology*, 25, 112, 1997.
11. Poupon R.E. et al. Polymorphism of alcohol dehydrogenase, alcohol and aldehyde dehydrogenase activities: implication in alcoholic cirrhosis in white patients. The French Group for Research on Alcohol and Liver. *Hepatology*, 15, 1017, 1992.
12. Tsutsumi M. et al. Genetic polymorphisms of cytochrome P4502E1 related to the development of alcoholic liver disease. *Gastroenterology*, 107, 1430, 1994.
13. Savolainen V.T. et al. Polymorphism in the cytochrome P4502E1 gene and the risk of alcoholic liver disease. *J. Hepatol.*, 26, 55, 1997.
14. Pirmohamed M. et al. Genetic polymorphism of cytochrome P4502E1 and risk of alcoholic liver disease in Caucasians. *Pharmacogenetics*, 5, 351, 1995.
15. Yamauchi M. et al. Association of a restriction fragment length polymorphism in the alcohol dehydrogenase 2 gene with Japanese alcoholic liver cirrhosis. *J. Hepatol.*, 23, 519, 1995.
16. Day C.P. et al. Alcohol dehydrogenase polymorphisms and predisposition to alcoholic cirrhosis. *Hepatology*, 18, 230, 1993.
17. Bellentani S. et al. Prevalence of chronic liver disease in the general population of northern Italy: the Dionysos Study. *Hepatology*, 20, 1442, 1994.
18. Corrao G. et al. Attributable risk for symptomatic liver cirrhosis in Italy. Collaborative Groups for the Study of Liver Diseases in Italy. *J. Hepatol.*, 28, 608, 1998.

19. Sorensen T.I. et al. Prospective evaluation of alcohol abuse and alcoholic liver injury in men as predictors of development of cirrhosis. *Lancet*, 2, 241, 1984.
20. Coates R.A. et al. Risk of fatty infiltration or cirrhosis of the liver in relation to ethanol consumption: a case-control study. *Clin. Invest. Med.*, 9, 26, 1986.
21. Klatsky A.L. et al. Alcohol and mortality. *Ann. Intern. Med.*, 117, 646, 1992.
22. Klatskin G. Alcohol and its relation to liver disease. *Gastroenterology*, 41, 443, 1961.
23. Lieber C.S. Alcohol and the liver: 1994 update. *Gastroenterology*, 106, 1085, 1994.
24. Becker U. et al. Prediction of risk of liver disease by alcohol intake, sex, and age: a prospective population study. *Hepatology*, 23, 1025, 1996.
25. Grant B.F. et al. Epidemiology of alcoholic liver disease. *Semin. Liver Dis.*, 8, 12, 1988.
26. Lelbach W.K. Cirrhosis in the alcoholic and its relation to the volume of alcohol abuse. *Ann. N.Y. Acad. Sci.*, 252, 85, 1975.
27. Bellentani S. and Tiribelli C. The spectrum of liver disease in the general population: lesson from the Dionysos study. *J. Hepatol.*, 35, 531, 2001.
28. Bellentani S. et al. Prevalence of and risk factors for hepatic steatosis in Northern Italy. *Ann. Intern. Med.*, 132, 112, 2000.
29. Ewusi-Mensah I. et al. The clinical nature and detection of psychiatric disorders in patients with alcoholic liver disease. *Alcohol Alcohol.*, 19, 297, 1984.
30. Sarin S.K. et al. Pattern of psychiatric morbidity and alcohol dependence in patients with alcoholic liver disease. *Dig. Dis. Sci.*, 33, 443, 1988.
31. Gronbaek M. et al. Population based cohort study of the association between alcohol intake and cancer of the upper digestive tract. *Br. Med. J.*, 317, 844, 1998.
32. Jang M. et al. Cancer chemopreventive activity of resveratrol, a natural product derived from grapes. *Science*, 275, 218, 1997.
33. Uenobe F. et al. Antimutagenic effect of resveratrol against Trp-P-1. *Mutat. Res.*, 373, 197, 1997.
34. Roizen R. et al. Cirrhosis mortality and per capita consumption of distilled spirits, United States, 1949–94: trend analysis. *Br. Med. J.*, 319, 666, 1999.
35. Becker U. et al. Lower risk for alcohol-induced cirrhosis in wine drinkers. *Hepatology*, 35, 868, 2002.
36. Guallar-Castillon P. et al. Consumption of alcoholic beverages and subjective health in Spain. *J. Epidemiol. Community Health*, 55, 648, 2001.
37. Tuyns A.J. and Pequignot G. Greater risk of ascitic cirrhosis in females in relation to alcohol consumption. *Int. J. Epidemiol.*, 13, 53, 1984.
38. Pares A. et al. Histological course of alcoholic hepatitis. Influence of abstinence, sex and extent of hepatic damage. *J. Hepatol.*, 2, 33, 1986.
39. Ashley M.J. et al. Morbidity in alcoholics. Evidence for accelerated development of physical disease in women. *Arch. Intern. Med.*, 137, 883, 1977.
40. Marshall A.W. et al. Ethanol elimination in males and females: relationship to menstrual cycle and body composition. *Hepatology*, 3, 701, 1983.
41. Frezza M. et al. High blood alcohol levels in women. The role of decreased gastric alcohol dehydrogenase activity and first-pass metabolism. *N. Engl. J. Med.*, 322, 95, 1990.
42. Villa E. et al. Susceptibility of chronic symptomless HBsAg carriers to ethanol-induced hepatic damage. *Lancet*, 2, 1243, 1982.
43. Schiff E.R. Hepatitis C and alcohol. *Hepatology*, 26, 39S, 1997.
44. Noda K. et al. Progression of type C chronic hepatitis to liver cirrhosis and hepatocellular carcinoma — its relationship to alcohol drinking and the age of transfusion. *Alcohol Clin. Exp. Res.*, 20, 95A, 1996.

45. Imbert-Bismut F. et al. Biochemical markers of liver fibrosis in patients with hepatitis C virus infection: a prospective study. *Lancet*, 357, 1069, 2001.
46. Lonardo A. et al. The bright liver syndrome. Prevalence and determinants of a "bright" liver echopattern. *Ital. J. Gastroenterol. Hepatol.*, 29, 351, 1997.
47. Nomura H. et al. Prevalence of fatty liver in a general population of Okinawa, Japan. *Jpn. J. Med.*, 27, 142, 1988.
48. Naveau S. et al. Excess weight risk factor for alcoholic liver disease. *Hepatology*, 25, 108, 1997.
49. Neuschwander-Tetri B.A. and Caldwell S.H. Nonalcoholic steatohepatitis: summary of an AASLD single topic conference. *Hepatology*, 37, 1202, 2003.
50. Reid A.E. Nonalcoholic steatohepatitis. *Gastroenterology*, 121, 710, 2001.
51. Falck-Ytter Y. et al. Clinical features and natural history of nonalcoholic steatosis syndromes. *Semin. Liver Dis.*, 21, 17, 2001.
52. Angulo P. Nonalcoholic fatty liver disease. *N. Engl. J. Med.*, 346, 1221, 2002.
53. Third Report of the National Cholesterol Education Program (NCEP) Expert Panel on Detection, Evaluation, and Treatment of High Blood Cholesterol in Adults (Adult Treatment Panel III) final report. *Circulation*, 106, 3143, 2002.
54. Marchesini G. et al. Nonalcoholic fatty liver, steatohepatitis, and the metabolic syndrome. *Hepatology*, 37, 917, 2003.
55. Marchesini G. et al. Nonalcoholic fatty liver disease: a feature of the metabolic syndrome. *Diabetes*, 50, 1844, 2001.
56. Pagano G. et al. Nonalcoholic steatohepatitis, insulin resistance, and metabolic syndrome: further evidence for an etiologic association. *Hepatology*, 35, 367, 2002.
57. Chitturi S. et al. NASH and insulin resistance: insulin hypersecretion and specific association with the insulin resistance syndrome. *Hepatology*, 35, 373, 2002.
58. Day C.P. Non-alcoholic steatohepatitis (NASH): where are we now and where are we going? *Gut*, 50, 585, 2002.
59. Day C. and James O. Steatohepatitis: a tale of two "hits"? *Gastroenterology*, 114, 842, 1998.
60. Chitturi S. et al. Serum leptin in NASH correlates with hepatic steatosis but not fibrosis: a manifestation of lipotoxicity? *Hepatology*, 36, 403, 2002.
61. Musso G. el al. Dietary habits and their relations to insulin resistance and postprandial lipemia in nonalcoholic steatohepatitis. *Hepatology*, 37, 909, 2003.

Section III

Alcohol and Heart Disease

6 Alcohol and Cardiovascular Disease

Dawn Warner Kershner, Patrick J. Skerrett, and J. Michael Gaziano

CONTENTS

6.1 ABSTRACT

While there is little debate that heavy alcohol consumption is harmful to the cardiovascular and other systems, the impact of light-to-moderate alcohol consumption is less certain. Numerous prospective studies suggest an inverse association between light-to-moderate alcohol intake and reduced risk of premature mortality and cardiovascular disease. For men, one to two alcoholic drinks per day appear to be optimal, while for women no more than one drink per day is optimal. Current evidence suggests that any cardiovascular benefits of alcohol consumption are due to the alcohol itself rather than to a particular beverage type. While strong data now exist supporting the benefit of light-to-moderate alcohol consumption in preventing cardiovascular disease, recommendations by clinicians should be given on an individual basis after a thorough review of each patient's history and risk profile.

6.2 INTRODUCTION

The effects of alcohol on the heart have been explored — and debated — for centuries. Ancient texts from Persia, China, Greece, and elsewhere describe alcohol's potential healthful and harmful cardiovascular effects. In the 18th century, William Heberden, the great English physician, recommended alcohol for patients with angina, while in the 19th century, alcohol was considered primarily a cardiac toxin. Today, researchers are still unraveling the complex relationship between alcohol and the heart.

There is little debate over the causal relationship between heavy alcohol intake and increased risk of all-cause mortality. At the same time, a large body of observational data supports an association between light-to-moderate alcohol intake and reduced risk of cardiovascular disease, particularly coronary heart disease (CHD). In this chapter, we summarize these data among individuals at usual and high risk of CHD, highlight recent research in this field, and discuss advice that clinicians can offer their patients.

6.3 ALCOHOL AND MORTALITY

Numerous studies suggest a U- or J-shaped association between alcohol consumption and all-cause mortality, with lowest risk among light-to-moderate drinkers and higher risk among heavy drinkers.[1-3] Results of several new studies examining this association have been reported. Data from the Japan Public Health Center cohort (19,231 men aged 40 to 59 years at baseline followed for 6 years),[4] the Physicians' Health Study enrollment cohort (89,299 initially healthy U.S. male physicians aged 40 to 84 years followed for 5.5 years),[5] a cross-sectional study of adult Germans,[6] and elderly New Zealanders in the Dubbo Study[7] all support a decreased all-cause mortality with light-to-moderate alcohol consumption. In contrast, among 5,766 Scottish men followed for 21 years, no decreased risk of all-cause mortality was observed among light-to-moderate drinkers.[8]

While the exact shape and nadir of the alcohol/mortality curve have yet to be determined, there is general agreement that the association between alcohol consumption and mortality results from summing cause-specific effects (Figure 6.1). The clear and consistent increase in mortality associated with heavy alcohol consumption is likely due to increased risk of liver disease, certain cancers, accidents, suicide, and cardiovascular diseases such as cardiomyopathy and stroke, both ischemic stroke and hemorrhagic stroke.[9-11] The lower risk of total mortality associated with light-to-moderate alcohol consumption appears to be due to a reduction in cardiovascular disease (CVD) mortality without dramatic increases in other causes of death.

6.4 ALCOHOL AND CORONARY HEART DISEASE

Observational studies conducted among diverse populations, including more than 60 prospective studies, point to an inverse association between light-to-moderate alcohol consumption and CHD. Structured reviews and meta-analyses of these

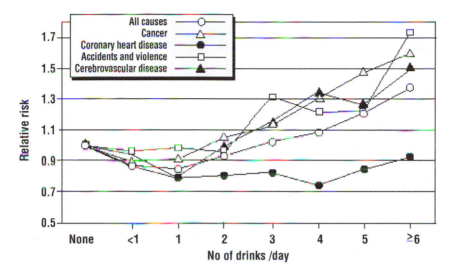

FIGURE 6.1 Alcohol consumption and relative risk of death over 12 years in American Cancer Society prospective study of 276,802 men aged 40 to 59. (From Marmot and Brunner. *Br. Med. J.*, 1991; 303: 565–568. With permission of BMJ Publishing Goup, London.)

studies describe the potential benefits in different ways. In a recent meta-analysis of 51 studies conducted between 1966 and 1998, pooled dose–response functions were derived from 28 high-quality cohort studies.[12] Consumption of 0 to 20 g/d of alcohol was associated with a decreased risk of CHD (RR, 0.80; 95% CI, 0.78 to 0.83) compared with no drinking, and a protective effect was evident at consumption up to 72 g/d (RR, 0.96; 95% CI, 0.92 to 1.00). Consumption ≥ 89 g/d, however, was associated with increased risk of CHD (RR, 1.05; 95% CI, 1.00 to 1.11). Rimm and colleagues took a different approach — examining experimental studies that assessed the effects of moderate alcohol intake on concentrations of high-density lipoprotein cholesterol (HDL-cholesterol), apolipoprotein A-1 (apoA1), fibrinogen, triglycerides, and other biological markers that have been associated with CHD risk.[13] Data from 42 eligible studies with information on change in these markers with alcohol consumption in subjects free of chronic disease indicate that an experimental dose of 30 g of ethanol a day increased concentrations of HDL-cholesterol by 3.99 mg/dl (95% CI, 3.25 to 4.73), apoA1 by 8.82 mg/dl (95% CI, 7.79 to 9.86), triglycerides by 5.69 mg/dl (95% CI, 2.49 to 8.89), and modestly affected several hemostatic factors related to a thrombolytic profile. From these data, the authors estimated that consumption of 30 g of alcohol a day would be associated with a 24.7% reduction in risk of CHD.

One limitation of many prior cohort studies is that alcohol exposure was measured at only one point in time. In the Physicians' Health Study, for example, baseline consumption of alcohol has been associated with decreased risk of myocardial infarction,[14,15] angina pectoris,[15] and peripheral arterial disease.[16] In this population, 7-year changes in alcohol consumption were assessed to determine if there was any association with the subsequent risk of CVD. Among men initially consuming one drink per week or less, those who reported moderate increases in alcohol consumption to between one and six drinks per week had a borderline significant (P, 0.05) 29% reduced risk of CVD compared with men not reporting changes in alcohol consumption.[17] No significant changes in CVD risk were observed with moderately increased consumption among men initially reporting one to six drinks per week, while a significant 63% increase in CVD risk was observed among men initially consuming one drink per day or more who reported increased alcohol consumption. However, in the Health Professionals Follow-up Study, a 12.5-g increase in alcohol consumption over 4 years of follow-up was associated with a decreased risk of myocardial infarction (MI) (RR, 0.78; 95% CI, 0.62 to 0.99).[18]

6.4.1 PATTERN OF ALCOHOL CONSUMPTION

The impact of pattern of drinking on CHD risk has also been relatively difficult to gauge in most studies, and drinking patterns may obscure the true association between light-to-moderate drinking and CVD risk, i.e., if some of those reporting six drinks per week take most of them in 1 d. Kauhanen and colleagues have examined this from several angles in the Kuopio Ischemic Heart Disease Risk Factor Study. They have found that men who report regularly drinking six or more bottles of beer per session had a 6.5-fold increased risk of fatal MI compared with those who drank three or fewer bottles[19]; men who reported at least one hangover per month had a 2.4-fold higher risk of cardiovascular death than men with fewer hangovers,[20] and binge drinkers had a more pronounced progression of carotid atherosclerosis, as measured by changes in maximum and mean intima-media thickness, than non-binge drinkers.[21] A careful review of pattern of alcohol use and CVD has been published by Puddey and colleagues stressing the importance of the pattern of alcohol intake on CHD outcomes.[22] Recently, Mukamal and colleagues examined drinking patterns, defined as the number of days per week alcohol was consumed, and CHD outcomes.[18] Their results showed that compared to men who consumed alcohol less than once a week, men who consumed alcohol three to four or five to seven times per week had decreased risks of CHD with an RR of 0.68 (95% CI, 0.55 to 0.84) and 0.63 (95% CI, 0.54 to 0.74), respectively. These RRs were similar among men who consumed <10 g of alcohol per drinking day and those consuming 30 g or more per day.

6.5 BEVERAGE TYPE

A lively controversy is currently under way regarding the possibility that some alcoholic beverages, particularly red wine, provide greater protection against cardiovascular disease than others. Flavonoids and antioxidants found in wine, but not beer and spirits, have been associated with reduced risk of CHD,[23] and the paradox of low CHD mortality in France and other Mediterranean countries has been attributed by some to their high consumption of wine.[24] In a recent Danish study, men and women who drank wine had a lower risk of CHD death (RR, 0.58; 95% CI, 0.47 to 0.72) than did drinkers of beer or liquor (RR, 0.76; 95% CI, 0.63 to 0.92),[25] and wine appeared to be more protective for ischemic stroke than spirits or beer in a case-control study of U.S. women.[26] In British men, a significantly lower risk of CHD was observed among regular beer and spirit drinkers compared with occasional drinkers, but not among wine drinkers.[27] However, men who reported wine drinking (either occasionally or regularly) had lower age-adjusted absolute rates of both major CHD events and all-cause mortality than those who reported drinking beer or spirits. A study of more than 1800 individuals whose alcohol consumption was assessed by a psychiatrist found that intake of wine once a week or more was associated with a relative risk ratio of 0.58 (95% CI, 0.40 to 0.84) for total mortality and 0.49 (95% CI: 0.27 to 0.90) for CVD mortality; consumption of beer or spirits was not associated with similar reductions in risk.[28]

While it is possible that antioxidants and other substances found in wine may account for the additional benefits observed with wine consumption, confounding may also explain the differences, as some evidence suggests that wine drinkers may smoke less and be of higher socioeconomic status than drinkers of other alcoholic beverages.[25] It is possible that wine tends to be consumed in modest amounts with meals, which may have metabolic advantages. Spirits, on the other hand, are often consumed at times other than meal times. More analytic data will be required to better answer this question, but at the present time it is felt that the ethanol content found in all alcoholic beverages is most likely responsible for the cardioprotective effects found with moderate alcohol consumption.

6.6 MECHANISMS

Establishing causal relationships in human disease where the size of the effect is small to moderate can be made much easier if mechanistic explanations for the association are available. A number of mechanisms have emerged from both experimental and observational epidemiologic studies of the past two decades that may explain the observed associations between alcohol consumption and cardiovascular disease. Alterations in plasma lipoproteins, particularly increases in HDL-cholesterol, represent the most plausible mechanism of the apparent protective effect of alcohol consumption on coronary heart disease. HDL-cholesterol is produced primarily in the liver and intestines and is released into the bloodstream. HDL binds with cholesterol and brings it back to the liver for elimination or reprocessing, thereby lowering total cholesterol levels in body tissues, including the arterial endothelium, and thus possibly reverses the atherosclerotic process.[29] In addition, HDL-cholesterol may play a role in rendering low-density lipoprotein-cholesterol less harmful by preventing it from becoming oxidized.[30]

Other potential mechanisms that may contribute to the cardioprotective effect of light-to-moderate alcohol consumption include alterations in the delicate balance between clot formation and clot dissolution in arterial blood. Studies suggest that light-to-moderate alcohol consumption may reduce levels of fibrinogen, clotting factor VII, platelet aggregability, and tissue plasminogen activator.[31-33] At the other end of the spectrum, acute ingestion of alcohol can prolong bleeding time and reduce platelet aggregation as well as inhibit fibrinolysis.[34,35] The extent to which alcohol's effects on thrombotic and fibrinolytic factors contributes to lower CHD risk beyond that of its effects on lipids remains unclear.

In a small case-control study of healthy volunteers, light-to-moderate alcohol consumption (10 to 30 g/d) was associated with enhanced insulin-mediated glucose uptake when compared to nondrinkers.[36] In the same study, light-to-moderate alcohol consumption was also associated with lower plasma glucose and insulin concentrations in response to an oral glucose load as well as higher HDL-cholesterol levels. This may be an important cardioprotective mechanism, especially in persons with diabetes.

Recently, Albert et al. demonstrated that individuals with moderate alcohol consumption (five to seven drinks per week) had lower levels of C-reactive protein (CRP) than those with light or occasional intake of alcohol.[37] This inverse association remained significant after adjusting for traditional risk factors for CVD including smoking status, systolic blood pressure, diabetes mellitus, body mass index, HDL-cholesterol levels, age, gender, and aspirin use. This relationship was present in both men and women not taking hormone replacement therapy, individuals with and without a history of CVD, and nonsmokers. This study suggests that moderate alcohol consumption may have an antiinflammatory mechanism as well. Similarly, Imhof et al. found a strong inverse association between alcohol consumption and CRP levels in both men and women, but the association was weaker among women.[38]

A recent genetic analysis of a polymorphism in the gene for alcohol dehydrogenase type 3 (ADH3) supports the hypothesis that slower metabolism of alcohol enhances its beneficial effect on cardiovascular disease. This polymorphism alters the rate of alcohol metabolism, with faster metabolism associated with the γ1 allele and slower metabolism associated with the γ2 allele. In a nested, case-control study, Hines and colleagues determined the ADH3 genotype in 396 men who had experienced a myocardial infarction and 770 matched controls.[39] Among men who were homozygous for the γ1 allele, those who consumed at least one drink per day had a relative risk of MI of 0.62 (95% CI, 0.34 to 1.13) compared with the risk among men who consumed less than one drink per week. Among men who were homozygous for the γ2 allele, those who consumed at least one drink per day had an even lower risk of MI (RR, 0.14; 95% CI, 0.04 to 0.45); they also had the highest plasma HDL-cholesterol levels. Interactions between the ADH3 genotype, level of alcohol consumption, and HDL-cholesterol levels were confirmed in a separate study of postmenopausal women.

6.7 HIGH-RISK GROUPS

Studies reported since 1999 generally support the inverse association between low-to-moderate alcohol consumption and CHD, and extend the possible benefits to several high-risk groups. They also suggest that low-to-moderate alcohol consumption may decrease the risk of sudden cardiac death,[40] intermittent claudication,[16] and heart failure.[41]

6.7.1 DIABETES MELLITUS

Among individuals with diabetes, age-adjusted rates for CHD are two to three times higher among men and three to seven times higher among diabetic women than among their counterparts without diabetes.[42] In fact, individuals with diabetes not diagnosed with CHD may have as high a risk of MI as nondiabetic individuals who have experienced a prior infarction.[43] Indeed, the most recent guidelines from the National Cholesterol Education Program's Adult Treatment Panel III now regard diabetes as a CHD equivalent.[44] The use of alcohol by diabetic patients has been controversial due to the potential of worsening neuropathy[45,46] and retinopathy[47] as well as the risk of hypoglycemia while drinking alcohol. Also, alcohol has no nutritional value and is counted as two fat exchanges for the diabetic patient. Several recent studies, however, suggest that similar magnitudes of CHD risk reduction are associated with light-to-moderate alcohol consumption among diabetic men and women as among healthy individuals. Data from the Wisconsin Epidemiologic Study of Diabetic Retinopathy showed a 55 to 75% reduction in CVD mortality in men and women with older onset diabetes who consumed >14 g of alcohol per day (approximately one drink per day).[48] Similar data were seen in the Nurses' Health Study with a greater than 50% reduction in CVD risk, both fatal and nonfatal MI, in female diabetics who consumed more than 5 g per day of alcohol.[49] More recently, Tanascau observed a 50% reduction in CVD in male diabetics in the Health Professionals' Follow-up Study who drank more than two alcoholic beverages per day after controlling for the traditional risk factors for CVD.[50] Previous data from the Physicians' Health Study Enrollment Cohort indicated that there was a similar reduction in CVD mortality in men both with and without diabetes.[51]

6.7.2 HYPERTENSION

Alcohol consumption has been shown in observational studies to have a strong positive association with elevated blood pressure.[52–54] In fact, a recent American Heart Association Science Advisory on wine consumption states "patients who are hypertensive should avoid alcohol,"[55] while the American Heart Association (AHA) dietary guidelines[56] and the Sixth Report of the Joint National Committee on Prevention, Detection, Evaluation, and Treatment of High Blood Pressure[57] recommend to limit alcohol to no more than two drinks per day in men and one drink per day for women for the prevention and treatment of hypertension. It has also been shown that a reduction in alcohol intake among heavy drinkers, persons drinking three or more drinks per day, can lower blood pressure in both normotensive and hypertensive men.[58,59]

Data from the Physicians' Health Study Enrollment Cohort suggest that light-to-moderate alcohol consumption is associated with a reduced risk of both CVD and total mortality in men with hypertension (in press).[60] There was a 45% reduction in CVD mortality for men who consumed one to two drinks per day after controlling for traditional CVD risk factors. In further analysis, this relationship between alcohol consumption and reduced CVD risk was similar for both controlled and uncontrolled blood pressure.

6.7.3 PREEXISTING CVD

Another high-risk group in whom light-to-moderate alcohol consumption may not be harmful and may offer some benefits are survivors of an acute MI. Among 1913 adults hospitalized with acute MI between 1989 and 1994, those who reported consuming <7 alcoholic drinks/week in the year prior to the event had a reduced risk of dying over 4 years of follow-up (hazard ratio, 0.79; 95% CI, 0.60 to 1.03), with an even lower risk among those who reported having seven or more drinks/week (hazard ratio, 0.68; 95% CI, 0.45 to 1.05; P for trend, 0.01), compared with abstainers and after adjusting for cardiovascular and other factors.[61] The association was similar for total and cardiovascular mortality, among both men and women, and among different types of alcoholic beverages. A similar reduction in post-myocardial infarction mortality was observed among U.S. male physicians over 5 years of follow-up with an RR of 0.72 (95% CI, 0.58 to 0.89) for those who reported consuming two to four drinks per week, 0.79 (95% CI, 0.64 to 0.96) for one drink per day, and 0.84 (95% CI, 0.55 to 1.26) for two or more drinks per day, compared with men who rarely or never drank alcohol.[62] In contrast, in the prospective British regional heart study, regular light-to-moderate alcohol consumption in men with established CHD was not associated with any significant benefit or deleterious effect for CHD, CVD, or all cause mortality, while higher levels of intake were associated with increased mortality in men with previous MI.[63]

CVD is the leading cause of death in both men and women in the U.S. and most other developed nations. The overwhelming body of evidence supports the association of moderate alcohol consumption and decreased risk of CVD in men and women in the general population, patients with diabetes mellitus and/or hypertension, and persons with preexisting CVD. After careful review of an individual's history, including prior alcohol dependence and consumption patterns, clinicians can provide individualized recommendations regarding alcohol consumption that may provide either primary or secondary prevention of CVD.

6.8 OTHER DISEASES

6.8.1 STROKE

The association between alcohol consumption and overall stroke risk is more complex than its association with CHD. Heavy consumption (≥30 g/d) increases blood pressure,[64] which would be expected to increase stroke risk, while the anticlotting effect of low-to-moderate alcohol consumption would be expected to decrease the risk of ischemic stroke and increase the risk of hemorrhagic stroke. Thus, it is important to examine the association with stroke types.

A 1999 review concluded that heavy alcohol intake appears to be an independent risk factor for all major subtypes of stroke, while data regarding the association between light-to-moderate drinking and stroke risk were inconclusive.[65] Since then, several reports on this topic have been published. During an average of 12.2 years of follow-up in the Physicians' Health Study, lower risks of total stroke (RR, 0.79; 95% CI, 0.66 to 0.94) and ischemic stroke (RR, 0.77; 95% CI, 0.63 to 0.94) were observed among men who consumed more than one alcoholic beverage per week compared to those who had less than one drink per week.[66] No statistically significant association was observed between alcohol consumption and hemorrhagic stroke. In a multiethnic population in New York City, consumption of up to two alcoholic drinks per day was associated with a reduced risk of ischemic stroke (RR, 0.51; 95% CI, 0.39 to 0.67), with the apparent protective effect observed among younger and older groups, in men and women, and in whites, blacks, and Hispanics.[67] Consumption of >5 drinks per day increased the risk of ischemic stroke, while consumption of two to five drinks per day was associated with an indeterminate risk. In a study of 224 women aged 15 to 44 years with a first cerebral infarction and 392 matched controls, light-to-moderate alcohol consumption was associated with a reduced risk of ischemic stroke.[26] The odds ratio of ischemic stroke was 0.57 (95% CI, 0.38 to 0.86) for consumption of <12 g/d in the past year, 0.38 (95% CI, 0.17 to 0.86) for consumption of 12 to 24 g/d, and 0.95 (95% CI, 0.43 to 2.10) for consumption of >24 g/d, compared with never drinking.

Fewer and less consistent data are available regarding the association between alcohol intake and risk of hemorrhagic stroke, with some earlier studies reporting an increased risk associated with light-to-moderate alcohol consumption[68,69] and others showing no such increase.[70] Studies reported in the past 3 years support the established relationship between heavy drinking and hemorrhagic stroke, and also tend to support the lack of association between light-to-moderate drinking and hemorrhagic stroke. Among male smokers in the Alpha-Tocopherol, Beta-Carotene Cancer Prevention (ATBC) Study, for example, the adjusted relative risk of sub-arachnoid hemorrhage was 1.0 in light drinkers, 1.3 in moderate drinkers, and 1.6 in heavy drinkers compared with nondrinkers, while the relative risks of intracerebral hemorrhage were 0.8 in light drinkers, 0.6 in moderate drinkers, and 1.8 in heavy drinkers; the respective risks of cerebral infarction were 0.9, 1.2, and 1.5.[71] In a community case-control study in Asturias, Spain, moderate alcohol consumption was not associated with intracerebral hemorrhage (odds ratio, 0.88; 95% CI, 0.44 to 1.74), but was associated with decreased risk of cerebral infarction.[72] No increase in risk of hemorrhagic stroke was observed among light to moderate drinkers in the Physicians' Health Study,[66] or in a study of 331 case-control pairs in Melbourne, Australia.[73] In the latter study, however, wine drinkers were apparently protected from intracerebral hemorrhage (odds ratio, 0.5; 95% CI, 0.2 to 0.9).

A recent meta-analysis is consistent with the above associations between alcohol consumption and risk of stroke.[11] The authors of the meta-analysis, including 19 cohort studies and 16 case-control studies, found a J-shaped relationship between alcohol consumption and total stroke and ischemic stroke, and a linear relationship between alcohol consumption and hemorrhagic stroke. Compared with abstainers, alcohol consumption of <12 g/d (approximately one drink) had an RR of 0.83, 0.80, and 0.79 for total, ischemic, and hemorrhagic stroke, respectively, while those consuming >60 g/d had an RR of 1.64, 1.69, and 2.18 for the same groups. These findings were similar for men and women, although the RRs were somewhat lower for the women in the light-to-moderate alcohol consumption categories.

Stroke is the third leading cause of death in the U.S.[74] as well as a leading causing of disability and health care expenditure.[75] Given the widespread consumption of alcohol in the general population, it is important as clinicians to give appropriate advice to our patients who consume alcohol. Based on the studies to date, advising those patients that drink heavily to dramatically decrease their alcohol consumption may be an important preventive measure to decrease their risk of stroke.

While moderate alcohol consumption appears to be protective for total and ischemic stroke, such advice should only be given on an individual basis after a careful review of the medical record.

6.8.2 PREVENTION OF DIABETES

Alcohol consumption and the risk of developing diabetes has been much debated over recent years. A reduced incidence of diabetes has been observed in light-to-moderate alcohol drinkers[76-80] while an increased incidence of diabetes has been observed in heavy drinkers.[79,81] More recently, it has been shown in the Health Professionals Follow-up Study, a cohort of 46,892 health professionals followed for 12 years, that compared with abstainers, consumption of 15 to 29 g/d of alcohol was associated with a 36% lower risk of developing diabetes (RR, 0.64, 95% CI 0.53 to 0.77).[82] This association remained significant if light drinkers were used as the referent group instead of abstainers (RR, 0.60, 95% CI 0.50 to 0.73). This inverse association persisted to those drinking ≥50 g/d of alcohol (RR, 0.60, 95% CI 0.43 to 0.84). Frequency of alcohol consumption was an important factor to this inverse relationship. Consumption of alcohol at least 5 d per week provided the greatest protection, even if less than one standard drink was consumed per day (RR, 0.48, 95% CI 0.27 to 0.86). For each additional day per week that alcohol was consumed, the risk of developing diabetes was reduced by 7% (95% CI 3 to 10%). This inverse relationship was seen with all types of alcoholic beverages, including beer, white and red wine, and spirits.

6.9 RECOMMENDATIONS

While the association of alcohol and CHD is likely to be causal, any individual or public health recommendations must consider the complexity of alcohol's metabolic, physiologic, and psychologic effects — the differences between daily intake of small-to-moderate quantities and larger quantities may be the difference between preventing and causing disease. A discussion of alcohol intake should be a part of routine preventive counseling, and this counseling must be individualized and take into account medical problems including coronary risk factors (particularly diabetes and hypertension), liver disease, tendency toward excess, and family history of alcoholism and possibly breast and colon cancer. In addition, the dose relationships in men and women appear to be different. Liver toxicities occur at lower levels among women compared to men, which does not appear to be entirely due to the difference in lean body weight. In addition, there is some evidence that consumption of ≥15g/d of alcohol increases the risk of breast cancer among women with low intake of folic acid.[83] Given the complex nature of alcohol/disease relationships, alcohol consumption should be viewed neither as a primary preventive strategy nor as an unhealthy behavior (depending on the individual).

Given the complex association of alcohol consumption and CHD, with heavy consumption increasing both total and cardiovascular mortality and moderate alcohol consumption decreasing CHD, the AHA published a science advisory on alcohol and heart disease.[84] After a careful review of the literature and strong consideration of the AHA advisory, we suggest the following guidelines for making recommendations to patients:

1. All patients should consult a physician regarding the risks and benefits of alcohol consumption.
2. Alcohol consumption, both use and patterns of use, should be reviewed with patients at least annually.
3. Review the risks and benefits of alcohol consumption periodically with patients, revising recommendations if necessary.
4. Clearly state that alcohol should never be consumed while operating heavy machinery or motor vehicles.
5. Consumption of moderate amounts of alcohol (one to two drinks per day) may be safe if no contraindications to consumption are present.
6. Adolescents and/or young adults should be educated about the potential harmful effects of alcohol consumption.

The AHA's Guidelines for Primary Prevention of Cardiovascular Disease and Stroke were updated in 2002 and recommend an overall healthy eating pattern that would limit alcohol intake to ≤2 drinks per day in men and ≤ one drink per day in women among those who drink.[85] Likewise, the AHA's Primary Prevention of Ischemic Stroke Scientific Statement also limits alcohol consumption in those who drink to the above limits.[86]

References

1. Rehm J and Bondy S. Alcohol and all-cause mortality: an overview. Novartis Found Symp 1998; 216: 223–32.
2. Fagrell B, De Faire U, Bondy S, Criqui M, Gaziano M, Gronbaek M, Jackson R, Klatsky A, Salonen J, and Shaper AG. The effects of light to moderate drinking on cardiovascular diseases. *J Intern Med* 1999; 246: 331–40.
3. Sasaki S. Alcohol and its relation to all-cause and cardiovascular mortality. *Acta Cardiol* 2000; 55: 151–6.
4. Tsugane S, Fahey MT, Sasaki S, and Baba S. Alcohol consumption and all-cause and cancer mortality among middle-aged Japanese men: seven-year follow-up of the JPHC study Cohort I. Japan Public Health Center. *Am J Epidemiol* 1999; 150: 1201–7.
5. Gaziano JM, Gaziano TA, Glynn RJ, Sesso HD, Ajani UA, Stampfer MJ, Manson JE, Hennekens CH, and Buring JE. Light-to-moderate alcohol consumption and mortality in the Physicians' Health Study enrollment cohort. *J Am Coll Cardiol* 2000; 35: 96–105.
6. Hoffmeister H, Schelp FP, Mensink GB, Dietz E, and Bohning D. The relationship between alcohol consumption, health indicators and mortality in the German population. *Int J Epidemiol* 1999; 28: 1066–72.
7. Simons LA, McCallum J, Friedlander Y, Ortiz M, and Simons J. Moderate alcohol intake is associated with survival in the elderly: the Dubbo Study. *Med J Aust* 2000; 173: 121–4.

8. Hart CL, Smith GD, Hole DJ, and Hawthorne VM. Alcohol consumption and mortality from all causes, coronary heart disease, and stroke: results from a prospective cohort study of Scottish men with 21 years of follow up. *Br Med J* 1999; 318: 1725–9.

9. Li G, Smith GS, and Baker SP. Drinking behavior in relation to cause of death among US adults. *Am J Public Health* 1994; 84: 1402–6.

10. Klatsky AL and Armstrong MA. Alcohol use, other traits, and risk of unnatural death: a prospective study. *Alc Clin Exp Res* 1993; 17: 1156–62.

11. Reynolds K, Lewis LB, Nolen JDL, Kinney GL, Sathya B, and He J. Alcohol consumption and risk of stroke: a meta-analysis. *JAMA* 2003; 289: 579–588.

12. Corrao G, Rubbiati L, Bagnardi V, Zambon A, and Poikolainen K. Alcohol and coronary heart disease: a meta-analysis. *Addiction* 2000; 95: 1505–23.

13. Rimm EB, Williams P, Fosher K, Criqui M, and Stampfer MJ. Moderate alcohol intake and lower risk of coronary heart disease: meta-analysis of effects on lipids and haemostatic factors. *Br Med J* 1999; 319: 1523–8.

14. Gaziano JM, Buring JE, Breslow JL, Goldhaber SZ, Rosner B, VanDenburgh M, Willett W, and Hennekens CH. Moderate alcohol intake, increased levels of high-density lipoprotein and its subfractions, and decreased risk of myocardial infarction. *N Engl J Med* 1993; 329: 1829–34.

15. Camargo CA, Jr., Stampfer MJ, Glynn RJ, Grodstein F, Gaziano JM, Manson JE, Buring JE, and Hennekens CH. Moderate alcohol consumption and risk for angina pectoris or myocardial infarction in U.S. male physicians. *Ann Intern Med* 1997; 126: 372–5.

16. Camargo CA, Jr., Stampfer MJ, Glynn RJ, Gaziano JM, Manson JE, Goldhaber SZ, and Hennekens CH. Prospective study of moderate alcohol consumption and risk of peripheral arterial disease in US male physicians. *Circulation* 1997; 95: 577–80.

17. Sesso HD, Stampfer MJ, Rosner B, Hennekens CH, Manson JE, and Gaziano JM. Seven-year changes in alcohol consumption and subsequent risk of cardiovascular disease in men. *Arch Intern Med* 2000; 160: 2605–12.

18. Mukamal KJ, Conigrave KM, Mittleman MA et al. Roles of drinking pattern and type of alcohol consumed in coronary heart disease in men. *N Engl J Med* 2003; 348: 109–18.

19. Kauhanen J, Kaplan GA, Goldberg DE, and Salonen JT. Beer binging and mortality: results from the Kuopio ischaemic heart disease risk factor study, a prospective population based study. *Br Med J* 1997; 315: 846–51.

20. Kauhanen J, Kaplan GA, Goldberg DD, Cohen RD, Lakka TA, and Salonen JT. Frequent hangovers and cardiovascular mortality in middle-aged men. *Epidemiology* 1997; 8: 310–4.

21. Kauhanen J, Kaplan GA, Goldberg DE, Salonen R, and Salonen JT. Pattern of alcohol drinking and progression of atherosclerosis. *Arterioscler Thromb Vasc Biol* 1999; 19: 3001–6.

22. Puddey IB, Rakic V, Dimmitt SB, and Beilin LJ. Influence of pattern of drinking on cardiovascular disease and cardiovascular risk factors — a review. *Addiction* 1999; 94: 649–63.

23. Hertog MG, Feskens EJ, Hollman PC, Katan MB, and Kromhout D. Dietary antioxidant flavonoids and risk of coronary heart disease: the Zutphen Elderly Study. *Lancet* 1993; 342: 1007–11.

24. Renaud S and de Lorgeril M. Wine, alcohol, platelets, and the French paradox for coronary heart disease. *Lancet* 1992; 339: 1523–6.

25. Gronbaek M, Becker U, Johansen D, Gottschau A, Schnohr P, Hein HO, Jensen G, and Sorensen TI. Type of alcohol consumed and mortality from all causes, coronary heart disease, and cancer. *Ann Intern Med* 2000; 133: 411–9.

26. Malarcher AM, Giles WH, Croft JB, Wozniak MA, Wityk RJ, Stolley PD, Stern BJ, Sloan MA, Sherwin R, Price TR, Macko RF, Johnson CJ, Earley CJ, Buchholz DW, and Kittner SJ. Alcohol intake, type of beverage, and the risk of cerebral infarction in young women. *Stroke* 2001; 32: 77–83.

27. Wannamethee SG and Shaper AG. Type of alcoholic drink and risk of major coronary heart disease events and all-cause mortality. *Am J Public Health* 1999; 89: 685–90.

28. Theobald H, Bygren LO, Carstensen J, and Engfeldt P. A moderate intake of wine is associated with reduced total mortality and reduced mortality from cardiovascular disease. *J Stud Alcohol* 2000; 61: 652–6.

29. von Eckardstein A, Nofer JR, and Assmann G. High density lipoproteins and arteriosclerosis. Role of cholesterol efflux and reverse cholesterol transport. *Arterioscler Thromb Vasc Biol* 2001; 21: 13–27.

30. Bonnefont-Rousselot D, Therond P, Beaudeux JL, Peynet J, Legrand A, and Delattre J. High density lipoproteins (HDL) and the oxidative hypothesis of atherosclerosis. *Clin Chem Lab Med* 1999; 37: 939–48.

31. Hendriks HF and van der Gaag MS. Alcohol, coagulation and fibrinolysis. Novartis Found Symp 1998; 216: 111–120.

32. Renaud SC, Beswick AD, Fehily AM, Sharp DS, and Elwood PC. Alcohol and platelet aggregation: the Caerphilly Prospective Heart Disease Study. *Am J Clin Nutr* 1992; 55: 1012–7.

33. Rubin R and Rand ML. Alcohol and platelet function. *Alc. Clin Exp Res* 1994; 18: 105–10.

34. Ridker PM, Vaughan DE, Stampfer MJ, Glynn RJ, and Hennekens CH. Association of moderate alcohol consumption and plasma concentration on endogenous tissue-type plasminogen activator. *JAMA*. 1994; 272: 929–33.

35. van de Wiel A, van Golde PM, Kraaijenhagen RJ, von dem Borne PA, Bouma BN, and Hart HC. Acute inhibitory effect of alcohol on fibrinolysis. *Eur J Clin Invest* 2001; 31: 164–70.

36. Facchini F, Chen YD, and Reaven GM. Light-to-moderate alcohol intake is associated with enhanced insulin sensitivity. *Diabetes Care* 1994; 17: 115–9.

37. Albert MA, Glynn RJ, and Ridker PM. Alcohol consumption and plasma concentration of C-reactive protein. *Circulation* 2003; 107: 443–447.

38. Imhof A, Froelich M, Brenner H et al. Effect of alcohol consumption on systemic markers of inflammation. *Lancet* 2001; 357: 763–767.

39. Hines LM, Stampfer MJ, Ma J, Gaziano JM, Ridker PM, Hankinson SE, Sacks F, Rimm EB, and Hunter DJ. Genetic variation in alcohol dehydrogenase and the beneficial effect of moderate alcohol consumption on myocardial infarction. *N Engl J Med* 2001; 344: 549–55.

40. Albert CM, Manson JE, Cook NR, Ajani UA, Gaziano JM, and Hennekens CH. Moderate alcohol consumption and the risk of sudden cardiac death among US male physicians. *Circulation* 1999; 100: 944–50.

41. Abramson JL, Williams SA, Krumholz HM, and Vaccarino V. Moderate alcohol consumption and risk of heart failure among older persons. *JAMA* 2001; 285: 1971–7.

42. Barrett-Connor EL, Cohn BA, Wingard DL, and Edelstein SL. Why is diabetes mellitus a stronger risk factor for fatal ischemic heart disease in women than in men? The Rancho Bernardo Study. *JAMA* 1991; 265: 627–31.

43. Haffner SM, Lehto S, Ronnemaa T, Pyorala K, and Laakso M. Mortality from coronary heart disease in subjects with type 2 diabetes and in nondiabetic subjects with and without prior myocardial infarction. *N Engl J Med* 1998; 339: 229–34.

44. Executive summary of the third report of the National Cholesterol Education Program (NCEP) expert panel on detection, evaluation, and treatment of high blood cholesterol in adults (Adult Treatment Panel III). *JAMA* 2001; 285: 2486–97.

45. McCullough DK, Campbell IW, Prescott RJ, and Clarke BF. Effect of alcohol intake on symptomatic peripheral neuropathy in diabetic men. *Diabetes Care* 1980; 3: 245–7.

46. Mitchell BD and Vinik IA. Alcohol consumption: a risk factor for diabetic neuropathy? *Diabetes Care* 1987; 36 suppl 1: 71A.

47. United Kingdom Prospective Diabetes Study, 30: Diabetic retinopathy at diagnosis of non-insulin dependent diabetes mellitus and associated risk factors. *Arch Ophthalmol* 1998; 116: 297–303.

48. Valmadrid CT, Klein R, Moss SE, Klein BE, and Cruickshanks KJ. Alcohol intake and the risk of coronary heart disease mortality in persons with older-onset diabetes mellitus. *JAMA* 1999; 282: 239–46.

49. Solomon CG, Hu FB, Stampfer MJ, Colditz GA, Speizer FE, Rimm EB, Willett WC, and Manson JE. Moderate alcohol consumption and risk of coronary heart disease among women with type 2 diabetes mellitus. *Circulation* 2000; 102: 494–9.

50. Tanasescu M, Hu FB, Willett WC et al. Alcohol consumption and risk of coronary heart disease among men with type 2 diabetes. *J Am Coll Cardiol* 2001; 38: 1836–42.

51. Ajani UA, Gaziano JM, Lotufo PA, Liu S, Hennekens CH, Buring JE, and Manson JE. Alcohol consumption and risk of coronary heart disease by diabetes status. *Circulation* 2000; 102: 500–5.

52. Stamler J, Caggiula AW, and Grandits GA. Relation of body mass and alcohol, nutrient, fiber, and caffeine intake to blood pressure in the special intervention and usual care groups in the Multiple Risk Factor Intervention Trial. *Circulation* 2000; 102: 2284–99.

53. Klatsky AL, Friedman JD, and Armstrong MA. The relationships between alcoholic beverage use and other traits to blood pressure: a new Kaiser Permanente study. *Circulation* 1986; 73: 628–36.

54. Klatsky AL, Armstrong MA, and Friedman JD. Risk of cardiovascular mortality in alcohol drinkers, ex-drinkers and nondrinkers. *Am J Med* 1991; 66: 1237–42.

55. Goldberg IJ, Mosca L, Piano MR, and Fisher EA. American Heart Association Science Advisory: wine and your heart: a science advisory for healthcare professionals from the Nutrition Committee, Council on Epidemiology and Prevention, and Council on Cardiovascular Nursing of the American Heart Association. *Circulation* 2001; 103: 472–5.

56. Krauss RM, Eckel RH, Howard B et al. American Heart Association Dietary Guidelines: revision 2000: a statement for healthcare professionals from the nutrition committee of the American Heart Association. *Circulation* 2000; 102: 2284–99.

57. The sixth report of the Joint National Committee on prevention, detection, evaluation, and treatment of high blood pressure. *Arch Intern Med* 1997; 157: 2413–46.

58. Puddey IB, Beilin LJ, Vandongen R, Rouse IL, and Rogers P. Evidence for a direct effect of alcohol consumption on blood pressure in normotensive men. A randomized controlled trial. *Lancet* 1985; 7: 707–13.

59. Puddey IB, Beilin LJ, and Vandongen R. Regular alcohol use raises blood pressure in treated hypertensive patients. A randomized controlled trial. *Lancet* 1987; 1: 647–51.

60. In press, *Arch Intern Med* 2003.

61. Mukamal KJ, Maclure M, Muller JE, Sherwood JB, and Mittleman MA. Prior alcohol consumption and mortality following acute myocardial infarction. *JAMA* 2001; 285: 1965–70.

62. Muntwyler J, Hennekens CH, Buring JE, and Gaziano JM. Mortality and light to moderate alcohol consumption after myocardial infarction. *Lancet* 1998; 352: 1882–1885.

63. Shaper AG and Wannamethee SG. Alcohol intake and mortality in middle aged men with diagnosed coronary heart disease. *Heart* 2000; 83: 394–9.

64. Keil U, Liese A, Filipiak B, Swales JD, and Grobbee DE. Alcohol, blood pressure and hypertension. Novartis Found Symp 1998; 216: 125–44.

65. Hillbom M, Juvela S, and Numminen H. Alcohol intake and the risk of stroke. *J Cardiovasc Risk* 1999; 6: 223–8.

66. Berger K, Ajani UA, Kase CS, Gaziano JM, Buring JE, Glynn RJ, and Hennekens CH. Light-to-moderate alcohol consumption and risk of stroke among U.S. male physicians. *N Engl J Med* 1999; 341: 1557–64.

67. Sacco RL, Elkind M, Boden-Albala B, Lin IF, Kargman DE, Hauser WA, Shea S, and Paik MC. The protective effect of moderate alcohol consumption on ischemic stroke. *JAMA* 1999; 281: 53–60.

68. Donahue RP, Abbott RD, Reed DM, and Yano K. Alcohol and hemorrhagic stroke. The Honolulu Heart Program. *JAMA* 1986; 255: 2311–4.

69. Stampfer MJ, Colditz GA, Willett WC, Speizer FE, and Hennekens CH. A prospective study of moderate alcohol consumption and the risk of coronary disease and stroke in women. *N Engl J Med* 1988; 319: 267–273.

70. Hansagi H, Romelsjo A, Gerhardsson de Verdier M, Andreasson S, and Leifman A. Alcohol consumption and stroke mortality. 20-year follow-up of 15,077 men and women. *Stroke* 1995; 26: 1768–73.

71. Leppala JM, Paunio M, Virtamo J, Fogelholm R, Albanes D, Taylor PR, and Heinonen OP. Alcohol consumption and stroke incidence in male smokers. *Circulation* 1999; 100: 1209–14.

72. Caicoya M, Rodriguez T, Corrales C, Cuello R, and Lasheras C. Alcohol and stroke: a community case-control study in Asturias, Spain. *J Clin Epidemiol* 1999; 52: 677–84.

73. Thrift AG, Donnan GA, and McNeil JJ. Heavy drinking, but not moderate or intermediate drinking, increases the risk of intracerebral hemorrhage. *Epidemiology* 1999; 10: 307–12.

74. American Heart Association. 2002 Heart and Stroke Statistical Update. Dallas, TX. American Heart Association; 2001.

75. Warlow CP. Epidemiology of stroke. *Lancet* 1998; 352(suppl 3): 1–4.

76. Rimm EB, Chan J, Stampfer MJ, Colditz GA, and Willett WC. Prospective study of cigarette smoking, alcohol use, and the risk of diabetes in men. *Br Med J* 1995; 310: 555–59.

77. Stampfer M, Colditz G, Willett WC, Manson JE, Arky RA, Hennekens C, and Speizer FE: a prospective study of moderate alcohol drinking and risk of diabetes in women. *Am J Epidemiol* 1988; 128: 549–58.

78. Perry E, Wannamethee SG, Walker MK, Thomson AG, Whincup PH, and Shaper AG. Prospective study of risk factors for development of non-insulin dependent diabetes in middle-aged British men. *Br Med J* 1995; 310: 560–64.

79. Tsumura K, Kayashi T, Suematsu C, Endo G, Fujii S, and Okada K. Daily alcohol consumption and the risk of type 2 diabetes in Japanese men: the Osaka Health Survey. *Diabetes Care* 1999; 22: 1432–37.

80. Ajani UA, Hennekens CH, Spelsberg A, and Manson JE. Alcohol consumption and risk of type 2 diabetes mellitus among US male physicians. *Arch Int Med* 2000; 160: 1025–30.

81. Holbrook TL, Barrett-Connor E, and Wingard DL. A prospective population-based study of alcohol use and non-insulin dependent diabetes mellitus. *Am J Epidemiol* 1990; 132: 902–09.

82. Conigrave KM, Hu FB, Camargo CA, Stampfer MJ, Willett WC, and Rimm EB. A prospective study of drinking patterns in relation to risk of type 2 diabetes among men. *Diabetes* 2001; 50: 2390–95.

83. Zhang S, Hunter DJ, Hankinson SE, Giovannucci EL, Rosner BA, Colditz GA, Speizer FE, and Willett WC. A prospective study of folate intake and the risk of breast cancer. *JAMA* 1999; 281: 1632–1637.

84. Pearson TA. Alcohol and heart disease. *Circulation* 1996; 94: 3023–25.

85. Pearson TA, Blair SN, Daniels SR et al. AHA guidelines for primary prevention of cardiovascular disease and stroke: 2002 update. *Circulation* 2002; 106: 388–391.

86. Goldstein LB, Adams R, Becker K et al. Primary prevention of ischemic stroke: A statement for healthcare professionals from the Stroke Council of the American Heart Association. *Circulation* 2001; 103: 163–82.

87. 10th Special Report to the US Congress on Alcohol and Health. Washington, DC: National Institute on Alcohol Abuse and Alcoholism; 2000.

7 Alcohol, Inflammation, and Coronary Heart Disease

Armin Imhof and Wolfgang Koenig

CONTENTS

7.1   INTRODUCTION

Moderate consumption of alcohol has been found to be consistently associated with reduced risk for fatal or nonfatal coronary heart disease (CHD) and consequently all-cause mortality.[1-3] Favourable effects on the lipid profile such as increased levels of high-density lipoprotein (HDL) cholesterol, and on haemostatic factors explain only about half of the beneficial effect of moderate alcohol consumption on CHD risk[4]; thus other mechanisms must be involved in mediating this risk reduction. Since atherosclerosis shows several features of an inflammatory disease, recently an anti-inflammatory action of moderate alcohol consumption has been suggested as contributing to the observed reduction in CHD morbidity and mortality.[5] Immunomodulatory effects of alcohol consumption have long been described.[6] Excessive and chronic alcohol consumption can lead to infections with various pathogens.[7] Moreover, alcoholic liver disease at different stages is associated with a complex immune response locally as well as systemically, such as immigration of inflammatory cells in the liver, increased levels of markers of the acute phase response and immunoglobulins, or alterations of the cytokine balance.[8–10]

This review summarizes the available evidence linking alcohol consumption with alterations of the immune system, focusing on recent findings and suggesting a causal link between moderate alcohol consumption and its effects on the immune system, cardiovascular disease morbidity, and mortality. Extensive overviews dealing specifically with the effects of alcohol on the immune system have been published elsewhere.[8,11–13]

7.2 ALCOHOL, "ALCOHOL-RELATED" DISEASES, AND ALL-CAUSE MORTALITY

Alcohol consumption is associated with all-cause mortality in a U- or J-shaped manner. That means, consumption of moderate amounts of alcohol is associated with lower all-cause mortality than abstention from alcohol or heavy drinking.[14–16] This reflects different overlaying morbidity and mortality rates of diseases of various organ systems in human beings. In a recently published meta-analysis of 200 studies on known or presumed alcohol-related diseases, alcohol consumption was associated with higher risk for liver cirrhosis, neoplasms of the upper respiratory and digestive track, hemorrhagic stroke, and injuries in a dose-dependent manner. Weaker but still significant associations were found with chronic pancreatitis, hypertension, and hepatocellular carcinoma.[17] There is also good evidence for an increased risk of cancers of the stomach, colon, rectum, female breast, and ovaries.[17–19]

7.3 ALCOHOL, PATTERN OF INTAKE, TYPE OF BEVERAGE, AND CORONARY HEART DISEASE MORBIDITY AND MORTALITY

Numerous epidemiological studies have shown that light to moderate drinkers of alcohol are at lower risk for fatal or nonfatal CHD than abstainers or heavy drinkers,[1,2] resulting in reduced all-cause mortality among these individuals. A recent meta-analysis including 51 studies (43 of them prospective) estimated a 20% risk reduction for consumption of 0 to 20 g of alcohol per day compared to nondrinkers and some risk reduction up to 72 g of alcohol per day[3] (see Figure 7.1). Besides the amount of alcohol consumed, drinking patterns seem to have an important effect on the association between alcohol and CHD.[20,21] Regular consumption of moderate amounts of alcohol has been found to be associated with lower risk estimates for CHD as well as for extension of atherosclerotic heart disease, whereas binge drinking does not seem to be beneficial or even exerts an adverse effect.[16,22–24] Some authors have suggested that, especially in the case of wine, other ingredients of alcoholic beverages than ethanol might at least in part

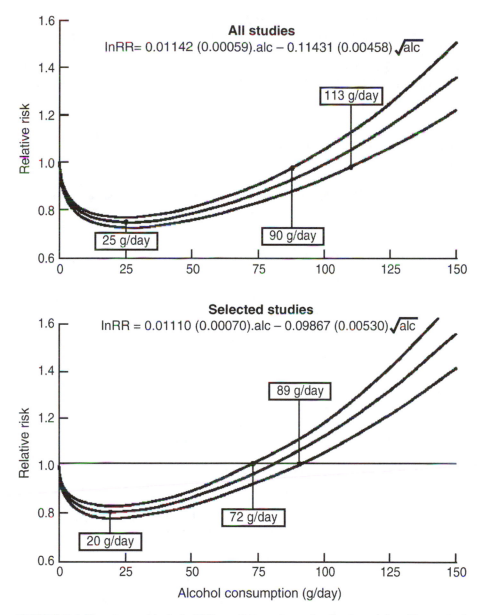

FIGURE 7.1 Functions with their 95% confidence intervals, fitted models with standard errors, and three critical exposure levels describing the dose–response relationship between alcohol consumption and the relative risk of coronary heart disease obtained by 51 pooled studies including 43 prospective ones and by 28 selected studies of highest quality. (From Corrao, G., Rubbiati, L., Bagnardi, V., Zambon, A., and Poikolainen, K. (2000) Alcohol and coronary heart disease: a meta-analysis, *Addiction*, 95, 1505–23. With permission.)

mediate the beneficial effects on CHD risk.[25-28] However, in several studies a reduced risk of CHD has been reported for moderate consumption of wine, as well as for beer and spirits.[4,28-30] Moreover, based on data from the Physicians' Health Study, a significant interaction among alcohol consumption, HDL-cholesterol, risk reduction for CHD, and a polymorphism in the gene coding for the alcohol dehydrogenase type 3 (ADH3) has been demonstrated, indicating that ethanol itself is largely responsible for the effect observed but also suggesting that genetic factors may play an important role.[31] The lower CHD risk in moderate drinkers has also been observed in a wide variety of patient populations including those with diabetes, hypertension, and prior myocardial infarction.[32] The consistency of these findings and the growing evidence that alcohol might protect against CHD via higher levels of HDL cholesterol, antithrombotic actions, or reduced insulin resistance argue for a causal protective effect of moderate alcohol consumption.[33-36]

7.4 ATHEROSCLEROSIS AND INFLAMMATION

Inflammatory processes play a pivotal role in the initiation, progression, and the final thrombotic complications of atherosclerosis. Atherosclerotic lesions contain immune cells such as macrophages and T cells in abundance. In addition, elevated plasma levels of several markers of the inflammatory cascade have been shown to predict future risk of plaque rupture. Several recent reviews provide excellent insight into the inflammatory characteristics of atherosclerosis on a molecular level, both locally and systemically, and from the clinical and epidemiological perspective.[37-40] Compelling evidence supports the notion that atherosclerosis is an inflammatory disease and links findings from epidemiological, interventional, and experimental studies bolstering the hypothesis that the association between alcohol consumption and CHD is at least in part mediated by immunomodulatory effects of alcohol.

7.4.1 ATHEROSCLEROSIS, ALCOHOL, AND THE SYSTEMIC INFLAMMATORY RESPONSE

A large number of epidemiological and clinical studies have consistently documented that increased levels of several systemic markers of the acute phase response including white blood cell count (WBC), IL-6, CRP, serum amyloid A (SAA), fibrinogen, selectins, tumor-necrosis-factor-α (TNF-α), cellular adhesion molecules (ICAM, VCAM), and lower levels of albumin — a negative marker of the acute phase response — are associated with cardiovascular endpoints (reviewed in Blake and Ridker[40] and Danesh et al.[41]). Of all markers, CRP, the classical acute-phase protein, has been most extensively investigated in clinical studies. Baseline levels of CRP are strong independent predictors of future risk of myocardial infarction, stroke, and peripheral vascular disease in initially healthy subjects from various populations, as well as in patients who already had suffered from atherosclerotic complications.[40] In a representative population-based sample of 1706 men and women aged 18 to 88 years, we found lower levels of several systemic markers of inflammation, including CRP, WBC, α-1 and α2-globulins, and higher concentrations of albumin among moderate consumers of alcohol compared to abstainers and heavy drinkers.[5] These findings have been confirmed by several authors. Albert et al. found lower levels of CRP with increasing self-reported alcohol intake among men and women in a large cross-sectional study of individuals with and without preexisting CHD.[42] In more than 5200 Japanese males aged 23 to 59 years, alcohol consumption was associated with WBC in a U-shaped manner, independently of several potential confounding factors.[43] Furthermore, in a cross-over study comprising 10 men and 9 women, Sierksma et al. could demonstrate a significant reduction of CRP concentrations and fibrinogen after 3 weeks of diet-controlled consumption of 4 (by men) or 3 (by women) glasses of beer equivalent to 40 and 30 grams of ethanol, respectively. Controls had received nonalcoholic beer underlining the assumption that ethanol itself rather than other ingredients of alcoholic beverages might be responsible for the observed effects on inflammatory markers.[44]

7.4.2 Inflammation at Different Stages of Atherosclerosis and Potential Interaction with Alcohol

7.4.2.1 Early Atherogenesis: Endothelial Dysfunction

Early atherogenesis is characterized by endothelial dysfunction with increased endothelial permeability for lipoproteins and other plasma components.[45,46] *In vitro*, modified lipoproteins such as oxidized low density lipoproteins (LDL) trigger the production of various mediators of the innate immune system.[47,48] Subsequently, upregulation of endothelial adhesion molecules, like vascular adhesion molecule-1 (VCAM-1), intercellular adhesion molecule-1 (ICAM-1), or E-selectin, and chemokine release from the endothelium and subendothelial cells mediate leukocyte recruitment and migration into the vessel wall.[49–52] Chemokines and cytokines are expressed in human atheroma and lead to the attraction of mainly monocytes and T-lymphocytes to these sites of inflammation. They include MCP-1, IL-1 (both CC-chemokines), as well as CXC chemokines like interferon-γ inducible protein-10 (IP-10), monokine induced by γ-interferon (MIG) and interferon (IFN)-inducible T-cell chemoattractant (I-TAC), IL-12, IL-18.[53–56]

Alcohol has been shown to significantly suppress the synthesis of proinflammatory cytokines and chemokines such as TNF-α, interleukin-1β (IL-1β), IL-6, IL-8, and monocyte chemoattractant protein-1 (MCP-1) both *in vivo* and/or *in vitro* in alveolar macrophages and human blood monocytes,[57–60] and thus may partly inhibit atherogenesis even at this very early stage.

7.4.2.2 The Early Stage: "Fatty Streak"

Once migrated into the vessel wall, monocytes begin to accumulate lipids, differentiate to macrophages, and release different inflammatory mediators such as TNF-α, IL-1, transforming growth factor-β (TGF-β), and several other growth factors.[37] Similarly, migrated T-cells release cytokines like IFN-γ, IL-2, TNF-α, or TNF-β.[61] The environment of inflammatory mediators leads to an activation of vascular smooth muscle cells (VSMC) and migration of medial VSMC into the developing lesion. Importantly, vascular endothelial (EC) and smooth muscle cells (SMC) not only respond to cytokines but also can produce large amounts of them. Both ECs and

SMCs respond to stimulation with IL-1 or TNF-α by producing large amounts of IL-6,[62] the major stimulating cytokine of the production of most acute phase proteins like C-reactive protein.[63] CRP is localized in the atheromatous plaque[64] and via opsonization of low density lipoprotein (LDL) also mediates LDL uptake by macrophages in the lesion which may represent an important mechanism in atherogenesis.[65]

These processes might be counteracted by effects of alcohol on the cell types involved. In isolated human monocytes *ex vivo* treated with ethanol, downregulation of nuclear transcription factor κB (NFκB) DNA binding attenuates lipopolysaccharide (LPS) stimulated expression of TNF-α and IL-1β.[66] Prevention of NFκB activity was also observed in monocytes from healthy volunteers 3, 6 and 9 h after consumption of moderate amounts of red wine but not after vodka intake.[67] Besides the effects on proinflammatory cytokines, alcohol intake affects production of antiinflammatory cytokines such as TGF-β and IL-10, both produced by macrophages and T lymphocytes. Alcohol induces production of TGF-β in monocytes and augments TGF-β production in response to a bacterial challenge *in vitro*.[68] Elevation of TGF-β may lead to inhibition of proinflammatory cytokine production by monocytes and other cells, inhibition of T cell proliferation and augmentation of Th2-type immune response. IL-10 is a typical Th2-type cytokine which inhibits cellular immune responses by downregulating the production of Th1 cytokines, antigen-specific T cell proliferation, and levels of proinflammatory cytokines.[69] Human monocyte IL-10 production is increased after alcohol exposure *in vitro*.[70]

As outlined before, moderate alcohol intake has been shown to be associated with lower levels of down-stream markers of the acute-phase response. However, no experimental studies have been reported so far linking these findings with inflammatory processes at this stage of atherogenesis.

7.4.2.3   The Advanced Lesion and the Unstable "Vulnerable" Plaque

Oxidized LDL, macrophage colony-stimulating factor (MCSF), and other mediators induce macrophage accumulation in the growing lesion and differentiation into foam cells.[37] Apoptosis, necrosis, and further lipid accumulation lead to the development of a necrotic lipid core in the center of the plaque.[37] At the same time a fibrous cap separating the plaque from circulating blood is built through further VSMC migration and synthesis of extracellular matrix.[71] The so-called stable plaque may transform into an unstable plaque mainly by two mechanisms: a decrease of extracellular matrix synthesis by VSMC and an increase in matrix degradation by proteolytic enzymes and matrix metalloproteinases (MMPs) from macrophages and foam cells in the shoulder region of the plaque. Whether or not alcohol intake might inhibit progression of stable atherosclerotic lesions and rupture of advanced plaques by an antiinflammatory action cannot be answered at present. However, epidemiologic studies indicate that regular moderate alcohol intake is also associated with reduced risk for recurrent coronary events.[32]

7.4.2.4   Atherosclerosis, Inflammation, and Alcohol: Future Perspectives

In light of the consistent association between alcohol intake and CHD risk in epidemiological and clinical studies, the modulatory effects of alcohol on the immune system described above and the compelling evidence for a major role of inflammation in atherosclerosis make an impact of alcohol on the various stages of atherogenesis a reasonable assumption. However, to the best of our knowledge, at present no experiment has specifically addressed the issue of potential antiinflammatory effects of alcohol in the vasculature.

Several questions concerning alcohol consumption and CHD via an immune-modulatory effect, dose-dependency, type of beverage, pattern of intake, and evidence for a net benefit, among others, possibly will not be answered definitely because they can only be addressed in long-term interventional trials which are not feasible for several reasons, including ethical concerns. However, since there is a strong evidence for a dose-dependent relationship, all studies in humans should consider drinking patterns and type of beverage when evaluating effects of alcohol on various components of the immune system and on cardiovascular diseases.

7.5   SUMMARY

Moderate alcohol intake is consistently associated with a reduced risk for fatal and nonfatal CHD. Inflammation plays a major role in both the initiation and progression of atherosclerosis. Systemic markers of inflammation including CRP, the classical acute phase protein, have been shown to predict cardiovascular events. Effects of alcohol consumption on the immune function are well known, but depend in part on the intensity, e.g., pattern, amount, and duration of alcohol consumption. Chronic alcohol consumption profoundly modulates various components of the immune system. Associations between moderate alcohol intake and lower levels of circulating markers of inflammation found in the general population, in patients with CHD, and in intervention studies are consistent with the hypothesis that antiinflammatory effects of moderate alcohol intake may represent a link to reduced cardiovascular morbidity and mortality. However, since long-term randomized controlled intervention trials are unfeasible for ethical reasons, to prove this hypothesis there is clearly a need for further observational epidemiological studies in other populations as well as for animal and experimental studies on the cellular and molecular level.

References

1. Fagrell, B., De Faire, U., Bondy, S. et al. (1999) The effects of light to moderate drinking on cardiovascular diseases, *J Intern Med*, 246, 331–40.
2. Maclure, M. (1993) Demonstration of deductive meta-analysis: ethanol intake and risk of myocardial infarction, *Epidemiol Rev*, 15, 328–51.
3. Corrao, G., Rubbiati, L., Bagnardi, V., Zambon, A., and Poikolainen, K. (2000) Alcohol and coronary heart disease: a meta-analysis, *Addiction*, 95, 1505–23.

4. Rimm, E. B. and Stampfer, M. J. (2002) Wine, beer, and spirits: are they really horses of a different color? *Circulation*, 105, 2806–7.
5. Imhof, A., Froehlich, M., Brenner, H. et al. (2001) Effect of alcohol consumption on systemic markers of inflammation, *Lancet*, 357, 763–7.
6. Kanagasundaram, N. and Leevy, C. M. (1981) Ethanol, immune reactions and the digestive system, *Clin Gastroenterol*, 10, 295–306.
7. MacGregor, R. R. and Louria, D. B. (1997) Alcohol and infection, *Curr Clin Top Infect Dis*, 17, 291–315.
8. Cook, R. T. (1998) Alcohol abuse, alcoholism, and damage to the immune system — a review, *Alcohol Clin Exp Res*, 22, 1927–42.
9. McClain, C. J., Barve, S., Deaciuc, I., Kugelmas, M., and Hill, D. (1999) Cytokines in alcoholic liver disease, *Semin Liver Dis*, 19, 205–19.
10. Tilg, H. and Diehl, A. M. (2000) Cytokines in alcoholic and nonalcoholic steatohepatitis, *N Engl J Med*, 343, 1467–76.
11. Diaz, L. E., Montero, A., Gonzalez-Gross, M. et al. (2002) Influence of alcohol consumption on immunological status: a review, *Eur J Clin Nutr*, 56 Suppl 3, S50–3.
12. Szabo, G. (1999) Consequences of alcohol consumption on host defence, *Alcohol Alcohol*, 34, 830–41.
13. Nelson, S. and Kolls, J. K. (2002) Alcohol, host defence and society, *Nat Rev Immunol*, 2, 205–9.
14. Gaziano, J. M., Gaziano, T. A., Glynn, R. J. et al. (2000) Light-to-moderate alcohol consumption and mortality in the Physicians' Health Study enrolment cohort, *J Am Coll Cardiol*, 35, 96–105.
15. Keil, U., Chambless, L. E., Doring, A., Filipiak, B., and Stieber, J. (1997) The relation of alcohol intake to coronary heart disease and all-cause mortality in a beer-drinking population, *Epidemiology*, 8, 150–6.
16. White, I. R. (1999) The level of alcohol consumption at which all-cause mortality is least, *J Clin Epidemiol*, 52, 967–75.
17. Corrao, G., Bagnardi, V., Zambon, A., and Arico, S. (1999) Exploring the dose-response relationship between alcohol consumption and the risk of several alcohol-related conditions: a meta-analysis, *Addiction*, 94, 1551–73.
18. Bagnardi, V., Blangiardo, M., La Vecchia, C., and Corrao, G. (2001) Alcohol consumption and the risk of cancer: a meta-analysis, *Alcohol Res Health*, 25, 263–70.
19. Smith-Warner, S. A., Spiegelman, D., Yaun, S. S. et al. (1998) Alcohol and breast cancer in women: a pooled analysis of cohort studies, *JAMA*, 279, 535–40.
20. Poikolainen, K. (1998) It can be bad for the heart, too — drinking patterns and coronary heart disease, *Addiction*, 93, 1757–9.
21. Mukamal, K. J., Conigrave, K. M., Mittleman, M. A. et al. (2003) Roles of drinking pattern and type of alcohol consumed in coronary heart disease in men, *N Engl J Med*, 348, 109–18.
22. Gruchow, H. W., Hoffmann, R. G., Anderson, A. J., and Barboriak, J. J. (1982) Effects of drinking patterns on the relationship between alcohol and coronary occlusion, *Atherosclerosis*, 43, 393–404.
23. Kauhanen, J., Kaplan, G. A., Goldberg, D. E., and Salonen, J. T. (1997) Beer binging and mortality: results from the Kuopio ischaemic heart disease risk factor study, a prospective population based study, *BMJ*, 315, 846–51.
24. Rehm, J., Sempos, C. T., and Trevisan, M. (2003) Average volume of alcohol consumption, patterns of drinking and risk of coronary heart disease — a review, *J Cardiovasc Risk*, 10, 15–20.

25. Bell, J. R., Donovan, J. L., Wong, R. et al. (2000) (+)-Catechin in human plasma after ingestion of a single serving of reconstituted red wine, *Am J Clin Nutr*, 71, 103–8.
26. Gronback, M., Becker, U., Johansen, D. et al. (2000) Type of alcohol consumed and mortality from all causes, coronary heart disease, and cancer, *Ann Intern Med*, 133, 411–9.
27. Renaud, S. and De Lorgeril, M. (1992) Wine, alcohol, platelets, and the French paradox for coronary heart disease, *Lancet*, 339, 1523–6.
28. Di Castelnuovo, A., Rotondo, S., Iacoviello, L., Donati, M. B., and De Gaetano, G. (2002) Meta-analysis of wine and beer consumption in relation to vascular risk, *Circulation*, 105, 2836–44.
29. Brenner, H., Rothenbacher, D., Bode, G. et al. (2001) Coronary heart disease risk reduction in a predominantly beer-drinking population, *Epidemiology*, 12, 390–5.
30. Gaziano, J. M., Hennekens, C. H., Godfried, S. L. et al. (1999) Type of alcoholic beverage and risk of myocardial infarction, *Am J Cardiol*, 83, 52–7.
31. Hines, L. M., Stampfer, M. J., Ma, J. et al. (2001) Genetic variation in alcohol dehydrogenase and the beneficial effect of moderate alcohol consumption on myocardial infarction, *N Engl J Med*, 344, 549–55.
32. Klatzky, A. (2001) Should patients with heart disease drink alcohol? *JAMA*, 285, 2004–6.
33. Langer, R. D., Criqui, M. H., and Reed, D. M. (1992) Lipoproteins and blood pressure as biological pathways for effect of moderate alcohol consumption on coronary heart disease, *Circulation*, 85, 910–5.
34. Rimm, E. B., Williams, P., Fosher, K., Criqui, M., and Stampfer, M. J. (1999) Moderate alcohol intake and lower risk of coronary heart disease: meta-analysis of effects on lipids and haemostatic factors, *BMJ*, 319, 1523–8.
35. Mukamal, K. J., Jadhav, P. P., D'Agostino, R. B. et al. (2001) Alcohol consumption and hemostatic factors: analysis of the Framingham Offspring cohort, *Circulation*, 104, 1367–73.
36. Mennen, L. I., Balkau, B., Vol, S., Caces, E., and Eschwege, E. (1999) Fibrinogen: a possible link between alcohol consumption and cardiovascular disease? DESIR Study Group, *Arterioscler Thromb Vasc Biol*, 19, 887–92.
37. Ross, R. (1999) Atherosclerosis — an inflammatory disease, *N Engl J Med*, 340, 115–26.
38. Hansson, G. K., Libby, P., Schonbeck, U., and Yan, Z. Q. (2002) Innate and adaptive immunity in the pathogenesis of atherosclerosis, *Circ Res*, 91, 281–91.
39. Rosenson, R. S. and Koenig, W. (2002) High-sensitivity C-reactive protein and cardiovascular risk in patients with coronary heart disease, *Curr Opin Cardiol*, 17, 325–31.
40. Blake, G. J. and Ridker, P. M. (2001) Novel clinical markers of vascular wall inflammation, *Circ Res*, 89, 763–71.
41. Danesh, J., Whincup, P., Walker, M. et al. (2000) Low grade inflammation and coronary heart disease: prospective study and updated meta-analyses, *BMJ*, 321, 199–204.
42. Albert, M. A., Glynn, R. J., and Ridker, P. M. (2003) Alcohol consumption and plasma concentration of C-reactive protein, *Circulation*, 107, 443–7.
43. Nakanishi, N., Yoshida, H., Okamoto, M. et al. (2003) Association of alcohol consumption with white blood cell count: a study of Japanese male office workers, *J Intern Med*, 253, 367–74.

44. Sierksma, A., Van Der Gaag, M. S., Kluft, C., and Hendriks, H. F. (2002) Moderate alcohol consumption reduces plasma C-reactive protein and fibrinogen levels; a randomized, diet-controlled intervention study, *Eur J Clin Nutr*, 56, 1130–6.
45. Napoli, C., D'Armiento, F. P., Mancini, F. P. et al. (1997) Fatty streak formation occurs in human fetal aortas and is greatly enhanced by maternal hypercholesterolemia. Intimal accumulation of low density lipoprotein and its oxidation precede monocyte recruitment into early atherosclerotic lesions, *J Clin Invest*, 100, 2680–90.
46. Skalen, K., Gustafsson, M., Rydberg, E. K. et al. (2002) Subendothelial retention of atherogenic lipoproteins in early atherosclerosis, *Nature*, 417, 750–4.
47. Witztum, J. L. and Berliner, J. A. (1998) Oxidized phospholipids and isoprostanes in atherosclerosis, *Curr Opin Lipidol*, 9, 441–8.
48. Rajavashisth, T. B., Andalibi, A., Territo, M. C. et al. (1990) Induction of endothelial cell expression of granulocyte and macrophage colony-stimulating factors by modified low-density lipoproteins, *Nature*, 344, 254–7.
49. Nelken, N. A., Coughlin, S. R., Gordon, D., and Wilcox, J. N. (1991) Monocyte chemoattractant protein-1 in human atheromatous plaques, *J Clin Invest*, 88, 1121–7.
50. Wang, J. M., Sica, A., Peri, G. et al. (1991) Expression of monocyte chemotactic protein and interleukin-8 by cytokine-activated human vascular smooth muscle cells, *Arterioscler Thromb*, 11, 1166–74.
51. Cybulsky, M. I., Iiyama, K., Li, H. et al. (2001) A major role for VCAM-1, but not ICAM-1, in early atherosclerosis, *J Clin Invest*, 107, 1255–62.
52. Dong, Z. M., Chapman, S. M., Brown, A. A. et al. (1998) The combined role of P- and E-selectins in atherosclerosis, *J Clin Invest*, 102, 145–52.
53. Gu, L., Okada, Y., Clinton, S. K. et al. (1998) Absence of monocyte chemoattractant protein-1 reduces atherosclerosis in low density lipoprotein receptor-deficient mice, *Mol Cell*, 2, 275–81.
54. Gosling, J., Slaymaker, S., Gu, L. et al. (1999) MCP-1 deficiency reduces susceptibility to atherosclerosis in mice that overexpress human apolipoprotein B, *J Clin Invest*, 103, 773–8.
55. Luster, A. D. (1998) Chemokines — chemotactic cytokines that mediate inflammation, *N Engl J Med*, 338, 436–45.
56. Gerdes, N., Sukhova, G. K., Libby, P. et al. (2002) Expression of interleukin (IL)-18 and functional IL-18 receptor on human vascular endothelial cells, smooth muscle cells, and macrophages: implications for atherogenesis, *J Exp Med*, 195, 245–57.
57. Nelson, S., Bagby, G. J., Bainton, B. G., and Summer, W. R. (1989) The effects of acute and chronic alcoholism on tumor necrosis factor and the inflammatory response, *J Infect Dis*, 160, 422–9.
58. Kolls, J. K., Xie, J., Lei, D. et al. (1995) Differential effects of *in vivo* ethanol on LPS-induced TNF and nitric oxide production in the lung, *Am J Physiol*, 268, L991–8.
59. Szabo, G., Mandrekar, P., and Catalano, D. (1995) Inhibition of superantigen-induced T cell proliferation and monocyte IL-1 beta, TNF-alpha, and IL-6 production by acute ethanol treatment, *J Leukoc Biol*, 58, 342–50.
60. Verma, B. K., Fogarasi, M., and Szabo, G. (1993) Down-regulation of tumor necrosis factor alpha activity by acute ethanol treatment in human peripheral blood monocytes, *J Clin Immunol*, 13, 8–22.
61. Frostegard, J., Ulfgren, A. K., Nyberg, P. et al. (1999) Cytokine expression in advanced human atherosclerotic plaques: dominance of pro-inflammatory (Th1) and macrophage-stimulating cytokines, *Atherosclerosis*, 145, 33–43.

62. Mach, F., Schonbeck, U., Sukhova, G. K. et al. (1997) Functional CD40 ligand is expressed on human vascular endothelial cells, smooth muscle cells, and macrophages: implications for CD40-CD40 ligand signaling in atherosclerosis, *Proc Natl Acad Sci USA*, 94, 1931–6.

63. Gabay, C. and Kushner, I. (1999) Acute-phase proteins and other systemic responses to inflammation, *N Engl J Med*, 340, 448–54.

64. Torzewski, J., Torzewski, M., Bowyer, D. E. et al. (1998) C-reactive protein frequently colocalizes with the terminal complement complex in the intima of early atherosclerotic lesions of human coronary arteries, *Arterioscler Thromb Vasc Biol*, 18, 1386–92.

65. Zwaka, T. P., Hombach, V., and Torzewski, J. (2001) C-reactive protein-mediated low density lipoprotein uptake by macrophages: implications for atherosclerosis, *Circulation*, 103, 1194–7.

66. Mandrekar, P., Catalano, D., and Szabo, G. (1999) Inhibition of lipopolysaccharide-mediated NF kappaB activation by ethanol in human monocytes, *Int Immunol*, 11, 1781–90.

67. Blanco-Colio, L. M., Valderrama, M., Alvarez-Sala, L. A. et al. (2000) Red wine intake prevents nuclear factor-kappaB activation in peripheral blood mononuclear cells of healthy volunteers during postprandial lipemia, *Circulation*, 102, 1020–6.

68. Szabo, G., Verma, B. K., Fogarasi, M., and Catalano, D. E. (1992) Induction of transforming growth factor-beta and prostaglandin E2 production by ethanol in human monocytes, *J Leukoc Biol*, 52, 602–10.

69. De Waal Malefyt, R., Yssel, H., and De Vries, J. E. (1993) Direct effects of IL-10 on subsets of human CD4+ T cell clones and resting T cells. Specific inhibition of IL-2 production and proliferation, *J Immunol*, 150, 4754–65.

70. Mandrekar, P., Catalano, D., Girouard, L., and Szabo, G. (1996) Human monocyte IL-10 production is increased by acute ethanol treatment, *Cytokine*, 8, 567–77.

71. Libby, P. (1995) Molecular bases of the acute coronary syndromes, *Circulation*, 91, 2844–50.

8 Deleterious Effects of Alcohol Intoxication on the Heart: Arrhythmias to Cardiomyopathies

Thomas C. Vary and Andrew Sumner

CONTENTS

0-8493-1680-4/04/$0.00+$1.50
© 2004 by CRC Press LLC

8.1 INTRODUCTION

Approximately two thirds of men and one third of women in Westernized countries, where no religious taboo associated with drinking exists, consume one form of alcoholic beverage or another. Within this large group of individuals, roughly 10 to 18% develop an alcohol abuse problem or become alcoholics.[83] Alcohol abuse and alcoholism have profound health consequences and are characterized by impaired control over drinking and an obsessive preoccupation with alcohol consistent with a drug dependency. Harmful drinking patterns characterized by overdrinking lead to repetitive problems such as loss of work or school truancy, frequent verbal and/or physical abuse of loved ones, and driving while intoxicated.[83]

Alcohol remains the most abused drug by adolescents. Surveys of junior and senior high school students indicate that a vast majority of students have experienced drinking alcohol. This behavior continues and in some cases worsens during college. For some, drinking alcohol is merely a right of passage to adulthood that loses its luster with time, but in the case of others the use of alcohol is excessive It places our youth in America at risk for harmful adverse consequences (such as automobile accidents and alcohol poisoning). For yet others, the pattern of heavy drinking continues into adulthood and results in an adult pattern of alcohol abuse.

The question becomes: how much alcohol is too much? In the U.S., a standard serving of alcohol contains approximately 12 g of ethanol. In terms of different libations and fluid amounts, 12 g of alcohol translates into 12 oz (340 ml) of beer (5% alcohol v/v), 5 oz (142 ml) of wine (12.5% alcohol v/v), and 1.5 fluid ounces (43 ml) of 80-proof spirits (40% alcohol v/v). Many individuals regularly exceed one standard serving per drink. National Institute on Alcoholism and Alcohol Abuse Guidelines recommend that men consume no more than 14 drinks per week and no more than four drinks per day. For women the amounts are lower, with no more than three drinks per day, and seven drinks per week. These estimates are higher than those considered "moderate drinking" by many health providers, which is one and two drinks a day for women and men, respectively. Light drinking appears to have beneficial effects on cardiovascular health through increases in high-density lipoprotein cholesterol, attenuation of inflammatory cascades, and/or changes in hemostatic factors. Heavy drinking, however, has profound adverse effects on the cardiovascular system, causing hypertension, left ventricular dysfunction, and cardiac arrhythmias. This chapter will focus on the detrimental effects of acute and chronic alcohol consumption on the myocardium.

8.2 ETHANOL-INDUCED ALTERATIONS IN MYOCARDIAL ELECTRICAL ACTIVITY

8.2.1 CARDIAC ARRHYTHMIAS FOLLOWING ACUTE ALCOHOL INTOXICATION

The regular beat of heart is a tightly controlled process essential for normal cardiac function and homeostasis. The initiation and propagation of the heartbeat is needed to allow proper filling of the ventricles and for synchronous contraction of the ventricular muscle to produce an adequate cardiac output. Acute ethanol intoxication can produce both atrial and ventricular arrhythmias. Arrhythmias are a disruption of the normal electrical activity of the heart, including disturbances in the initiation of the electrical depolarization, interference in the propagation of the electrical signal, and alterations in the normal path and sequence in the electrical excitation and subsequent repolarization. Arrhythmias may involve either irregular beating of the heart (dysrhythmias) or asynchronous contractions of cardiac muscle cells (fibrillation).

In the general population, atrial fibrillation is the most common cardiac arrhythmia occurring in 2 to 4% of persons aged 60 years and older.[106] In alcoholic subjects, acute alcohol ingestion induces atrial arrhythmias in up to 60% of binge drinkers.[22,23,35,51] The arrhythmia occurs in individuals with or without underlying alcoholic cardiomyopathy or other cardiac disease. Arrhythmias are considered to be a prime factor contributing to cardiac dysfunction in people who consume large quantities of alcohol.[19,72]

Atrial fibrillation is characterized by (1) rapid and irregular atrial fibrillatory waves at a rate of 350 to 600 discharges/min and (2) an irregularly irregular ventricular response of 90 to 170 beats/min. These features typically produce an electrocardiogram in which P waves are absent; fibrillating waves of varying amplitude, morphology, and intervals are present; and R-R intervals are irregularly irregular.

Atrial fibrillation is potentially life-threatening for several reasons. First, rapid ventricular rates and loss of atrioventricular synchrony may compromise cardiac output, resulting in hypotension and pulmonary congestion. Second, atrial fibrillation promotes blood stasis in the atria, which increases the risk of thrombus formation and embolic stroke.[106] Third, rapid ventricular rates can also induce a tachycardia-induced cardiomyopathy.

The pioneering work of Ettinger and colleagues firmly established the correlation between alcohol consumption and atrial fibrillation.[23] Because most of the arrhythmias occurred during the weekend, the authors termed this type of alcohol-dependent arrhythmia "holiday heart."[23] The "holiday heart arrhythmia" designation is applied to arrhythmias associated with binge drinking, and occurs even in subjects who do not abuse alcohol.[97] Atrial fibrillation induced by binge drinking usually resolves within 24 h after stopping ethanol ingestion or following treatment with β-blockers.[43,50] However, irregular binge drinking in Eastern European men predisposes the myocardium to alterations in the conduction system and reduces the threshold for ventricular fibrillation.[56]

The mechanisms responsible for generating atrial fibrillation following alcohol intoxication remain unresolved. Atrial fibrillation is most likely the result of multiple, wandering reentry circuits in the atrium. In addition to intrinsic effects of ethanol on cardiac muscle, alcohol can interfere with regulation of heart rate and impulse conduction by neurohormones released by the autonomic system.[12,107] Alcohol causes an increase in the release of catecholamines, a well-known risk factor in development of arrhythmias, and may reduce vagal nerve activity and decrease heart rate variability,[80] a factor known to predispose the myocardium to arrhythmias. During withdrawal phase, both hypokalemia and hypomagnesemia increase the risk for development of arrhythmias.

Although acute alcohol abuse most commonly causes atrial arrhythmias, it can also increase the risk of ventricular arrhythmias, a prime factor precipitating sudden cardiac death in people who consume large quantities of alcohol.[19,72] Cardiac arrest resulting from ventricular fibrillation is the most common cause of sudden cardiac death. Even with early cardiopulmonary resuscitation and defibrillation, only 25 of the cases out of hospital ventricular fibrillation survive to leave the hospital.[21]

8.2.2 CARDIAC ARRHYTHMIAS FOLLOWING CHRONIC ALCOHOL ABUSE

Atrial fibrillation can also occur following chronic alcohol abuse. Mechanisms for atrial fibrillation in chronic alcohol abuse include those produced by acute alcohol intoxication plus structural changes in the atria and ventricles as a consequence of the pathological processes involved in alcoholic cardiomyopathy. The myotrophic ventricular functions at a higher ventricular end-diastolic volume, contributing to increased atrial pressure and atrial size. Both of these functions can beget atrial fibrillation.

Chronic, heavy alcohol consumption also increases the risk of sudden cardiac death. Alcohol can induce structural changes in cardiac muscle that not only predispose the myocardium to ventricular arrhythmias but can trigger them as well. Induction of ventricular tachycardia can be facilitated by acute alcohol ingestion in men who drink chronically.[35] QT prolongation is one possible mechanism for this phenomenon. Prolonged QT interval indicates heterogeneity with respect to repolarization and is a risk factor for malignant ventricular arrhythmias and sudden death. Nonhomogeneous ventricular repolarization means that regions of the ventricular myocardium have varying refractory periods, a phenomenon known to initiate reenterant tachyarrhythmias. Interestingly, a prolongation of the QT interval is observed in persons with signs of alcoholic liver disease.[19] Furthermore, prolongation of QT interval is especially prominent in women and predicts a worse prognosis over time.[19] The mechanism for these ventricular arrhythmias is complex and most likely involves reentry mechanisms as a result of underlying structural heart disease and altered automaticity.

8.3 CHRONIC ALCOHOL-INDUCED ALTERATIONS IN CARDIAC MUSCLE

8.3.1 ETHANOL-INDUCED CARDIOMYOPATHY — GENERAL CONSIDERATIONS

Heart failure, as well as cirrhosis, is an important cause of mortality in chronic alcoholics. In fact, textbooks of medicine have described for more than 100 years that the progressive and excessive intake of alcohol brings about myocardial lesions. Excessive alcohol consumption is the leading cause of a nonischemic, dilated cardiomyopathy. Cardiomyopathies are classified by the dominant pathophysiology, or if possible by the etiologic/pathogenetic factor.[77] Consequently, alcoholic cardiomyopathy is considered a dilated and a specific cardiomyopathy that occurs in patients for whom the sole causative agent is excessive and prolonged alcohol consumption (>80 g of ethanol a day for >10 years).[77] An alcoholic cardiomyopathy is also frequently referred to as alcoholic heart muscle disease (AHMD). Approximately 20 to 50% of all cases of dilated cardiomyopathy have chronic alcohol abuse as an underlying causative agent. However, only a small percentage of persons with chronic alcohol abuse develop alcoholic cardiomyopathy.

Patients with alcoholic cardiomyopathy typically present with symptoms and physical findings similar to patients with dilated cardiomyopathies of any etiology. Symptoms of left heart failure, such as dyspnea, orthopnea, and paroxysmal nocturnal dyspnea may develop insidiously or be present in an acute fashion. Physical examination usually reveals cardiomegaly with laterally displaced left ventricle apical pulsations, and often protodiastolic (S3) and presystolic (S4) gallops.

The diagnosis of alcoholic cardiomyopathy is suspected in individuals who have clinical findings of congestive heart failure coupled with a long history of alcohol abuse.[93] Noninvasive testing, typically using echocardiography, confirms the myocardial dysfunction. Chronic alcohol abuse can produce both systolic and diastolic dysfunction. The degree of cardiac dysfunction is proportional to the duration and severity of alcohol consumption.[101] Alcoholic cardiomyopathy is rarely produced by short-term ethanol administration, thus necessitating a more prolonged exposure to alcohol. The effects of alcohol on the heart in middle-aged men are dose dependent. The myocardial lesion induced by chronic alcohol ingestion leads to cardiac enlargement and dilation with progressive congestive heart failure, and in most cases minimal coronary artery disease is present.

Chronic alcohol consumption causes derangements in either systolic or diastolic function or both. The deleterious effects of chronic alcohol consumption on systolic function lead to a reduced ejection fraction (<50%). Diastolic dysfunction is observed in one third of the alcoholics without any evidence of cardiomyopathy, compared with two thirds of patients with overt evidence of cardiomyopathy.[26] Furthermore, asymptomatic alcoholic patients show left ventricular dilation with preservation of ejection fraction while exhibiting impaired left ventricular relaxation. Deterioration of diastolic function correlates with alcohol consumption.

The major pathologic features revealed through biopsy or postmortem examination include generalized enlargement of the heart, including both ventricles, thinning of the ventricular wall with evidence of fibrosis and endocardial fibroelastic thickening, myocyte degeneration, interstitial edema, and focal areas of necrosis within the ventricular wall.[9,28,39] Microscopic examination of biopsy specimens obtained from humans reveals a thinning of the ventricular wall, myocyte degeneration, loss of striations, and myofilament dissolution, consistent with alterations in structural and myofibrillar proteins.[3,4,9,39] An *in vitro* study using myocytes has shown that ethanol reduces the number and uniformity of the myofibrils.[2] It therefore appears that in alcoholic heart disease the performance of the heart as a pump is seriously compromised mechanically by loss of contractile elements or their functional impairment by fragmentation and disarrangement.

8.3.2 Etiology of Disease

The exact pathogenesis of alcoholic cardiomyopathy remains unknown and most likely is multifactorial. To this end, animal models have provided a wealth of information regarding potential mechanisms involved in the pathogenesis and development of alcoholic cardiomyopathy. These studies provide invaluable information concerning the acute and long-term effects of alcohol consumption on the myocardium. In general the histological and cellular changes induced by alcohol ingestion can be described in terms of myocyte loss, subcellular organelle dysfunction, loss or change of contractile proteins, and calcium dyshomeostasis. There are several possible contributors to the development of this disease process, and these are discussed in the following sections.

8.3.3 Chronic Ethanol Exposure and Protein Synthesis

As alcoholic cardiomyopathy is associated with reduced contractility and derangements in myofibrillar architecture, it follows that one explanation for these changes is that the integrity of cellular proteins may be compromised by ethanol toxicity. In view of the prolonged time required for manifestation of the histologic changes in the alcoholic heart, it is very important to evaluate protein turnover following ethanol exposure. Indeed, one of the metabolic hallmarks of chronic alcohol abuse is the negative nitrogen balance resulting from the net catabolism of muscle protein.[46,64,65,68–70] This imbalance in protein metabolism, when prolonged, leads to the erosion of lean body mass and the proximal myopathy commonly observed in alcoholics. These effects most likely result from ethanol *per se*. Early work indicated that chronic ethanol consumption led to a decreased association of actin and myosin *in vitro*,[79] and it was suggested that persistent changes in some proteins may have occurred and may have been related to an inhibition of protein synthesis.

The dynamic balance of proteins in the myocardium is dependent upon both protein synthesis and protein degradation. Alcohol consumption increases lysosomal cathepsin D and B activities in hearts from alcohol-fed rats, suggesting that degradation may be accelerated.[88] However, at least one study has indicated that feeding ethanol was without effect on the rate of breakdown of myofibrillar and sarcoplasmic proteins.[99] In contrast to protein degradation, the effect of ethanol on protein synthesis varies with the duration of exposure. Chronic feeding of ethanol for 6 weeks is associated with a reduced heart size and total protein per heart. However, no impairment in ventricular protein synthesis was observed.[64,65,67]

Because of the long time required for evolution of changes in myocytes in humans, 6 weeks may not be sufficiently long enough to induce changes in protein metabolism. With longer exposure to ethanol (12 to 14 weeks), a decreased heart size, loss of cardiac protein mass, and diminished rate in the synthesis of cardiac proteins is observed.[48,104] Likewise, hearts from guinea pigs fed ethanol for 11 weeks and perfused *in vitro* showed a depressed rate of protein synthesis.[85] Thus, the effect of alcohol on protein synthesis worsens with the long duration of alcohol abuse needed to produce alcoholic cardiomyopathy. Alterations in myocardial protein balance as evidenced by the loss of myocardial mass and protein content may be responsible for the histological changes characteristic of alcohol-induced cardiomy-opathy.

Chronic alcohol consumption involves the consumption of alcohol on a daily basis. Therefore, the chronic effects of ethanol consumption may merely reflect the changes in heart function observed in response to a daily alcohol load. Indeed, acute alcohol misuse, i.e., binge drinking, leads to a syndrome described as the "holiday heart,"[23,35] characterized by abnormal cardiac rhythm and changes in other biochem-ical and ultrastructural indices of myocardial function and metabolism. With regards to protein metabolism, there are conflicting reports describing the effects of acute ethanol intoxication upon cardiac protein synthesis. Early work failed to demonstrate the effect of ethanol on protein synthesis in the heart.[84] However, more recent studies have indicated that acute administration of ethanol depresses protein synthesis in cardiac muscle.[45,65,67,70,98]

8.3.3.1 Specific Proteins Affected by Chronic Ethanol Consumption

Most of the studies outlined above measure the rate of incorporation of radioactivity into mixed proteins within the cell. They do not differentiate between protein syn-thesis in different subcellular fractions or individual proteins. Indeed studies inves-tigating the effect of ethanol on subcellular fractions or individual proteins are scanty. Evaluation of the steady state protein content of various myocardial proteins was examined by two-dimensional gel electrophoresis following administration of eth-anol for 6 weeks.[62] Chronic alcohol feeding caused significant decreases in heat shock protein (HSP) 60, HSP 70, and desmin, but contractile proteins were unaf-fected. The synthesis of actin was significantly reduced following feeding of guinea pigs a diet supplemented with 10% ethanol in drinking water for 40 weeks.[86] In the same animals the synthesis of other contractile proteins such as myosin heavy chains, myosin light chains, and tropomyosin were reduced but did not attain a significant difference.

Shifts in the expression of the isoforms of myosin heavy chains, protein involved in the contractile apparatus, are associated with alterations in cardiac function and isometic force production. Changes in the expression of myosin isoforms alter the myosin ATPase, a measure of the ability of the muscle to shorten. Chronic alcohol ingestion causes a shift in the myosin heavy chain isoforms from alpha to beta following 13 weeks of ethanol feeding.[57] A functional consequence of the transition in myosin heavy chain isoforms is significant because a decrease in the myofibrillar and myosin ATPase activities induces a slower velocity of shortening. As the velocity of shortening is a measure of the contractile activity of the muscle, a shift in the isoform would be consistent with a reduced force of contraction, which would be manifested in the heart by a reduced ejection fraction. With acute alcohol intoxica-tion, the synthesis of both proteins in both myofibrillar and nonmyofibrillar fractions of the heart are equally (~20%) depressed.[66] These observations suggest that the inhibition of protein synthesis involves the contractile proteins, but does not rule out the possibility that other proteins necessary for normal ventricular function are also affected by chronic ethanol consumption.

Desmin is a muscle-specific protein that forms a lattice around the Z-discs, interconnects them together, and links the entire contractile sarcomere, the sarcolemmal cytoskeleton, cytoplasmic organelles, and the nucleus.[11] Removal of desmin leads to development of cardiac hypertrophy (as evidenced by increase in heart weight to body weight ratio) which later leads dilation with compromised systolic function.[58] There is generally no increase in heart size and no increase in ventricular wall thickness. The defects identified in cardiac muscle of desmin null mice appear similar to those observed in some familial desminopathies.[6] Thus alteration in expression of desmin with prolonged alcohol ingestion may contribute to development of alcoholic cardiomyopathy.

8.3.4 MECHANISMS REGULATING MYOCARDIAL PROTEIN SYNTHESIS DURING ACUTE AND CHRONIC ETHANOL ADMINISTRATION

8.3.4.1 Translational Control of Protein Synthesis

Synthesis of proteins in eukaryotic cells is achieved through a complex series of discrete reactions. The process involves the association of the 40S and 60S ribosomal subunits, messenger RNA (mRNA), initiator methionyl-tRNA (met-tRNA$_i^{met}$), other amino acyl-tRNAs, cofactors (i.e., GTP; ATP), and protein factors [collectively known as eukaryotic initiation factors (eIF), elongation factors (eEF), and releasing factors (RF)] through a series of reactions resulting in the translation of mRNA into proteins. Translation of mRNA on the ribosome is composed of three phases: (1) initiation, whereby met-tRNA$_i^{met}$ associates with mRNA bound to 40S ribosomal subunit, and subsequent binding of the 40S ribosomal subunit to the 60S subunit, to form a ribosome complex capable of translation; (2) elongation, during which tRNA-bound amino acids are incorporated in growing polypeptide chains according to the mRNA template; and (3) termination, where the completed protein is released from the ribosome (Figure 8.1).

Regulation of protein synthesis occurs through changes in the abundance of ribosomes, translational efficiency, and/or concentration of translatable mRNA. Because approximately 80% of the RNA in muscle is ribosomal RNA, changes in total RNA content presumably reflect changes in the number of ribosomes. Alternatively, the amount of 15S and 18S RNA can be analyzed. The RNA content of hearts from alcohol-fed rats is not different compared with controls.[48] Therefore, alterations in the relative abundance of ribosomes are not responsible for inhibition in myocardial protein synthesis from rats chronically fed a diet containing alcohol. The efficiency of translation, calculated by dividing the protein synthesis rates by the total RNA content, provides an index of how rapidly the existing ribosomes synthesize protein. The translational efficiency is diminished by approximately 50% in animals chronically fed a diet containing alcohol.[48] Thus, alcohol feeding induces an inhibition of protein synthesis by reducing the translational efficiency.

The reduced translational efficiency following chronic alcohol feeding may result from an inhibition of peptide-chain initiation, elongation/termination, or both. Relative rates of translation initiation and elongation can be assessed by the measurement of incorporation of phenylalanine and analysis of the relative abundance of

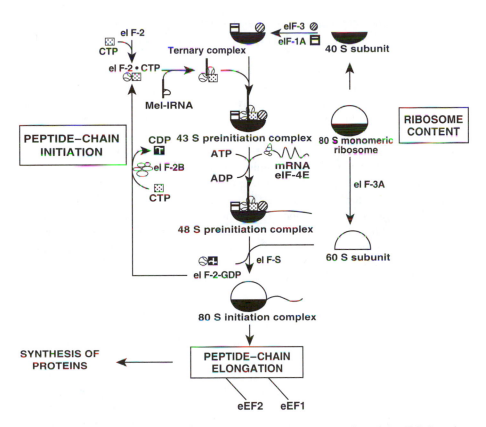

FIGURE 8.1 Regulation of protein synthesis in the heart. (Adapted from Vary, T.C. Regulation of skeletal muscle protein turnover in sepsis. *Curr. Opin. Clin. Nutr. Metab. Care* 1: 217–224, 1998. With permission.)

free ribosomal subunits. The amount of RNA in free ribosomal subunits is reflective of the balance between the rates of peptide-chain initiation and elongation/termination (for reviews see References 15, 46, and 102). Thus, a decrease in the rate of peptide-chain initiation relative to elongation/termination means the free ribosomal subunits are entering polysomes at a slower rate (initiation), whereas they are moving along mRNA (elongation) and exiting (termination) at the same rate. With a decrease in peptide-chain initiation relative to elongation, the abundance of free ribosomal subunits increases. If the abundance of free ribosomal subunits remains unchanged, despite a diminished rate of protein synthesis, such a finding would indicate that both translation initiation and elongation are affected proportionately.

Prolonged ethanol intoxication limits the ability of isolated ribosomes to carry out protein synthesis.[71] The steps of the translation process are affected following chronic alcohol feeding by examining the distribution of ribosomal subunits between free (i.e., free ribosomal subunits not associated with polysomes) and polysome-associated states.[15,46,102] Analysis of the ribosomal subunits from the hearts from animals chronically fed a diet containing alcohol revealed no significant differences in the ribosomal subunits compared with control rats.[48,104] Hence, feeding rats a diet containing alcohol chronically decreases the rate of protein synthesis in cardiac muscle through a relatively equal inhibition of both translation initiation and elongation.

Both acute and chronic alcohol intoxication induces derangements in the peptide-initiation phase of protein synthesis. Acute alcohol ingestion limits myocardial protein synthesis through a greater impairment in translation initiation than elongation.[45] Acute ethanol intoxication is associated with an increase in myocardial content of free 40S and 60S ribosomal subunits in conjunction with an inhibition in protein synthesis. However, a block in peptide-chain elongation develops as the length of ethanol exposure increases, further limiting protein synthesis.

The process of peptide-chain initiation involves essentially four major steps (for reviews see References 15, 46, and 102): (1) dissociation of the 80S ribosome into 40S and 60S ribosomal subunits; (2) formation of the 43S preinitiation complex with binding of initiator met-tRNA$_i^{met}$ to the 40S subunit; (3) binding of mRNA to the 43S preinitiation complex; and (4) association of the 60S ribosomal subunit to form an active 80S ribosome (Figure 8.1).

Two of the steps involved in translation initiation appear important as major regulatory points in the overall control of protein synthesis in the heart. The first step controlling initiation is the binding of met-tRNA$_i^{met}$ to the 40S ribosomal subunit to form the 43S preinitiation complex. This reaction is mediated by eukaryotic initiation factor 2 (eIF2) and is regulated by the activity of another initiation factor, eIF2B. The second regulatory step in translation initiation involves the binding of mRNA to the 43S preinitiation complex, which is mediated by eIF4F, a complex of several subunits. One of the subunits, eIF4E, binds the 7-methylguanosine 5′triphosphate (m^{7}GTP) cap structure present at the 5′-end of eukaryotic mRNAs to form an eIF4E·mRNA complex.[75] During translation initiation, the eIF4E·mRNA complex binds to eIF4G and eIF4A to form the active eIF4F complex.[75,76,91] Formation of the active eIF4F complex allows initiation to proceed. The binding of eIF4E to eIF4G is controlled in part by the translation repressor proteins 4E-BP1, 4E-BP2, and 4E-BP3. Binding of 4E-BPs to eIF4E is hypothesized to limit eIF4E availability for formation of the active eIF4E·eIF4G complex. The binding of 4E-BP1 to eIF4E is regulated, in part, by phosphorylation of 4E-BP1 (for a review see Reference 29).

As discussed above, both acute alcohol intoxication and chronic alcohol consumption impair translational efficiency in cardiac muscle. The cellular mechanisms by which this response occurs has only recently been investigated. The combined efforts of eIF2 and eIF2B regulate an early step in peptide-chain initiation (Figure 8.1). However, our studies detected no difference in the amount of eIF2α protein, the fraction of eIF2α in the phosphorylated form, total eIF2B protein content, or eIF2B activity after acute alcohol intoxication. In contrast to the eIF2 system, eIF4E availability in cardiac muscle appears markedly altered by ethanol and may represent an important site of regulatory control.[45,46] Acute alcohol administration dramatically decreased the amount of 4E-BP1 in the γ-phosphorylated form. Reduced phosphorylation of 4E-BP1 would be expected to enhance the ability of 4E-BP1 to bind to eIF4E. Indeed, acute alcohol more than doubled the amount of the translational repressor molecule 4E-BP1 bound to eIF4E (Figure 8.2). There was also a concomitant decrease in the amount of active eIF4E·eIF4G complex in skeletal muscle. This decrease in eIF4E associated with eIF4G did not result from a reduction in the total amount of eIF4E or eIF4G. These results are consistent with competition between 4E-BPI and eIF4G for eIF4E because of the known shared binding motif for eIF4E on 4E-BP1 and eIF4G. Hence, an impairment in eIF4F function secondary to a decrease in eIF4E availability appears to represent, at least in part, a likely explanation for the acute effects of alcohol on muscle protein synthesis. Finally, posttranslational modification of eIF4E can also influence translation initiation. The phosphorylation of eIF4E increases the ability of this initiation factor to bind to the cap mRNA several-fold, thereby stimulating protein synthesis. However, we have failed to detect any significant effect of alcohol on eIF4E phosphorylation.[45,46,104] A comparison of the changes in the eIF2 and eIF4F system induced by either acute or chronic alcohol is provided in Table 8.1.

Rats maintained on a nutritionally complete alcohol-containing diet for 14 to 16 weeks demonstrate qualitatively similar changes in cardiac muscle[48,104] with regard to translational control as seen in the acute studies described above.[45] The amount of inactive 4EBP1 eIF4E complex was increased, the amount of the active eIF4E·eIF4G complex was decreased, and the amount of 4E-BP1 in the γ-phosphorylated form was decreased, compared to pair-fed control animals (Figure 8.2).

Chronically feeding rats a diet containing ethanol reduces elongation relative to peptide-chain initiation. The elongation phase of protein synthesis is dependent upon two protein factors, elongation factor 1 (eEF1A) and eEF2 (Figure 8.1). During elongation, the aminoacyl-tRNA associates with the A-site on the ribosome, forming a tertiary complex with eEF1A and GTP. Following hydrolysis of the GTP to GDP,

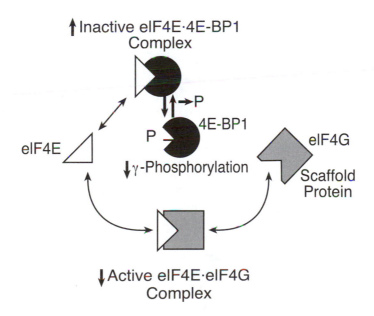

FIGURE 8.2 Regulation by alcohol of formation of active eIF4E/EIF4G complex through competition with 4E-BP1.

TABLE 8.1

Comparison of Changes in eIF2, eIF4F, eEF1, and eEF2 in Control of Protein Synthesis in Response to Either Acute Intoxication or Chronic Alcohol Feeding

		Acute Intoxication	Chronic Alcohol Feeding
Initiation			
	eIF2α Content	↔	↔
	eIF2α Phosphorylation	↔	↔
	eIF2B Activity	↔	↔
	eIF2B Content	↔	↔
	4E-BP1·eIF4E Complex	↑	↑
	4E-BP1 Phosphorylation	↓	↓
	eIF4G·eIF4E Complex	↓	↓
	eIF4E Complex	↔	↔
	eIF4E Phosphorylation	↔	↔
Elongation			
	eEF1A Content	↔	↓
	eEF2 Content	↔	↓
	eEF2 Phosphorylation	↔	↔

Note: Significant changes in components of the initiation and elongation systems in cardiac muscle obtained from rats either after acute intoxication (2.5 h) or after feeding rats a diet containing alcohol for 14 to 16 weeks, relative to values obtained in pair-fed animals. Data obtained from References 45, 48, 104, and 105. ↔ No changes induced by alcohol; ↑ increased compared with controls; ↓ decreased compared with controls.

the eEF1A-GDP complex leaves the ribosome and a peptide bond between the nascent peptide-chain on the ribosomal P-site and aminoacyl-tRNA is formed. eEF2 catalyzes the translocation of the elongated peptidyl-tRNA from the A-site to the P-site on the ribosome and the ejection of the deacylated tRNA from the P-site. The eEF2-dependent translocation is accompanied by the hydrolysis of GTP. The ribosome is then ready to accept the next aminoacyl-tRNA into the A-site. The process repeats itself until the mRNA reaches a stop codon for translation and the newly synthesized protein becomes released from the ribosome.

By 16 weeks of alcohol feeding, the eEF1A and eEF2 content in cardiac muscle were significantly reduced by 25 and 39%, respectively, compared with pair-fed control rats.[105] Northern blot analysis of RNA isolated from hearts of alcohol-fed rats showed no diminution in the steady-state amount of eEF1A and eEF2 mRNA. Hence, the decreased amount of eEF1A and eEF2 protein in rats fed an alcohol-containing diet presumably does not result from a reduced abundance of eEF1A and eEF2 mRNA, and suggests that alcohol may alter the half-life of these particular mRNAs or accelerate the degradation of the protein. Reductions in elongation factor(s) content may contribute to the inhibition in protein synthesis in chronic alcoholism.[105]

8.3.5 ALCOHOL-INDUCED ALTERATIONS IN MYOCARDIAL Ca^{2+} HOMEOSTASIS

When contractile function is depressed in patients with alcoholic cardiomyopathy, abnormalities in excitation–contraction coupling are typically present. The process of excitation–contraction coupling entails the transmission of the signal generated by the action potential on the sarcolemma membrane to induce contraction of the myofibrillar protein. This process involves the movement of ions, particularly calcium. Calcium homeostasis is essential for normal cardiac function. The cardiac action potential depolarizes the cardiac sarcolemmal membrane causing L-type voltage-gated Ca 2+ channels to open, resulting in Ca^{2+} influx into the cytosol. This inward current through cardiac L-type Ca^{2+} channels (Ica) serves to activate, or "trigger" Ca release channels (ryanodine receptors, RyRs) located in the terminal cisternae of the sarcoplasmic reticulum (SR). The result is the flow of Ca^{2+} from concentrated storage in the SR out into the cytoplasm where it activates myofilaments to produce contraction. These processes are often referred to as calcium-induced calcium-release. Ca^{2+} released by the sarcoplasmic reticulum is smoothly graded and closely regulated by sarcolemmal membrane potential. Relaxation of cardiac muscle occurs upon Ca^{2+} removal from the cytosol, following both Ca^{2+} reuptake into the SR catalyzed by a Ca^{2+}-ATPase in the vicinity of the myofilaments, and by extrusion of Ca^{2+} out of the myocyte via the sarcolemmal Na–Ca exchanger and Ca^{2+}-ATPase. The repetition of this excitation–contraction–relaxation cycle underlies the contraction of the heart.

Cardiac function is reduced following administration of alcohol through at least two modes. First, alcohol induces an indirect positive inotropic and chronotropic effect secondary to enhanced sympathetic activation, and subsequent release of catecholamines. The ethanol-induced increase in sympathetic activation is the likely cause of downregulation of β-adrenergic receptors observed in the heart when cardiomyopathy develops into chronic heart failure.[94] Second, alcohol has a direct negative inotropic effect on the heart. The latter property is often obscured during acute ethanol exposure by the enhanced sympathetic reflex activity.[78,82,107] When unmasked by sympathetic/autonomic blockade, the acute negative inotropic effects of alcohol become apparent, including reductions in cardiac contractility, cardiac output, and left ventricle ejection fraction.

The alcohol-induced negative inotropic effects are ultimately the result of interference with the some or all of the individual steps underlying cardiac excitation–contraction coupling: (1) ion channels and pumps that contribute to the cardiac action potential; (2) the processes involved in the Ca^{2+} regulation of sarcoplasmic reticulum Ca^{2+}-release and the intracellular Ca^{2+} transient; (3) the cardiac contractile proteins themselves; and (4) the molecular entities involved in removal of Ca^{2+} from the cytoplasm, through extrusion from the cell across the sarcolemmal membrane or reuptake into the sarcoplasmic reticulum.

Alcohol has minimal effects on the cardiac action potential, indicating that ethanol has little effect on the channels that contribute to the action potential in cardiac muscle. ATP-dependent Ca^{2+}-uptake by the sarcoplasmic reticulum is only slightly affected by alcohol, even under conditions where phospholamban is phosphorylated.[38,74,95] However, alcohol can inhibit ATP-dependent sarcoplasmic reticulum Ca^{2+}-uptake by increasing the rate at which Ca^{2+} "passively leaks" from the sarcoplasmic reticulum.[40,96]

In contrast to the modest effects on inward Ca^{2+} current of the action potential and sarcoplasmic reticulum Ca^{2+} uptake, a more likely mechanism responsible for the negative inotropic action of alcohol involves suppression of sarcoplasmic reticulum Ca^{2+} release and of Ca^{2+} transients. Acute exposure to moderate-to-high concentrations of ethanol (0.4 to 0.6%) caused a concentration-dependent suppression of Ca^{2+} transients, resulting in a 30% reduction in peak amplitude, a 40% decrease in the rate of Ca^{2+} increase (dCa^{2+}/dt) and a 25% increase in the half-time for Ca^{2+} decay in isolated rat ventricular myocytes, all of which were reversible.[18,96] Several additional studies reported that moderate concentrations of alcohol (0.2 to 0.3%) inhibited contractions in the absence of detectable changes in Ca^{2+} transients, suggesting a reduction in Ca^{2+} sensitivity of the contractile proteins.[18,36,78,95] Under more physiological conditions, however, low ethanol concentrations (0.05%) caused both significant decreases in the extent and rate of myocyte shortening and lengthening in the absence of changes in total contraction duration. These results are consistent with alcohol decreasing sarcoplasmic reticulum Ca^{2+}-release, without changing the timing or magnitude of the Ca^{2+} trigger.[20] This latter finding suggests that the most sensitive targets for alcohol most likely include sarcoplasmic reticulum Ca^{2+}-release and calcium-induced Ca^{2+} release.

In this regard, changes in the stabilization of the ryanodine receptor are implicated in the development of heart failure.[54] The ryanodine receptor forms a channel that is approximately 10 times larger than voltage-gated Ca^{2+} and Na^+-channels. When the channel opens, the cytosolic concentration of Ca^{2+} increases 10-fold, causing activation of the contractile apparatus. The ryanodine receptor is a complex of proteins including protein kinase A and its anchoring protein, protein phosphatases PP1 and PP2A, sorcin, calmodulin, and FK506 binding protein. The assembly of the multiprotein complex implies that the ryanodine receptor is regulated by protein:protein interactions. Phosphorylation of ryanodine receptor dissociates FKBP12.6 from the channel, altering channel function.[55] The net effect of this alteration on cardiac function is twofold. First, activity of the channel (open probability) is increased. The increased sensitivity is associated with destabilization of the channel. Second, dissociation of FKBP12.6 from the channel uncouples multiple ryanodine receptors and disturbs coupled gating. Coupled gating allows adjacent ryanodine receptors to open and close in a coordinated manner. With uncoupling, not all the ryanodine receptors in a given area would open and close simultaneously during systole and diastole. Some of the ryanodine receptors would remain open and thereby give rise to the diastolic leak from the sarcoplasmic reticulum.[53] Overexpression of FKBP12.6 in myocytes reduces Ca^{2+} leak from sarcoplasmic and promotes Ca^{2+} release during activation of ryanodine receptor.[63a] Unfortunately, there are scant data relating to the effects of ethanol on this process.

8.3.5.1 Role of Acetate and Acetaldehyde in the Pathogenesis of Alterations in Translational Control

After years of study, the specific etiology responsible for the alcohol-induced inhibition of translation efficiency remains unresolved. The question remains as to whether the alcohol-induced inhibition in protein synthesis was mediated by factors other than ethanol. Ethanol is metabolized in the liver to acetylaldehyde and acetate and these compounds are released into the circulation. The plasma concentration of both these metabolites rises after ingesting ethanol. Both ethanol and its active metabolites acetate and acetaldehyde may be involved in the pathogenesis of alcoholic cardiomyopathy[64,84] during ethanol intoxication. It is unlikely that the effects of ethanol are mediated by acetate because this compound actually stimulates myocardial protein synthesis[89] and protects the ischemic myocardium from injury.[103]

Unlike acetate, acetaldehyde is reported to disrupt many cellular processes. However, the role of acetaldehyde in pathogenesis of myocardial dysfunction *in vivo* is not as well established. Acetaldehyde exerts biphasic chronotrophic and inotrophic effects on the heart. At low concentrations there is a positive component consisting of increases in heart rate, coronary blood flow, cardiac output, and left-ventricular pressure consistent with a stimulation of the β-adrenergic system. At high concentration, the negative inotropic effects are believed to be a direct toxic effect on the myocardium, independent of cholingeric or purinergic input.

Acetaldehyde is the major metabolite of ethanol. The concentration of acetaldehyde in the blood is fairly constant despite widely different plasma ethanol concentrations and appears more dependent upon the nature of the alcoholic beverage (i.e., bourbon vs. grain alcohol) consumed rather than on the amount.[52] The plasma concentration of acetaldehyde following ethanol consumption ranges from 0.04 to 0.15 mg/dl (0.008 to 0.03 mM). Short-term exposure of cardiomyocytes to acetaldehyde depresses ventricular function through changes in relaxation duration which may be related to metabolism of ethanol through the cytochrome P450 oxidase 2E1.[1] Acetaldehyde (0.8 mM) inhibits myocardial protein synthesis in a perfused system.[64] Therefore, *in vitro* studies using higher doses may reflect pharmacological response. In this regard, chronic administration of acetaldehyde vapors does not depress the synthesis of myocardial proteins *in vivo* although its inotrophic effects are observed.[7]

Other approaches to answering the question concerning the role of acetaldehyde in modulating cardiac protein synthesis are generated from the use of inhibitors of ethanol metabolism or genetic manipulations of the mouse genome. Overexpression of alcohol dehydrogenase to elevate cardiac exposure to acetaldehyde results in a fourfold elevation in myocardial acetaldehyde content.[49] Chronic alcohol ingestion in these animals produced many characteristics of alcoholic cardiomyopathy observed in humans, such as reduced contractility, ultrastructural changes, and biochemical alterations.[49] These results support the concept that acetaldehyde may have a role in the development of alcoholic cardiomyopathy.

The formation of acetaldehyde is blocked by inhibition of alcohol dehydrogenase with 4-methylpyrazole.[87] When 4-methylpyrazole and ethanol are administered acutely, a depression of cardiac protein synthesis is observed. Thus, ethanol *per se* can inhibit protein synthesis in cardiac muscle independent of acetaldehyde formation. These findings provide evidence for a direct effect of ethanol on protein metabolism, but do not preclude a role for acetaldehyde. When acetaldehyde degradation is inhibited with cyanamide, raising the acetaldehyde concentration results in a larger effect than of ethanol alone. Thus, ethanol and acetaldehyde both can cause an inhibition of protein synthesis in cardiac muscle.

8.3.5.2 Mitochondrial Failure Does Not Account for Ventricular Dysfunction Following Elevation of Acetaldehyde

The potential mechanism by which acetaldehyde may inhibit protein synthesis remains unknown. Acetaldehyde has been suggested to interfere with mitochondrial function by interfering with oxygen consumption and ATP production, thereby lowering the energy charge [ATP/(ATP+ADP+AMP)] of myocytes.[39] Rates of protein synthesis decrease as the energy charge falls. Indeed, mitochondrial ultrastructural changes are observed following acute and chronic alcohol ingestion.[3,39,81] However, energy metabolism shows no significant depression of oxygen consumption.[32,33] Likewise, feeding rats with an alcohol-containing diet chronically does not depress the myocardial content of high-energy phosphates (ATP or creatine phosphate).[104] Thus, decreased translation efficiency probably does not result from diminished oxidative energy metabolism secondary to mitochondrial dysfunction.

8.3.6 ALCOHOL-INDUCED APOPTOSIS

In many organ systems, including the heart, myocyte loss or cell death may be an important component of organ dysfunction and pathology.[37] A significant loss of myocytes is observed in the left ventricle from rats fed ethanol in their drinking water for 8 months.[10] Cell death can result from either necrosis or apoptosis (programmed cell death) (for a review see Reference 42). Ethanol-induced apoptosis is probably a critical mechanism underlying ethanol-induced disorders such as fetal alcohol syndrome. There are several early reports in humans with alcoholic cardiomyopathy and animal models of cardiomyopathy that support a role for myocyte loss as a mechanism underlying alcohol-induced cardiac dysfunction. A histopathologic examination of hearts of patients with the diagnosis of alcoholic cardiomyopathy showed that myocytes lost their cross-striated appearance and had pyknotic nuclei.[39] The latter, a reduction in the size of the nucleus, can be a characteristic of apoptosis.

Alcohol potentiates the apoptotic effect of serum withdrawal (as measured by DNA acid fragmentation).[13] In addition, alcohol increases the protein levels of the pro-apoptotic protein Bax and increases caspase-3 enzyme activity (the latter is a member of a family of intracellular proteases activated in apoptosis). The concentrations of alcohol used in these studies are very high (500 mg/dl can be associated with respiratory depression and death); however, lower concentrations of alcohol, 200 mg/dl, potentiate the effects of serum withdrawal on apoptosis. In contrast, apoptosis is not accelerated following an acute infusion of alcohol (500 mg/dl for 150 min), but acute alcohol intoxication increases the p21 mRNA content.[41] p21 is an inhibitor of cyclin-dependent kinases, and it may be one of the many proteins involved in the hypertrophic response.

Interestingly, the application of insulin-like growth factor (IGF)-1 attenuates the apoptotic effects of ethanol on serum withdrawal.[13] IGF-1 has multiple effects on the cell; some which include cell proliferation and differentiation, whereas activation of signaling components downstream to the IGF receptor are linked to the development of hypertrophy.

8.3.7 FACTORS AFFECTING PATHOGENESIS OF ALCOHOLIC CARDIOMYOPATHY

8.3.7.1 Nutritional Factors and Other Micronutrients

Originally, the development of the myocardial lesion induced by chronic alcohol ingestion was suggested to result from nutritional imbalances. In particular the correlation between thiamine deficiency and alcoholic cardiomyopathy led to the suggestion of vitamin deficiency as a causative agent. However, thiamine deficiency occurs in only a small proportion of chronic alcohol abusers. In such cases, derangements in myocardial function respond to treatment with thiamine. However, both animal and clinical studies where the overall nutritional status was evaluated by examination of the diet or by analysis of specific markers of thiamine deficiency indicate that development of the alcoholic heart muscle disease *per se* is independent of nutritional deficiencies.[17,59,101] Furthermore, when alcoholics develop a dilated cardiomyopathy without a history of significant malnutrition, the patients do not improve their clinical course with thiamine supplementations.[14] Thus, while malnutrition *per se* does not induce the myopathy, certainly alterations in the nutritional status may exacerbate the disease.[16]

In addition to nutritional deficiencies, additives to alcoholic beverages, such as cobalt, may exert a toxic effect on the myocardium. However, this is a relatively rare event.[5]

8.3.7.2 Angiotensin-Converting Enzyme Gene Polymorphism

Another possibility leading to the development of alcoholic cardiomyopathy could involve the genetic makeup of the individual. In this regard, polymorphism of the angiotensin-converting enzyme (ACE) has been implicated in development of cardiac dysfunction in various pathological conditions. The ACE genotype of the individual in other forms of cardiac dysfunction has been correlated with the progression of the disease. Hence, one would expect that the ACE genotypes of alcoholics who have a cardiomyopathy to differ from those who do not present with symptoms of cardiac dysfunction. The DD ACE genotype is present in 57% of alcoholics with left ventricular ejection fraction less than 0.50 and only in 7% of those with normal cardiac function. Compared with those with an I allele, the odds ratio for development of left ventricular dysfunction in alcoholic persons with the DD genotype was 16.4. These observations suggest that the possible development of cardiomyopathy among those persons chronically abusing alcohol may be partially genetically predetermined by the presence of the ACE DD genotype. Despite the association, the potential cause for development of cardiomyopathy remains unresolved by this type of analysis simply on the basis of polymorphism of ACE genotypes.

8.3.7.3 Alcohol-Induced Changes in IGF-I System

IGF-I is important in maintaining normal cardiac structure and function in an adult animal. It can modulate metabolism functioning as a classical hormone and as an autocrine:paracrine mediator. IGF-I has specific cardiac effects as well as growth-promoting properties. Elevations in IGF-I result in stimulation of protein synthesis in cardiac muscle,[8,31] whereas inhibition of IGF-I action diminishes protein synthesis. IGF-I improves myocardial function in normal adult rats and healthy humans, in rats after myocardial infarction, and in patients with heart failure (for a review see Reference 73). Part of this enhanced cardiac performance following IGF-I may be mediated by enhanced contractility secondary to increases in Ca^{2+} transients.[30] Furthermore, IGF-I enhances dihydropyridine-sensitive Ca^{2+} channel activity through a PKC-dependent pathway.[90] IGF-I may also decrease apoptosis induced in cardiac muscle by a number of pathological conditions through increased expression of antiapoptotic Bcl-2 protein.[61]

Chronic alcohol consumption in rats markedly reduces the concentration of IGF-I in the blood compared to pair-fed control animals.[44,92] Acute alcohol intoxication leads to impairment in IGF-I signaling in the heart.[47] Alcohol exposure prevents the IGF-I-induced changes in Ca^{2+} channel activity and stimulation of protein synthesis.[63] The failure of IGF-I to stimulate these processes involved in normal cardiac structure and function may result from alcohol-induced alterations in the signal transduction pathway for IGF-I.[47,63] Ultimately, these changes may contribute to the development of alcoholic cardiomyopathy.

8.4 GENDER DIFFERENCES IN RESPONSE TO ETHANOL

Alcohol-related complications afflict both male and female alcoholics. Approximately one third of all alcoholics in the U.S. are women. There is a general impression that few female alcoholics develop alcoholic cardiomyopathy, even adjusting for the lower incidence of alcoholism in women. However, the cardiotoxicity of ethanol does not spare the female heart. Like men, about one third of all the asymptomatic women have evidence of cardiomyopathy.[100] Despite the significant number of women presenting with alcoholic cardiomyopathy, there are very few studies examining the incidence, pathophysiology, or clinical outcome in woman who abuse alcohol. The incidence, presentation, clinical features, and evolution of several cardiomyopathies possess gender-related differences (for a review see Reference 27).

Females appear more susceptible to alcoholic liver injury, brain disorders, and myopathies of skeletal and cardiac muscle. Similar to men, long-term alcohol consumption is also associated with the development of alcoholic cardiomyopathy. Among cases for alcoholic cardiomyopathies, men represent the largest percentage and death rates are higher in men than in women. Furthermore, death rates in African-American men and women are greater than in Caucasians diagnosed with alcoholic cardiomyopathy. The pathologic changes in cardiac muscle occur despite the amount of ethanol consumed by females being generally only 60% of that consumed by their male counterparts. Thus, the threshold dose for the development of cardiomyopathy is lower in women than in men.

In terms of the pathophysiology of etiology of alcohol-induced heart disease, women metabolize alcohol differently from men. Women generally have a smaller volume of distribution per unit weight because of greater proportion of body fat. One consequence of this phenomenon is that women attain a higher mean blood alcohol level than men. In addition, women have a lower gastric alcohol dehydrogenase content, which means that there is a reduction in first pass ethanol metabolism leading to higher blood alcohol concentrations.

When symptomatic, the clinical presentation of alcoholic cardiomyopathy resembles that observed in men and includes a dilated left ventricle and systolic dysfunction.[25,27] Furthermore, the threshold dose for the development of cardiomyopathy was considerably less in women than in men, and the decline in the ejection fraction with increasing alcohol dose was significantly steeper ($P < 0.001$) for women compared with men.[100] The fact that women have the same prevalence of cardiomyopathies as men despite consuming less alcohol is strong evidence for a greater propensity of alcohol-induced cardiac damage in females. Urbano-Marquez and colleagues[100] suggested that a 55-kg woman who consumes approximately 9 fl oz (270 ml) of spirits (or its equivalent of 1 liter of wine) per day for 20 years has a risk for development of alcoholic cardiomyopathy. There appear to be distinct pathophysiological mechanisms leading to a higher sensitivity to alcohol-induced cardiac damage in that it takes less consumption of alcohol to produce alcoholic cardiomyopathy in women compared with men.

8.5 TREATMENT OF ALCOHOLIC HEART DISEASE

8.5.1 Treatment of Cardiac Arrhythmias

Treatment of atrial and ventricular arrhythmias in patients with alcoholic cardiomyopathies begins with abstinence from alcohol. Additional treatment recommendations follow ACC/AHA practice guidelines. In patients with atrial fibrillation, treatment is focused on three major areas: ventricular rate control, appropriate use of anticoagulants, and chemically or electrically restoring sinus rhythm.

Sudden cardiac death resulting from ventricular arrhythmias can be reduced in patients with left ventricular systolic dysfunction by treating such patients with angiotensin-converting enzyme inhibitors and β-adrenergic blockers. Amioderone, a class III antiarrhythmic drug, is safe in patients with heart failure. It is, however, of uncertain benefit in this patient population. The role of implantable cardiac defibrillators (ICD) in patients with heart failure remains unclear as well. Though ICDs may have a role in high-risk patients, this is not recommended for routine prophylactic therapy.

8.5.2 Treatment of Left Ventricular Dysfunction

Patients presenting with heart failure with systolic dysfunction should be treated based on standard therapeutic regimens for heart failure. First-line therapy approaches include angiotensin-converting enzyme inhibitors and β-adrenergic blockers that reduce mortality in symptomatic and asymptomatic patients with left ventricular systolic dysfunction. Diuretics reduce symptoms of congestion but have no beneficial effects on mortality. Cardiac glycosides also have a neutral effect on mortality but do reduce hospitalization as a result of congestive heart failure. Treatment in the presence of continued alcohol consumption does not reduce mortality.[24,34] Abstinence after development of mild heart failure can arrest the progression and potentially reverse the symptoms.[60] Prognosis is good even in patients with New York Heart Association class IV heart failure caused by cardiomyopathy following complete abstinence. Improvement in left ventricular ejection fraction can be seen within 1 year and continual improvement is observed going forward. Interestingly, patients who reduced their ethanol consumption from 100 to about 50 g of ethanol (about four drinks) per day show a comparable improvement in left ventricular function.[60]

References

1. Aberle N S, II, and J Ren. Short-term acetaldehyde exposure depresses ventricular myocyte contraction: role of cytochrome P450 oxidase, xanthine oxidase, and lipid peroxidation. *Alcohol Clin. Exp. Res.* 27: 577–583, 2003.
2. Adickes, E, T Mollner, and S Lockwood. Ethanol induced morphologic alterations during growth and maturation of cardiac myocytes. *Alcohol Clin. Exp. Res.* 14: 827–831, 1990.
3. Alexander, C S. Electron microscopic observations in alcoholic heart disease. *Br. Heart J.* 29: 200–206, 1966.
4. Alexander, C S. Idiopathic heart disease. II. Electron microscopic examination of myocardial biopsy specimens in alcoholic heart disease. *Am. J. Med.* 41: 229–234, 1966.
5. Alexander, C S. Cobalt-beer cardiomyopathy: a clinical and pathological study of twenty-eight cases. *Am. J. Med.* 53: 395–417, 1972.
6. Ariza, A, J Coll, M T Fernandez-Figureras, M D Lopez, J L Mate, O Garcia, A Fernandaz-Vasalo, and J J Navas-Palacios. Desmin myopathy: a multisystem disorder involving skeletal, cardiac and smooth muscle. *Hum. Pathol.* 26: 1032–1037, 1995.
7. Auton, W P and L C Ward. Acetaldehyde and cardiac protein synthesis in the rat *in vivo*. *Int. J. Biochem.* 18: 289–292, 1986.
8. Bark, T H, M A McNurlan, C H Lang, and P J Garlick. Increased protein synthesis after acute IGF-I or insulin infusion is localized to muscle in mice. *Am. J. Physiol. Endocrinol Metabol.* 275: E118–E123, 1998.
9. Bulloch, R T, M B Pearce, M L Murphy, B J Jenkins, and J L Davis. Myocardial lesions in idiopathic and alcoholic cardiomyopathy. *Am. J. Cardiol.* 29: 15–25, 1972.
10. Capasso, J M, P Li, and G Giuideri. Myocardial mechanical, biochemical and structural alterations induced by chronic ethanol ingestion in rats. *Circ. Res.* 71: 346–356, 1992.

11. Capetanaki, Y and D J Milner. Desmin cytoskeleton in muscle integrity and function. *Subcell. Biochem.* 31: 463–495, 1998.

12. Caryl, O R, A Gallardo-Carpentier, and R G Carpentier. Cardiac chronotropic effects of nicotine and ethanol in the rat. *Alcohol* 9: 103–107, 1991.

13. Chen, D B, L Wang, and P H Wang. Insulin-like growth factor I retards apoptotic signaling induced by ethanol in cardiomyocytes. *Life Sci.* 67: 1683–1693, 2000.

14. Constant, J. The alcoholic cardiomyopathies — genuine and pseudo. *Cardiology* 91: 92–95, 1999.

15. Cooney, R N, S R Kimball, and T C Vary. Regulation of skeletal muscle protein turnover during sepsis: mechanisms and mediators. *Shock* 7: 1–16, 1997.

16. Cummingham, R K and P I Spach. Alcoholism and the myocardium energy metabolism. *Alcohol Clin. Exp. Res.* 18: 132–137, 1994.

17. Dancy, M, J M Bland, G Leech, M K Gaitonde, and J D Maxwell. Preclinical left ventricular abnormalities in alcoholics are independent of nutritional status, cirrhosis, and cigarette smoking. *Lancet* 1122–1125, 1985.

18. Danzinger, R S, M Sakai, M C Capogrossi, H A Spurgeon, R Hansford and E G Lakatta. EtOH acutely and reversibly suppresses excitation-contraction coupling in cardiac myocytes. *Circ. Res.* 68: 1660–1668, 1991.

19. Day, C P, O F W James, T J Butler, and R W F Campbell. QT prolongation and sudden cardiac death inpatients with alcoholic liver disease. *Lancet* 341(8858): 1423–1428, 1993.

20. Delbridge, L M, P J Connell, P J Harris, and T O Morgan. Ethanol effects on cardiomyocyte contractility. *Clin. Sci.* 98: 401–407, 2000.

21. Demirovic, J and R J Myerburg. Epidemiology of sudden cardiac death: an overview. *Prog. Cardiovasc. Dis.* 37: 39–48, 1994.

22. Engel, T R and J C Luck. Effect of whiskey on atrial vulnerability and "holiday heart." *J. Am. Coll. Cardiol.* 1: 816–820, 1983.

23. Ettinger, P O, C F Wu, C de la Cruz Jr., A B Weisse, S S Ahmed, and T J Regan. Arrhythmias and the holiday heart: alcohol associated cardiac rhythm disorders. *Am. Heart J.* 95: 555–562, 1978.

24. Fauchier, L, D Babuty, P Poret, D Cosset-Senon, M L Autret, P Cosney, and J P Fauchier. Comparison of long-term outcome of alcoholic and idiopathic dilated cardiomyopathy. *Eur. Heart J.* 21: 306–314, 2000.

25. Fernandaz-Sola, J, R Estruch, J M Nicolas-Arfelis et al. Comparison of alcoholic cardiomyopathy in women compared with men. *Am. J. Cardiol.* 80: 481–485, 1997.

26. Fernandaz-Sola, J, J M Nicolas, J C Pare, E Sacanella, F Fatjo, M Cofan, and R Estruch. Diastolic function impairment in alcoholics. *Alcohol Clin. Exp. Res.* 24: 1830–1835, 2000.

27. Fernandaz-Sola, J and J M Nicolas-Arfelis. Gender differences in alcoholic cardiomyopathy. *J. Gender-Specific Med.* 5: 41–47, 2002.

28. Ferrans, V J, L M Buja, and W C Roberts. Cardiac morphological changes produced by ethanol. In: *Alcohol and Abnormal Protein Biosynthesis*, Rothschild MA, Oratz M, and Schreiber SS (Eds.). New York: Pergamon Press, 1975, pp. 139–185.

29. Flynn, A and C G Proud. The role of eIF-4 in cell proliferation. *Cancer Surg.* 27: 162–166, 1996.

30. Freestone, N S, S Ribaric, and W T Mason. The effect of insulin-like growth factor I on adult contractility. *Mol. Cell. Biochem.* 163: 223–229, 1996.

31. Fuller, S J, J R Mynett, and P H Sugden. Stimulation of cardiac protein synthesis by insulin like growth factor. *Biochem. J.* 282: 85–90, 1992.

32. Gailis, L and M Verdy. The effects of ethanol and acetaldehyde on metabolism and vascular resistance in perfused heart. *Can. J. Biochem.* 49: 227–233, 1971.

33. Ganz, V. The acute effect of alcohol on the circulation and oxygen metabolism of the heart. *Am. Heart J.* 56: 494–500, 1963.

34. Gavazzi, A, R De Maria, M Parolini, and M Porcu. Alcohol abuse and cardiomyopathy in men. *Am. J. Cardiol.* 85: 1114–1118, 2000.

35. Greenspon, A J and S F Scheal. The "holiday heart": electrophysiologic studies of alcohol effects in alcoholics. *Ann. Intern. Med.* 98: 135–139, 1983.

36. Guarmieri, T and E G Lakatta. Mechanism of myocardial contractile depression by clinical concentrations of EtOH. *J. Clin. Invest.* 85: 1462–1467, 1990.

37. Hamstetter, A and S Izumo. Apoptosis: basic mechanisms and implications for cardiovascular disease. *Circulation* 82: 1111–1129, 1998.

38. Hara, K and M Kasai. The mechanism of increase in the ATPase activity of sarcoplasmic reticulum vesicles treated with n-alcohol. *J. Biochem.* 82: 1005–1007, 1977.

39. Hibbs, R G, V J Ferrans, W C Black, D G Weilbaecher, J J Walsh, and G E Burch. Alcohol cardiomyopathy. An electron microscopic study. *Am. Heart J.* 69: 766–779, 1965.

40. Horton, J W and D J White. Cardiac contractile and sarcoplasmic reticulum function after acute EtOH consumption. *J. Surg. Res.* 64: 132–138, 1996.

41. Jankala, H, K K Eklund, J O Kokkonen et al. Ethanol infusion increases ANP and p21 gene expression in isolated perfed rat heart. *Biochem. Biophys. Res. Comm.* 281: 328–333, 2001.

42. Kang, P M and S Izumo. Apoptosis and heart failure: a critical review of the literature. *Circ. Res.* 86: 1107–1113, 2000.

43. Koskinen, P and M Kupari. Alcohol and cardiac arrhythmias. *Br. Med. J.* 304: 1394–1399, 1992.

44. Lang, C H, J Fan, B P Lipton, B J Potter, and K H McDonough. Modulation of the insulin-like growth factor system by chronic alcohol feeding. *Alcohol Clin. Exp. Res.* 22: 823–829, 1998.

45. Lang, C H, R A Frost, V Kumar, and T C Vary. Impaired myocardial protein synthesis induced by acute alcohol intoxication is associated with changes in eIF4F. *Am. J. Physiol. Endocrinol. Metab.* 279: E1029–E1038, 2000.

46. Lang, C H, S R Kimball, R A Frost, and T C Vary. Alcohol myopathy: impairment of protein synthesis and translation initiation. *Int. J. Biochem. Cell Biol.* 33: 457–473, 2001.

47. Lang, C H, V Kumar, X Liu, R A Frost, and T C Vary. IGF-I induced phosphorylation of S6K1 and 4E-BP1 in heart is impaired by acute alcohol intoxication. *Alcohol Clin. Exp. Res.* 27: 485–494, 2003.

48. Lang, C H, D Wu, R A Frost, L Jefferson, S Kimball, and T Vary. Inhibition of muscle protein synthesis by alcohol is associated with modulation of eIF2B and eIF4E. *Am. J. Physiol. Endocrinol. Metabol.* 277: E268–E276, 1999.

49. Liang, Q, E C Carlson, A J Borgerding, and P N Epstein. A transgenic model of acetaldehyde overproduction accelerates alcohol cardiomyopathy. *J. Pharmacol. Exp. Ther.* 291: 766–772, 1999.

50. Lowenstein, S R, P A Gabow, J Cramer, P B Oliva, and K Ratner. The role of alcohol in new-onset atrial fibrillation. *Arch. Intern. Med.* 143: 1882–1885, 1983.

51. Luca, C. Electrophysiological properties of right heart and atrio-ventricular conducting system in patients with alcoholic cardiomyopathy. *Br. Heart J.* 42: 274–278, 1979.

52. Majchrowicz, E and J H Mendelson. Blood concentrations of acetaldehyde and ethanol in chronic alcoholics. *Science* 1100–1102, 1970.

53. Marx, S O, J Gaburjakova, M Gaburjakova, C Henrikson, K Ondriask, and A R Marks. Coupled gating between calcium release channels (ryanodine receptors). *Circ. Res.* 88: 1151–1158, 2001.

54. Marx, S O and A R Marks. Regulation of the ryanodine receptor in heart failure. *Basic Res. Cardiol.* 97 Suppl. 1: I49–I51, 2002.

55. Marx, S O, S Reiken, Y Hisamatsu, T Jayaraman, D Burkoff, N Rosenblit, and M A R. PKA phosphorylation dissociates FKBP12.6 from the calcium release channel (ryanodine receptor): defective regulation in failing heart. *Cell* 101: 365–376, 2000.

56. McKee, M and A Britton. The positive relationship between alcohol and heart disease in eastern Europe: potential physiological mechanisms.[comment]. *J. R. Soc. Med.* 91: 402–407, 1998.

57. Meehan, J, M R Piano, R J Solarao, and J M Kennedy. Heavy long-term ethanol consumption induces an alpha- to beta-myosin heavy chain isoform transition in rat. *Basic Res. Cardiol.* 94: 481–488, 1999.

58. Milner, D J, G E Taffet, X Wang, T Pham, T Tamura, C Hartley, A M Gerdes, and Y Capetanaki. The absence of desmin leads to cardiomyocyte hypertrophy and cardiac dilation with compromised systolic function. *J. Mol. Cell. Cardiol.* 31: 2063–2076, 1999.

59. Nicolas, J M, R Estruch, E Antunez, E Scanella, and V Urbano-Marquez. Nutritional status in chronically alcoholic men from middle socioeconomic class and its relation to ethanol intake. *Alcohol Alcohol.* 28: 559–569, 1993.

60. Nicolas, J M, J Fernandaz-Sola, R Estruch, J C Pare, E Sacanella, V Urbano-Marquez, and E Rubin. The effect of controlled drinking in alcoholic cardiomyopathy. *Ann. Intern. Med.* 136: 192–200, 2002.

61. Parrizas, M and D LeRoith. Insulin-like growth factor I inhibits apoptosis is associated with increased expression of bcl-xL gene product. *Endocrinology* 138: 1355–1358, 1997.

62. Patel, V B, J M Corbett, M J Dunn, V R Winrow, B Portman, P J Richardson, and V R Preedy. Protein profiling in cardiac tissue in response to chronic effects of alcohol. *Electrophoresis* 18: 2788–2794, 1997.

63. Pecherskaya, A, E Rubin, and M L Solem. Alterations in insulin-like growth factor-I signaling in cardiomyocytes from chronic alcohol-exposed rats. *Alcohol Clin. Exp. Res.* 26: 995–1002, 2002.

64. Preedy, V R, V B Patel, II J F Why, J M Corbett, M J Dunn, and P J Richardson. Alcohol and the heart: biochemical alterations. *Cardiovascular Res.* 31: 139–147, 1996.

65. Preedy, V R and T J Peters. The acute and chronic effects of ethanol on cardiac muscle protein synthesis in the rat *in vivo*. *Alcohol* 7: 97–102, 1990.

66. Preedy, V R and T J Peters. Synthesis of subcellular protein fractions in the rat heart *in vivo* in response to chronic feeding. *Cardiovascular Res.* 23: 730–736, 1989.

67. Preedy, V R and T J Peters. Changes in protein, RNA, and DNA and rates of protein synthesis in muscle-containing tissues of the mature rat in response to ethanol feeding: a comparative study of heart, small intestine and gastrocnemius muscle. *Alcohol Alcohol.* 25: 489–498, 1990.

68. Preedy, V R and T J Peters. Protein metabolism in alcoholism. In: *Nutrition and Alcohol*, Watson RR and Watzl B, (Eds.) Boca Raton, FL: CRC Press, 1992, pp. 143–189.

69. Preedy, V R, T J Peters, V B Patel, and J P Miell. Chronic alcoholic myopathy: transcription and translational alterations. *FASEB J.*, 1994.

70. Preedy, V R, T Siddiq, H Why, and P J Richardson. The deleterious effects of alcohol on the heart: involvement of protein turnover. *Alcohol Alcohol.* 29: 141–147, 1994.

71. Rawat, A K. Inhibition of cardiac protein synthesis by prolonged ethanol administration. *Res. Comm. Chem. Path. Pharma.* 25: 89–102, 1979.

72. Regan, T J. Alcohol and the cardiovascular system. *JAMA* 264: 377–381, 1990.

73. Ren, J, W K Samson, and J R Sowers. Insulin-like growth factor I as a cardiac hormone: physiological and pathological implications in heart disease. *J. Mol. Cell. Cardiol.* 31: 2049–2061, 1999.

74. Retig, J N, M A Kirchberger, E Rubin, and A M Katz. Effects of EtOH on calcium transport by microsomes phosphorylated by cyclic AMP-dependent protein kinase. *Biochem. Pharmacol.* 26: 393–396, 1977.

75. Rhoads, R E. Regulation of eukaryotic protein synthesis by initiation factors. *J. Biol. Chem.* 268: 3017–3020, 1993.

76. Rhoads, R E, S Joshi-Barve, and W B Minich. Participation of initiation factors in recruitment of mRNA to ribosomes. *Biochimie* 76: 831–838, 1994.

77. Richardson, P J. Report of the 1995 World Health Organization/International Society and Federation of Cardiology Task Force on the definition and classification of cardiomyopathies. *Circulation* 93: 841–842, 1995.

78. Riff, D P, A C Jain, and J T Doyle. Acute hemodynamic effects of EtOH on normal human volunteers. *Am. Heart J.* 78: 592–597, 1969.

79. Rubin, E, A M Katz, C S Lieber, E P Stein, and S Puszki. Muscle damage produced by chronic alcohol consumption. *Am. J. Pathol.* 83: 499–516, 1976.

80. Ryan, J M and L G Howes. Relations between alcohol consumption, heart rate, and heart rate variability in men. *Heart* (British Cardiac Society) 88: 641–642, 2002.

81. Sarma, J S M, S Ikeda, R Fischer, Y Maruyama, R Weishaar, and R J Bing. Biochemical and contractile properties of heart muscle after prolonged alcohol administration. *J. Mol. Cell. Cardiol.* 8: 951–972, 1976.

82. Schoppet, M and B Maisch. Alcohol and the heart. *Herz* 26: 3345–3352, 2001.

83. Schorling, J B and D G Buscbaum. Screening for alcohol and drug abuse. *Med. Clin. N. Am.* 81: 845–861, 1997.

84. Schreiber, S S, K Briden, M Oratz, and M A Rothschild. Ethanol, acetaldehyde and myocardial protein synthesis. *J. Clin. Invest.* 51: 2820–2826, 1972.

85. Schreiber, S S, C D Evans, F Reff, M A Rothschild, and M Oratz. Prolonged feeding of the young growing guinea pig: I. The effects on protein synthesis in afterloaded right ventricle measured *in vitro*. *Alcohol. Clin. Exp. Res.* 6: 384–390, 1982.

86. Schreiber, S S, F Reff, C D Evans, M A Rothschild, and M Oratz. Prolonged feeding of ethanol to young growing guinea pig. III. Effect on synthesis of myocardial contractile proteins. *Alcohol Clin. Exp. Res.* 10: 531–534, 1986.

87. Siddiq, T, P J Richardson, W Mitchell, J Teare, and V R Preedy. Ethanol-induced inhibition of ventricular protein synthesis *in vivo* and possible role of acetylaldehyde. *Cell Biochem. Function* 11: 45–54, 1993.

88. Siddiq, T, D K Shori, G B Proctor, C Luckhaus, P J Richardson, and V R Preedy. The activities of cathespin B,D and H in hearts treated with ethanol. *Biochem. Soc. Trans.* 22: 171S, 1994.

89. Smith, D M, S J Fuller, and P H Sugden. The effects of lactate, acetate, glucose, insulin, starvation and alloxan diabetes on protein synthesis in perfused rat hearts. *Biochem. J.* 236: 543–547, 1986.

90. Solem, M L and A P Thomas. Modulation of cardiac Ca^{2+} channels by IGF-I. *Biochem. Biophys. Res. Comm.* 252: 151–155, 1998.

91. Sonenberg, N. Regulation of translation and cell growth by eIF-4E. *Biochimie* 76: 839–846, 1994.
92. Sonntag, W E and R L Boyd. Chronic ethanol feeding inhibits plasma levels of insulin-like growth factor-I. *Life Sci.* 43: 1325–1330, 1988.
93. Spies, C D, M Sander, K Stangl, J Fernandaz-Sola, V R Preedy, E Rubin, S Andreasson, E Z Hanna, and W J Knox. Effects of alcohol on the heart. *Curr. Opin. Crit. Care* 7: 337–343, 2001.
94. Strasser, R, I Nutcher, B Rauch, R Marquetant, and H Seitz. Changes in cardiac signal transduction systems in chronic EtOH treatment preceding the development of cardiomyopathy. *Herz* 21: 323–240, 1996.
95. Swartz, M H, D I Repke, A M Katz, and E Rubin. Effects of EtOH on calcium binding and calcium uptake by cardiac microsomes. *Biochem. Pharmacol.* 23: 2369–2376, 1974.
96. Thomas, A P, D J Rozanski, D C Renard, and E Rubin. Effects of ethanol on the contractile function of the heart. A review. *Alcohol Clin. Exp. Res.* 18: 121–131, 1994.
97. Thorton, J R. Atrial fibrillation in healthy non-alcoholic people after an alcohol binge. *Lancet* 2: 1013–1014, 1984.
98. Tierman, J M and J C Ward. Acute effects of ethanol on protein synthesis in the rat. *Alcohol Alcohol.* 21: 171–179, 1986.
99. Tierman, J M, J C Ward, and W G E Cooksley. Inhibition by ethanol of cardiac protein synthesis in the rat. *Int. J. Biochem.* 17: 793–798, 1985.
100. Urbano-Marquez, A, R Estruch, J Fernandez-Smith, J M Nicolas, J Carlos, and E Rubin. The greater risk of alcoholic cardiomyopathy and myopathy in women compared with men. *JAMA* 274: 149–154, 1995.
101. Urbano-Marquez, V, R Estruch, F Navarro-Lopez, J M Grau, L Mont, and E Rubin. The effects of alcoholism on skeletal and cardiac muscle. *New Engl. J. Med.* 320: 409–415, 1989.
102. Vary, T C. Regulation of skeletal muscle protein turnover in sepsis. *Curr. Opin Clin. Nutr. Metab. Care* 1: 217–224, 1998.
103. Vary, T C, E T Angelakos, and S W Schaffer. Relationship between adenine nucleotide metabolism and irreversible ischemic tissue damage in isolated perfused rat heart. *Circ. Res.* 45: 218–225, 1979.
104. Vary, T C, C J Lynch, and C H Lang. Effects of chronic alcohol consumption on regulation of myocardial protein synthesis. *Am. J. Physiol. Heart Circ. Physiol.* 281: H1242–H1251, 2001.
105. Vary, T C, A C Nairn, G Deiter, and C H Lang. Differential effects of alcohol consumption on eukaryotic elongation factors in heart, skeletal muscle and liver. *Alcohol Clin. Exp. Res.* 26: 1794–1802, 2002.
106. Wolf, P A, R D Abbott, and W B Kannel. Atrial fibrillation: a major contributor to stroke in the elderly. *Arch. Intern. Med.* 147: 1561–1566, 1987.
107. Zakhari, S. Vulnerability to cardiac disease. *Recent Dev. Alcoholism* 9: 225–262, 1991.

Section IV

Alcohol: Metabolism and Metabolites

9 Alcohol, Nutrition, and Recovery of Brain Function

*Adrian B. Bonner, Allan D. Thomson,
and Christopher C.H. Cook*

CONTENTS

9.1 ABSTRACT

This review considers the role of nutrition in the development of alcohol-related brain dysfunction. Particular attention is paid to the serotonergic modulation of brain function and the role of tryptophan metabolism, including the dynamic relationship between the neurotoxic and neuroprotective effects of tryptophan metabolism, via the kynurenine pathway. The mechanisms of thiamine deficit-related brain disease are also reviewed, and commonalities between these cytotoxic mechanisms and the neurotoxicity/neuroprotection effects of tryptophan metabolism are discussed. The potential for therapeutic approaches of manipulating and providing dietary supplementation is explored by reference to existing and new strategies which might be developed to support the behavioral therapies employed to help in the rehabilitation of alcohol misusers. These issues are considered within the context of nutritional deficiencies and developmental challenges, which occur in socially excluded populations and include a commentary on the utility of automated neuropsychological assessments.

9.2 INTRODUCTION

A complex relationship exists among alcohol, nutrition, and brain function due to the interplay among a wide range of biological, psychological, and social factors linked to the development of alcohol dependency. It is well established that chronic ethanol misuse is associated with impaired nutrition, primarily as a consequence of the disadvantaged socioeconomic lifestyles, the perturbations in nutrient handling resulting in reduced absorption, and metabolism in chronic alcohol abusers. Thiamine deficiency has been proposed as a causal mechanism in the pathological development of brain-damage leading, if untreated, to Korsakoff's psychosis.[1] Nicotinic acid, pyridoxine, and vitamin B_{12} are important dietary components necessary for normal central nervous system (CNS) activity, and functional deficits may present in the development of brain damage. The devastating complications and brain changes leading to atrophy due to excessive ingestion of the macronutrient alcohol include impaired cognitive function, reflected in reduced quality of life with corresponding increases in morbidity and mortality. Many factors have been proposed to account for these defects including increased apoptosis,[2] free radical injury,[3] disturbances of protein synthesis,[4] DNA damage,[5,6] and effects on protein formation via derangements of RNA metabolism. More recently, attention has focused on the possibility that transcription factors such as intermediate early genes and heat shock or stress proteins play a key role in the pathogenesis of alcohol-induced brain dysfunction. A candidate gene, heat shock protein HSP[7] has been implicated in this process.

However, the intervening steps between the gene activation and the development of presenting features have not been established. The signals responsible for alcohol-induced brain damage are not fully understood. Increased production of corticotrophin, resulting in elevations of circulating ACTH, causes raised cortisol[8] and catecholamine concentrations[9] and is thought to contribute to alcohol induced brain-damage.[10–13]

9.3 NUTRITION AND ETHANOL IN EARLY DEVELOPMENT

It would appear that the roots of alcohol dependence, alcoholic brain damage, and related problems are laid down in the early developmental stages, and the effects on the brain of cumulative damage, resulting from a series of insults, make a person more vulnerable to further damage by changing behavior, memory, or encouraging malnutrition — all of which add to the vicious circle of events leading through alcohol misuse to dependence and alcohol-related brain damage. The maximum rate of brain growth occurs during the first two years of life. Although the basic brain infrastructure is genetically preprogrammed, giving an overproduction of neurons in some regions such as the olfactory and hippocampal regions, the fine structure is tuned by the "pruning" of axons, dendrites, and synapses which are not utilized. The concept of neural Darwinism[14] provides an explanation, based on the principles of natural selection, of the way in which neurons are influenced by stimulation of the brain in the course of sensory inputs from the environment, a process described as learning. Learning perceived as a behavioral output originates from neurobiological mechanisms at cellular and molecular levels. *Long term potential* (LTP) provides a useful conceptual framework for understanding the cellular basis of learning[15] and the possible effects of ethanol on this important basis of learned behavior via the NMDA receptors (see Section 9.5.4). Emotional behavior, a specific form of learning, results from sensory inputs, which are assimilated and processed in association with existing memories within the limbic system. Prenatally and postnatally, the development and maintenance of this neuronal infrastructure is significantly influenced by the internal biochemical status of the brain. In discussing the interference of ethanol with cellular protein synthesis, Krebs[16] has pointed to the biochemical adaptation of the enzymes which degrade the amino acids tryptophan and tyrosine. These essential amino acids must be conserved when the diet is low in protein and must be removed when in excess in order to prevent the formation of the physiologically destabilizing compounds such as tyramine and tryptamine. In this respect, ethanol inhibits the capacity of the tissues to adapt and maintain a homeostatic state. Within this internal environment the presence of growth factors[17] (e.g., interleukin 1), hormones (e.g., cortisol), neurotoxic compounds (e.g., nicotine and ethanol), and nutrients (e.g., amino acids and vitamins) will have major influence in this early development period. These internal factors can be affected by external stimulation as evidenced by the early death of preprogrammed neurones in one-day-old rats, deprived of their mothers. This maternal deprivation and subsequent death is attributed to decreased levels of neurotrophic factors in the hippocampus of the infant rats.[18] An important conclusion from the concept of neuronal Darwinism, as noted above, is that metabolic changes in brain cells throughout life, recognized or not, may predispose the individual to brain damage. A critical issue here relates to which changes are positive adaptations and which are detrimental in the ontogenetic development of the individual.

Postnatally, the family environment has significant influences on the developing child through inadequate parenting, nutrition, stress, and abuse mediated by neuroendocrine responses. Thiamine deficiency due to medically derived malnutrition has been found in children and can lead to Wernicke encephalopathy if untreated.[19] The biochemical outcome of chronic stress and abuse includes elevated cortisol production, which can chronically result in suppressed cognitive development due to damage to the hippocampus, a region of the brain concerned with learning and memory.[20] Stress in this early period is thought to lead to late-life psychiatric problems.[21] Optimal development, therefore, depends upon a subtle interaction between behavioral events — in particular, mother–infant interactions — and molecular phenomena which require appropriate concentrations of precursors for synthesizing structural and enzymatic proteins required for brain structures, supplemented by a wide array of neurotrophic compounds and cofactors. When alcohol and other drugs are present in the pre- and postnatal environment, this complex set of interactions becomes destabilized due to effects on cellular membranes and receptor-signaling processes.

Studies on fetal alcohol syndrome (FAS) are relevant here in that mechanisms of cellular damage resulting from heavy drinking in pregnant females may provide an insight into the more subtle effects on the nervous system, perhaps unrecognized, of lower levels of consumption which may predispose the individual to alcohol misuse/or damage in later life.[22] A large literature has shown the confounding effect of ethanol on morphological development giving rise to fetal alcohol syndrome[23–25] and brain damage in premature infants.[26,27] Nutritional factors are important during the development of the fetus when the embryonic nervous system is being laid down.

Earlier studies suggested that the neurological problems of FAS were caused by reductions in blood flow leading to hypoxia and acidosis. These events were related to problems in cell replication, cell growth, and cell death, the latter being specifically due to overstimulation of NMDA receptors with consequential excitotoxicity and cell death.[24] This issue will be considered in relation to nutrition factors in Section 9.5.3. In chick embryos and in chronic studies on postnatal development in the rat, chronic ethanol brain protein synthesis is significantly affected. Such major perturbations in tissue formation possibly relate to a multiple systems cascade involving disruptions of protein synthesis, prostaglandins, gangliosides, hypoxia, and free radical damage. Protein synthesis and the expression of various regulatory proteins such as c-Fos and heat shock protein-70 are thought be primarily effected in alcohol-related tissue damage.[7] Various brain regions are differentially damaged by alcohol and here the synthesis of proteins is significantly affected by oxidative stress.[28]

These molecular events impact on the functional capacity of the brain. Cognitive dysfunction has been demonstrated in males, females, and abstinent children of alcohol misusers who lack a P300 wave.[29–34] This neuropsychological response is indicative of frontal lobe problems in the children of alcoholic parents and might be due to genetic factors. Conversely, this dysfunction may originate from a combination of alcohol, nutritional, and hormonal factors, which adversely affect pre-, peri-, or postnatal development.

Cognitive impairment in alcoholics frequently takes the form of frontal lobe dysfunction and may be relatively subtle, requiring a neuropsychological examination for diagnosis. Signs of cognitive impairment may precede those of alcohol-related neurological disorders by more than 10 years.[35]

9.4 COGNITIVE DYSFUNCTION IN ALCOHOL DEPENDENCY

Alcohol consumption impairs information processing and cognitive performance on a range of tasks[36,37] and chronic misuse of ethanol is associated with mild to severe neuro-cognitive deficits compared to controls that are nonusers of alcoholic beverages.[38] Social drinkers, drinking most heavily, perform less well on tests of memory and abstract thinking compared to peers drinking at lower levels.[39] A well-known severe form of brain damage in alcohol misusers is Wernicke's encephalopathy. This acute brain syndrome is associated with neurocognitive impairment, — severe short-term amnesia, mental confusion, eye movement abnormalities, and poor muscular coordination.[40] If treated inadequately, this acute syndrome may lead to the chronic deficit state of Korsakoff's psychosis, characterized by impairment of short-term memory and confabulation.[41] Aside from this severe form of alcoholic brain damage there is a much less severe and general overall pattern of neurocognitive deficits seen in statistically significant numbers in the general population of alcohol-misuse patients. Typically, patients with extensive histories of alcohol dependence display relatively preserved verbal reasoning and verbal learning skills, but they have measurable deficits on tests of verbal problem solving, conceptual shifting, perceptual–spatial and abstracting abilities, motor speed, information-processing speed, and memory.[42] Because the therapeutic and educational components of most alcohol treatment programs rely heavily on auditory and visual presentations of material, the presence of cognitive impairment may restrict patients' abilities to receive, encode, and integrate the newly introduced information, thereby limiting impaired patients' capabilities to make substantive behavioral changes in response to therapy.[43] Cognitive impairment appears to be a significant predictor of treatment outcome.[39]

9.4.1 ASSESSMENT OF BRAIN DAMAGE

In view of the potential treatment implications of impaired cognitive status among alcohol misuse patients, several authors[35,44,45] have argued for more widespread use of neuropsychological testing in substance misuse treatment programs. However, evaluation with comprehensive neuropsychological test batteries, such as the Halstead–Reitan Neuropsychological Test Battery,[46] is costly in terms of administration and scoring time (approximately 3 to 10 h), making their routine use impractical in most settings. Short-version neuropsychological instruments emphasizing the assessment of known deficit areas of alcoholics have been introduced but none show high correlation to deficits found in more robust and comprehensive instruments. In light of recent technological advancements in the computer industry, a new alternative has become available to researchers and clinicians in the field of addiction medicine.

Computer-based assessment has become an attractive alternative to traditional assessment procedures in psychological testing. Computer-assisted assessment packages have gradually progressed from software that merely scores item responses to comprehensive programs that administer the test, then immediately compute the scores, and generate the interpretative reports that summarize the test results.

A relatively new, brief, neuropsychological assessment device that addresses the related alcohol deficit areas of verbal problem solving, conceptual shifting, perceptual–spatial and abstracting abilities, motor speed, information-processing speed, and memory has recently been developed as a computer-based instrument. It is called The Bexley, Maudsley Automated Psychological Screening Test (BMAPS), derived from the well-known paper-and-pencil instrument used by Acker and Shaw. This is a collection of psychological screening tests based on original research and designed for automated presentation by computer. It was originally developed for the Commodore Pet computer by William and Clare Acker.[47] The current version has been updated to run on an IBM-compatible computer using Microsoft Windows 95 or Windows NT. The theoretical emphasis of the BMAPS test is toward nonverbal skills because these abilities can be identified only by testing and are found in spite of intact verbal intelligence. Therefore, nonverbal deficits are easy to overlook unless specific means of assessment are available. The tests included are ones that have been used for distinguishing between alcoholic and other psychological problems.

Presently, normative and clinical values of the PC version of BMAPS are being determined for a range of clinical applications.[48] By providing an insight into the severity of cognitive dysfunction, the effectiveness of interventions may be measured with the ultimate objective of improving cognitive performance.

9.5 BRAIN DYSFUNCTION: MALADAPTATION OR NEUROTOXICITY?

Human brains have been subjected to selective pressures since the dawn of humankind. Brains evolved to be responsive to experience but the degree of tolerance to maltreatment and physiological stressors such as malnutrition must have limits. When these limits are exceeded, behavioral dysfunction and pathological states appear. An insight into these issues is provided by the destabilization of behavioral and physiological homeostasis brought about by chronic alcohol consumption.[21,49]

9.5.1 BEHAVIOR, NEUROTRANSMISSION, AND NUTRITION

During development and in the adult, a number of interactions between neurotransmitter and peptidergic systems are important in modulating behavior. For example, noradrenergic neurons are principally involved in activation via the ascending reticular activation system (ARAS). Dopaminergic neurons form the circuitry of the mesolimbic dopamine reward system (MDRS). Disorders of function of serotonin (5-HT) innervation of a number of brain systems are linked to a wide range of neuropsychiatric and related conditions including depression, insomnia, aggression and anxiety, eating disorders, hypertension, behavioral disinhibition,[50–52] pathological and suicidal aggression, aggression,[53] and delirium.[54–56]

There is substantial evidence that 5-HT is involved in the control of mood and cognitive performance.[57,58] Brain 5-HT is dependent on the availability of the amino acid precursor tryptophan (Trp), which competes with other large neutral amino acids (LNAA's) for transport into the brain via the blood–brain barrier[59]. Mental performance is significantly affected by changes in the Trp/LNAA ratio.[60–62] This ratio is decreased following consumption of ethanol over a 2- to 3-h time period.[63]

Excitatory amino acids (glutamate, aspartate) provide major activation and inhibitory (GABA) influences on brain function. There are two types of glutamate receptors, alpha-amino-3-hydroxy-5-methyl-4-isoxazole-proprionate (AMPA) and *N*-methyl-D-aspartate (NMDA), which are found in neurons within the hippocampus and facilitate memory function and learning. This is the cellular basis of learning called LTP.[15] discussed in Section 9.3.

These neurotransmitter and neuromodulatory systems provide the psychopharmacological substrate through which behaviors, including those related to problems of alcohol and other drug dependencies, are expressed. Significant changes in biogenic amine transmitter systems and tryptophan metabolism occur within the first year of life.[64] These changes are thought to be important in the regulation of 5-HT synthesis, possibly indicating a role for this compound not only as a neurotransmitter but also a neuromodulator influencing neurodifferentiation in certain regions of the brain.[65]

In addition to the above mechanisms, phosphate esters of thiamine have been implicated in neural transmission. However, limited evidence is presently available to support this hypothesis.[66]

9.5.2 REWARD-MEDIATED BEHAVIOR

Acute and chronic effects of ethanol intoxication and withdrawal have been associated with a number of neurotransmitters which condense with acetaldehyde, the primary metabolite of ethanol, to form tetrahydroisoquinolines (TIQs). TIQs have similar properties and function as opioids.[67] Furthermore, opioids and ethanol appear to act on a similar receptor systems, providing an explanation for enhanced ethanol drinking in rodents, and the possibility that the opioid-like properties of TIQs compensate for a deficiency in opioid activity.

Evidence of this has been obtained from studies of laboratory bred genetic strains of mice, C57BL and DBA, which are alcohol- and water-preferring, respectively.[51] This suggests a genetic basis to alcohol-seeking behavior which is underpinned by an opioid-linked metabolic response to ethanol. Chronic administration of ethanol has been shown to decrease opioid concentrations in the brain and pituitary,[68] with 50% or more decreases in hypothalamic and hippocampal levels of dynorphin and alpha neo-endorphin.[51] Genazzani et al.[69] found a threefold reduction of beta-endorphin in the CSF of chronic alcoholics, compared to controls. It is interesting to speculate on the relevance of the studies described in Section 9.3. Here the endocrine-related consequences of high levels of stress in children and deficits in the opioid-linked system are correlated with dysfunctional mother–infant bonding.[20] An interesting question arises as to whether this disrupted developmental progression should be considered to be *brain damage* per se or a *maladaptive behavior.* No matter which description is used, the reality of the irreversibility of this process strongly suggests the overwhelming influence of child abuse on later-life behaviors and antecedents of psychiatric morbidity.[70]

Opioids and ethanol, therefore, appear to have common modes of action by modifying the responsiveness of the mesolimbic–dopamine reward system and other parts of the limbic system, the outcomes of which are expressed in terms of craving and behaviors associated with withdrawal. A molecular explanation for some of these actions has been proposed by Blum,[71] with reference to the reward cascade. The cascade is thought to be initiated in the hypothalamus where neurons secrete serotonin (5-HT), causing the activation of methionine enkephalin, an opioid peptide. This peptide, produced in the substantia nigra by inhibiting GABA receptors, controls the production of dopamine (DA) from the ventral tegmental area (VTA). Increased DA then has both a direct effect on neurones in the nucleus accumbens and an indirect effect on CA_1 cells in the hippocampus. Both of these regions act as target messengers of reward. This homeostatically regulated system could be dysregulated by a dysfunctioning neurotransmitter (e.g., 5-HT) or neuromodulator (e.g., an opioid peptide) resulting in a change in affect (emotional) or overt behavior. Such perturbations could originate from neuroendocrine stress-related changes, changes in immune system status, drug-induced changes, genetically inherited neurotranmitter defects and nutritional imbalances.

The concentration of 5-HT in the brain, therefore, has a significant influence on mental state. Furthermore, in contrast to other neurotransmitters, brain 5-HT is dependent on the availability of its dietary precursor, tryptophan.

9.5.3 Ethanol and Serotonergic Modulation of Brain Function

From the previous sections it will be noted that many of the effects of ethanol on behavior will involve perturbations of 5-HT and related systems either by direct impact of ethanol causing the degeneration of 5-HT axons and axon terminals[72] or via other aspects of the metabolism of tryptophan, the precursor of 5-HT. Acutely, ethanol depletes brain serotonin in normal subjects, which may explain alcohol-induced aggression[53] in susceptible individuals and also the incidence of depression in alcohol misusers.[73]

Tryptophan availability to the brain is increased before the appearance of the alcohol-withdrawal syndrome (AWS) in humans, raising the possibility that the associated behavioral disturbances seen in AWS are related to this metabolic domain.[74–76] Tryptophan metabolism is also implicated in the predisposition to becoming alcohol dependent.[77]

These effects of tryptophan metabolism in the brain do not solely involve 5-HT; instead a major effect on tryptophan metabolism results from enzymes involved in the conversion of tryptophan into kynurenine-related compounds (see Figure 9.1).

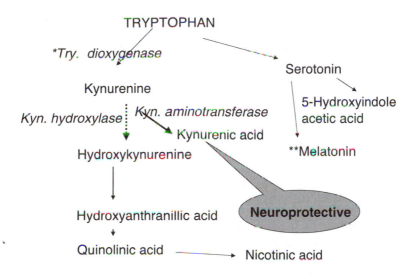

FIGURE 9.1 Metabolism of tryptophan. * = hepatic inducible enzyme; ** = free radical scavenger.

9.5.4 TRYPTOPHAN METABOLISM AND NEUROTOXICITY

The principal enzyme involved in the diversion of tryptophan from 5-HT synthesis into kynurenine and its metabolites is tryptophan-dioxygenase (TDO, or tryptophan pyrrolase) located in the liver (see Figure 9.1). Molecular studies using cDNA encoding, isolation, and protein characterization have revealed that the TDO gene contains glucocorticoid-responsive elements. Furthermore, glucocorticoid administration increases TDO formation in the liver, suggesting a link between cortisol production (stress related) and the induction of the TDO gene. This will result in a decrease in blood levels of tryptophan which, following TDO enzyme induction, will divert circulating tryptophan into the kynurenine pathway and cause a subsequent reduction in the pool of tryptophan for synthesis into 5-HT in the brain. This reduction of brain 5-HT synthesis will be exacerbated by the competition between kynurenine and Trp for the same transporters through the blood–brain barrier.[78] The consequences of reduced brain 5-HT have been outlined above. Furthermore glucocorticoid administration increases TDO formation in the liver, the induction of which is responsible for mood changes in patients chronically treated with glucocorticoids due to reduced tryptophan catabolism in the liver and increase in the brain. TDO gene regulation may be an important biological determinant of the ethanol withdrawal syndrome.[74]

A second mechanism which results in the formation of kynurenine is via the enzyme indoleamine 2,3-dioxygenase (IDO). High concentration of kynurenine are excreted in the urine of patients with rheumatoid arthritis, tuberculosis, leukemia, Hodgkin's disease, and bladder tumors. IDO production is induced by interferons and other proinflammatory cytokines leading to the suggestion that cellular deprivation of tryptophan results in the antiproliferation effects of interferon.[79] IDO induction plays a role in immunological tolerance between mother and fetus and might have relevance where poor health due to social exclusion and inequalities is associated with high consumption of alcohol and other drugs.

The kynurenine metabolite quinolinic acid has been implicated in neurologic diseases and neurodegeneration including Huntingdon's disease, temporal lobe epilepsy, glutaric aciduria, hepatic encephalopathy, and coma.[55] Quinolinic acid (QA) destroys neuronal cell bodies. Cortical cells with NMDA receptors are particularly sensitive to QA. Elevated QA concentrations have been found in viral infections, forebrain global ischemia, and spinal trauma.[80] In autopic Huntington's disease patients, 3OH-anthranilate-3,4-dioxygenase required for the formation of QA appears to be increased.[81]

NMDA receptors mediate the actions of many of the excitatory amino acids such as glutamate. This is central to memory function and learning via LTP. Quinolinic acid is a selective excitant (agonist) of the NMDA receptor. Kynurenic acid is an antagonist,[55] having a neuroprotective role.

Neurotoxicity induced by quinolinic acid primarily occurs in the hippocampus, striatum, and neocortex brain areas particularly affected by the disorders mentioned above. Animal studies suggest that quinolinic acid causes axon-sparing lesions.[82] Excitotoxicity results in overstimulation of NMDA receptors in the hippocampus affecting LTP and the cellular basis of learning (see Section 9.3 and Section 9.5.1). 3OH-kynurenine, the precursor of quinolinic acid, can bring about neuronal apoptosis and necrosis.[83]

The link with ethanol consumption stems from observation of increased sensitivity of NMDA receptors in alcohol withdrawal,[75,84] excitotoxic damage due to neural compensation for sustained alcohol levels, and nutritional deficits underlying alcohol-related brain damage. The specific nutritional deficit here is thiamine.[85] Other studies have demonstrated the role of reduced hippocampal glutamate decarboxylase (GAD) in cell death occurring during ethanol dependence.[86] The development of brain damage in binge drinkers is more likely due to increased vulnerability of the brain to these neurotoxic mechanisms.[87]

9.5.5 TRYPTOPHAN METABOLISM AND NEUROPROTECTION

While one component of the kynurenine pathway is implicated in neurotoxicity, there is substantial evidence that an alternative pathway involving kynurenic acid (KA) is important in providing neuro-protection. KA is an antagonist of the excitatory amino acid receptor NMDA.[88] It can be synthesized in the brain and can also be transported through the blood–brain barrier and taken up by glia cells. KA causes an increased expression and synthesis of growth factors.[89] Shifting the balance of kynurenine metabolism from 3-hydroxykynurenine, which leads to quinolinic acid, to KA reduces glutamate receptor activation and excitotoxic or ischemic neuronal damage.[82]

In the development of neuroprotective agents, pharmacological compounds designed as KA prodrugs and KA analogues are being produced. These compounds are presently being investigated in a number of clinical trials focusing on neurodegenerative disorders.

Clinical trials for stroke, Alzheimer's disease, Parkinson's disease, and related disorders are underway. Further studies into cerebral ischemia, HIV, Parkinson's disease, schizophrenia, epilepsy, and depression are being pursued.[90] Commercially produced compounds include KA derivatives, designed as NMDA antagonists (e.g., L705022, L701324) and pro-drugs of KA (e.g., SC49468, 4,6-dichlorokynurenine) have been developed. Modulators of QA and KA concentrations (e.g., 540C91) lower the concentrations of TDO and NCR631 and inhibit 3-hydroxyanthranilic acid, reducing the loss of hippocampal cells.

Despite this extensive work on pharmacologically designed neuroprotectants, therapeutic trials have yet to be been undertaken on patients with alcohol-related brain damage. With regard to the rehabilitation of alcohol misusers, a pharmacological approach is probably not the most appropriate strategy where the possibility of substitute dependencies might arise. A more realistic way forward is to support behavioral and physiological change during addiction rehabilitation by more naturalistic methods such as dietary interventions. The success of this approach will depend on how much and when, during the diurnal cycle, the supplement should be given. The ability of the patient to absorb the nutrients will relate to the degree of malabsorption, i.e., pathological stage of the gut, and will determine whether oral or parenteral therapy will be effective.

9.5.6 Thiamine Deficiency and Neurological Responses

Chronic alcohol consumption when an individual has adequate nutrition results in subtle brain damage in cortical and subcortical regions.[91] However, it has been well established that major neurological symptoms occur in cases of thiamine deficiency. In 1881, Wernicke[92] described behavioral and pathological signs of an acute superior hemorrhagic polioencephalitis (Wernicke's encephalopathy) afflicting alcoholics. The most frequent indications of this condition include lethargy, fatigue, apathy, impaired awareness, loss of equilibrium, disorientation, difficulty concentrating, retrograde amnesia, ophthalmoplegia, anorexia, muscle weakness, peripheral numbness, paresthesia, and ataxia. Korsakoff's psychosis was later identified as including disorientation, hallucinations, confabulation, memory loss, perceptual impairments, impaired linguistic processing, anterograde amnesia, and global intellectual impairment similar to presenile dementia or dementia of Alzheimer's disease.[40,92] Witt[93] has demonstrated bilaterally symmetrical lesions in a range of animal species, particularly in the hypothalamus, periventricular regions of the thalamus, the mammillary bodies, the midbrain, brainstem, and cerebellum. Metabolic, neurophysiological, and genetic mechanisms have been proposed to explain these selective vulnerabilities. For instance, the thiamine-utilizing enzyme transketolase and its cofactor thiamine pyrophosphate (TPP) possibly provide the differential selectivity of the various brain tissues.[91] Oxidative stress (i.e., abnormal metabolism of free radicals) contributes to this process of neurodegeneration in that reductions in thiamine and thiamine-dependent processes promote neurodegeneration and cause oxidative stress.[94] However, the spectrum of pathological changes observed depended on the number of deprivation and recovery periods.[93] While inadequate thiamine intake and general malnutrition are primary deficiencies, secondary effects are caused by ethanol-induced destruction of intestinal mucosa, inhibiting the absorption of thiamine by as much as 90% in chronic alcohol misusers. They include persistent vomiting and chronic diarrhea. Liver damage will further reduce thiamine metabolism and storage. Folic acid and magnesium deficiencies may induce signs of thiamine deficiency. Furthermore, gastrointestinal carcinoma, AIDS, anorexia, rapid parenteral carbohydrate loading, and multiple organ failure syndrome may give rise to polyneuropathies similar to Wernicke's/Korsakoff's psychosis (WP).[40] Chronic alcohol misusers with liver disease have a limited ability to absorb folates, thiamine, and B_6, and appear to absorb pantothenate and riboflavin.[95]

Wernicke's encephalopathy (WE), leading to Korsakoff's psychosis (KP), is perhaps the most widely known and best understood neuropsychiatric disorder associated with long-term alcohol misuse, the mechanisms of which might be considered to be *alcohol neurotoxicity* or *thiamine malnutrition*.[96] Results from the animal model with induced thiamine deficiency encephalopathy (TDE) have pointed to the role of glutamate neurotoxicity (or excitotoxicity) as the primary cause of TDE. Although seizure-like movements and opisthotonus are found in both TDE and WKS, there are some neurological differences between the animal and human situations. Nevertheless, a blockade of NMDA-type glutamate receptors by MK-801 provides significant protection against TDE, suggesting a mechanism as follows: Glutamate concentrations increase in the third and fourth ventricles which causes an increase of this excitatory amino acid in the cerebral spinal fluid (CSF). Ventricular CSF then diffuses into the periventricular and peraqueductal brain loci, thereby causing lesions of WE. It appears that brain lesions found in WE and TDE do not result from decreased energy metabolism but are caused by a significant reduction of glutamic acid decarboxylase (GAD), a consequence of thiamine-deficient tissue status.[97] A model showing the impact of thiamine (B_1), vitamin B_2, and B_6 deficiencies on cellular energy metabolism and glutamate accumulation leading to neurotoxicity and cell death has been presented by Thomson et al.[1] (see Figure 9.2).

9.5.7 THIAMINE DEFICIENCY AND TRYPTOPHAN METABOLISM

Both thiamine deficiency and abnormal tryptophan metabolism give rise to symptoms in alcohol withdrawal. This suggests that brain damage may also be compounded by these two factors. The explanation for this is as follows: Alcohol withdrawal (AWS) is caused primarily by an imbalance between neuroexcitability and neuroinhibition. GABA is the major inhibitory neurotransmitter in the CNS. Both GABA and its receptor are downregulated by chronic alcohol misuse. The downregulation persists after cessation of alcohol and contributes significantly to the AWS. Chronic alcohol misuse inhibits activity in the glutamate neurotransmitter system. Abstention reverses it and adds to the symptomatology of the AWS.

GABA and glutamate production are managed by conversion of Alpha-ketoglutarate to glutamate, glutamate to GABA, and GABA to succinate, i.e., the GABA shunt that bypasses the rate-limiting step in the TCA cycle of alpha-ketoglutarate to succinate, which is facilitated by alpha-ketoglutarate reductase, a thiamine dependent enzyme (see Figure 9.2). The conversion of glutamate to GABA requires the

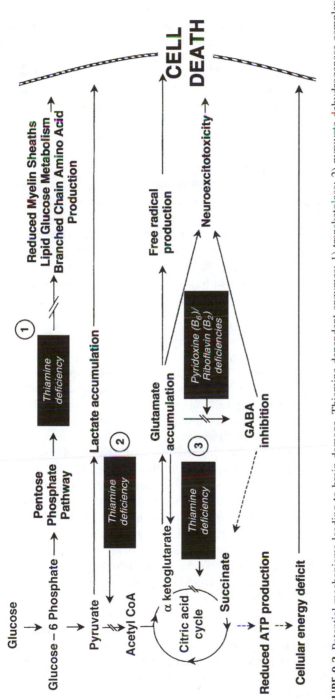

FIGURE 9.2 Potential mechanisms leading to brain damage. Thiamine-dependent enzymes: 1) transketolase; 2) pyruvate dehydrogenase complex; 3) α-ketoglutarate dehydrogenase complex. (From Thomson, A.D., Cook, C.C., Touquet, R., and Henry, J.A. The Royal College of Physicians report on alcohol: guidelines for managing Wernicke's encephalopathy in the accident and emergency department. *Alcohol Alcohol.*, 37: 513–521; 2002. With permission.)

presence of glutamic acid decarboxylase (GAD). For GAD to function it must bind to pyridoxal 5 phosphate (P5P) which is produced from pyridoxine and requires the presence of riboflavin. It appears, therefore, that production of adequate supplies of GABA during alcohol withdrawal — and, importantly, reductions in glutamate levels — both require adequate supplies of P5P and thus adequate supplies of B_6 and B_2.

During alcohol withdrawal one would expect this situation to become worse if thiamine deficiency was also present, as this would force a greater production of activity through the GABA shunt. In these circumstances there would be no problem if there were sufficient P5P to bind to GAD. In the case of B_6 and B_2 deficiency the conversion of glutamate to GABA would be impeded, resulting in an imbalance in favor of neuroexcitation. This raises the question as to whether the imbalance can be improved by high doses of B_1, B_2, and B_6.

In addition to specific and perhaps critical factors such as glutamate activity, the cumulative effect of many factors indicated in Figure 9.2 may also be important contributory factors.

Studies of cognition in older persons suggest that plasma vitamin C and carotene concentrations are good predictors of memory function.[98] These results add to the evidence that oxidative stress plays a significant role in neurodegeneration, a gradual process which precedes the clinical manifestation of Alzheimer's disease, Parkinson's disease, and perhaps WE and KP.

9.5.8 RELATIONSHIP OF AWS TO WE

There are a number of factors in common between AWS and WE. First, free radical production and excitotoxicity caused by excess glutamate has been proposed as a major factor in the development of WE. Presumably, the lack of GABA would contribute to cell death by increasing cell vulnerability to excitation. B_1 deficiency pushes metabolism through the GABA shunt which, if overloaded due to lack of B_2 and B_6, would result in an excess of glutamate.

Some evidence for this is suggested by the work of Shaw[99] who showed the reduction in withdrawal delirium and incidence of fitting were achieved using benzodiazepines, but there were no significant changes seen in symptoms in a group of highly dependent alcohol misusers over 8 days (see Figure 9.3). This is an important observation as WE occurring in detoxification is often overlooked. WE and AWS share the same symptoms. The only sign of WE may be confusion. In view of the relatively low incidence (16%) of the classic triad of WE, an interesting question is how frequently this is observed in patients undergoing detoxification.

Subclinical episodes of WE may occur and the presentation of incipient WE is varied and difficult to diagnose. If, however, AWS is created by the same problem, i.e., multiple vitamin B deficiencies plus abnormal tryptophan, then these patients should be treated with adequate supplementation. This idea suggests strong support for the administration of parenteral vitamins to "revolving door" alcoholics in casualty or elsewhere. A common mechanism affected by thiamine deficiency and tryptophan disturbance during withdrawal is probably related to NMDA receptors and exocytotoxic neuronal death.[100]

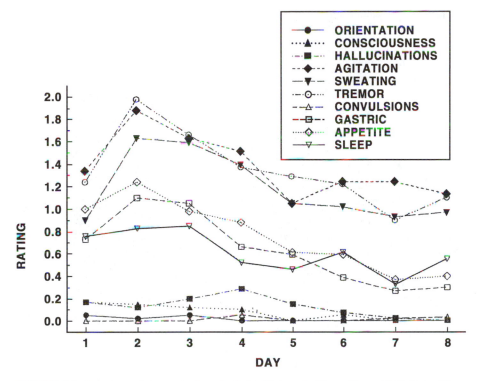

FIGURE 9.3 Symptom changes during alcohol withdrawal. (From Shaw, G.K. Detoxification: the use of benzodiazepines. *Alcohol Alcohol.*, 30: 765; 1995. With permission.)

9.6 NUTRITIONAL APPROACHES TO MINIMIZING ALCOHOL-RELATED BRAIN DAMAGE

Structural and functional damage due to long-term alcohol consumption results in neuropsychological impairment, mood disorders, and personality changes. Damage is normally located in temporal and prefrontal areas, regions which are specialized for memory, working memory, strategic planning, goal selection, and response inhibition. Interference with these cognitive functions will undoubtedly mitigate against good outcomes in alcohol rehabilitation programmes.[43,101] Current treatments aim to change behavior and develop skills to prevent relapse and enhance psychosocial adaptation. Clearly attempts to arrest and hopefully reverse cognitive decline, and to improve quality of life should be central to the strategy of rehabilitation, thereby increasing a sense of meaning and belonging in previously socially excluded individuals. Relapse occurs frequently in "rehabilitated" clients and high-order measurements such as length of tenancy or social connectivity might not be the best indicators of the appropriate treatment regime, as attempted by Project MATCH. The ideas developed in this chapter suggest that the principal outcomes of long-term drinking will be cognitive deficits, ranging from severe memory problems in WE/KP to more subtle impairments which may be assessed using the approach discussed in

Section 9.4.1. Behavioral therapies employing practice can lead to improved performance. More generalized approaches can be employed by cognitive behavior therapy (CBT). However, these methods are likely to be limited in their effectiveness if cellular mechanisms of brain function are compromised by neurotoxic factors, which mainly emanate from nutritional imbalances. Section 9.5, above, suggests a number of possibilities for developing nutritional strategies which might be used as adjuncts to cognitive and behavioral therapies.

9.6.1 NUTRITIONAL STRATEGIES AIMED AT REWARD-MEDIATED BEHAVIORS

Litten and Allen[102] have reviewed animal studies in which dietary interventions have been aimed at influencing alcohol intake. While consistent results have been obtained when dietary proteins were manipulated, more variable findings were obtained from research on fats and/or carbohydrates. Carbohydrates may reduce available thiamine. The most likely explanation for this observation is that high carbohydrate will result in an insulin surge which will cause large neutral amino acids (LNAAs) to be absorbed into muscle, reducing competition for transport of tryptophan across the blood–brain barrier and permitting enhanced synthesis of central 5-HT. Raised brain 5-HT is known to reduce drinking behavior. This suggestion is supported by McBride et al.[103] who found a 68% reduction in alcohol consumption with i.p. administration of D,L-5-hydroxytryptophan in alcohol-preferring rats. Similar results were obtained by others.[104–106] However, in contrast to these observations, an alternative explanation is that acetaldehyde produced from oxidation of ethanol may mediate these dietary effects as demonstrated by higher levels of acetaldehyde in alcohol-avoiding strains of rats compared to alcohol-preferring rats.[107]

In Section 9.5.1 evidence was provided that common brain reward-mediated behaviors involve (1) opiates, presumed to influence the reward circuits via opiate receptor-mediated activation of the mesolimbic dopamine system, (2) alcohol by the formation of condensation products (TIQs) which are thought to interact with opioid receptors, thereby stimulating catecholamine systems, and (3) alcohol through a cascade of events in which 5-HT, endogenous opioids and dopamine activate the norepinephrine neurones of the mesolimbic circuitry. From this theoretical perspective Blum[108] has developed a dietary supplement which includes amino acids and vitamins that are designed to assist in neurochemical restoration. The rationale here is to raise brain neurotransmitter levels and affect behavior and opioid degradation inhibition to reduce drug-seeking behavior. SAAVE contains D-phenylanine which is thought to inhibit enkephalinase, and was developed primarily for alcohol and opiate misusers by purportedly increasing levels of endogenous opioids. Tropamine was designed as an adjunct for the treatment of cocaine abuse. A double-blind placebo-controlled study of SAAVE and an open clinical trial with tropamine provided evidence of the effectiveness of these supplements. Improvements in craving, reduced withdrawal tremors, reduced stress levels (by skin conductance), increased behavioral, emotional, social, spiritual, and physical scores were found in the inpatient treatment of alcoholics, cocaine abusers, and polydrug users.[108] In reviewing the work of Blum, Litten and Allen[102] point out that this work did not examine the role of individual amino acids and, as the physical and BESS scores are subjective, it is likely that the subjects in the trial were able to discriminate between the dietary formulation and the placebo.

Despite some inconsistencies in the literature the prospect of nutritional therapy to modify neurotransmitters in the brain and thus modify drinking behavior suggests the importance of amino acid supplements which include *l*-glutamine, *l*-tryptophan, L-5-hydroxytryptophan and *l*-phenylanine, which are precursors for neurotransmitters thought to alter ethanol consumption. Additionally, iodine, zinc, and sodium have been implicated in alcohol seeking in experimental animal studies.[102] The nature and dosage of the nutritional supplement should be researched in relation to the nutritional requirements of alcohol misusers.

9.6.2 VITAMIN SUPPLEMENTATION IN THE MANAGEMENT OF ALCOHOL-RELATED BRAIN DAMAGE

Supplementation of thiamine has been employed and shown to have a therapeutic benefit in alcohol-dependent subpopulations without severe KP as shown in the first reported randomized, double-blind, multidose study by Ambrose et al.[109] Increased alcohol consumption has been found in thiamine and B complex deficient rats.[110,111] However these early studies have not been substantiated.

Thomson et al.[112] found a significant decrease in thiamine absorption in alcoholic patients by measuring radioactivity in the femoral artery, hepatic vein, and umbilical vein. Using ^{35}S-thiamine together with a nonradioactive flushing dose of thiamine, Thomson showed that the cumulative urinary radioactivity over a 72-h period was a measure of the amount of thiamine originally absorbed. This model provided evidence that absorption in alcohol misusers was significantly reduced, and that very significant improvements in absorption occurred in malnourished patients after treatment with a nutritious diet, a situation which was rapidly reversed after oral or parenteral ethanol in one third of the patients.[112] Applying enzyme kinetic mathematics to ^{35}S-thiamine and flushing doses of nonradioactive doses of thiamine, Thomson and Leevy[113] showed that this vitamin is absorbed by a saturable mechanism with a maximum absorption of approximately 4.5 to 5.6 mg of thiamine hydrochloride after a single dose of this compound, and that the number of effective receptor sites may be reduced by malnutrition or intestinal resection.[114] Work by Heap and Pratt et al.[115] has highlighted the importance of the thiamine-dependent enzyme transketolase in vulnerability to alcohol-induced cognitive deficit and KP, and the existence of subgroups of alcohol misusers who have elevated requirements for thiamine in addition to abnormal transketolase protein. These discoveries led to a number of studies into the effectiveness of dosing regimes and the optimization of nutritional support for chronic alcohol abusing patients.[116] Guidelines for the management of WE patients in accident and emergency departments have recently been published.[117] Building on the evidence and mechanism of alcoholic brain damage caused by thiamine deficiency in chronic alcohol misusers, the principal recommendation of this paper is that patients suspected of having a poor diet should be treated as soon as possible with intravenous or intramuscular injections of B vitamins. This recommendation is based on evidence that 30 to 80% of alcohol misusing patients have low circulating levels of thiamine,[41] intestinal absorption of thiamine being reduced by 70% in these patients, then another 50% by ethanol consumption. This work suggests that total absorption of thiamine from three oral doses of 100 mg each would be reduced to one third or less of that in healthy subjects (i.e., 5 mg in 24 h). Conversely, in healthy subjects, an oral dose of 30 mg will achieve maximum plasma concentration due to rate-limiting enzymes, and would be adequate for healthy subjects with mild deficiency.

To overcome the problems of intestinal absorption, oral administration of lipid soluble allithiamines (thiamine propyl disulfide, TPD, and thiamine tetrahydrofurfuryl disulfide, TTHD) has been used. TPD is absorbed from the intestine by diffusion and provides blood concentrations similar to IV thiamine administration.[118] TPD absorption is not impaired in alcohol misusers and no toxic effects were found after 3 to 6 months of continuously high doses of TPD.[119,120] A formulation called ThiaSure, manufactured by Recovery Pharmaceuticals, contains 50 mg of TPD plus other nutrients such as folic acid, vitamins B_{12}, B_6, and magnesium. TPD has been widely used in Japan since the 1950s and a similar product has been available in Germany. ThiaSure is sold in the U.S. as a dietary supplement; however, it is not recommended where IV administration of thiamine is indicated in the absence of clinical trials to determine its efficacy.

Further research is required into genetic markers in order to indicate individuals who have transketolase deficiencies[115] and also into B vitamin absorption measurements for those who have problems with intestinal malabsorption as indicated above. However, the latter is not practical due to ethical reasons. In view of the problems of identifying those at most risk of developing WE, more research is needed to develop neuropsychological tools for the early detection of functional deficits.

9.6.3 Tryptophan Supplementation in Alcohol Withdrawal

The review of tryptophan metabolism above presents the possibility of tryptophan supplementation in minimizing the side effect of alcohol withdrawal in patients with alcoholism. Dietary manipulation of brain 5-HT is possible as the conversion of the dietary amino acid tryptophan is regulated by the enzyme tryptophan hydroxylase. This enzyme is unsaturated and thus increased availability of the precursor tryptophan leads to an increased synthesis of 5-HT dietary.[78,121] Increases in the Trp/LNAA ratio influence the transport of Trp across the blood–brain barrier facilitating an increase in the synthesis of brain serotonin.[122] The potential benefits of facilitating brain serotonin by enhancing tryptophan metabolism in recovering alcohol-dependent individuals has been previously reviewed indicating that Trp metabolism is implicated in the predisposition to becoming alcohol dependent. Additionally, alcohol has a major effect on tryptophan metabolism by its perturbation of enzymes involved in the conversion of tryptophan into kynurenine-related compounds. Work by one of the authors (ABB) of this chapter indicates that changes in tryptophan metabolism during detoxification probably contribute to alcohol withdrawal syndrome.[123] Elevations of kynurenine metabolites in the early stages of withdrawal have been previously noted by the present authors.

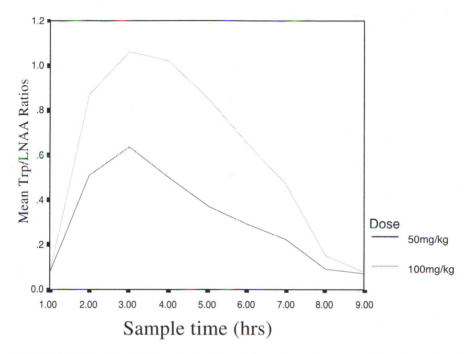

FIGURE 9.4 Mean Trp/LNAA ratios in nine abstinent alcohol misusers, at two doses of oral Trp: 50 mg/kg and 100 mg/kg.

The potential for dietary manipulation of Trp solely of carbohydrates and proteins in the absence of supplements is unlikely to result in significant behavioral changes.[124] In a pilot study to develop a tryptophan supplementation strategy, plasma tryptophan and tryptophan metabolite profiles have been studied in nine abstinent alcohol-misusing patients. Responses to *two* different dietary tryptophan loads were investigated to establish the most efficacious dose and frequency of administration of the supplement. In this study, tryptophan levels remained significantly elevated for up to 6 h and up to 10 h for the 50 and 100 mg/kg doses, respectively. This was reflected in the Trp/LNAA ratio (see Figure 9.4).

As elevation of the tryptophan/LNAA ratio demonstrated here suggests, the therapeutic possibility of self-medication via dietary manipulation could be employed by appropriately motivated individuals. The potential benefits in the treatment of alcohol dependency include reducing craving, reducing anxiety and depression, ameliorating memory loss, and an overall neuroprotection since tryptophan metabolism is central to each of these issues.[51,55] The results from these preliminary experiments provide evidence that not only is there a lack of significant change in the concentrations of the neurotoxic metabolite 3-HK but the concentrations of the neuroprotectant KA are significantly elevated. This is an important finding in view of the increased cytotoxic damage which is associated with alcohol withdrawal, and linked with alcohol withdrawal-induced seizures.

9.7 CONCLUSION

A review of the literature suggests that the development of alcohol-related brain damage results from an accumulation of critical events and circumstances which begin prenatally. Genetic predisposition is multifactorial and includes polymorphisms in tryptophan metabolism (Trp dioxygenase), B vitamin enzymes (in particular transketolase) and dopamine (DRD2 and DRD4 receptors), providing a combination of physiological and behavioral influences which increase vulnerability to alcohol consumption and later brain damage in some individuals. Postnatally inadequate caregiving will contribute to this vulnerability by inappropriate nutrition. A stressful/abusive childhood will compromise the optimal development of the nervous system by nutritional deficiencies and chronic production of the neuronal-damaging stress hormone cortisol. As the individual begins to consume alcohol, interaction of ethanol with endorphin, serotonergic, and other brain systems will not only exacerbate drinking behavior but will adversely affect behavioral performance as a result of accruing neuropsychological deficits. These behavioral problems will limit social success and increase the possibility of social exclusion. Nutritional factors confound the effect of alcohol in disadvantaged populations.[125] Reduced intake of thiamine and other vitamins due to poor nutrition, increased requirements of these vitamins with increasing alcohol misuse, vomiting, diarrhea, and steatorrhea, and reduced intestinal absorption of vitamins will all contribute to the 20% weight loss and signs of malnutrition in the chronic alcohol misuser.

These nutritional factors will result in oxidative stress in the absence of adequate levels of antioxidants and the depletion of vitamin stores, especially thiamine, and lead to damage of tissues including muscles, liver, and brain. Specific damage to brain areas results from less responsive or abnormal apoenzymes, causing reduced cellular energy production and excitotoxicity in NMDA mediated neurons in the hippocampus. These cellular changes in learning and memory underlie the behavioral changes in early stages of WE. Malnutrition and malabsorption of essential vitamins become intensified as the individual becomes confused and shows increasing tendencies to DTs and seizures. After losing 30% of muscle weight and the development of liver cirrhosis, a wide range of metabolic perturbancies will prevail, including disruption of the tryptophan metabolism and the inability to store and process vitamins, which are required as cofactors in a wide range of metabolic functions. These events and circumstances will lead to WE and KP and result in 1.4% of general hospital postmortems showing evidence of WE damage. It has been estimated that 7 to 40% of all acute, nonaccident, and emergency hospital patients are alcohol misusers, the greatest number presenting in acute, unselected medical admissions.[126] This emphasizes the economic load on community health resources and also the extent of neuropsychologically damaged individuals in the population. From the ideas developed in this review, the following suggestions are offered to encourage the development of strategies which use dietary manipulation and supplementation to underpin behavioral approaches in the treatment of alcohol misusers (see Figure 9.5a and Figure 9.5b). An understanding of the role of neurotransmitter precursors and, in particular, the potential for elevating the Trp/LNAA ratio

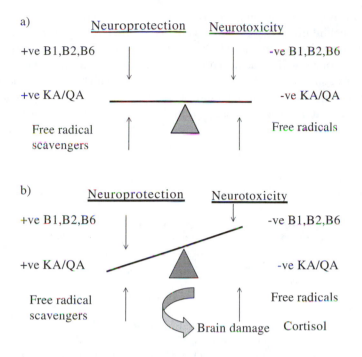

FIGURE 9.5 a) The balance between neuroprotection and neurotoxicity. B1, B2, B6: vitamins. KA/QA; ratio of kynurenic/quinolinic acids. b) B1, B2, B6: vitamins. KA/QA; ratio of kynurenic/quinolinic acids. Cortisol: chronic elevated levels.

should be explored within the wider nutritional background including oxidative status. Optimizing the availability of free radical scavengers by, for example, vitamins E and C is important but attention should also be paid to the most effective free radical scavenger, melatonin. This tryptophan metabolite is only produced in the dark phase of the light–dark cycle and again underlines the importance of chronobiological dimensions of tryptophan metabolism and the sleep–wake cycle. Neuroprotective aspects of nutritional supplementation include shifting the balance of tryptophan metabolism from quinolinic acid production (an NMDA agonist) in favor of kynurenic acid (an NMDA antagonist). Deficits in thiamine availability should be addressed by effective dosing regimes which include high concentrations of oral thiamine and IV doses where significant risks indicate an immediate need to address this deficiency. The possibility of lipid soluble allithiamines provides a less invasive approach, but this needs further investigation.

The efficacy of dietary manipulation and supplementation will depend on a range of general medical conditions including the presence of diabetes, hypertension, and liver disease. Further work is required to exploit the clinical utility of computer-based neuropsychological assessments in monitoring the progression of deficits in a brain area known to be particularly susceptible to damage in chronic alcohol misusers. In developing a case-managed approach to patients undergoing alcohol rehabilitation, the potential benefits of dietary supplementation as an adjunct to behavior therapy need to be further researched. However, it is clear that the best outcomes will be achieved by appropriate monitoring of neurocognitive assessments and nutritional status. Supplementation which takes into account the need for neuroprotection will facilitate personal empowerment by self-medication and hopefully help those who are especially vulnerable to alcohol-related brain damage. This approach provides a practical approach to socially deprived communities.

References

1. Thomson, A.D., Cook, C.C., Touquet, R., and Henry, J.A. The Royal College of Physicians report on alcohol: guidelines for managing Wernicke's encephalopathy in the accident and emergency department. *Alcohol Alcohol.*, 37: 513–521; 2002.
2. Freund, G. Apoptosis and gene expression: perspectives on alcohol-induced brain damage. *Alcohol*, 11: 385; 1994.
3. Gonthier, B., Jeunet, A., and Barret, L. Electron spin resonance study of free radicals produced from ethanol and acetaldehyde after exposure to a Fenton system or to brain and liver microsomes. *Alcohol*, 8: 369; 1991.
4. Bonner, A.B., Marway, J.S., Swann, M., and Preedy, V.R. Brain nucleic acid composition and fractional rates of protein synthesis in response to chronic ethanol feeding: comparison with skeletal muscle. *Alcohol*, 13: 581; 1996.
5. Renis, M., Calabrese, V., Russo, A. et al. Nuclear DNA strand breaks during ethanol-induced oxidative stress in rat brain. *FEBS Lett.*, 390: 153; 1996.
6. Mansouri, A., Demeilliers, C., Amsellem, S. et al. Acute ethanol administration oxidatively damages and depletes mitochondrial dna in mouse liver, brain, heart, and skeletal muscles: protective effects of antioxidants. *J. Pharmacol. Exp. Ther.*, 298: 737; 2001.
7. Nakahara, T., Hirano, M., Uchimura, H. et al. Chronic alcohol feeding and its influence on c-Fos and heat shock protein-70 gene expression in different brain regions of male and female rats. *Metabolism*, 51: 1562; 2002.
8. Emsley, R.A., Roberts, M.C., Aalbers, C. et al. Endocrine function in alcoholic Korsakoff's syndrome. *Alcohol Alcohol.*, 29: 187; 1994.
9. Mair, R.G., Anderson, C.D., Langlais, P.J., and Mcentee, W.J. Thiamine deficiency depletes cortical norepinephrine and impairs learning processes in the rat. *Brain Res.*, 360: 273; 1985.
10. Hellevuo, K., Kiianmaa, K., and Kim, C. Effect of ethanol on brain catecholamines in rat lines developed for differential ethanol-induced motor impairment. *Alcohol*, 7: 159; 1990.
11. Brown, L.M., Trent, R.D., Jones, T.W. et al. Alcohol inhibition of NMDA-stimulated catecholamine efflux in aging brain. *Alcohol*, 9: 555; 1992.
12. Lin, A.M., Freund, R.K., and Palmer, M.R. Ethanol potentiation of GABA-induced electrophysiological responses in cerebellum: requirement for catecholamine modulation. *Neurosci. Lett.*, 122: 154; 1991.
13. Shafik, E.N., Aiken, S.P., and McArdle, J.J. Regional catecholamine levels in brains of normal and ethanol-tolerant long-sleep and short-sleep mice. *Brain Res.*, 563: 44; 1991.

14. Edelman, G.M. *Neural Darwinism.* New York: Basic Books, 1987: 331.
15. Okada, T., Yamada, N., Tsuzuki, K. et al. Long-term potentiation in the hippocampal CA1 area and dentate gyrus plays different roles in spatial learning. *Eur. J. Neurosci.*, 17: 341; 2003.
16. Krebs, H. The affects of alcohol on metabolic processes. In: Richter, D. (Ed.), *Addiction and Brain Damage.* Baltimore: Croom Helm, 1980: 11.
17. Bartfai, T. and Schultzberg, M. Cytokines in neuronal cell types. *Neurochem. Int.*, 22: 435; 1993.
18. Zhang, L.X., Levine, S., Dent, G. et al. Maternal deprivation increases cell death in the infant rat brain. *Brain Res. Dev. Brain Res.*, 133: 1; 2002.
19. Seear, M., Lockitch, G., Jacobson, B. et al. Thiamine, riboflavin, and pyridoxine deficiencies in a population of critically ill children. *J. Pediatr.*, 121: 533; 1992.
20. Kalin, N.H. The neurobiology of fear. *Sci. Am.*, 268: 94; 1993.
21. Teicher, M.H. Scars that won't heal: the neurobiology of child abuse. *Sci. Am.*, 286: 68; 2002.
22. Sokol, R.J. Alcohol and abnormal outcomes of pregnancy. *CMA J.*, 125: 143; 1981.
23. Halliday, H.L., Reid, M., and McClure, G. Results of heavy drinking in pregnancy. *Br. J. Obstet. Gynaecol.*, 89: 892; 1982.
24. Michaelis, E.K. Fetal alcohol exposure: cellular toxicity and molecular events involved in toxicity. *Alc. Clin. Exp. Res.*, 14: 819; 1990.
25. Randall, C.L., Ekblad, U., and Anton, R.F. Perspectives on the pathophysiology of fetal alcohol syndrome. *Alc. Clin. Exp. Res.,* 14: 807; 1990.
26. Holzman, C., Paneth, N., Little, R., and Pinto-Martin, J. Perinatal brain injury in premature infants born to mothers using alcohol in pregnancy. Neonatal Brain Hemorrhage Study Team. *Pediatrics*, 95: 66; 1995.
27. West, J.R., Chen, W.J., and Pantazis, N.J. Fetal alcohol syndrome: the vulnerability of the developing brain and possible mechanisms of damage. *Metab. Brain Dis.*, 9: 291; 1994.
28. Bonner, A.B., Dalwai, S., Marway, J.S., and Preedy, V.R. Acute exposure to the nutritional toxin alcohol reduces brain protein synthesis *in vivo. Metabolism*, 52: 389; 2003.
29. Rodriguez Holguin, S., Porjesz, B., Chorlian, D.B. et al. Visual P3a in male subjects at high risk for alcoholism. *Biol. Psychiatry*, 46: 281; 1999.
30. Rangaswamy, M., Porjesz, B., Chorlian, D.B. et al. Beta power in the EEG of alcoholics. *Biol. Psychiatry*, 52: 831; 2002.
31. Prabhu, V.R., Porjesz, B., Chorlian, D.B. et al. Visual p3 in female alcoholics. *Alc. Clin. Exp. Res.*, 25: 531; 2001.
32. Hada, M., Porjesz, B., Chorlian, D.B. et al. Auditory P3a deficits in male subjects at high risk for alcoholism. *Biol. Psychiatry*, 49: 726; 2001.
33. Begleiter, H. and Porjesz, B. What is inherited in the predisposition toward alcoholism? A proposed model. *Alc. Clin. Exp. Res.*, 23: 1125; 1999.
34. Hesselbrock, V., Begleiter, H., Porjesz, B. et al. P300 event-related potential amplitude as an endophenotype of alcoholism — evidence from the collaborative study on the genetics of alcoholism. *J. Biomed. Sci.*, 8: 77; 2001.
35. Tuck, R.R. and Jackson, M. Social, neurological and cognitive disorders in alcoholics. *Med. J. Aust.*, 155: 225; 1991.
36. Koelega, H.S. Alcohol and vigilance performance: a review. *Psychopharmacology* (Berlin), 118: 233; 1995.

37. Maylor, E.A., Rabbitt, P.M., James, G.H., and Kerr, S.A. Effects of alcohol, practice, and task complexity on reaction time distributions. *Q. J. Exp. Psychol. A*, 44: 119; 1992.

38. Glenn, S.W., Errico, A.L., Parsons, O.A. et al. The role of antisocial, affective, and childhood behavioral characteristics in alcoholics' neuropsychological performance. *Alc. Clin. Exp. Res.*, 17: 162; 1993.

39. Shaw, G.K. and Spence, M. Psychological impairment in alcoholics. *Alcohol Alcohol.*, 20: 243; 1985.

40. Anonymous. Thiamin addition to alcohol: American Medical Association, 1996.

41. Cook, C.C., Hallwood, P.M., and Thomson, A.D. B Vitamin deficiency and neuropsychiatric syndromes in alcohol misuse. *Alcohol Alcohol.*, 33: 317; 1998.

42. Errico, A.L., King, A.C., and Parsons, O.A. The influence of depressive symptomatology on alcoholics' locus of control: a methodological note and a correction. *J. Clin. Psychol.*, 47: 600; 1991.

43. McCrady, B.S. and Smith, D.E. Implications of cognitive impairment for the treatment of alcoholism. *Alc. Clin. Exp. Res.*, 10: 145; 1986.

44. Goldman, M.J., Grinspoon, L., and Hunter-Jones, S. Ritualistic use of fluoxetine by a former substance abuser. *Am. J. Psychiatr.*, 147: 1377; 1990.

45. Miller, L. Neuropsychological assessment of substance abusers: review and recommendations. *J. Subst. Abuse Treat.*, 2: 5; 1985.

46. Reitan, R.M. and Wolfson, D. A selective and critical review of neuropsychological deficits and the frontal lobes. *Neuropsychol. Rev.*, 4: 161; 1994.

47. Acker, W. and Acker, C. Bexley Maudsley Automated Psychological Screening and Bexley Maudsley Category Sorting Test Manual NFER-Nelson, Windsor 1982.

48. Martin, C., Bonner, A., and Cook, C. Development of the PC version of the Bexley-Maudsley automated psychological screening test. *Proc. Br. Psychol. Soc.*, 2002.

49. Fadda, F., and Rossetti, Z.L. Chronic ethanol consumption: from neuroadaptation to neurodegeneration. *Prog. Neurobiol.*, 56: 385; 1998.

50. Mulder, R.T. and Joyce, P.R. Relationship of temperament and behavior measures to the prolactin response to fenfluramine in depressed men. *Psychiatr. Res.*, 109: 221; 2002.

51. Badawy, A.A. The neurobiological background to the study of addiction. In: Bonner, A.B. and Waterhouse, J. (Eds.), *Addictive Behavior: Molecules to Mankind*. Basingstoke: Macmillan Press, 1996: 41.

52. Lemarquand, D.G., Benkelfat, C., Pihl, R.O. et al. Behavioral disinhibition induced by tryptophan depletion in nonalcoholic young men with multigenerational family histories of paternal alcoholism. *Am. J. Psychiatr.*, 156: 1771; 1999.

53. Pihl, R.O., Young, S.N., Harden, P. et al. Acute effect of altered tryptophan levels and alcohol on aggression in normal human males. *Psychopharmacology* (Berlin), 119: 353; 1995.

54. Van Der Mast, R.C. and Fekkes, D. Serotonin and amino acids: partners in delirium pathophysiology? *Semin. Clin. Neuropsychiatry*, 5: 125; 2000.

55. Freese, A., Swartz, K.J., During, M.J., and Martin, J.B. Kynurenine metabolites of tryptophan: implications for neurologic diseases. *Neurology*, 40: 691; 1990.

56. Cleare, A.J. and Bond, A.J. Relationship of plasma tryptophan and blood serotonin to aggression, mood and anxiety in males. *J. Serotonin Res.*, 2: 77; 1995.

57. Altman, H.J. and Normile, H.J. What is the nature of the role of the serotonergic nervous system in learning and memory: prospects for development of an effective treatment strategy for senile dementia. *Neurobiol. Aging*, 9: 627; 1988.

58. Maes, M., Scharpe, S., Verkerk, R. et al. Seasonal variation in plasma L-tryptophan availability in healthy volunteers. Relationships to violent suicide occurrence. *Arch. Gen. Psychiatry*, 52: 937; 1995.

59. Fernstrom, J.D., and Wurtman, R.J. Brain serotonin content: physiological regulation by plasma neutral amino acids. *Obes. Res.*, 5: 377; 1997.

60. Bellisle, F., Blundell, J.E., Dye, L. et al. Functional food science and behavior and psychological functions. *Br. J. Nutr.*, 80 Suppl. 1: S173; 1998.

61. Markus, C.R., Olivier, B., and De Haan, E.H. Whey protein rich in alpha-lactalbumin increases the ratio of plasma tryptophan to the sum of the other large neutral amino acids and improves cognitive performance in stress-vulnerable subjects. *Am. J. Clin. Nutr.*, 75: 1051; 2002.

62. Rosenthal, N.E., Genhart, M.J., Caballero, B. et al. Psychobiological effects of carbohydrate- and protein-rich meals in patients with seasonal affective disorder and normal controls. *Biol. Psychiatry*, 25: 1029; 1989.

63. Badawy, A.A., Morgan, C.J., Lovett, J.W. et al. Decrease in circulating tryptophan availability to the brain after acute ethanol consumption by normal volunteers: implications for alcohol-induced aggressive behavior and depression. *Pharmacopsychiatry*, 28 Suppl 2: 93; 1995.

64. Yamamoto, H. Changes in CSF neurotransmitters during the first year of life. *Pediatric Neurol.*, 7: 406; 1991.

65. Battie, C. and Verity, M.A. Presence of kynurenine hydroxylase in developing rat brain. *J. Neurochem.*, 36: 1308; 1981.

66. Iwata, H. Possible role of thiamine in the nervous system. *Trends Pharmacol. Sci.*, 171; 1982.

67. Cohen, G. and Collins, M. Alkaloids from catecholamines in adrenal tissue: possible role in alcoholism. *Science*, 167: 1749; 1970.

68. Seizinger, B.R., Hollt, V., and Herz, A. Effects of chronic ethanol treatment on the *in vitro* biosynthesis of pro-opiomelanocortin and its posttranslational processing to beta-endorphin in the intermediate lobe of the rat pituitary. *J. Neurochem.*, 43: 607; 1984.

69. Genazzani, A.R., Nappi, G., Facchinetti, F. et al. Central deficiency of beta-endorphin in alcohol addicts. *J. Clin. Endocrinol. Metab.*, 55: 583; 1982.

70. Teichner, G., Donohue, B., Crum, T.A. et al. The relationship of neuropsychological functioning to measures of substance use in an adolescent drug abusing sample. *Int. J. Neurosci.*, 104: 113; 2000.

71. Blum, K. and Trachtenberg, M. New insights into the causes of alcoholism. *Prof. Counsellor*, 33; 1987.

72. Halliday, G., Baker, K., and Harper, C. Serotonin and alcohol-related brain damage. *Metab. Brain Dis.*, 10: 25; 1995.

73. Meyer, S.E., Chrousos, G.P., and Gold, P.W. Major depression and the stress system: a life span perspective. *Dev. Psychopathol.*, 13: 565; 2001.

74. Badawy, A.A., Rommelspacher, H., Morgan, C.J. et al. Tryptophan metabolism in alcoholism. Tryptophan but not excitatory amino acid availability to the brain is increased before the appearance of the alcohol-withdrawal syndrome in men. *Alcohol Alcohol.*, 33: 616; 1998.

75. Oretti, R.G., Bano, S., Azani, M.O. et al. Rat liver tryptophan pyrrolase activity and gene expression during alcohol withdrawal. *Alcohol Alcohol.*, 35: 427; 2000.

76. Oretti, R., Bano, S., Morgan, C.J. et al. Prevention by cycloheximide of the audiogenic seizures and tryptophan metabolic disturbances of ethanol withdrawal in rats. *Alcohol Alcohol.*, 31: 243; 1996.

77. Badawy, A.A. Tryptophan metabolism in alcoholism. *Adv. Exp. Med. Biol.*, 467: 265; 1999.

78. Young, S.N. Mechanism of decline in rat brain 5-hydroxytryptamine after induction of liver tryptophan pyrrolase by hydrocortisone: roles of tryptophan catabolism and kynurenine synthesis. *Br. J. Pharmacol.*, 74: 695; 1981.

79. Takikawa, O., Habara-Ohkubo, A., and Yoshida, R. Induction of indoleamine 2,3-dioxygenase in tumor cells transplanted into allogeneic mouse: interferon-gamma is the inducer. *Adv. Exp. Med. Biol.*, 294: 437; 1991.

80. Heyes, M.P., Chen, C.Y., Major, E.O., and Saito, K. Different kynurenine pathway enzymes limit quinolinic acid formation by various human cell types. *Biochem. J.*, 326 (Pt 2): 351; 1997.

81. Schwarcz, R., Tamminga, C.A., Kurlan, R., and Shoulson, I. Cerebrospinal fluid levels of quinolinic acid in Huntington's disease and schizophrenia. *Ann. Neurol.*, 24: 580; 1988.

82. Schwarcz, R., Whetsell, W.O., Jr., and Mangano, R.M. Quinolinic acid: an endogenous metabolite that produces axon-sparing lesions in rat brain. *Science*, 219: 316; 1983.

83. Guilarte, T.R. Effect of vitamin B-6 nutrition on the levels of dopamine, dopamine metabolites, dopa decarboxylase activity, tyrosine, and GABA in the developing rat corpus striatum. *Neurochem. Res.*, 14: 571; 1989.

84. Nagy, J. and Laszlo, L. Increased sensitivity to NMDA is involved in alcohol-withdrawal induced cytotoxicity observed in primary cultures of cortical neurones chronically pre-treated with ethanol. *Neurochem. Int.*, 40: 585; 2002.

85. Lovinger, D.M. Excitotoxicity and alcohol-related brain damage. *Alc. Clin. Exp. Res.*, 17: 19; 1993.

86. Davidson, M.D., Wilce, P., and Shanley, B.C. Increased sensitivity of the hippocampus in ethanol-dependent rats to toxic effect of *N*-methyl-D-aspartic acid *in vivo. Brain Res.*, 606: 5; 1993.

87. Hunt, W.A. Are binge drinkers more at risk of developing brain damage? *Alcohol*, 10: 559; 1993.

88. Stone, T.W., Perkins, M.N. Quinolinic acid: a potent endogenous excitant at amino acid receptors in CNS. *Eur. J. Pharmacol.*, 72: 411; 1981.

89. Dong-Ruyl, L., Sawada, M., and Nakano, K. Tryptophan and its metabolite, kynurenine, stimulate expression of nerve growth factor in cultured mouse astroglial cells. *Neurosci. Lett.*, 244: 17; 1998.

90. Stone, T.W. Development and therapeutic potential of kynurenic acid and kynurenine derivatives for neuroprotection. *Trends Pharmacol. Sci.*, 21: 149; 2000.

91. Cala, L.A., Mastaglia, F.L., Jones, B., and Wiley, B. The effects of alcohol in social drinkers. *J. Stud. Alcohol*, 43: 614; 1982.

92. Wernicke, C. Die acute haemorrhagische polioencephalitis superior. In: Fischer, T. (Ed.), *Lehbuch der Gehirnkrankheiten fur Aerzte und Studierende*. Berlin: Theodor Fischer, 1881: 229.

93. Witt, E.D. Neuroanatomical consequences of thiamine deficiency: a comparative analysis. *Alcohol Alcohol.*, 20: 201; 1985.

94. Gibson, G.E. and Zhang, H. Interactions of oxidative stress with thiamine homeostasis promote neurodegeneration. *Neurochem. Int*, 40: 493; 2002.

95. Baker, H., Frank, O., Zetterman, R.K. et al. Inability of chronic alcoholics with liver disease to use food as a source of folates, thiamin and vitamin B6. *Am. J. Clin. Nutr.*, 28: 1377; 1975.

96. Joyce, E.M. Aetiology of alcoholic brain damage: alcoholic neurotoxicity or thiamine malnutrition? *Br. Med. Bull.*, 50: 99; 1994.

97. McEntee, W.J. Wernicke's encephalopathy: an excitotoxicity hypothesis. *Metab. Brain Dis.*, 12: 183; 1997.

98. Stahelin, H. Vitamins. In: Grimley Evans, J., Franklin Williams, T., Lynn Beattie, B. et al. (Eds.), *Oxford Textbook of Geriatric Medicine*. Oxford: Oxford University Press, 2000.

99. Shaw, G.K. Detoxification: the use of benzodiazepines. *Alcohol Alcohol.*, 30: 765; 1995.

100. Hoffman, P.L. and Tabakoff, B. The role of the NMDA receptor in ethanol withdrawal. *Exs*; 71: 61; 1994.

101. Roehrich, L. and Goldman, M.S. Experience-dependent neuropsychological recovery and the treatment of alcoholism. *J. Consult. Clin. Psychol.*, 61: 812; 1993.

102. Litten, R.Z. and Allen, J.P. Dietary factors and alcohol consumption. In: Watson R.R. and Watzl B. (Eds.) *Nutrition and Alcohol*. Boca Raton, FL: CRC Press, Inc., 1992: 39.

103. McBride, W.J., Murphy, J.M., Lumeng, L., and Li, T.K. Serotonin, dopamine and GABA involvement in alcohol drinking of selectively bred rats. *Alcohol*, 7: 199; 1990.

104. Zabik, J.E. and Roache, J.D. 5-hydroxytryptophan-induced conditioned taste aversion to ethanol in the rat. *Pharmacol. Biochem. Behav.*, 18: 785; 1983.

105. Gellert, J. and Lieber, C.S. Effects of acute ethanol administration and chronic ethanol feeding on mixed function oxidation in deermice lacking ADH. *Alcohol*, 2: 13; 1985.

106. Walters, J.K. Effects of PCPA on the consumption of alcohol, water and other solutions. *Pharmacol. Biochem. Behav.*, 6: 377; 1977.

107. Eriksson, C.J. Factors affecting voluntary alcohol intake of rats. *Ann. Zool. Fenn*; 16: 227; 1969.

108. Blum, K. A commentary on neurotransmitter restoration as a common mode of treatment for alcohol, cocaine and opiate abuse. *Integr. Psychiatry*, 199; 1989.

109. Ambrose, M.L., Bowden, S.C., and Whelan, G. Thiamin treatment and working memory function of alcohol-dependent people: preliminary findings. *Alc. Clin. Exp. Res.*, 25: 112; 2001.

110. Brady, R.A. and Westerfield, W.W. The effect of B-complex vitamins on voluntary consumption alcohol by rats. *Q. J. Stud. Alcohol*, 7: 499; 1947.

111. Mirone, L. Effect of vitamins in single dose on liver of mice on prolonged ethanol intake. *Life Sci.*, 5: 317; 1966.

112. Thomson, A.D., Baker, H., and Leevy, C.M. Patterns of 35S-thiamine hydrochloride absorption in the malnourished alcoholic patient. *J. Lab. Clin. Med.*, 76: 34; 1970.

113. Thomson, A.D. and Leevy, C.M. Observations on the mechanism of thiamine hydrochloride absorption in man. *Clin. Sci.*, 43: 153; 1972.

114. Thomson, A.D. and Majumdar, S.K. The influence of ethanol on intestinal absorption and utilization of nutrients. *Clin. Gastroenterol.*, 10: 263; 1981.

115. Heap, L.C., Pratt, O.E., Ward, R.J. et al. Individual susceptibility to Wernicke-Korsakoff syndrome and alcoholism-induced cognitive deficit: impaired thiamine utilization found in alcoholics and alcohol abusers. *Psychiatr. Genet.*, 12: 217; 2002.

116. Thomson, A.D. Mechanisms of vitamin deficiency in chronic alcohol misusers and the development of the Wernicke–Korsakoff syndrome. *Alcohol Alcohol.*, 35 Suppl. 1: 2; 2000.

117. Thomson, A.D., Cook C.C.H., Toughet, R., and Henry, J.A. The Royal College of Physicians report on alcohol: guidelines for managing Wernicke's encephalopathy in the accident and emergency department. *Alcohol Alcohol.*, 37: 513; 2002.

118. Thomson, A.D., Frank, O., Baker, H., and Leevy, C.M. Thiamine propyl disulfide: absorption and utilization. *Ann. Int. Med.*, 74: 529; 1971.
119. Baker, H. and Frank, O. Absorption, utilization and clinical effectiveness of allithiamines compared to water-soluble thiamines. *J. Nutr. Sci. Vitaminol.* (Tokyo), 22 Suppl. 63; 1976.
120. Kitamori, N., and Itokawa, Y. Pharmacokinetics of thiamin after oral administration of thiamin tetrahydrofurfuryl disulfide to humans. *J. Nutr. Sci. Vitaminol.* (Tokyo), 39: 465; 1993.
121. Wurtman, R.J. Nutrients affecting brain composition and behavior. *Integr. Psychiatry*, 5: 226; 1987.
122. Markus, C.R., Panhuysen, G., Tuiten, A. et al. Does carbohydrate-rich, protein-poor food prevent a deterioration of mood and cognitive performance of stress-prone subjects when subjected to a stressful task? *Appetite*, 31: 49; 1998.
123. Bano, S., Oretti, R.G., Morgan, C.J. et al. Effects of chronic administration and subsequent withdrawal of ethanol-containing liquid diet on rat liver tryptophan pyrrolase and tryptophan metabolism. *Alcohol Alcohol.*, 31: 205; 1996.
124. Martin, C.R. and Bonner, A.B. A pilot investigation of the effect of tryptophan manipulation on the affective state of male chronic alcoholics. *Alcohol Alcohol.*, 35: 49; 2000.
125. Adams, W.R., Kiefer, S.W., and Badia-Elder, N. Tryptophan deficiency and alcohol consumption in rats as a model for disadvantaged human populations: a preliminary study. *Med. Anthropol.*, 16: 175; 1995.
126. Anonymous. Alcohol — can the NHS afford it? London: Royal College of Physicians, 2001: 14.

10 Nutritional Modulation of the Expression of Alcohol and Aldehyde Dehydrogenases and Alcohol Metabolism

Min You and David Crabb

CONTENTS

10.1 INTRODUCTION

The activities of alcohol and aldehyde dehydrogenases are believed to be important determinants of responses to ethanol. The strongest evidence for this assertion is the finding, replicated by many laboratories in many countries, that the inheritance of alcohol dehydrogenase (ADH) alleles encoding high activity enzymes are associated with lower prevalence of alcoholism and, conversely, that inheritance of the dominant negative mitochondrial aldehyde dehydrogenase (ALDH2) allele (*ALDH2*2*) is associated with a marked reduction in the risk of alcoholism.[1,2] Although it has been postulated that the activity of these enzymes might also affect the risk of developing alcoholic liver disease, considerably less data support this notion.[3] Given that the activity of these enzymes as determined by their isozyme type affects the risk of alcoholism, it is natural to ask if other influences on the activity of these enzymes might also affect responses to alcohol. Considerable interest has centered on the possibility that nutritional factors may affect the expression of these enzymes.

Review of the experimental literature reveals an important source of confusion. Much of the older literature utilized measurement of enzyme activity in liver extracts following nutritional modifications. The enzyme activity in units (typically 1 unit = 1 μmol NADH generated per minute) was often normalized to the protein concentration of the extract (and this number was called the specific activity) or to the wet weight of liver from which the extract was made. Both such measurements are subject to changes in liver weight or protein content induced by the nutritional perturbation. The overall effect of changes in ADH or ALDH2 activity on alcohol metabolism depends on the change in total enzyme activity in the liver. For example, with fasting, the liver becomes smaller and the protein content falls. ADH activity expressed per mg protein or gram of liver remains nearly constant, but because of the reduction in liver mass, total liver ADH activity is reduced as is the rate of alcohol metabolism, discussed in detail in Lumeng et al.[4] An alternative denominator is the DNA content of the liver sample, which is less likely to be altered by nutritional changes. Where these data are available, they are discussed. A further problem, which is nearly impossible to recognize in reading the literature, is the presence of multiple isozymes for ADH and ALDH2. These enzyme activities may be only partly discriminated by differences in substrate preference or K_m; hence, the reported enzyme activity may reflect the sum of activities of several isozymes. Investigators interested in further studies on nutritional effects on these enzymes are urged to take these suggestions into consideration.

10.2   ALCOHOL DEHYDROGENASE

The alcohol dehydrogenase (ADH) gene family encodes enzymes that metabolize a wide variety of substrates, including ethanol, retinal, other aliphatic alcohols, hydroxysteroids, and lipid peroxidation products. Human ADH is a dimeric protein consisting of two subunits with a molecular weight of 40 kDa each. The proteins contain catalytic and structural zinc atoms. So far, seven ADH genes and subunits have been identified in humans.[5,6]

Various human ADH forms can be divided into five major classes (I to V). However, the ADH isoforms that are important for ethanol metabolism are the Class I, Class II, and Class IV isozymes. Class I isozymes are formed by random dimeric association of the three types of polypeptide subunits, α, β, and γ encoded by three separate genes, *ADH1*, *ADH2*, and *ADH3*, respectively.[7] Recently, the nomenclature for ADH was modified to relate the gene name to the structural similarity of the proteins; hence, these three genes, which appear to have evolved by gene duplication, are now named ADH1A, ADH1B, and ADH1C.[8] These isoenzymes belong to the low K_m (<4 mM) forms found at highest activity in liver, and play a major role in ethanol metabolism. The ADH1B and ADH1C genes have allelic variants: ADH1B1, ADH1B2, and ADH1B3, encoding β1, 2, and 3 isozymes, respectively. ADH1C1 and ADH1C2 encode γ1 and 2 peptides. An additional form, ADH1Cpro361Thr, was reported based on sequencing studies.[8] The effect of nutrition on differential expression of the isozymes has not been studied, and it is assumed that potential effects on transcription, translation, and degradation will be the same for all members of each gene type, since at the present time it is thought that the promoters for each allele are identical. It remains possible that the differences in protein and mRNA sequences alter the half-life of these molecules.

The Class II ADH, encoded by the ADH4 (now renamed ADH2) gene, is a single homodimeric enzyme ππ found in liver. A class III enzyme (now ADH3) has long been known, and may represent the most ancient precursor of the ADH family. The class IV enzyme is a single homodimeric enzyme σσ encoded by ADH7 (now renamed ADH4) gene found primarily in the stomach.[9] This isoenzyme is moderately active with ethanol and with retinol.

Most work has been done on the ADH1 family of genes. Their promoter structures were determined largely by the laboratories of Edenberg and Duester, and this has been reviewed in detail.[7,10,11] Of note, the ADH1C promoter contains a retinoid response element that may be influenced by dietary vitamin A sufficiency. Nutritional studies have largely dealt with the effect of fasting, protein restriction, alteration in dietary fat content and composition, and the content of vitamins and zinc in the diet. Unless otherwise noted, the studies described below refer to liver ADH expression.

10.2.1 FASTING

It is well established that fasting reduces the liver content of ADH (units per liver).[12,13] Lumeng and Crabb found that the reduction in enzyme activity was paralleled by a reduction in alcohol elimination rate,[14] which can be accurately estimated from the steady-state concentrations of substrates and products plus the maximal activity (reflecting total enzyme content of the liver) using steady-state rate equations.[13] Bosron's laboratory[12,15] measured the effect of 72 h of fasting on rat liver ADH using isotopic methods that permitted the calculation of synthesis and degradation rate constants. His study showed that the synthetic rate fell during fasting, and the degradation rate increased substantially. Lakshman's group further investigated the hormonal control of this shift in rates of synthesis. He reported that fasting reduced ADH activity by 50%, and that insulin was able to increase the activity in fasted rats within 2 h of administration. Diabetic rats had reduced ADH activity, further indicating a dependence of ADH expression on insulin. Surprisingly, refeeding or meal feeding the rats a high carbohydrate, fat-free diet resulted in a reduction in total ADH activity in the liver,[16] suggesting that fat content of the diet could contribute to expression of ADH (see following text). Maly and Sasse[17] have argued that the reduction in ADH activity (expressed per unit of dry weight) is the result of the reduction in liver size with fasting, but others found reduced ADH per mg

DNA in short-term fasted rats, arguing that the amount of enzyme per liver cell was indeed decreased. These findings can be reconciled by noting that ADH may simply be reduced in proportion to the overall reduction in liver protein mass; this in turn suggests that ADH is catabolized by the same systems that handle bulk cytosolic protein turnover, namely lysosomal and proteosomal systems.

It is interesting to note that fasting also reduces the activity of gastric ADH, expressed per mg gastric mucosal protein.[18] Since first-pass metabolism of ethanol likely involves both a gastric and hepatic contribution, individuals drinking after fasting will be predicted to have considerably higher blood alcohol levels.

Food restriction also affects ADH activity, and may be more relevant to human malnutrition than prolonged fasting. Food-restricted animals are deficient in both calories and in amino acids. Rats restricted in diet had reduced ADH activity and alcohol elimination rates.[4]

10.2.2 PROTEIN RESTRICTION

Heavy drinkers are prone to marginal or deficient nutrition; protein malnutrition is common among alcoholics, and almost universal among individuals suffering from alcoholic hepatitis. ADH enzyme activity (units/g liver) is reduced in protein-restricted rats,[19–21] and this has been found to be associated with reduced abundance of ADH mRNA.[22] Blood ethanol and acetaldehyde levels were elevated in animals maintained on low protein (5%) diets.[21] This has also been observed after feeding diets deficient in essential amino acids, and in the latter experiment, the reduced ADH activity resulted in a reduced rate of alcohol clearance.[23] An unexpected finding was that when protein-deficient animals were administered ethanol in the diet, the ADH activity levels were not as depressed as in protein deficient rats not consuming ethanol.[20] This was attributed to reduced testosterone levels in the former. Castration has been well established to induce liver ADH activity.

10.2.3 EFFECT OF FAT CONTENT OR COMPOSITION OF DIET

The effect of the fat content of the diet is of considerable interest to alcohol researchers. Models of alcoholic liver disease in rodents have shown a dependence of the degree of liver injury on the type of fat fed: high polyunsaturated fatty acid (PUFA) diets (enriched with corn or fish oil) are associated with greater degrees of inflammation and fatty liver, while saturated fat or medium chain triglycerides prevented the development of fatty liver during ethanol consumption.[24–29] Fisher et al.[30] reported that while supplementation of a liquid alcohol-containing diet (containing up to 37% of calories as ethanol) with carbohydrate or fat (at the expense of water) improved weight gain in rats, changes in diet composition did not affect liver ADH activity. This study reported ADH activity as units/g liver; thus, if the alcohol or high fat feeding increased liver size (not reported), there could have been an effect on total liver ADH activity that was overlooked.

10.2.4 EFFECT OF ETHANOL ON ADH ACTIVITY

It has long been held that ethanol consumption *per se* did not affect hepatic ADH activity[31,32] while it clearly induces the CYP2E1 enzyme. This conclusion needs to be tempered by issues related to the gender of the animals studied, the dose of ethanol, and duration of the treatment. We know little about the effect of heavy alcohol use in humans prior to the development of liver injury.

The doses of ethanol that can be delivered to adult rats or mice via the use of liquid diets have not had significant effects on liver ADH.[33] One group has reported decreased liver ADH activity (units/g protein) in alcohol-consuming pregnant rats that was not explained by zinc deficiency.[34] However, higher ethanol doses, such as those that can only be achieved by intragastric delivery of ethanol (the Tsukamoto–French model), induced liver ADH activity. This was recently shown to result from induction of the transcription factor C/EBPβ and suppression of C/EBPγ and a truncated, inhibitory form of C/EBPβ called LIP.[35] Since this alcohol-feeding regimen approximates the percentage of calories taken in the diet by human alcoholic patients, similar effects may occur in humans.

One additional factor may play a role in the effects of ethanol on liver ADH activity. Chronic ethanol feeding using gastric infusion increases portal vein endotoxin and sensitizes the liver to endotoxin actions.[36–39] Mezey's group[40] recently showed that endotoxin can induce ADH mRNA, protein (units/mg cytosolic protein), and activity. They found that endotoxin increased the binding of upstream stimulatory factor (USF) to the ADH promoter, which may mediate the effect of endotoxin. Thus, we need to be aware of differences in effects of ethanol on the expression of liver ADH or ALDH2 that may be dependent on the dose and route of administration or that may be influenced by factors such as endotoxinemia.

10.2.5 Effects of Vitamins

The effects of vitamin A have been investigated in some detail because of the report of a retinoid response element in the ADH1C promoter, and because ADH may participate in the oxidation of retinol to retinal.[41] Duester's group[42] has used knockout mice to determine that the mouse Adh1 enzyme (a class I, low K_m form analogous to the ADH1 family of human ADHs) plays a major role in the clearance of vitamin A when it is given in large doses, and Adh3 (a ubiquitously expressed ADH with glutathione-dependent formaldehyde dehydrogenase activity) but not Adh4 (the isozyme expressed at high levels in the stomach mucosa) made a secondary contribution to metabolism of retinol to retinal. In fact, it appears that ADH1 may play a role in protecting against vitamin A toxicity. Of interest, ethanol and retinol are competitive substrates; hence, the presence of ethanol interferes with the ability of these enzymes to generate retinal (and, therefore, retinoic acid) from retinal.[43] In early embryogenesis, it appears that the Adh4 enzyme is the main form involved in retinal generation, and may be a site at which ethanol interferes with development (and hence be important in the pathogenesis of fetal alcohol syndrome). Further, heavy alcohol use depletes the liver of vitamin A.[31,44,45] Grummer reported that while alcohol feeding depleted the liver of vitamin A stores, neither vitamin A supplementation nor the alcohol diet affected ADH activity. Our group also found no effect of severe vitamin A deficiency on ADH protein levels, assessed by Western blots normalized to liver protein content. The deficient animals had reduced alcohol elimination rates that were explained by a reduction in liver size.[46]

Experimental thiamine deficiency maintained for 4 weeks was reported to decrease ADH activity in rats.[47] Moreover, blood ethanol levels were increased in these animals 1 h after a dose of ethanol, suggesting impaired alcohol elimination. There is no obvious explanation for this finding.

The dietary supplement carnitine (in the form of acetylcarnitine) has been reported to inhibit ADH activity with a Ki (competitive with NAD+) of 135 µM.[48] While this concentration is somewhat higher than physiologically found for a given acylcarnitine, it may be that each species of acylcarnitine additively inhibits ADH. This raises the possibility that this supplement or conditions in which acylcarnitines are elevated (e.g., high fat diets) may reversibly inhibit ADH activity *in situ*. Cha and Sachan[49] provide support for this notion through studies in which high saturated fat (10% coconut oil) diets reduced ethanol elimination rates and raised plasma acylcarnitines, compared to diets high in polyunsaturated fat (10% corn oil), without affecting liver ADH activity. This fascinating observation needs to be extended by enzyme inhibition studies on purified human isozymes.

10.2.6 MISCELLANEOUS DIETARY EFFECTS

ADH has long been a model for the study of metalloenzymes. As expected, dietary zinc deficiency has been reported to reduce the activity of hepatic ADH.[50,51] Since ADH may contribute to the conversion of retinol to retinoic acid, a reduction in ADH activity could explain an increase in hepatic vitamin A stores in zinc-deficient rats. However, one study that used pair feeding for different degrees of zinc deficiency showed no difference in the ADH activity between zinc-deficient animals and the pair-fed controls.[52] This suggests that global effects of zinc deficiency on food intake may in part be responsible for a reduction in ADH activity. Zinc supplementation was shown to restore gastric ADH activity (and increase first-pass metabolism of ethanol which is in part a result of gastric ADH activity in animals fed a liquid, alcohol-containing diet.[53] Dietary isoflavones may have an effect on human ADH. The gamma ADH isozyme is inhibited *in vitro* by daidzen, genistein, and their 4-methoxy derivatives (formononetin and biochanin A, respectively). This appears to be relatively selective for the gamma isoenzymes.[54] It is possible that ingestion of these compounds (naturally found in kudzu root) would reduce alcohol clearance rates but this has not been studied.

10.3 ALDEHYDE DEHYDROGENASES

Aldehyde dehydrogenases (ALDHs; EC 1.2.1.3) are a group of NAD(P)+-dependent enzymes that catalyze the oxidation of a wide variety of endogenous and exogenous aliphatic and aromatic aldehydes including retinaldehyde.[55] So far, there are 16 ALDH genes and three pseudogenes that have been identified in the human genome at distinct chromosomal locations. However, only class I and class II isozymes, encoded by *ALDH1* and *ALDH2*, respectively, are important for acetaldehyde metabolism.[56]

ALDH1 is the cytosolic enzymes ubiquitously distributed in various tissues including the lens of the eye, brain, and red blood cells, but at highest levels in liver.

It has relatively low catalytic efficiency (k_{cat}/K_m) for acetaldehyde oxidation. The ALDH1 enzyme has high affinities for all-*trans*- and 9-*cis* retinal (K_m <0.1 μM) and acetaldehyde (K_m 50 to 100 μM).[56]

ALDH2 is the mitochondrial enzyme expressed in most tissues, with the highest level in the liver, kidney, muscle, and heart.[57] It exhibits high catalytic efficiency for acetaldehyde oxidation (with a K_m for acetaldehyde in the submicromolar range). It plays a major role for acetaldehyde oxidation *in vivo*, based on the fact that individuals with the dominant negative *ALDH2*2* allele are deficient in enzyme activity and exhibit the "alcohol flushing" syndrome due to elevated blood acetaldehyde after drinking alcohol.[56,58] Since deficiency of ALDH2 activity is protective against alcoholism,[1,2] it is of interest to learn if environmental factors such as nutritional status also affect its activity.

Both human liver ALDH1 and ALDH2 are homotetrameric and contain 500 amino acid residues in each subunit with a molecular weight of 54 kDa each. Although ALDH1 and ALDH2 are expressed constitutively in many tissues, there is substantial variation in the level of expression in each tissue. The molecular basis for this variation is unknown. This review will focus on the nutritional control of ALDH2 expression.

Regulation of ALDH2 expression is incompletely understood. Its promoter contains a CCAAT box that is bound by NF-Y, a trimeric CCAAT box-binding protein.[59] This factor does not appear to mediate regulated expression. Upstream from this site is a nuclear receptor response element that has been shown to bind the peroxisome proliferator activated receptor (PPAR), retinoic acid receptors (RAR/RXR heterodimers), hepatocyte nuclear factor 4 (HNF4), and the orphan receptors chicken ovalbumin upstream promoter transcription factor (COUP-TF), ARP-1, and Ear2.[60–62] HNF4 and the retinoid receptors have been shown to activate promoter–reporter constructs *in vitro* and the orphan receptors suppress expression.[63] These findings have led to testing effects of retinoids and peroxisome proliferators on ALDH2 expression.

10.3.1 FASTING

Recently, we demonstrated that in the mouse, fasting significantly reduced ALDH2 protein levels in liver and kidney, but not in heart. This may be explained by the effect of elevated cAMP on the liver and kidney transcription factor HNF4. The ability of HNF4 to bind its cognate response element in the ALDH2 promoter was reduced in cells treated cAMP, and fasting is well known to increase hepatic cAMP. Heart, on the other hand, lacks this transcription factor.[63] Thus, the response of ALDH2 to fasting may be limited to tissues in which ALDH2 expression is dependent on HNF4.

10.3.2 PROTEIN RESTRICTION

It has been reported that ALDH2 activity is decreased by protein-deficient diets. Feeding rats for 8 weeks on a low-protein, high-carbohydrate diet (5% and 80% of calorie content, respectively) caused a significant reduction of both alcohol and aldehyde dehydrogenase activities expressed per gram of liver.[64,19,21] The results suggest that chronic consumption of a protein-deficient diet may derange acetaldehyde metabolism. The rate of alcohol elimination in these animals was decreased, yet blood acetaldehyde levels were increased after ethanol dosing. This suggests that the reduction in ALDH2 activity was greater than the reduction in ethanol oxidizing enzymes. Such an effect of a protein-deficient diet has not been established in humans but might be predicted to cause alcohol-induced flushing. Chen and Yu reported that mitochondrial ALDH2 was decreased with aging in rats, and that this decline could be prevented by dietary restriction of calories.[65]

10.3.3 EFFECT OF FAT CONTENT OR COMPOSITION OF DIET

In hepatoma cells, arachidonic acid supplementation increased levels of ALDH2 mRNA and protein as well as activity. The authors of that study suggested that this resulted from increased PPAR gene expression,[66] based on the report of a PPAR binding site in the *ALDH2* promoter.[60] However, our group was unable to demonstrate induction of ALDH2 in rats treated with peroxisome proliferating drugs, and ALDH2 expression was not impaired in PPARα knockout mice. Further, these results cannot necessarily be extrapolated to the liver *in vivo*. Our laboratory has examined the effect of feeding high carbohydrate, high saturated fat and high polyunsaturated fat diets to mice for 4 weeks, and found no effect of the diet on levels of ALDH2 protein.[67]

10.3.4 EFFECT OF ETHANOL ON ALDH2 ACTIVITY

Tomita et al.[68] reported that 1 week of alcohol feeding of mice reduced mitochondrial ALDH activity dramatically but that the level returned to normal after 4 weeks of feeding. It is possible that this observation related to the usual reduction in food intake that accompanies presenting ethanol-containing diets to mice. Other groups have reported that chronic ethanol feeding, in the quantities that can be accepted in liquid diets, did not affect mitochondrial ALDH2 in mice.[32] However, one group reported that specific activities (units per mg mitochondrial protein) of high-K_m ALDH and low-K_m ALDH were both increased after the prolonged administration of ethanol to rats.[69] Since the effects of alcohol feeding on mitochondrial protein were not studied, it is possible that this change relates to an alteration in protein synthesis in the cytosol or to mitochondrial damage in the alcohol-fed animals, resulting in protein leakage during isolation.

ALDH2 activity is reported to be decreased in alcoholic liver disease (especially cirrhosis),[70–72] and to decrease as the liver disease becomes more severe. This reduction was also seen in liver disease of other etiologies, suggesting that it is not simply a result of heavy drinking but rather of the other pathogenic responses of the liver to alcohol, such as oxidative stress or mitochondrial injury. Since the liver stores of retinol are commonly depleted in cirrhosis, the role of retinoids in ALDH2 expression has been examined (see following text).

10.3.5 EFFECTS OF VITAMINS

Heavy alcohol use is known to both deplete hepatic vitamin A stores and to reduce the activity of low K_m ALDH2, suggesting that vitamin A metabolites such as retinoic acid are important for the expression of ALDH2, presumedly acting through the retinoid response element in the promoter.[61] Dietary vitamin A deficiency modestly reduced ALDH2 protein expression level in the rat liver.[73] Another study showed that a 2-week period of chronic ethanol intake increased the activity of aldehyde dehydrogenase, and this effect was potentiated by feeding a vitamin E–deficient diet.[74] To the contrary, liver aldehyde dehydrogenase activity (unit/mg protein) was found to increase significantly by feeding rats a vitamin E-deficient diet for 5 to 8 weeks.[75]

10.3.6 MISCELLANEOUS DIETARY EFFECTS

ALDH enzymes contain a reactive cysteine at their active site, and hence are subject to inhibition by compounds that may react with them. The most famous such compound is cyanamide, found to be a contaminant of calcinated bone meal in some brands of rat chow.[76] Cyanamide markedly inhibits ALDH2 and causes accumulation of acetaldehyde after alcohol administration. The isothiocyanates found in cruciferous vegetables have been demonstrated to inhibit mitochondrial ALDH2.[77] Citral (3,7-dimethyl-2,6-octadienal), a flavoring and fragrance agent, was similarly noted to inhibit the mitochondrial enzyme.[78] An isoflavone, prunetin, has been shown to inhibit ALDH2.[79] Potential food contaminants, including the fungicide benomyl and the herbicide S-ethyl N,N-dipropylthiocarbamate, have also been shown to inhibit ALDH2. Whether one could ingest sufficient amounts of these vegetables or compounds to affect enzyme activity *in vivo* and to affect ethanol metabolism has not been determined.

10.4 CONCLUSIONS

This review demonstrates that the activities of ADH and ALDH2 can vary under different nutritional states, but the mechanisms responsible for these changes remain uncertain. Fasting is the most common nutritional state shown to affect the activity of each enzyme. The results of past studies are limited by the different ways enzyme activity has been reported and the presence of multiple isozymes of both ADH and ALDH which can confound measurement of enzyme activity in liver homogenates. We suggest that future studies will incorporate measurement of mRNA levels, and possibly nuclear run-on rates to determine if the rate of synthesis of the enzymes is altered. Further, the level of protein or enzyme activity should take into account potential dietary effects on liver size, weight, and protein content. Expression of the enzyme activity per total volume of liver may be the most relevant to predicting effects of dietary perturbations on alcohol elimination rates.

ACKNOWLEDGMENTS

The authors are supported by AA 07611 (the Indiana Alcohol Research Center), AA 06434, and AA 13623.

References

1. Agarwal, D.P. Genetic polymorphisms of alcohol metabolizing enzymes, *Pathol. Biol. (Paris)*, 49, 703, 2001.
2. Ferguson, R.A. and Goldberg, D.M. Genetic markers of alcohol abuse, *Clin. Chim. Acta*, 257, 199, 1997.
3. Crabb, D.W. Ethanol oxidizing enzymes: roles in alcohol metabolism and alcoholic liver disease, *Prog. Liver Dis.*, 13, 151, 1995.
4. Lumeng. L., Bosron, W.F., and Li, T.K. Quantitative correlation of ethanol elimination rates *in vivo* with liver alcohol dehydrogenase activities in fed, fasted and food-restricted rats, *Biochem. Pharmacol.*, 28, 1547, 1979.
5. Ramchandani, V.A., Bosron, W.F., and Li TK. Research advances in ethanol metabolism, *Pathol. Biol. (Paris)*, 49, 676, 2001.
6. Edenberg, H.J. and Bosron, W.F., *Biotransformation*, Guengerich, New York, 1997, 119.
7. Edenberg, H.J. Regulation of the mammalian alcohol dehydrogenase genes, *Prog. Nucleic Acid Res. Mol. Biol.*, 64, 295, 2000.
8. Duester, G. et al. Recommended nomenclature for the vertebrate alcohol dehydrogenase gene family, *Biochem. Pharmacol.*, 58, 389, 1999.
9. Seitz, H.K. and Oneta, C.M. Gastrointestinal alcohol dehydrogenase, *Nutr. Rev.*, 56, 52, 1998.
10. Goate, A.M. and Edenberg, H. J. The genetics of alcoholism, *Curr. Opin. Genet. Dev.*, 8, 282, 1998.
11. Duester, G. Genetic dissection of retinoid dehydrogenases, *Chem. Biol. Interact.*, 130, 469, 2001.
12. Bosron, W. F. et al. Effect of fasting on the activity and turnover of rat liver alcohol dehydrogenase, *Alcohol. Clin. Exp. Res.*, 8, 196, 1984.
13. Crabb, D.W., Bosron, W.F., and Li, T.K. Steady-state kinetic properties of purified rat liver alcohol dehydrogenase: application to predicting alcohol elimination rates *in vivo*, *Arch. Biochem. Biophys.*, 224, 299, 1983.
14. Lumeng, L. and Crabb, D.W. Rate-determining factors for ethanol metabolism in fasted and castrated male rats, *Biochem. Pharmacol.*, 33, 2623, 1984.
15. Bosron, W.F., Crabb, D.W., and Li, T.K. Relationship between kinetics of liver alcohol dehydrogenase and alcohol metabolism, *Pharmacol. Biochem. Behav.*, 18 Suppl. 1, 223,1983.
16. Lakshman, M.R. et al. Roles of hormonal and nutritional factors in the regulation of rat liver alcohol dehydrogenase activity and ethanol elimination rate *in vivo*, *Alcohol. Clin. Exp. Res.*, 12, 407, 1988.
17. Maly, I.P. and Sasse, D. The effects of starving and refeeding on the intra-acinar distribution pattern of alcohol-dehydrogenase activity in rat liver, *Histochemistry*, 86, 275, 1987.
18. Mezey, E. et al. Sex differences in gastric alcohol dehydrogenase activity in Sprague-Dawley rats, *Gastroenterology*, 103, 1804, 1992.
19. Lindros, K.O., Pekkanen, L., and Koivula, T. Enzymatic and metabolic modification of hepatic ethanol and acetaldehyde oxidation by the dietary protein level, *Biochem. Pharmacol.*, 28, 2313, 1979.
20. Wilson, J.S., Korsten, M.A., and Lieber, C.S. The combined effects of protein deficiency and chronic ethanol administration on rat ethanol metabolism, *Hepatology*, 6, 823, 1986.

21. Yang, S.C. et al. Comparative study of alcohol metabolism in stroke-prone spontaneously hypertensive rats and Wistar-Kyoto rats fed normal or low levels of dietary protein, *J. Nutr. Sci. Vitaminol. (Tokyo)*, 40, 547, 1994.

22. Straus, D.S. et al. Protein restriction specifically decreases the abundance of serum albumin and transthyretin nuclear transcripts in rat liver, *J. Nutr.*, 124, 1041, 1994.

23. Sachan, D.S. and Mynatt, R.L. Wheat gluten-based diet retarded ethanol metabolism by altering alcohol dehydrogenase and not carnitine status in adult rats, *J. Am. Coll. Nutr.*, 12, 170, 1993.

24. Polavarapu, R. et al. Increased lipid peroxidation and impaired antioxidant enzyme function is associated with pathological liver injury in experimental alcoholic liver disease in rats fed diets high in corn oil and fish oil, *Hepatology*, 27, 1317, 1998.

25. Nanji, A.A., Sadrzadeh, S.M., and Dannenberg, A.J. Liver microsomal fatty acid composition in ethanol-fed rats: effect of different dietary fats and relationship to liver injury, *Alcohol. Clin. Exp. Res.*, 18, 1024, 1994.

26. Amet, Y., Adas, F., and Nanji, A.A. Fatty acid omega- and (omega-1)-hydroxylation in experimental alcoholic liver disease: relationship to different dietary fatty acids, *Alcohol. Clin. Exp. Res.*, 22, 1493, 1998.

27. Mezey, E. Dietary fat and alcoholic liver disease, *Hepatology*, 28, 901, 1998.

28. Nanji, A.A. et al. Dietary saturated fatty acids down-regulate cyclooxygenase-2 and tumor necrosis factor alfa and reverse fibrosis in alcohol-induced liver disease in the rat, *Hepatology*, 26, 1538, 1997.

29. French, S.W. Nutrition in the pathogenesis of alcoholic liver disease, *Alcohol Alcohol.*, 28, 97, 1993.

30. Fisher, H. et al. Diet composition, alcohol utilization, and dependence, *Alcohol*, 13, 195, 1996.

31. Grummer, M.A. and Erdman, J.W. Jr. Effect of chronic alcohol consumption and moderate fat diet on vitamin A status in rats fed either vitamin A or beta-carotene, *J. Nutr.*, 113, 350, 1983.

32. Kishimoto, R. et al. Changes in hepatic enzyme activities related to ethanol metabolism in mice following chronic ethanol administration, *J. Nutr. Sci. Vitaminol. (Tokyo)*, 41, 527, 1995.

33. Zimatkin, S.M., Pronko, P.S., and Grinevich, V.P. Alcohol action on liver: dose dependence and morpho-biochemical correlations, *Cas. Lek. Cesk.*, 136, 598, 1997.

34. Traves, C., Camps, L., and Lopez-Tejero, D. Liver alcohol dehydrogenase activity and ethanol levels during chronic ethanol intake in pregnant rats and their offspring, *Pharmacol. Biochem. Behav.*, 52, 93, 1995.

35. He, L., Ronis, M.J., and Badger, T.M. Ethanol induction of class I alcohol dehydrogenase expression in the rat occurs through alterations in CCAAT/enhancer binding proteins beta and gamma, *J. Biol. Chem.*, 277, 43572, 2002.

36. Yin, M. et al. Reduced early alcohol-induced liver injury in CD14-deficient mice, *J. Immunol.*, 166, 4737, 2001.

37. Enomoto, N. et al. Kupffer cell sensitization by alcohol involves increased permeability to gut-derived endotoxin, *Alcohol. Clin. Exp. Res.*, 25, 51S, 2001.

38. Enomoto, N. et al. Long-term alcohol exposure changes sensitivity of rat Kupffer cells to lipopolysaccharide, *Alcohol. Clin. Exp. Res.*, 25, 1360, 2001.

39. Uesugi, T. et al. Toll-like receptor 4 is involved in the mechanism of early alcohol-induced liver injury in mice, *Hepatology*, 34, 101, 2001.

40. Potter, J.J., Rennie-Tankersley, L., and Mezey, E. Endotoxin enhances liver alcohol dehydrogenase by action through upstream stimulatory factor but not by nuclear factor-kB, *J. Biol. Chem.*, 278, 4353, 2003.

41. Hoffmann, I., Ang, H.L., and Duester, G. Alcohol dehydrogenases in *Xenopus* development: conserved expression of ADH1 and ADH4 in epithelial retinoid target tissues, *Dev. Dyn.*, 213, 261, 1998.

42. Molotkov, A. et al. Distinct retinoid metabolic functions for alcohol dehydrogenase genes Adh1 and Adh4 in protection against vitamin A toxicity or deficiency revealed in double null mutant mice, *J. Biol. Chem.*, 277, 13804, 2002.

43. Molotkov, A. and Duester, G. Retinol/ethanol drug interaction during acute alcohol intoxication in mice involves inhibition of retinol metabolism to retinoic acid by alcohol dehydrogenase, *J. Biol. Chem.*, 277, 22553, 2002.

44. Leo, M.A. and Lieber, C.S. Alcohol, vitamin A, and beta-carotene: adverse interactions, including hepatotoxicity and carcinogenicity, *Am. J. Clin. Nutr.*, 69, 1071, 1999.

45. Lieber, C.S. Alcohol, liver, and nutrition, *J. Am. Coll. Nutr.*, 10, 602, 1991.

46. Pinaire, J. et al. Effects of vitamin A deficiency on rat liver alcohol dehydrogenase expression and alcohol elimination rate in rats, *Alcohol. Clin. Exp. Res.*, 24, 1759, 2000.

47. Abe, T., Okamoto, E., and Itokawa, Y. Biochemical and histological studies on thiamine-deficient and ethanol-fed rats, *J. Nutr. Sci. Vitaminol. (Tokyo)*, 25, 375, 1979.

48. Sachan, D.S. and Cha, Y.S. Acetylcarnitine inhibits alcohol dehydrogenase, *Biochem. Biophys. Res. Commun.*, 203, 1496, 1994.

49. Cha, Y.S. and Sachan, D.S. Opposite effects of dietary saturated and unsaturated fatty acids on ethanol-pharmacokinetics, triglycerides and carnitines, *J. Am. Coll. Nutr.*, 13, 338, 1994.

50. Das, I., Burch, R.E., and Hahn, H.K. Effects of zinc deficiency on ethanol metabolism and alcohol and aldehyde dehydrogenase activities, *J. Lab. Clin. Med.*, 104, 610, 1984.

51. Boron, B. et al. Effect of zinc deficiency on hepatic enzymes regulating vitamin A status, *J. Nutr.*, 118, 995, 1988.

52. Indo, Y. Effects of dietary zinc deficiency on hepatic ornithine carbamoyltransferase and alcohol dehydrogenase activities in rats, *J. Pediatr. Gastroenterol. Nutr.*, 4, 268, 1985.

53. Caballeria, J. Zinc administration improves gastric alcohol dehydrogenase activity and first-pass metabolism of ethanol in alcohol-fed rats, *Alcohol. Clin. Exp. Res.*, 21, 1619, 1997.

54. Keung, W.M. Biochemical studies of a new class of alcohol dehydrogenase inhibitors from *Radix puerariae*, *Alcohol. Clin. Exp. Res.*, 17, 1254, 1993.

55. Lindahl, R. Aldehyde dehydrogenases and their role in carcinogenesis, *Crit. Rev. Biochem. Mol. Biol.*, 27, 283, 1992.

56. Yoshida, A. et al. Human aldehyde dehydrogenase gene family, *Eur. J. Biochem.*, 251, 549, 1998.

57. Stewart, M.J., Malek, K., and Crabb, D.W. Distribution of messenger RNAs for aldehyde dehydrogenase 1, aldehyde dehydrogenase 2, and aldehyde dehydrogenase 5 in human tissues, *J. Investig. Med.*, 44, 42, 1996.

58. Ambroziak, W., Izaguirre, G., and Pietruszko, R. Metabolism of retinaldehyde and other aldehydes in soluble extracts of human liver and kidney, *J. Biol. Chem.*, 274, 33366, 1999.

59. Stewart, M. et al. The role of nuclear factor NF-Y/CP1 in the transcriptional regulation of the human aldehyde dehydrogenase 2-encoding gene, *Gene*, 173, 155, 1996.

60. Crabb, D.W. et al. Peroxisome proliferator-activated receptors (PPAR) and the mitochondrial aldehyde dehydrogenase (ALDH2) promoter *in vitro* and *in vivo*, *Alcohol. Clin. Exp. Res.*, 25, 945, 2001.

61. Pinaire, J. et al. The retinoid X receptor response element in the human aldehyde dehydrogenase 2 promoter is antagonized by the chicken ovalbumin upstream promoter family of orphan receptors, *Arch. Biochem. Biophys.*, 380, 192, 2000.

62. Stewart, M.J. et al. Binding and activation of the human aldehyde dehydrogenase 2 promoter by hepatocyte nuclear factor 4, *Biochim. Biophys. Acta,* 1399, 181, 1998.

63. You, M. et al. Transcriptional control of the human aldehyde dehydrogenase 2 promoter by hepatocyte nuclear factor 4: inhibition by cyclic AMP and COUP transcription factors, *Arch. Biochem. Biophys.*, 398, 79, 2002.

64. Lindros, K.O., Pekkanen, L., and Koivula, T. Effect of a low-protein diet on acetaldehyde metabolism in rats, *Acta. Pharmacol. Toxicol. (Copenhagen)*, 40, 134, 1977.

65. Chen, J.J. and Yu, B.P. Detoxification of reactive aldehydes in mitochondria: effects of age and dietary restriction, *Aging (Milano)*, 8, 334, 1996.

66. Canuto, R.A. et al. Increase in class 2 aldehyde dehydrogenase expression by arachidonic acid in rat hepatoma cells, *Biochem. J.*, 357, 811, 2001.

67. Fischer, M. et al. unpublished data, 2002.

68. Tomita, Y. et al. Effects of chronic ethanol intoxication on aldehyde dehydrogenase in mouse liver, *Alcohol Alcohol.*, 27, 171, 1992.

69. Aoki, Y. and Itoh, H. Effects of alcohol consumption on mitochondrial aldehyde dehydrogenase isoenzymes in rat liver, *Enzyme*, 41, 151, 1989.

70. Ricciardi, B.R. et al. Hepatic ADH and ALDH isoenzymes in different racial groups and in chronic alcoholism, *Pharmacol. Biochem. Behav.*, 18 Suppl. 1, 61, 1983.

71. Nilius, R., Zipprich, B., and Krabbe, S. Aldehyde dehydrogenase (E.C. 1.2.1.3) in chronic alcoholic liver diseases, *Hepatogastroenterology*, 30, 134, 1983.

72. Pares, A. et al. Hepatic alcohol and aldehyde dehydrogenases in liver disease, *Alcohol Alcohol.*, Suppl. 1, 513, 1987.

73. Crabb, D.W. et al. Unpublished data, 2002.

74. Tyopponen, J.T. and Lindros, K.O. Combined vitamin E deficiency and ethanol pretreatment: liver glutathione and enzyme changes, *Int. J. Vitam. Nutr. Res.*, 56, 241, 1986.

75. Yoshino, K. et al. Studies on the formation of aliphatic aldehydes in the plasma and liver of vitamin E-deficient rats, *Chem. Pharm. Bull. (Tokyo)*, 38, 2212, 1990.

76. Tottmar, O., Marchner, H., and Karlsson, N. The presence of an aldehyde dehydrogenase inhibitor in animal diets and its effects on the experimental results in alcohol studies, *Br. J. Nutr.*, 39, 317, 1978.

77. Lindros, K.O. et al. Phenethyl isothiocyanate, a new dietary liver aldehyde dehydrogenase inhibitor, *J. Pharmacol. Exp. Ther.*, 275, 79, 1995.

78. Boyer, C.S. and Petersen, D.R. The metabolism of 3,7-dimethyl-2,6-octadienal (citral) in rat hepatic mitochondrial and cytosolic fractions. Interactions with aldehyde and alcohol dehydrogenases, *Drug Metab. Dispos.*, 19, 81, 1991.

79. Sheikh, S. and Weiner, H. Allosteric inhibition of human liver aldehyde dehydrogenase by the isoflavone prunetin, *Biochem. Pharmacol.*, 53, 471, 1997.

11 Genetic Aspects of Alcohol Metabolism

Vijay A. Ramchandani

CONTENTS

11.1 INTRODUCTION

Ethanol (also referred to as alcohol in this chapter) is probably the most widely investigated drug in the world, not only because of its ubiquitous use and its widespread abuse, but also because of its unique pharmacological properties. Following administration, systemic concentrations of alcohol are a consequence of the absorption and metabolism of alcohol, which display unique characteristics and demonstrate substantial interindividual variability.[1] As the pharmacological effects of alcohol depend on its systemic concentrations, variability in the pharmacokinetics of alcohol can have a significant impact on its pharmacodynamic effects. Following oral ingestion, alcohol is absorbed by passive diffusion, primarily from the small intestine.[2,3] The rate of absorption depends on several factors, both genetic and environmental, and is highly variable.[1] Some of these factors include the volume, concentration and nature of the alcoholic beverage,[2,4,5] the rate of drinking,[4] the fed or fasted state,[6] the nature and composition of food,[6,7] rate of gastric emptying,[8,9] gender differences in first-pass metabolism,[10,11] and other drugs including histamine

(H1) receptor antagonists like cimetidine and ranitidine.[12,13] Ethanol is a small polar molecule and its volume of distribution is comparable to total body water.[3] No plasma protein binding has been reported for alcohol. Elimination of alcohol occurs primarily through metabolism with small fractions of the administered dose being excreted in the breath (0.7%), sweat (0.1%), and urine (0.3%).[3] Alcohol metabolism occurs mainly via hepatic oxidation and is governed by the catalytic properties of the alcohol metabolizing enzymes, alcohol dehydrogenase (ADH), and aldehyde dehydrogenase (ALDH). The cytochrome P450 enzymes (CYP2E1) and catalase also contribute to alcohol metabolism and alcohol-related cytotoxicity in specific circumstances.[14]

Alcohol metabolic rates show a considerable degree of interindividual and ethnic variability, in part due to allelic variants of the genes encoding ADH and ALDH producing functionally different isozymes.[15–17] Functional polymorphisms of the *ADH1B* and *ALDH2* genes have been shown to increase the variance in alcohol metabolism among individuals. Additionally, a multitude of environmental factors can influence the metabolic regulation of alcohol metabolism, which results in a large threefold to fourfold variance in the alcohol elimination rate in humans.[18] Factors that have been shown to be important determinants of alcohol metabolism include age,[19,20] gender,[21,22] ethnicity and genetics,[21,23–26] and body mass and liver size,[27] as well as environmental factors such as food intake.[28]

This chapter will focus on genetic variation in the alcohol metabolizing enzymes and its impact on the metabolism of alcohol.

11.2 ALCOHOL METABOLIZING ENZYMES AND GENETIC ASPECTS

11.2.1 ALCOHOL DEHYDROGENASE

The alcohol dehydrogenase (*ADH*) gene family encodes oxidative enzymes that metabolize a wide variety of alcohols including ethanol, retinol, other aliphatic alcohols, hydroxysteroids, and lipid peroxidation products.[15] Currently, seven human ADH genes have been identified and organized into five classes based on amino acid sequence alignments, catalytic properties and patterns of tissue-specific expression.[29] Human ADH is a dimeric molecule, arising from the association of different subunits expressed by the seven genes. Thus, there are over 20 ADH isozymes that vary greatly with regard to the types of alcohols they preferentially metabolize and the maximal rate at which they oxidize ethanol.[15] The five classes of ADH are divided according to their subunit and isozyme composition (Table 11.1).

The Class I isozymes are found in liver, and consist of homo- and hetero-dimeric forms of the three subunits (i.e., αα, αβ, ββ, βγ, γγ, etc.). Classes II, III, and IV enzymes are homodimeric forms of the π, χ, and σ subunits, respectively. All the Class I ADHs metabolize ethanol and are inhibited by pyrazole derivatives.[30] The ADH1 subunits share about 94% sequence identity. The relative order of catalytic efficiency (k_{cat}/K_m) for ethanol oxidation at ethanol concentrations of about 100 mg% and saturating coenzyme NAD$^+$ concentration (0.5 mM) is: β2 > β1 > γ1 > γ2 ≈ σ

TABLE 11.1
Nomenclature for Alcohol Dehydrogenase Genes

ADH Class	New Gene Nomenclature	Former Gene Nomenclature	Enzyme Subunit Nomenclature	K_m for Ethanol (mM)
I	ADH1A	ADH1	α	4.0
I	ADH1B*1	ADH2*1	β1	0.05
I	ADH1B*2	ADH2*2	β2	0.9
I	ADH1B*3	ADH2*3	β3	40
I	ADH1C*1	ADH3*1	γ1	1.0
I	ADH1C*2	ADH3*2	γ2	6.0
II	ADH4	ADH4	π	30
III	ADH5	ADH5	χ	>1000
IV	ADH7	ADH7	σ	30
V	ADH6	ADH6	Not identified	?

Note: Human Genome Organization Gene Nomenclature Committee, Official gene nomenclature for ADH, http://www.gene.ucl.ac.uk/nomenclature/genefamily/ADH.shtml, 2001.

>> β3 > α >>π. However, the relative order of k_{cat} at saturating concentrations of both ethanol and NAD$^+$ is σ > β3 ≈ β2 > γ1 > γ2 ≈ π > β1. Thus, the relative contributions of each of the ADH isozymes to ethanol oxidation changes with the hepatic concentration of alcohol.[31]

The human ADH genes are differentially expressed in different tissues, and this is a very important determinant of the physiological consequences of alcohol metabolism in specific cells and tissues.[30,32] The liver contains a large amount of ADH (about 3% of soluble protein) and expresses the widest number of different isozymes. ADH4 (π-ADH) is solely expressed in liver. Only ADH7 (σ-ADH) is not highly expressed in liver. ADH5 (χ-ADH) is ubiquitously expressed in human tissues. ADH1C, ADH4, ADH5, and ADH7 are expressed in gastrointestinal tissues. The expression of ADH5 in humans and its role in ethanol metabolism remain to be elucidated. Also, the expression of ADH in other tissues such as skeletal muscle, and the quantitative significance of muscle ADH metabolism (because of the large proportion of muscle mass in the body), remains to be determined.[16]

In addition to ethanol, alcohol dehydrogenases also oxidize several "physiological" alcohols with high catalytic efficiency including retinol, ω-hydroxy fatty acids, hydroxy steroids, and hydroxy derivatives of dopamine and epinephrine metabolites.[30,33] Oxidation of these alcohols can be inhibited by ethanol, and therefore the role of ethanol substrate competition is an important issue in alcohol-related toxicology. Another important issue is the regional expression of ADHs in the brain and their potential role in the local formation of acetaldehyde, which may be psychoactive, possessing stimulant as well as sedative/hypnotic effects.[34–36]

11.2.1.1 Genetic Polymorphisms

Genetic polymorphism occurs at the *ADH1B* and *ADH1C* loci.[15,37] Variant alleles of *ADH1B* result in the β1, β2, and β3 subunits, while variants of *ADH1C* result in the γ1 and γ2 subunits. The resulting subunits have different catalytic activities for ethanol (see Table 11.1). Additionally, the *ADH1B* alleles appear with different frequencies in different racial groups, with the *ADH1B*1* form predominating in white and black populations, and *ADH1B*2* predominating in East Asian populations (e.g., Chinese and Japanese), and also found in about 25% of white subjects with Jewish ancestry. The *ADH1B*3* form is found in about 25% of black subjects. With respect to the *ADH1C* polymorphism, *ADH1C*1* and *ADH1C*2* appear with about equal frequency in white populations, but *ADH1C*1* predominates in black and East Asian populations.[18,38]

Recently, a novel single nucleotide polymorphism was identified in *ADH1C*. This polymorphism results in an allele that codes for a subunit with a proline → threonine substitution in position 351.[39] This variant is found to occur primarily in Native Americans with frequencies as high as 26%. However, the catalytic activity of the isozyme coded by this variant and its effect on the overall elimination of alcohol remain to be established.

11.2.2 ALDEHYDE DEHYDROGENASE

Acetaldehyde is the first metabolic product of ethanol metabolism, and is itself metabolized via oxidation by the NAD^+-dependent aldehyde dehydrogenase (ALDH). Several isozymes of ALDH, differing in kinetic properties and tissue distribution, have been detected in human organs and tissues.[15] Currently, 17 functional ALDH genes have been identified in the human genome.[40] However, only the *ALDH1* (*ALDH1A1*) and *ALDH2* genes encode the class I and class II isozymes that are involved in acetaldehyde oxidation. ALDH1 is the cytosolic form distributed ubiquitously in tissues including brain. It exhibits relatively low catalytic activity ($K_m \sim 30$ μM) for acetaldehyde oxidation. ALDH2 is the mitochondrial enzyme that is highly expressed in liver and stomach.[41] It exhibits high catalytic activity ($K_m \sim 3$ μM) for acetaldehyde oxidation and is primarily responsible for acetaldehyde oxidation *in vivo*.

11.2.2.1 Genetic Polymorphisms

There is one known functionally significant genetic polymorphism of the *ALDH2* gene. The allelic variants are *ALDH2*1* and *ALDH2*2*, encoding for the high activity and low activity forms of the subunits respectively. The low activity form arises from a single amino acid exchange (glutamine to lysine substitution at position 487) at the coenzyme binding site of the enzyme subunit.[15] This results in a 100-fold increase in the K_m for NAD^+.[42] This very prominent variant allele has been seen in about half of the East Asian populations studied (including the Han Chinese, Taiwanese, and Japanese).[43,44] It has not been observed in populations of Caucasian origin. It exhibits virtually no acetaldehyde oxidizing activity *in vitro*, and represents the "deficient" phenotype seen in these Asian populations.[45] Individuals who are heterozygous or homozygous for *ALDH2*2* show the characteristic sensitivity reaction (facial flushing, increased skin temperature and heart rate) following alcohol intake.[26,46]

11.2.3 MICROSOMAL ETHANOL OXIDIZING SYSTEM (MEOS)

A small fraction of an ingested dose of ethanol is metabolized by enzymes other than ADH. Metabolism of ethanol by microsomal enzymes, particularly the cytochrome P450 enzymes, accounts for the major non-ADH system. The cytochrome P450 isoform, P4502E1 (CYP2E1), is the major alternative system that catalyzes the NADPH- and O_2-dependent oxidation of ethanol to form acetaldehyde, $NADP^+$, and water. As many as 13 different *CYP2E1* polymorphisms have been identified.[15] A polymorphism has been reported in the 5'-flanking region of the *CYP2E1* gene. This polymorphism is differentially expressed in different racial populations, and the rare mutant allele (*c2* allele) has been found to be associated with higher transcriptional activity, protein levels, and enzyme activity than the common wild-type *c1* allele.[15,47] The influence of *CYP2E1* genotypes on alcohol elimination was examined in one study in Japanese alcoholics and control, and indicated that the presence of the *c2* allele (heterozygous or homozygous) may be associated with higher alcohol metabolic rates but only at blood alcohol levels greater than 0.25% (g/dl).[48]

While MEOS accounts for a much smaller fraction of ethanol oxidation than the ADH system under normal conditions, it represents a major adaptive response of alcohol metabolism with chronic ethanol consumption.[14] This is due to the direct effect of chronic ethanol consumption on the expression of hepatic CYP2E1. In humans, there is an induction of CYP2E1 with chronic alcohol consumption that can be followed by a decrease in activity associated with generalized hepatic injury and loss of function. There are two mechanisms postulated for CYP2E1 induction: (1) a posttranslational mechanism involving mRNA stabilization and protection of the expressed protein against degradation and (2) a direct transcriptional regulation of CYP2E1 expression, generally following high exposures to ethanol. The expression of CYP2E1 is influenced by factors such as diet (lipids, carbohydrates) and hormones (thyroid hormones, glucocorticoids, steroids, pituitary hormones). However, much work needs to be done to understand mechanisms for transcriptional and posttranslational regulation of the MEOS genes, and their role in alcohol metabolism and alcohol-related liver disease.[14]

11.2.4 CATALASE

Catalase is an enzyme that catalyzes the H_2O_2-dependent oxidation of ethanol yielding acetaldehyde and two molecules of water. It is found in the cytosol and mitochondria but its main expression and function is in peroxisomes. Most studies indicate that it contributes very little to total ethanol elimination because of the limited availability of hydrogen peroxide.[14,49] However, the activation of peroxisomal catalase by increased generation of hydrogen peroxide via peroxisomal β-oxidation leads to a hypermetabolic state and a swift increase in alcohol metabolism.[50] This state may contribute to alcohol-related inflammation and necrosis in alcoholic liver disease.

11.3 ADH AND ALDH POLYMORPHISMS: INFLUENCE ON ALCOHOL METABOLISM

Functional polymorphisms of the alcohol metabolizing enzymes ADH and ALDH2, and differences in the prevalence of the polymorphic alleles in different ethnic populations, have resulted in several studies examining ethnic differences in alcohol metabolism and the influence of *ADH1B*, *ADH1C*, and *ALDH2* genotypes. The isozymes encoded by the polymorphic alleles have very different catalytic properties *in vitro*,[30,31] and would be expected to exert influences on an individual's alcohol metabolic rate.

One of the first studies examining the influence of *ADH* and *ALDH* polymorphisms on alcohol metabolism was done by Mizoi et al.[23] in 68 healthy Japanese subjects. Subjects were genotyped for *ADH1B* as well as *ALDH2* polymorphisms and alcohol disappearance rates (mg/ml/h) and elimination rates (mg/kg/h) were compared among the groups classified, based on zygosities of both *ADH1B* (*ADH1B*1/*1*, *ADH1B*1/*2* and *ADH1B*2/*2*), and *ALDH2*. Results indicated that there were no differences in alcohol metabolism among the *ADH1B* genotypes; however, there were marked differences among the *ALDH2* genotypes with regard to alcohol metabolism. This is discussed further below.

In another study, Neumark et al.[51,52] found differences in alcohol elimination rates in Jewish subjects with different *ADH1B* genotypes following alcohol administration using the alcohol clamp method.[53,54] The authors found significantly higher alcohol elimination rates in subjects carrying the *ADH1B*2* allele (heterozygotes and homozygotes) compared with *ADH1B*1* homozygotes. As the Jewish do not show polymorphisms of the *ALDH2* genes, this appears to be a direct effect of *ADH1B* genotypes on alcohol metabolism.

Thomasson et al.[21] examined the influence of the other *ADH1B* polymorphism (*ADH1B*3*) on alcohol metabolism in a sample of 112 African-American subjects selected by genotype. In this study, subjects received an oral dose of alcohol and alcohol disappearance rates were determined from the slope of the pseudo-linear portion of the blood ethanol concentration vs. time curves. Results revealed that subjects who had β3-containing ADH isozymes showed a higher alcohol disappearance rate (mg% per h) compared to those with β1β1-ADH isozymes. A study in Native Americans also showed that subjects with *ADH1B*3* alleles had a trend toward higher alcohol elimination rates than subjects with *ADH1B*1*.[24] However, this difference was not statistically significant probably because of the small number of subjects possessing the *ADH1B*3* genotype in the study and the low frequency of occurrence of this genotype (~7%) in this ethnic group. Earlier studies in Native Americans had also demonstrated higher alcohol elimination rates compared to those reported in Caucasians; however, *ADH* genotypes were not determined in these studies.[55–57]

The influence of *ALDH2* polymorphisms on alcohol metabolism has been studied more extensively, although almost exclusively in Asian subjects, mainly because of the high frequency of the polymorphism in this population. Most of these studies have compared peak concentrations of alcohol and acetaldehyde as well as peak responses on subjective and cardiovascular measures and flushing across *ADH1B* and *ALDH2* genotypes, with generally consistent results. In general, individuals who are heterozygous or homozygous for *ALDH2*2* show increased acetaldehyde levels following alcohol administration.[25,26,46,58–60] Some studies have also demonstrated significant increases in ethanol concentrations and area under the ethanol concentration time curves,[46,60] possibly due to product inhibition of ADH activity by acetaldehyde. However, other studies have shown accumulation of acetaldehyde in subjects carrying the *ALDH2*2* allele without any alterations in alcohol concentrations or elimination rates.[25,26]

There are only a few studies that have actually estimated and compared alcohol disappearance rates (beta-60) or elimination rates among *ADH1B* and/or *ALDH2* genotypes.[23,25,61] A study in Chinese men indicated that the presence of the *ALDH2*2* allele was associated with slower alcohol metabolism following oral administration.[61] In the study by Mizoi et al.[23] described above, peak acetaldehyde levels, alcohol disappearance rates (mg/ml/h), and elimination rates (mg/kg/h) were compared among subjects classified into groups based on zygosities of both *ADH1B* and *ALDH2* (*ALDH2*1/*1*, *ALDH2*1/*2*, and *ALDH2*2/*2*). Results indicated that subjects homozygous for *ALDH2*1/*1* showed no increase in acetaldehyde levels regardless of their *ADH1B* genotype. There was a progressive increase in peak acetaldehyde levels in subjects with the *ALDH2*1/*2* and *ALDH2*2/*2* genotypes. Both alcohol disappearance rates and elimination rates showed significant differences among the *ALDH2* genotypes and decreased in the following order: *ALDH2*1/*1 > ALDH2*1/*2 > ALDH2*2/*2*.

Thus, genetic polymorphisms of *ADH* and *ALDH* result in alterations in the metabolism of alcohol and/or acetaldehyde. Polymorphisms in *ADH* result in variants (*ADH1B*2* and *ADH1B*3*) that code for isozymes that tend to show a faster rate of alcohol metabolism, while the *ALDH2*2* polymorphism results in a "deficient" form of ALDH2 that causes an accumulation of acetaldehyde and its associated physiological effects.

11.4 ADH AND ALDH POLYMORPHISMS: ASSOCIATION WITH ALCOHOL DEPENDENCE

Functional polymorphisms of the alcohol metabolizing enzymes ADH and ALDH2 can also exert important effects on the biological effects of alcohol.[62] In fact, *ADH* and *ALDH* are the only genes which have been firmly established to influence vulnerability to alcohol dependence or alcoholism.[38] Studies have demonstrated unequivocally that the allele frequencies of *ADH1B*2*, *ADH1B*3*, and *ALDH2*2* are significantly decreased in subjects diagnosed with alcohol dependence as compared with the general population of East Asians, including the Japanese, Han Chinese, and Koreans.[43,44,63–67] The *ALDH2*2* allele and the *ADH1B*2* allele also significantly influence drinking behavior in nonalcoholic individuals. Association between reduced alcohol consumption or reduced risk of alcohol dependence and the *ADH1B*2* variant allele has recently been found in other ethnic groups that do not carry the *ALDH2*2* allele, including Europeans,[68–70] Jews in Israel,[71,72] as well as Mongolians in China,[44] and the Atayal natives of Taiwan.[73] A recent study has also shown a protective association between the *ADH1B*3* allele and alcohol dependence in Native Americans.[74] Finally, studies have indicated that the *ADH1B*3* allele may be protective against alcohol-related problems in children born to African-American mothers who may have consumed alcohol during pregnancy.[75–78]

11.5 SUMMARY

There has been substantial progress in the field of alcohol pharmacogenetics to characterize differences in alcohol metabolism in subjects exhibiting polymorphic genotypes of the alcohol metabolizing enzymes. Studies are, however, needed to further evaluate these genetic determinants of alcohol metabolism, particularly differences arising from the polymorphisms of *ADH1C* and *ALDH2*.

Recent studies have characterized the genetic polymorphisms in different racial and ethnic groups, but large differences in alcohol elimination rates still exist between individuals within the various ethnic groups. Of potential significance in this regard may be the recent discovery of polymorphisms in the promoter regions of *ALDH2*[79,80] and *ADH4*,[81] as well as the recently identified *ADH1C*351Thr* polymorphism.[39] Studies are needed to evaluate the influence of these polymorphisms on the activity of ADH and ALDH and on alcohol levels and elimination rates in individuals, as well as on the physiological response to alcohol consumption and alcoholism.

Studies in monozygotic and dizygotic twins have shown that the heritability (i.e., genetic component of variance) of alcohol metabolic rates is about 50%.[82,83] Further evaluation of the factors, both genetic and environmental, regulating the rates of alcohol and acetaldehyde metabolism will help improve our understanding of the metabolic basis and consequences of alcohol's effects, including the risk and consequences of alcohol-related organ damage and developmental problems, as well as alcohol dependence.

ACKNOWLEDGMENTS

The author wishes to thank Dr. Ting-Kai Li, National Institute on Alcohol Abuse and Alcoholism, Bethesda, MD, and Dr. William F. Bosron, Indiana University School of Medicine, Indianapolis, IN.

References

1. Norberg, A., Jones, W.A., Hahn, R.G., and Gabrielsson, J.L., Role of variability in explaining ethanol pharmacokinetics: research and forensic applications, *Clin. Pharmacokinet.*, 42, 1–31, 2003.
2. Wilkinson, P.K., Sedman, A.J., Sakmar, E., Kay, D.R., and Wagner, J.G., Pharmacokinetics of ethanol after oral administration in the fasting state, *J. Pharmacokinet. Biopharm.*, 5, 207–224, 1977.
3. Holford, N.H.G., Clinical pharmacokinetics of ethanol, *Clin. Pharmacokinet.*, 13, 273–292, 1987.

4. O'Neill, B., Williams, A., and Dubowski, K.M., Variability in blood alcohol concentrations, *J. Stud. Alcohol.*, 44, 222–230, 1983.

5. Dubowski, K.M., Absorption, distribution and elimination of alcohol: highway safety aspects, *J. Stud. Alcohol.*, Suppl., 10, 98–108, 1985.

6. Sedman, A., Wilkinson, P.K., Sakmar, E., Weidler, D.J., and Wagner, J.G., Food effects on absorption and metabolism of alcohol, *J. Stud. Alcohol.*, 37, 1197–1214, 1976.

7. Jones, A.W., Jonsson, K.A., and Kechagias, S., Effect of high-fat, high-protein and high-carbohydrate meals on the pharmacokinetics of a small dose of ethanol, *Br. J. Clin. Pharmacol.*, 44, 521–526, 1997.

8. Mushambi, M.C., Bailey, S.M., Trotter, T.N., Chadd, G.D., and Rowbotham D.J., Effect of alcohol on gastric emptying in volunteers, *Br. J. Anaesth.*, 71, 674–676, 1993.

9. Kalant, H., Effects of food and of body composition on blood alcohol curves, *Alc. Clin. Exp. Res.*, 24, 413–414, 2000.

10. Frezza, M., Di Padova, C., Pozzato, G., Maddalena, T., Baraona, E., and Lieber, C.S., High blood alcohol levels in women. The role of decreased gastric alcohol dehydrogenase activity and first-pass metabolism, *N. Engl. J. Med.*, 322, 95–99, 1990.

11. Ammon, E., Schafer C., Hofmann, U., and Klotz, U., Disposition and first-pass metabolism of ethanol in humans: is it gastric or hepatic and does it depend on gender? *Clin. Pharmacol. Ther.*, 59, 503–513, 1996.

12. Gupta, A.M., Baraona, E., and Lieber, C.S., Significant increase of blood alcohol by cimetidine after repetitive drinking of small alcohol doses, *Alc. Clin. Exp. Res.*, 19, 1083–1087, 1995.

13. Arora, S., Baraona, E., and Lieber, C.S., Alcohol levels are increased in social drinkers receiving ranitidine, *Am. J. Gastroenterol.*, 95, 208–213, 2000.

14. Lieber, C.S., Microsomal ethanol-oxidizing system (MEOS): the first 30 years (1968–1998) — a review, *Alc. Clin. Exp. Res.*, 23, 991–1007, 1999.

15. Agarwal, D.P., Genetic polymorphisms of alcohol metabolizing enzymes, *Pathol. Biol.*, 49, 703–709, 2001.

16. Ramchandani, V.A., Bosron, W.F., and Li, T.-K., Research advances in ethanol metabolism, *Pathol. Biol.*, 49, 676–682, 2001.

17. Hurley, T.D., Edenberg, H.J., and Li, T.-K., Pharmacogenomics of alcoholism, in: Licinio, J. and Wong, M.-L. (Eds.), *Pharmacogenomics: The Search for Individualized Therapeutics*, Wiley-VCH, Weinheim, Germany, 2002, 417–441.

18. Eckardt, M.J., File, S.E., Gessa, G.L., Grant, K.A., Guerri, C., Hoffman, P., Kalant, H., Koob, G., Li, T,.K., and Tabakoff, B., Effects of moderate alcohol consumption on the central nervous system, *Alc. Clin. Exp. Res.*, 22, 998–1007, 1998.

19. Vestal, R., McGuire, E.A., Tobin, J.D., Andres, R., Norris, A.H., and Mezey, E., Aging and ethanol metabolism, *Clin. Pharmacol. Ther.*, 21, 343–354, 1977.

20. Jones, A.W. and Neri, A., Age-related differences in blood alcohol parameters and subjective feelings of intoxication in healthy men, *Alcohol Alcohol.*, 20, 45–52, 1985.

21. Thomasson, H.R., Beard, J.D., and Li, T.-K., ADH2 gene polymorphisms are determinants of alcohol pharmacokinetics, *Alc. Clin. Exp. Res.*, 19, 1494–1499, 1995.

22. Thomasson, H.R., Alcohol elimination: faster in women? *Alc. Clin. Exp. Res.*, 24, 419–420, 2000.

23. Mizoi, Y., Yamamoto, K., Ueno, Y., Fukunaga, T., and Harada, S., Involvement of genetic polymorphism of alcohol and aldehyde dehydrogenases in individual variation of alcohol metabolism, *Alcohol Alcohol.*, 29, 707–710, 1994.

24. Wall, T.L., Garcia-Andrade, C., Thomasson, H.R., Cole, M., and Ehlers, C., Alcohol elimination in Native American Mission Indians: an investigation of inter-individual variation, *Alc. Clin. Exp. Res.*, 20, 1159–1164, 1996.

25. Wall, T.L., Peterson, C.M., Peterson, K.P., Johnson, M.L., Thomasson, H.R., Cole, M., and Ehlers, C.L., Alcohol metabolism in Asian-American men with genetic polymorphisms of aldehyde dehydrogenase, *Ann. Intern. Med.*, 127, 376–379, 1997.

26. Peng, G.S., Yin, J.H., Wang, M.F., Lee, J.T., Hsu, Y.D., and Yin, S.J., Alcohol sensitivity in Taiwanese men with different alcohol and aldehyde dehydrogenase genotypes, *J. Formos. Med. Assoc.*, 101, 769–774, 2002.

27. Kwo, P.Y., Ramchandani, V.A., O'Connor, S., Amann, D., Carr, L.G., Sandrasegaran, K., Kopecky, K., and Li, T.-K., Gender differences in alcohol metabolism: Relationship to liver volume and effect of adjusting for lean body mass, *Gastroenterology*, 115, 1552–1557, 1998.

28. Ramchandani, V.A., Kwo, P.Y., and Li, T.-K., Influence of food and food composition on alcohol elimination rates in healthy men and women, *J. Clin. Pharmacol.*, 41, 1345–1350, 2001.

29. Duester, G., Farres, J., Felder, M., Holmes, S., Hoog, J.O., Pares, X., Plapp, B., Yin, S.J., and Jornvall, H., Recommended nomenclature for the vertebrate alcohol dehydrogenase gene family, *Biochem. Pharmacol.*, 58, 389–395, 1999.

30. Edenberg, H.J. and Bosron, W.F., Alcohol dehydrogenases, in: Guengerich, F.P. (Ed.), *Biotransformation*, Pergamon, New York, 1997, 119–131.

31. Bosron, W.F., Ehrig, T., and Li, T.-K., Genetic factors in alcohol metabolism and alcoholism. *Semin. Liver Dis.*, 13, 126–135, 1993.

32. Edenberg, H.J., Regulation of the mammalian alcohol dehydrogenase genes, *Prog. Nucleic Acid Res. Mol. Biol.*, 64, 295–341, 2000.

33. Boleda, M.D., Saubi, N., Farres, J., and Pares, X., Physiological substrates for rat alcohol dehydrogenase classes: aldehydes of lipid peroxidation, omega-hydroxy fatty acids, and retinoids, *Arch. Biochem. Biophys.*, 307, 85–90, 1993.

34. Hunt, W.A., Role of acetaldehyde in the actions of ethanol on the brain — a review, *Alcohol*, 13, 147–151, 1996.

35. Zimatkin, S.M., Liopo, A.V., and Deitrich, R.A., Distribution and kinetics of ethanol metabolism in rat brain, *Alc. Clin. Exp. Res.*, 22, 1623–1627, 1998.

36. McBride, W.J., Li, T.-K., Deitrich, R.A., Zimatkin, S., Smith, B.R. and Rodd-Henricks, Z.A., Involvement of acetaldehyde in alcohol addiction, *Alc. Clin. Exp. Res.*, 26, 114–119, 2002.

37. Yin, S.J. and Li, T.-K., Genetic polymorphism and properties of human alcohol and aldehyde dehydrogenases: implications for ethanol metabolism and toxicity, in: Sun, G.Y., Rudeen, P.K., Wood, W.G., Wei, Y.H., and Sun, A.Y. (Eds.), *Molecular Mechanisms of Alcohol: Neurobiology and Metabolism*, Humana Press, Clifton, NJ, 1989, 227–247.

38. Li, T.-K., Pharmacogenetics of responses to alcohol and genes that influence alcohol drinking, *J. Stud. Alcohol.*, 61, 5–12, 2000.

39. Osier, M.V., Pakstis, A.J., Goldman, D., Edenberg, H.J., Kidd, J.R., and Kidd, K.K., A proline–threonine substitution in codon 351 of ADH1C is common in Native Americans, *Alc. Clin. Exp. Res.*, 26, 1759–1763, 2002.

40. Sophos, N.A. and Vasiliou, V., Aldehyde dehydrogenase gene superfamily: the 2002 update, *Chem. Biol. Interact.*, 143 and 144, 5–22, 2003.

41. Yoshida, A., Rzhetsky, A., Hsu, L.C., and Chang, C.-P., Human aldehyde dehydrogenase gene family, *Eur. J. Biochem.*, 251, 549–557, 1998.

42. Steinmetz, C.G., Xie, P., Weiner, H., and Hurley, T.D., Structure of mitochondrial aldehyde dehydrogenase: the genetic component of alcohol aversion, *Structure*, 5, 701–711, 1997.

43. Thomasson, H.R., Edenberg, H.J., Crabb, D.W., Mai, X.-L., Jerome, R.E., Li, T.-K., Wang, S.-P., Lin, Y.-T., Lu, R.-B., and Yin, S.-J., Alcohol and aldehyde dehydrogenase genotypes and alcoholism in Chinese men, *Am. J. Hum. Genet.*, 48, 677–681, 1991.

44. Shen, Y.C., Fan, J.H., Edenberg, H.J., Li, T.-K., Cui, Y.H., Wang, Y.F., Tian, C.H., Zhou, C.F., Zhou, R.L., Wang, J., Zhao, Z.L., and Xia, G.Y., Polymorphism of ADH and ALDH genes among four ethnic groups in China and effects upon the risk for alcoholism, *Alc. Clin. Exp. Res.*, 21, 1272–1277, 1997.

45. Crabb, D.W., Edenberg, H.J., Bosron, W.F., and Li, T.-K., Genotypes for aldehyde dehydrogenase deficiency and alcohol sensitivity. The inactive ALDH2(2) allele is dominant, *J. Clin. Invest.*, 83, 314–316, 1989.

46. Peng, G.S., Wang, M.F., Chen, C.Y., Luu, S.U., Chou, H.C., Li, T.-K., and Yin, S.J., Involvement of acetaldehyde for full protection against alcoholism by homozygosity of the variant allele of mitochondrial aldehyde dehydrogenase gene in Asians, *Pharmacogenetics*, 9, 463–476, 1999.

47. Hayashi, S., Watanabe, J., and Kawajiri, K., Genetic polymorphisms in the 5′-flanking region change transcriptional regulation of the human cytochrome P450IIE1 gene, *J. Biochem. (Tokyo)*, 110, 559–65, 1991.

48. Ueno, Y., Adachi, J., Imamichi, H., Nishimura, A., and Tatsuno, Y., Effect of the cytochrome P-450IIE1 genotype on ethanol elimination rate in alcoholics and control subjects, *Alc. Clin. Exp. Res.*, 20 (1 Suppl.), 17A–21A, 1996.

49. Crabb, D.W., Ethanol oxidizing enzymes: roles in alcohol metabolism and alcoholic liver disease, *Prog. Liv. Dis.*, 13, 151–172, 1995.

50. Bradford, B.U., Enomoto, N., Ikejima, K., Rose, M.L., Bojes, H.K., Forman, D.T., and Thurman, R.G., Peroxisomes are involved in the swift increase in alcohol metabolism, *J. Pharmacol. Exp. Ther.*, 288, 254–259, 1998.

51. Neumark, Y.D., Friedlander, Y., O'Connor, S., Ramchandani, V.A., Carr, L., and Li, T.-K., The influence of alcohol dehydrogenase polymorphisms on alcohol metabolism among Jewish males in Israel, *Alc. Clin. Exp. Res.*, 25, 126A (abstract), 2001.

52. Neumark, Y.D., unpublished data, 2003.

53. O'Connor, S., Morzorati, S., Christian, J., and Li, T.-K., Clamping breath alcohol concentration reduces experimental variance: application to the study of acute tolerance to alcohol and alcohol elimination rate, *Alc. Clin. Exp. Res.*, 22, 202–210, 1998.

54. Ramchandani, V.A., Bolane, J., Li, T.-K., and O'Connor, S., A physiologically-based pharmacokinetic (PBPK) model for alcohol facilitates rapid BrAC clamping, *Alc. Clin. Exp. Res.*, 23, 617–623, 1999.

55. Farris, J.J. and Jones, B.M., Ethanol metabolism and memory impairments in American Indian and white women social drinkers, *J. Stud. Alcohol.*, 39, 1975–1979, 1978.

56. Farris, J.J. and Jones, B.M., Ethanol metabolism in male American Indians and Whites, *Alc. Clin. Exp. Res.*, 2, 77–81, 1978.

57. Reed, T.E., Kalant, H., Gibbins, R.J., Kapur, B.M., and Rankin J.G., Alcohol and acetaldehyde metabolism in Caucasians, Chinese and Amerinds, *Can. Med. Assoc. J.*, 115, 851–855, 1976.

58. Meier-Tackmann, D., Leonhardt, R.A., Agarwal, D.P., and Goedde, H.W., Effect of acute ethanol drinking on alcohol metabolism in subjects with different ADH and ALDH genotypes, *Alcohol*, 7, 413–418, 1990.

59. Enomoto, N., Takase, S., Yasuhara, M., and Takada, A., Acetaldehyde metabolism in different aldehyde dehydrogenase-2 genotypes, *Alc. Clin. Exp. Res.*, 15, 141–144, 1991.

60. Luu, S.U., Wang, M.F., Lin, D.L., Kao, M.H., Chen, M.L., Chiang, C.H., Pai, L., and Yin, S.J., Ethanol and acetaldehyde metabolism in Chinese with different aldehyde dehydrogenase-2 genotypes, *Proc. Natl. Sci. Counc. Repub. China B.*, 19, 129–136, 1995.

61. Thomasson, H.R., Crabb, D.W., Edenberg. H.J., and Li, T.-K., Alcohol and aldehyde dehydrogenase polymorphisms and alcoholism, *Behav. Genet.*, 23, 131–136, 1993.

62. Eriksson, C.J., Fukunaga, T., Sarkola, T., Chen, W.J., Chen, C.C., Ju, J.M., Cheng, A.T., Yamamoto, H., Kohlenberg-Muller, K., Kimura, M., Murayama, M., Matsushita, S., Kashima, H., Higuchi, S., Carr, L., Viljoen, D., Brooke, L., Stewart, T., Foroud, T., Su, J., Li, T.-K., and Whitfield, J.B., Functional relevance of human ADH polymorphism, *Alc. Clin. Exp. Res.*, 25 (5 Suppl ISBRA), 157S–163S, 2001.

63. Chen, W.J., Loh, E.W., Hsu Y.-P., Chen, C.-C., Yu, J.-M., and Cheng, A.T.A., Alcohol-metabolizing genes and alcoholism among Taiwanese Han men, *Br. J. Psychiatry*, 1996, 168, 762–767.

64. Chen, C.C., Lu, R.B., Chen, Y.C., Wang, M.F., Chang, Y.C., Li, T.-K., and Yin, S.J., Interaction between the functional polymorphisms of the alcohol-metabolism genes in protection against alcoholism. *Am. J. Hum. Genet.*, 65, 795–807, 1999.

65. Higuchi, S., Matsushita, S., Murayama, M., Takagi S., and Hayashida, M., Alcohol and aldehyde dehydrogenase polymorphisms and the risk for alcoholism, *Am. J. Psychiatry*, 1995, 152, 1219–1221.

66. Muramatsu, T., Wang, Z.C., Fang, Y.R., Hu, K.B., Yan, H., Yamada, K., Higuchi, S., Harada, S., and Kono, H., Alcohol and aldehyde dehydrogenase genotypes and drinking behavior of Chinese living in Shanghai, *Hum. Genet.*, 96, 151–154, 1995.

67. Nakamura, K., Iwahashi, K., Matsuo, Y., Miyatake, R., Ichikawa, Y., and Suwaki, H., Characteristics of Japanese alcoholics with the atypical aldehyde dehydrogenase 2*2. I. A comparison of the genotypes of ALDH2, ADH2, ADH3, and cytochrome P-4502E1 between alcoholics and nonalcoholics, *Alc. Clin. Exp. Res.*, 20, 52–55, 1996.

68. Whitfield, J.B., Meta-analysis of the effects of alcohol dehydrogenase genotype on alcohol dependence and alcoholic liver disease, *Alcohol Alcohol.*, 32, 613–619, 1997.

69. Whitfield, J.B., Nightingale, B.N., Bucholz, K.K., Madden, P.A.F., Heath, A.C., and Martin, N.G., ADH genotypes and alcohol use and dependence in Europeans, *Alc. Clin. Exp. Res.*, 22, 1463–1469, 1998.

70. Borràs, E., Coutelle, C., Rosell, A., Fernández-Muixi, F., Broch, M., Crosas, B., Hjelmqvist, L., Lorenzo, A., Gutiérrez, C., Santos, M., Szczepanek, M., Heilig, M., Quattrocchi, P., Farrés, J., Vidal, F., Richart, C., Mach, T., Bogdal, J., Jörnvall, H., Seitz, H.K., Couzigou, P., and Parés, X., Genetic polymorphism of alcohol dehydrogenase in Europeans: the ADH2*2 allele decreases the risk for alcoholism and is associated with ADH3*1, *Hepatology*, 31: 984–989, 2000.

71. Neumark, Y.D., Friedlander, Y., Thomasson, H.R., and Li, T.-K., Association of the ADH2*2 allele with reduced ethanol consumption in Jewish men in Israel: a pilot study, *J. Stud. Alcohol.*, 59, 133–139, 1998.

72. Hasin, D., Aharonovich, E., Liu, X., Mamman, Z., Matseoane, K., Carr, L., and Li, T.-K., Alcohol and ADH2 in Israel: Ashkenazis, Sephardics, and recent Russian immigrants, *Am. J. Psychiatry*, 159(8): 1432–1434, 2002.

73. Thomasson, H.R., Crabb, D.W., Edenberg, H.J., Li, T.-K., Hwu, H.-G., Chen, C.-C., Yeh, E.-K., and Yin, S.-J., Low frequency of the ADH2*2 allele among Atayal natives of Taiwan with alcohol use disorders, *Alc. Clin. Exp. Res.*, 18, 640–643, 1994.

74. Wall, T.L., Carr, L.G., and Ehlers, C.L., Protective association of genetic variation in alcohol dehydrogenase with alcohol dependence in Native American Mission Indians, *Am. J. Psychiatry*, 160, 41–46, 2003.

75. McCarver, D.G., Thomasson, H.R., Martier, S.S., Sokol, R.J., and Li, T.-K., Alcohol dehydrogenase-2*3 allele protects against alcohol-related birth defects among African-Americans. *J. Pharmacol. Exp. Ther.*, 283, 1095–1101, 1997.

76. McCarver, D.G., ADH2 and CYP2E1 genetic polymorphisms: risk factors for alcohol-related birth defects, *Drug Metab. Dispos.*, 29, 562–565, 2001.

77. Jacobson, S.W., Chiodo, L., Jester, J., Carr, L., Sokol, R., Jacobson, J., and Li, T.-K., Protective effects of ADH2*3 in African-American infants exposed prenatally to alcohol, *Alc. Clin. Exp. Res.*, 24, 28A (abstract), 2000.

78. Viljoen, D.L., Carr, L.G., Foroud, T.M., Brooke, L., Ramsay, M., and Li, T.-K., Alcohol dehydrogenase-2*2 allele is associated with decreased prevalence of fetal alcohol syndrome in the mixed-ancestry population of the Western Cape Province, South Africa, *Alc. Clin. Exp. Res.*, 25, 1719–1722, 2001.

79. Chou, W.Y., Stewart, M.J., Carr, L.G., Zheng, D., Stewart, T.R., Williams, A., Pinaire, J., and Crabb D.W., An A/G polymorphism in the promoter of mitochondrial aldehyde dehydrogenase (ALDH2): effects of the sequence variant on transcription factor binding and promoter strength, *Alc. Clin. Exp. Res.*, 23, 963–968, 1999.

80. Harada, S., Okubo, T., Nakamura, T., Fujii, C., Nomura, F., Higuchi, S., and Tsutsumi, M., A novel polymorphism (-357 G/A) of the ALDH2 gene: linkage disequilibrium and an association with alcoholism, *Alc. Clin. Exp. Res.*, 23, 958–962, 1999.

81. Edenberg, H.J., Jerome, R.E., and Li, M., Polymorphism of the human alcohol dehydrogenase 4 (AHD4) promoter affects gene expression, *Pharmacogenetics*, 9, 25–30, 1999.

82. Kopun, M. and Propping, P., The kinetics of ethanol absorption and elimination in twins and supplementary repetitive experiments in singleton subjects, *Eur. J. Clin. Pharmacol.*, 111, 337–344, 1977.

83. Martin, N.G., Perl, J., Oakeshott, J.G., Gibson, J.B., Starmer, G.A., and Wilks, A.V., A twin study of ethanol metabolism, *Behav. Genet.*, 15, 93–109, 1985.

12 Measuring Energy Intake in Alcohol Drinkers

Jianjun Zhang and Hugo Kesteloot

CONTENTS

A growing body of epidemiological evidence suggests that nutrition plays a predominant role in differences in incidence and mortality of major chronic diseases both within and between populations.[1-4] Many epidemiological studies showed that a diet high in saturated fat and red meat was associated with an increased risk of coronary heart disease[1] and cancers of the female breast, prostate, colon, and rectum.[3,4] Conversely, a high intake of vegetables and fruits, a rich source of antioxidants, was found to protect against these diseases.[1-4] Salt intake in Korea, China, and Japan is among the highest in the world, which offers a reasonable explanation for the excessive risk of stomach cancer and stroke in these countries.[5,6] Migrant studies lend further support to the importance of nutrition in the risk and pattern of diseases. After people in Asian countries immigrate to North America and gradually adopt the Western diet, they experience a decrease in incidence of stomach and liver cancers and an increase in incidence of female breast, prostate, colon, and rectal cancers.[7,8]

A fundamental prerequisite for any epidemiological studies on the relation between diet and disease is an accurate assessment of dietary intake of energy and nutrients in dietary surveys. Alcohol consumption is a common lifestyle habit in many populations worldwide. Alcohol intake itself has been linked to all-cause, cardiovascular, and cancer mortality in a number of epidemiological studies.[9,10] However, it is still unclear whether alcohol drinkers adequately report their energy intake in dietary surveys, an issue that is critical for validating and interpreting the findings obtained from epidemiological studies on nutrition and disease among alcohol drinkers.

12.1 PREVALENCE AND AMOUNT OF ALCOHOL CONSUMPTION WORLDWIDE

The amount and prevalence of alcohol consumption in adult populations (15 years and older) in 43 countries is shown in Table 12.1. Data of alcohol consumption were derived from the World Health Organization (WHO).[11] The inclusion criteria were mainly based on the availability of data. Twenty countries were included because they had the highest per capita alcohol consumption in the world. It can be seen from Table 12.1 that the amount of alcohol consumption is generally positively proportional to the level of socioeconomic development. Alcohol consumption varies considerably among the countries compared. The highest alcohol consumption (liter/year/adult) was observed in Slovenia (15.15), South Korea (14.40), and Luxembourg (14.35) and the lowest in Papua New Guinea (1.02), Guatemala (1.99), and Bolivia (3.35). Alcohol beverages are seldom consumed in the east Mediterranean countries (mean: 0.30) due to the strong influence of Islam on the region. The status of alcohol consumption in Africa is obscure. A small amount of data gathered mostly from sub-Saharan and Anglophone areas suggest a very low level of alcohol consumption in this continent (mean: 1.37). The amount of alcohol consumption in developed countries peaked in 1979 and then gradually declined, whereas it has been steadily increasing since 1970 in developing countries. The annual drinking prevalence of all the countries included in Table 12.1 was over 64% in men (except Jamaica) and over 31% in women (except Papua New Guinea and Jamaica). Alcohol consumption is always more common in men than in women. This sex difference was more pronounced in developing countries than in developed countries. It should be noted that the drinking prevalence showed in Table 12.1 was derived from alcohol surveys conducted in a population sample that might not be representative of the entire population in some countries. Of the countries included in Table 12.1, Estonia had the highest drinking prevalence in both sexes but its amount of alcohol consumption was relatively low, which also suggests that caution should be exercised when interpreting the WHO alcohol data.

TABLE 12.1
Amount and Prevalence of Alcohol Consumption in Adult[a] Populations Worldwide[b]

Country (n = 43)	Pure Alcohol Consumption in 1996 (Liter/Year/Person)	Annual Prevalence (%)		
		Year Reported	Men	Women
Australia	9.55	1996	80.0	72.0
Austria	11.90	—	—	—
Bahamas	12.09	—	—	—
Belgium	10.94	—	—	—
Bolivia	3.35	—	76.2	60.4
Canada	7.52	1997	78.1	66.7
Chile	7.06	1996	68.7	53.6

-continued

TABLE 12.1 (continued)
Amount and Prevalence of Alcohol Consumption in Adult[a] Populations Worldwide[b]

Country (n = 43)	Pure Alcohol Consumption in 1996 (Liter/Year/Person)	Annual Prevalence (%)		
		Year Reported	Men	Women
China	5.39	1997	87.3	31.5
Croatia	11.75	—	—	—
Czech Republic	14.35	—	—	—
Denmark	12.15	—	—	—
Dominican Republic	5.90	1992	64.8	46.0
Estonia	8.07	1991	97.0	86.0
Finland	8.26	1995	90.0	82.0
France	13.37	—	—	—
Germany	11.67	—	—	—
Greece	10.41	1987	93.4	77.8
Guatemala[c]	1.99	1990	65.9	48.3
Guyana	14.03	—	—	—
Haiti[c]	6.55	1991	60.3	56.4
Hungary	12.85	1987	93.4	78.6
Ireland	11.90	—	—	—
Jamaica	3.90	1994	45.0	20.0
Japan	7.85	1993	85.0	53.0
Korea[d]	14.40	1998	83.0	44.6
Luxembourg	14.35	—	—	—
Mexico	5.04	1997	73.0	37.0
Netherlands	9.80	1997	88.4	76.3
New Caledonia	11.26	—	—	—
New Zealand	8.85	1996	89.0	85.0
Norway	4.97	1997	89.9	80.3
Panama	5.74	1992	72.1	37.9
Papua New Guinea[c]	1.02	1997	78.0	13.5
Paraguay[c]	9.71	1997	88.0	75.0
Poland	7.93	1997	93.8	84.1
Portugal	13.57	—	85.2	66.8
Slovenia	15.15	—	—	—
Slovakia	13.00	—	—	—
Spain	11.09	1987	90.0	80.0
Sweden	6.04	1997	90.0	75.0
Switzerland	11.27	1993	90.0	77.0
Yugoslavia	13.17	—	—	—
USA	8.90	1996	70.0	60.2

[a] 15 years and older.

[b] Data were derived from World Health Organization.[11]

[c] Prevalence refers to lifetime prevalence.

[d] Prevalence refers to monthly prevalence.

12.2 PREVAILING METHODS FOR VALIDATING REPORTED ENERGY INTAKE IN DIETARY SURVEYS

Dietary assessment is an essential part of nutritional epidemiology. Dietary survey methods can be classified into two broad categories: dependent and independent upon memory.[12] The first category includes a food frequency questionnaire, dietary history, and 24-h dietary recall, while the second category refers to dietary record with and without weighing. Theoretically, there are three main sources of measurement errors in dietary surveys: precision and reproducibility of an assessment instrument, accuracy of reporting or recording of food intake by study participants, and variation in diet over time.[12] However, it has long been assumed that data collected from dietary surveys are a reflection of actual dietary intake in studies investigating the relation between nutrition and disease. Recently researchers began to realize that this assumption is often violated in dietary surveys.[13,14] A substantial body of evidence shows that subjects who are female, obese, older, and more health conscious tend to underreport their energy intake [15,16] but lean subjects tend to overreport their energy intake[15]

The existence of dietary measurement errors justifies the validation of data gathered from dietary surveys. Validating dietary assessments is testing the truth of the energy and nutrient intake reported by participants. Performing a validation requires a gold standard (reference measure) with which other dietary assessment methods can be compared. To date, four validating methods have been used in nutritional epidemiological studies that are described below.

The most commonly used method to evaluate the relative validity of dietary assessment is to compare data on energy and nutrient intake obtained from one dietary instrument with those from another instrument that is judged to be superior.[17] As the food frequency questionnaire is less costly, easy to administer, and capable of capturing usual dietary intake in a large population sample, it has been selected as dietary assessment method in many epidemiological studies. Dietary record or 24-h dietary recall is often employed as the reference measure to validate data gathered from a food frequency questionnaire.[17] To allow for daily variation in diet, several days of dietary records or several 24-h dietary recalls need to be administered in validation studies. Dietary record is well recognized to be better than 24-h dietary recall for this purpose. This is because dietary record is independent of measurement errors inherent in a food frequency questionnaire that include restriction imposed by a fixed list of food items, reliance on memory, and the subject's ability to perceive portion sizes.[17] In some epidemiological studies, 24-h dietary recall is used as the reference measure due to its simplicity and good compliance from participants.[18] The main limitation of 24-h dietary recall is that it shares some measurement error (e.g., recall bias) with a food frequency questionnaire.[17] All dietary assessment methods are subject to measurement errors. Even if dietary assessments from the method being validated and the reference method agree, it is not clear whether both methods are reliable or have the same degree of measurement errors (i.e., correlation error). The reproducibility or consistency of a dietary assessment instrument is usually evaluated by administering the same instrument more than one time to the same persons at different times.[17] The problem with this approach is that if the two methods disagree, it is uncertain whether the dietary measurement instrument used has a low reproducibility or the dietary intake of subjects has changed during the time interval between two administrations.

Under a condition of stable body weight, energy expenditure is equal to energy intake. Therefore, measuring energy expenditure provides an alternative approach to validate reported energy intake in dietary surveys. The main advantage of the doubly labeled water technique (DLW) is that it can accurately measure total energy expenditure in free-living subjects.[19–21] Briefly, a weighed dose of $^2H_2^{18}O$ is given to subjects who are then asked to collect their timed urine samples over an extended period of 7 to 21 d. The deuterium labels the water pool and the oxygen labels the water and carbon dioxide pools in the human body. Carbon dioxide production is determined by the difference in the turnover of water pool and carbon dioxide plus water pool. Energy expenditure is thus calculated from carbon dioxide production using classical indirect calorimetric equations.[19–21] The accurate and objective measurement of energy expenditure by DLW allows to identify misreporters and to assess how much they misreport their energy intake. Since the advent of DLW, it has been widely accepted as the gold standard for validating reported energy intake in dietary surveys.[19–21] The availability of DLW has greatly promoted the research in this field and increased awareness of researchers about the existence and magnitude of measurement errors in dietary assessment. However, DLW is too costly, time-consuming, and technically demanding, and thus impractical to apply in large epidemiological studies.[19–21]

Energy expenditure can be partitioned into three components: basal metabolic rate, the thermogenic effect of food, and energy spent on physical activity. Basal metabolic rate is mainly determined by age, sex, and body weight.[22,23] For a given person, the amount of energy intake primarily depends on the level of physical activity (PAL).[24] In 1991, Goldberg et al.[25] proposed to use a ratio of energy intake to basal metabolic rate (EI/BMR or PAL) to evaluate the validity of reported energy intake in nutritional studies. This method uses energy balance principles to define minimum cut-off limits for the ratio EI/BMR below which a person of given age, sex, and body weight could not maintain a long-term energy balance and thus a long-term survival. The calculated cutoff limit for a dietary survey depends on its sample size, duration of measurement, and means PAL of its participants. For example, the 1985 FAO/WHO/UNU report[24] suggested that a PAL of 1.27 is the minimum requirement for survival. In the same report, a PAL of 1.55 is considered to be necessary for persons to live a sedentary lifestyle. Black et al.[13] evaluated the validity of data from dietary surveys published from 1975 to 1991 using this method and found that the EI/BMR of most studies was below the study-specific cutoff value, suggesting underreporting of energy intake. Since basal metabolic rate can be estimated from the established regression equations based on sex, age, and body weight, the Goldberg method has been used in many epidemiological studies.[15,16] However, this method has two limitations. In the calculation of the cut-off limit for the ratio TEI/BMR, it arbitrarily assumes that all individuals in a population have the same level of PAL.[13] In addition, basal metabolic rate is overestimated from most regression equations available, including the most widely used Schofield equation.[22,26]

Validating dietary assessments against biochemical markers is a promising and attractive approach. Measurement errors of biomarkers are not correlated to those of dietary assessment instruments.[17] For example, the biochemical measurement of biomarkers is independent of the errors related to recall, perception of portion sizes, and under- or overreporting of food intake. Therefore, a modest or strong correlation between dietary intake of a nutrient and its biomarker provides unquestionable evidence of validity. According to the temporal relation to dietary intake, biomarkers can be divided into two categories: short-term and medium/long-term indicators.[27] Short-term biomarkers refer to the biochemical determination of nutrients in the blood, urine, and feces, while medium- and long-term biomarkers are mainly obtained from the biochemical measurement of nutrients in blood cells, adipose tissue, hair, and nails. For example, serum lipids and fatty acid composition in adipose tissue are short and medium/long-term biomarkers of dietary fat intake, respectively. For the time being, reliable and commonly used biomarkers are urinary excretion of total nitrogen and urea for protein intake and of sodium for salt intake.[27] Measuring urinary excretion of sodium is especially important in investigating the role of salt intake in health and disease since it is difficult to accurately measure the discretionary use of salt added to food during cooking and at the table.[28] To date, no reliable biochemical indicators are available for some nutrients of main interest: total fat, total carbohydrate, and fiber.[17]

In four 7-d balance studies,[29] one in each season of the year, 24-h urinary excretion of potassium and sodium accounted for on average 86 and 77% of their dietary intake, respectively. In a large Belgian study, significant positive associations existed between dietary intake and urinary excretion of potassium and sodium.[30] The findings mentioned above indicate that 24-h urinary potassium and sodium are direct biomarkers of their dietary intake but an excretion delay should be taken into account. Potassium and sodium are present in the majority of raw or processed food items. The food sources of potassium are more diverse than nitrogen.[31] For instance, vegetables and fruits are rich in potassium but poor in nitrogen. Therefore, 24-h urinary potassium and sodium may reasonably be considered as indirect but objective biomarkers of total energy intake and thus be used to evaluate the validity of reported energy intake in dietary surveys. Using this methodology, we have demonstrated that the amount and prevalence of underreporting of energy intake were positively associated with the degree of adiposity,[32] a finding that was consistent and extended previous studies using DLW as the reference measure.[19,21]

Although validating dietary assessments against nutrient biomarkers has advantages over other methods, this approach also has several limitations. The levels of biochemical indicators are affected by between-person variation in the absorption and metabolism of most nutrients, difference in the bioavailability of various foods, and technical errors related to laboratory determination of nutrients.[17,27]

12.3 VALIDITY OF REPORTED ALCOHOL INTAKE IN DIETARY SURVEYS

Before discussing the validity of reported energy intake in dietary surveys among alcohol drinkers, it is necessary to understand how they report their alcohol intake.

Several methods have been employed to validate data on reported alcohol intake, although none of them is accepted as the gold standard. Like the validation of reported energy intake, the most widely used approach is to compare alcohol estimates between two assessment instruments.[33,34] For example, alcohol data collected from a food frequency questionnaire are often validated against those from a dietary record.[33] It has been frequently reported that alcohol drinkers tend to underreport the amount of the alcohol beverages consumed.[34–36] Underreporting is more common among persons who are male, unmarried, or heavy drinkers.[34,36] However, the findings obtained from the studies using this validation method should be interpreted with caution because of its limitations discussed previously.

Several studies[37,38] compared the amount of alcohol consumption reported by residents in a defined geographical area with its alcohol sales data and showed that self-reported alcohol intake in surveys usually accounted for only 40 to 70% of the amount sold. Although these studies strongly suggest underreporting of alcohol intake, these findings may be in part confounded by the following factors. Sampling errors may play a role since heavy drinkers may be less likely to participate in surveys. Illegal production and import of alcohol beverages cannot be reflected in sales data.[37] One possible exception is a study conducted in the Norwegian island of Spitzbergen, Svalbard.[37] Because of the low prices of alcohol beverages, counterfeit production and smuggling did not exist in this island, thus making complete registration of all sources of alcohol possible. In addition, participants in this study did not differ from nonparticipants in age and sex distribution. This unique study showed that reported alcohol intake only covered 38.7% of the alcohol sold and that underreporting was more serious for liquor (27.6%) than for beer (54.6%) and wine (54.9%).

Serum gamma-glutamyltransferase (GGT), an indicator of liver damage, has been found to correlate with alcohol intake and is sometimes used as a biomarker of alcohol intake.[39,40] A few epidemiological studies[33,41] showed that serum high-density lipoprotein cholesterol (HDL-C) levels were positively associated with alcohol intake, suggesting that the serum HDL-C level could also be used as an indicator of alcohol intake. Serum GGT levels are elevated in obstructive liver disease and in the subjects taking medications influencing hepatic metabolism.[39] Substantial epidemiological evidence exists that serum HDL-C concentrations are affected by dietary intake of fat and carbohydrate[42,43] and by sex.[42] Therefore, the specificity and validity of serum GGT and HDL-C taken as the reference measures to validate alcohol intake are uncertain and deserve further investigation.

12.4 VALIDITY OF REPORTED ENERGY INTAKE IN DIETARY SURVEYS AMONG ALCOHOL DRINKERS

Many studies have investigated the effect of alcohol consumption on dietary intake of energy and nutrients. The population characteristics and main results of these studies are summarized in Table 12.2. All studies in this field have two general objectives. As alcohol is a substantial source of energy intake for moderate and heavy drinkers, the question arises whether energy derived from alcohol is added to or replaces energy derived from food. Another objective of these studies is to examine the difference in dietary habits between alcohol drinkers and nondrinkers.

According to the principles of energy physiology, obesity develops if energy intake exceeds energy expenditure during a prolonged time period. Of 14 studies[41,44–56] included in Table 12.2, 13 studies[41,44–53,55,56] showed that alcohol drinkers had a higher total energy intake than nondrinkers. Seven studies[41,48–52,56] also reported data on nonalcoholic energy intake and five of these studies[41,48,50,51,56] revealed that drinkers also digested more energy from food than nondrinkers. Body mass index, computed as body weight (kg) divided by body height (m^2), is an indicator of adiposity widely used in epidemiological studies. Nine[41,44,45,49,51–54,56] of the 14 studies had data available on body mass index, and all but one[49] found that body mass index was similar between drinkers and nondrinkers or even lower in drinkers. Physical activity is a considerable component of energy expenditure in persons who live an active lifestyle.[24] However, the lack of data on physical activity from most of the studies on alcohol intake and diet published thus far makes it impossible to evaluate the validity of reported energy intake in dietary surveys among alcohol drinkers.

The relation between alcohol intake and diet was examined in 72,904 women, aged 40 to 65 years, who were members of the French cohort of the European Prospective Investigation into Cancer and Nutrition (EPIC).[56] All women were classified into nondrinkers and drinkers and the latter were further divided into six categories in terms of the amount of alcohol consumption. Total energy and food-derived energy intakes were higher in drinkers than in nondrinkers. Among drinkers, both energy indices increased progressively with the increasing level of alcohol consumption. No striking difference in body mass index was observed between drinkers and nondrinkers and across the six categories of alcohol intake. Subjects who drank more tended to have a lower intake of carbohydrate but a higher intake of lipids and protein. Another study conducted in 216 French men yielded similar results.[48] In addition, this study showed that moderate and heavy drinkers had a lower intake of vegetables and fruits than light drinkers. In a pooled analysis of the Nurses' Health Study and the Health Professionals Follow-up Study,[52] total energy intake was positively associated with alcohol intake but energy derived from food appeared to be not related to alcohol intake. Women who drank more alcoholic beverages were leaner than those who drank less and nondrinkers. Alcohol intake did not have an influence on adiposity in men. The authors of the studies mentioned above, however, suggested that alcoholic energy was added to nonalcoholic energy.

Conversely, the authors of the following studies provided evidence that alcoholic energy replaced nonalcoholic energy. The first National Health and Nutrition Examination Survey (HANES I)[45] showed that total energy intake increased but nonalcoholic energy decreased with alcohol intake. There was no difference in the levels of physical activity and adiposity between drinkers and nondrinkers and between the three categories of alcohol intake. In a study including 179 middle-class men in Pullman, WA,[46] total energy intake correlated positively with alcohol intake. An increase in alcohol consumption was associated with a decrease in percent of energy derived from fat, protein, and carbohydrate and the number of meals eaten per week.

TABLE 12.2
A Summary of Studies on the Relationship between Alcohol Consumption and Diet

Author, Year (Reference)	Location	Population	Major Findings
Jones, 1982[44]	Southern California	132 men and 209 women aged 30–90 years	Alcohol drinkers had higher TEI than nondrinkers and percentage of subjects exercising regularly was similar between nondrinkers and drinkers. Drinkers were not more obese than nondrinkers. AEI was added to NAEI.
Gruchow, 1985[45]	HANES I	4276 men and 6152 women aged 18–74 years	Drinkers had higher TEI than nondrinkers. Among drinkers, NAEI decreased as alcohol intake increased. No differences in the levels of physical activity and adiposity existed between drinkers and nondrinkers. AEI replaced NAEI (mainly carbohydrate) in moderate and heavy drinkers.
Hillers, 1985[46]	Pullman, Washington	179 men, ages not reported	TEI increased and percentage of energy from fat, protein, and carbohydrate decreased with increasing alcohol intake. Moderate and heavy drinkers ate less food and skipped meals. AEI replaced NAEI.
Fisher, 1985[47]	10 populations in U.S. and Canada	2269 men and 2105 women aged 20–59 years	TEI was higher in drinkers than in nondrinkers in women but this difference did not exist in men. Drinkers weighed less than would be expected from their TEI. Drinkers derived less energy from carbohydrate than nondrinkers. AEI was added to NAEI.
Herbeth, 1988[48]	Nancy–Vandoeuvre, France	216 men aged 18–44 years	Both TEI and NAEI were higher in moderate and heavy drinkers than in light drinkers. Moderate and heavy drinkers consumed more fat, protein, and meats and less carbohydrate, vegetables, and fruits than light drinkers. AEI was added to NAEI.

-- continued

TABLE 12.2 (continued)
A Summary of Studies on the Relationship between Alcohol Consumption and Diet

Author, Year (Reference)	Location	Population	Major Findings
Ferro—Luzzi, 1988[49]	Seven areas, Italy	188 men and 205 women aged 65–90 years	In both sexes, TEI was higher in heavy drinkers than in light drinkers but opposite results were found for NAEI. Heavy drinkers were slightly more obese than light drinkers. AEI replaced NAEI. Folate malnutrition occurred in heavy drinkers.
Thomson, 1988[50]	Scotland	164 middle—aged Scottish men	Alcohol intake was associated with a decrease in intake of carbohydrate, total fat, saturated fat, and monounsaturated fat. Light drinkers had a higher intake of fiber and polyunsaturated fat. AEI replaced NAEI.
Toniolo, 1991[51]	North—western Italy	499 middle—aged women	Both TEI and NAEI increased but BMI and percentage of blue—collar workers decreased with increasing categories of alcohol intake. When intake of nutrients and foods were expressed as percentage EI, dietary habits of moderate and heavy drinkers were similar to those of non and light drinkers. Increasing alcohol intake decreased intake of fruits, fiber, vitamin C, and β-carotene.
Colditz, 1991[52]	NHS and HPFS	48,493 men and 89,538 women aged 30–75 years	TEI increased with alcohol intake and NAEI varied little with alcohol intake. Alcohol intake was not associated with BMI in men but was inversely associated with BMI in women. Carbohydrate (mainly sucrose) decreased with alcohol intake.
Veenstra, 1993[53]	DNFCS, the Netherlands	1145 men and 1171 women aged 22–49 years	Alcohol intake was positively correlated with TEI and had no relation to body mass index. Dietary intake of nutrients was similar among non-, moderate, and heavy drinkers on weekdays. On weekend days, intake of total fat was higher in male moderate drinkers and intake of cholesterol was higher in female drinkers. AEI was added to NAEI.

Männistö, 1997[54]	Four areas, Finland	863 men and 985 women aged 25–64 years	TEI was similar between drinkers and nondrinkers but drinkers generally were leaner than nondrinkers. Drinkers had higher intake of fat (% EI) and lower intake of carbohydrate (% EI) than nondrinkers. Except for spirit drinkers, AEI replaced NAEI in both sexes.
Ma, 2000[55]	CSFII	3701 men and 3037 women aged 19 years and older	TEI was higher in heavy drinkers than in non-, light and moderate drinkers, but the opposite finding was observed for the intake of carbohydrate, protein, and fat (all in % EI) in men and women. No marked difference in TEI and micronutrient intake existed between nondrinkers and light and moderate drinkers.
Kesse, 2001[56]	The French cohort of EPIC	72,904 women aged 40–65 years	Both TEI and NAEI increased with alcohol intake. BMI was similar between nondrinkers and drinkers and across six categories of alcohol intake. Alcohol intake was associated positively with percentage of energy from fat and protein and inversely with percentage of energy from carbohydrate and intake of β-carotene.
Zhang, 2001[41]	BIRNH, Belgium	2124 men and 1998 women aged 25–74 years	Moderate and heavy drinkers had higher intake of TEI and NAEI than nondrinkers. BMI was almost identical among three groups in men but was lower in heavy drinkers than in nondrinkers in women. Alcohol intake was associated with high fat intake but did not have effect on protein and carbohydrate intake. AEI replaced NAEI.

Notes: TEI, total energy intake; AEI, energy intake from alcohol; NAEI, nonalcoholic energy intake; HANES I, the first National Health and Nutrition Examination Survey; BMI, body mass index; NHS, the Nurses' Health Study; HPFS, the Health Professional Follow-Up Study; DNFCS, the Dutch National Food Consumption Survey; CSFII, the Continued Survey of Food Intakes by Individuals; EPIC, the European Prospective Investigation into Cancer and Nutrition; BIRNH, the Belgian Interuniversity Research on Nutrition and Health.

The effect of total alcohol intake and types of alcoholic beverages on diet was examined in a Finnish study.[54] Although no striking differences in total energy intake and physical activity level existed between drinkers and nondrinkers, drinkers were leaner than nondrinkers in both sexes except for women who preferred to drink spirits. Energy from beer, wine, and mixed drinks, but not spirits, appeared to substitute energy from food sources.

A common limitation in the studies debating upon whether alcohol intake is added to or replaces energy from food is that energy intake reported by alcohol drinkers was assumed to be accurate in these studies. Although underreporting of energy intake among obese and health-conscious individuals is a well-recognized epidemiological phenomenon, it is still largely unclear whether alcohol drinkers correctly report their energy intake in dietary surveys. To date, only one study[41] conducted by our group using data from the BIRNH study has addressed this crucial issue in nutritional epidemiology.

The Belgian Interuniversity Research on Nutrition and Health (BIRNH) is a Belgian nationwide cohort study on nutrition and health that started in 1981 and is now still in progress.[41] Diet of the participants was assessed by a one-day dietary record. A unique advantage of this study is that 2124 men and 1998 women aged 25 to 74 years collected their 24-h urine samples at the baseline. The 24-h urinary excretion of sodium, potassium, and other cations for all urine samples was measured in only one laboratory,[41] which eliminated difference in the precision of chemical measurements among different laboratories. The availability of data on the 24-h urinary excretion of potassium and sodium from the BIRNH study provided us with a good opportunity to evaluate the validity of reported energy intake among alcohol drinkers. As discussed previously, 24-h urinary potassium and sodium may be considered as indirect but objective biomarkers of energy intake. In our study, five ratios were calculated: dietary potassium/urinary potassium (D-K/U-K), dietary sodium/urinary sodium (D-Na/U-Na), total energy intake/urinary potassium (TEI/U-K), nonalcoholic energy intake/urinary sodium (NAEI/U-Na), and total energy intake/basal metabolic rate (TEI/BMR). Sex-specific BMR was estimated from the Schofield equations based on age and weight.[23] Potassium concentrations in alcoholic beverages are approximately equal to those in various food items but sodium concentrations were much lower in alcoholic beverages.[31] Urinary sodium excretion predominately reflects energy intake from food sources, especially snacks and processed food products. Therefore, the NAEI/U-Na was employed as a measure of misreporting of nonalcoholic energy intake. Since data on urinary excretion of potassium and sodium are independent of dietary measurement errors, an increase in the ratios D-K/U-K, D-Na/U-Na, and TEI/U-K and the ratio NAEI/U-Na in drinkers as compared with nondrinkers is a suggestion of the overreporting of total energy intake and nonalcoholic energy intake, respectively.

Our study[41] showed that TEI, NAEI, the ratios D-K/U-K, D-Na/U-Na, TEI/U-K, and NAEI/U-Na were much higher in heavy drinkers than in nondrinkers in both sexes. Similar but less marked differences were observed between moderate drinkers and nondrinkers. These results are further illustrated in Figure 12.1 that was made from our own published data.[41] The adjustment for age, body mass index, smoking, and educational level did not materially alter the findings mentioned above. The

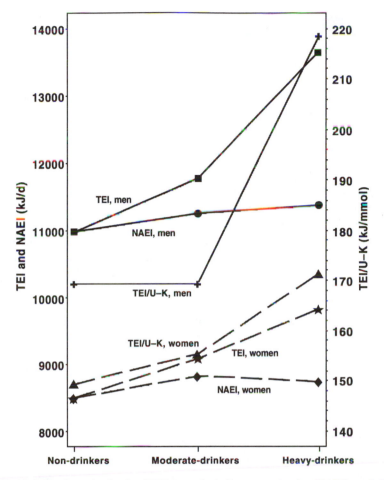

FIGURE 12.1 Total energy intake (TEI), nonalcoholic energy intake (NAEI), and the ratio of total energy intake to 24-h urinary excretion of potassium (TEI/U-K) by alcohol-drinking status in both sexes. (Data from Zhang, J., Temme, E.H., and Kesteloot, H. Alcohol drinkers overreport their energy intake in the BIRNH study: evaluation by 24-h urinary excretion of cations. Belgian Interuniversity Research on Nutrition and Health. *J. Am. Coll. Nutr.* 20, 510, 2001.)

ratio TEI/BMR, a multiple of BMR, was used by the FAO/WHO/UNU[24] to estimate the age- and sex-specific energy requirements for persons with the different levels of physical activity. In the age group of 60 years and younger, 1.55, 1.78, and 2.10 of BMR were suggested for men who perform light, moderate, and heavy physical activity, respectively. The corresponding values for women were 1.56, 1.64, and 1.82.[24] In our study, mean TEI/BMRs for nondrinkers, moderate drinkers, and heavy drinkers were 1.57, 1.69, and 1.95 in men and 1.51, 1.60, and 1.74 in women. The mean values of the ratio in moderate and heavy drinkers in both sexes were similar to the FAO/WHO/UNU criteria of energy requirements for persons with moderate and heavy physical activity, respectively. To date, however, no epidemiological studies have showed that alcohol drinkers were generally more physically active than nondrinkers. The proportion of subjects who exercised regularly was similar between drinkers and nondrinkers in a study conducted in Southern California.[44] No significant difference in the physical activity index, calculated from the intensity and duration of each professional and recreational activity, was found between consumers of beer, wine, spirits, and mixed beverages and nondrinkers in a Finnish study.[54] As alcohol drinkers were not more obese or even leaner than nondrinkers in women in our study (mean body mass index for non-, moderate, and heavy drinkers: 25.9, 26.0, and 26.1 in men and 26.4, 26.0, and 25.2 in women),[41] the most probable and reasonable explanation for high energy intake in drinkers was that drinkers, especially male heavy drinkers, overreported their energy intake. It was estimated by our study[41] that heavy drinkers overreported their energy intake by 27.8% in men and 13.7% in women. Considering the fact that alcohol drinkers tended to underreport their alcohol intake, the real degree of overreporting of energy intake would have been even greater than our estimation. Our study provided evidence that reported higher energy intake in alcohol drinkers relative to nondrinkers was not true and that energy from alcohol replaced, rather than added to, energy from food sources.

If alcohol drinkers overreport their total energy intake, the next question is what food items or nutrients they tend to overreport. Most studies showed that drinkers had an increased intake of fat[41,48,53,54,56] and a reduced intake of carbohydrate,[45–48,50,52,54–56] vegetables, and fruits.[48,51] This suggests that drinkers are most likely to overreport their fat intake in dietary surveys.

12.5 CONCLUSIONS

Alcoholic beverages are regularly consumed in most parts of the world. Moderate alcohol consumption may protect against coronary heart disease, whereas heavy drinking has been associated with an increased risk of liver cirrhosis, hypertension, certain cancers, and traffic accidents.[9,10,57] In view of the widespread exposure and tremendous public health implications of alcohol consumption, it is important to elucidate how drinkers behave in dietary surveys. The primary reason for the long-lasting debate upon whether alcoholic energy is added to or replaces nonalcoholic energy intake is that the majority of the previous studies examining the relation between alcohol and diet did not validate the energy intake reported by drinkers against independent reference measures. Using the 24-h urinary potassium and sodium as indirect but objective biomarkers of alcohol intake, we revealed that alcohol drinkers generally overreported their energy intake and that energy derived from alcohol replaced energy from food sources in a large Belgian population sample. Our findings need to be confirmed by future studies conducted in populations with different habits of dietary intake and alcohol consumption. It is suggested that overreporting of energy intake in alcohol drinkers should be considered in future studies examining the effect of alcohol consumption on diet and disease.

References

1. Kesteloot, H. Nutrition and health. *Eur. Heart J.* 13, 120, 1992.
2. Hu, F.B. and Willett, W.C. Optimal diets for prevention of coronary heart disease. *JAMA* 288, 2569, 2002.
3. Key, T.J. et al. The effect of diet on risk of cancer. *Lancet* 360, 861, 2002.
4. Cummings, J.H. and Bingham, S.A. Diet and the prevention of cancer. *BMJ* 317, 1636, 1998.
5. Joossens, J.V. et al. Dietary salt, nitrate and stomach cancer mortality in 24 countries. European Cancer Prevention (ECP) and the INTERSALT Cooperative Research Group. *Int. J. Epidemiol.* 25, 494, 1996.
6. Sasaki, S., Zhang, X.H., and Kesteloot, H. Dietary sodium, potassium, saturated fat, alcohol, and stroke mortality. *Stroke* 26, 783, 1995.
7. Zhang, J., Suzuki, S., and Sasaki, R. Cancer incidence among native Chinese and Chinese residing in Hong Kong, Singapore and the United States. *J. Aichi Med. Univ. Assoc.* 23, 427, 1995.
8. Flood, D.M. et al. Colorectal cancer incidence in Asian migrants to the United States and their descendants. *Cancer Causes Control* 11, 403, 2000.
9. Gronbaek, M. Alcohol, type of alcohol, and all-cause and coronary heart disease mortality. *Ann. N.Y. Acad. Sci.* 957, 16, 2002.
10. Tsugane, S. et al. Alcohol consumption and all-cause and cancer mortality among middle-aged Japanese men: seven-year follow-up of the JPHC study Cohort I. Japan Public Health Center. *Am. J. Epidemiol.* 150, 1201, 1999.
11. World Health Organization. *Global Status Report on Alcohol.* Geneva, World Health Organization, 1999.
12. Nelson, M. and Bingham, S.A. Assessment of food consumption and nutrient intake, in *Design Concepts in Nutritional Epidemiology.* Margetts, B.A. and Nelson, M., Eds. Oxford University Press, Oxford, U.K., 1997, pp. 123–169.
13. Black, A.E. et al. Critical evaluation of energy intake data using fundamental principles of energy physiology: 2. Evaluating the results of published surveys. *Eur. J. Clin. Nutr.* 45, 583, 1991.
14. Zhang, J., Temme, E.H., and Kesteloot, H. Sex ratio of total energy intake in adults: an analysis of dietary surveys. *Eur. J. Clin. Nutr.* 53, 542, 1999.
15. Johansson, L. et al. Under- and overreporting of energy intake related to weight status and lifestyle in a nationwide sample. *Am. J. Clin. Nutr.* 68, 266, 1998.
16. Pryer, J.A. et al. Who are the "low energy reporters" in the dietary and nutritional survey of British adults? *Int. J. Epidemiol.* 26, 146, 1997.
17. Willett, W. and Lenart, E. Reproducibility and validity of food-frequency questionnaire, in *Nutritional Epidemiology.* Willet, W., Ed. Oxford University Press, New York, 1998, pp. 101–147.
18. Wengreen, H.J. et al. Comparison of a picture-sort food-frequency questionnaire with 24-hour dietary recalls in an elderly Utah population. *Public Health Nutr,* 4, 961, 2001.
19. Johnson, R.K., Soultanakis, R.P., and Matthews, D.E. Literacy and body fatness are associated with underreporting of energy intake in U.S. low-income women using the multiple-pass 24-hour recall: a doubly labeled water study. *J. Am. Diet. Assoc.* 98, 1136, 1998.
20. Prentice, A.M. et al. High levels of energy expenditure in obese women, *Br. Med. J. (Clin. Res. Ed.)* 292, 983, 1986.

21. Schoeller, D.A., Bandini, L.G., and Dietz, W.H. Inaccuracies in self-reported intake identified by comparison with the doubly labelled water method. *Can. J. Physiol. Pharmacol.* 68, 941, 1990.

22. Taaffe, D.R. et al. Accuracy of equations to predict basal metabolic rate in older women. *J. Am. Diet. Assoc.* 95, 1387, 1995.

23. Schofield, W.N. Predicting basal metabolic rate, new standards and review of previous work. *Hum. Nutr. Clin. Nutr.* 39 (Suppl 1), 5, 1985.

24. FAO/WHO/UNU: *Energy and Protein Requirements. Report of a Joint FAO/WHO/UNU Expert Consultation.* Technical Report Series 724. Geneva, World Health Organization, 1985.

25. Goldberg, G.R. et al. Critical evaluation of energy intake data using fundamental principles of energy physiology: 1. Derivation of cut-off limits to identify under-recording. *Eur. J. Clin. Nutr.* 45, 569, 1991.

26. Piers, L.S. et al. The validity of predicting the basal metabolic rate of young Australian men and women. *Eur. J. Clin. Nutr.* 51, 333, 1997.

27. Bates, C.J., Thurnham, D.I., and Bingham, S.A. Biochemical markers of nutrient intake, in *Design Concepts in Nutritional Epidemiology.* Margetts, B.A. and Nelson, M., Eds. Oxford University Press, Oxford, U.K., 1997, pp. 170–240.

28. Liu, K. et al. Assessment of the association between habitual salt intake and high blood pressure: methodological problems. *Am. J. Epidemiol.* 110, 219, 1979.

29. Holbrook, J.T. et al. Sodium and potassium intake and balance in adults consuming self-selected diets. *Am. J. Clin. Nutr.* 40, 786, 1984.

30. Kesteloot, H. and Joossens, J.V. The relationship between dietary intake and urinary excretion of sodium, potassium, calcium and magnesium: Belgian Interuniversity Research on Nutrition and Health. *J. Hum. Hypertens.* 4, 527, 1990.

31. Holland, B. et al. *McCance and Windowson's The Composition of Foods.* The Royal Society of Chemistry, London, 1991.

32. Zhang, J. et al. Under- and overreporting of energy intake using urinary cations as biomarkers: relation to body mass index. *Am. J. Epidemiol.* 152, 453, 2000.

33. Giovannucci, E. et al. The assessment of alcohol consumption by a simple self-administered questionnaire. *Am. J. Epidemiol.* 133, 810, 1991.

34. Corti, B. et al. Comparison of 7-day retrospective and prospective alcohol consumption diaries in a female population in Perth, Western Australia — methodological issues. *Br. J. Addict.* 85, 379, 1990.

35. Feunekes, G.I. et al. Alcohol intake assessment: the sober facts. *Am. J. Epidemiol.* 150, 105, 1999.

36. Midanik, L.T. Comparing usual quantity/frequency and graduated frequency scales to assess yearly alcohol consumption: results from the 1990 U.S. National Alcohol Survey. *Addiction* 89, 407, 1994.

37. Hoyer, G. et al. The Svalbard study 1988–89: a unique setting for validation of self-reported alcohol consumption. *Addiction* 90, 539, 1995.

38. Lemmens, P., Tan, E.S., and Knibbe, R.A. Measuring quantity and frequency of drinking in a general population survey: a comparison of five indices. *J. Stud. Alcohol* 53, 476, 1992.

39. Whitfield, J.B. Gamma glutamyl transferase. *Crit. Rev. Clin. Lab. Sci.* 38, 263, 2001.

40. Anton, R.F., Lieber, C., and Tabakoff, B. Carbohydrate-deficient transferrin and gamma-glutamyltransferase for the detection and monitoring of alcohol use: results from a multisite study. *Alcohol Clin. Exp. Res.* 26, 1215, 2002.

41. Zhang, J., Temme, E.H., and Kesteloot, H. Alcohol drinkers overreport their energy intake in the BIRNH study: evaluation by 24-hour urinary excretion of cations. Belgian Interuniversity Research on Nutrition and Health. *J. Am. Coll. Nutr.* 20, 510, 2001.
42. Kesteloot, H., Geboers, J., and Pietinen, P. On the within-population relationship between dietary habits and serum lipid levels in Belgium. *Eur. Heart J.* 8, 821, 1987.
43. Sacks, F.M. and Katan, M. Randomized clinical trials on the effects of dietary fat and carbohydrate on plasma lipoproteins and cardiovascular disease. *Am. J. Med.* 113 (Suppl 9B), 13S, 2002.
44. Jones, B.R. et al. A community study of calorie and nutrient intake in drinkers and nondrinkers of alcohol. *Am. J. Clin. Nutr.* 35, 135, 1982.
45. Gruchow, H.W. et al. Alcohol consumption, nutrient intake and relative body weight among U.S. adults. *Am. J. Clin. Nutr.* 42, 289, 1985.
46. Hillers, V.N. and Massey, L.K. Interrelationships of moderate and high alcohol consumption with diet and health status. *Am. J. Clin. Nutr.* 41, 356, 1985.
47. Fisher, M. and Gordon, T. The relation of drinking and smoking habits to diet: the Lipid Research Clinic's Prevalence Study. *Am. J. Clin. Nutr.* 41, 623, 1985.
48. Herbeth, B. et al. Dietary behavior of French men according to alcohol drinking pattern. *J. Stud. Alcohol* 49, 268, 1988.
49. Ferro-Luzzi, A. et al. Habitual alcohol consumption and nutritional status of the elderly. *Eur. J. Clin. Nutr.* 42, 5, 1988.
50. Thomson, M. et al. Alcohol consumption and nutrient intake in middle-aged Scottish men. *Am. J. Clin. Nutr.* 47, 139, 1988.
51. Toniolo, P., Riboli, E., and Cappa, A.P. A community study of alcohol consumption and dietary habits in middle-aged Italian women. *Int. J. Epidemiol.* 20, 663, 1991.
52. Colditz, G.A. et al. Alcohol intake in relation to diet and obesity in women and men. *Am. J. Clin. Nutr.* 54, 49, 1991.
53. Veenstra, J. et al. Alcohol consumption in relation to food intake and smoking habits in the Dutch National Food Consumption Survey. *Eur. J. Clin. Nutr.* 47, 482, 1993.
54. Mannisto, S. et al. Alcohol beverage drinking, diet and body mass index in a cross-sectional survey. *Eur. J. Clin. Nutr.* 51, 326, 1997.
55. Ma, J., Betts, N.M., and Hampl, J.S. Clustering of lifestyle behaviors: the relationship between cigarette smoking, alcohol consumption, and dietary intake. *Am. J. Health Promot.* 15, 107, 2000.
56. Kesse, E. et al. Do eating habits differ according to alcohol consumption? Results of a study of the French cohort of the European Prospective Investigation into Cancer and Nutrition (E3N-EPIC). *Am. J. Clin. Nutr.* 74, 322, 2001.
57. Thun, M.J. et al. Alcohol consumption and mortality among middle-aged and elderly U.S. adults. *N. Engl. J. Med.* 337, 1705, 1997.

13 The Effect of Diet on Protein Modification by Ethanol Metabolites in Tissues Damaged in Chronic Alcohol Abuse

Simon Worrall

CONTENTS

13.1 GENERAL INTRODUCTION

Alcohol (ethanol) is the most commonly abused drug in Western societies and is a major cause of morbidity and mortality, leading to major social and economic costs. Despite many years' intensive research, the mechanism(s) by which ethanol exerts its toxic actions are not well understood. The main tissues pathologically affected by long-term chronic alcohol abuse include the brain, cardiac muscle, skeletal muscle, and the liver. What has recently become clear is that the etiology of most tissue damage in alcohol abuse is probably multifactorial with genetic and dietary factors, as well as gender, being important. Furthermore, there is now a growing body of evidence that modification of cellular macromolecules such as proteins may be involved in the etiology of some, if not all, types of alcohol-related tissue injury.

0-8493-1680-4/04/$0.00+$1.50
© 2004 by CRC Press LLC

This chapter will focus on protein modification by metabolites of ethanol, particularly in the liver, and show that there is growing evidence that at least some types of modification are affected by dietary constituents, particularly antioxidants.

13.2 ALCOHOL-RELATED TISSUE INJURY

The chronic abuse of alcohol results in injury to many tissues and organs, with the main targets being the liver, skeletal and cardiac muscle, and the brain. Alcoholic liver disease can be divided into three main stages based on histological observations.[1] Initially, long-term excessive drinking leads to alcoholic steatosis, a relatively benign condition, whose etiology can be explained in terms of metabolic changes induced by the alterations in the redox state of the hepatocytes. This condition is reversible if drinking ceases. Continued heavy drinking leads to the induction of alcoholic hepatitis, which is characterized by centrilobular foci of necrotic and ballooning hepatocytes with an associated neutrophil infiltrate, and the formation of intracellular keratin-containing Mallory bodies. Alcoholic hepatitis is generally thought of as the transition lesion between steatosis and cirrhosis since continued drinking generally leads to irreversible liver damage whereas cessation of drinking generally leads to full recovery. The end-stage form of alcoholic liver disease is alcoholic cirrhosis. This is characterized by small regenerating nodules of liver cells surrounded by bands of fibrous tissue. Alcoholic hepatitis is often superimposed on cirrhosis and indicates continued excessive drinking. Despite many years extensive research effort, we still do not have a full understanding of the mechanisms responsible for the progression from reversible liver damage (steatosis and hepatitis) to irreversible damage (cirrhosis). However, evidence now suggests that aberrant immunological responses may play a critical role in disease progression.[2]

Skeletal muscle myopathy occurs as a result of prolonged ethanol misuse and is characterized by atrophy of type II muscle fibers. Type I fibers are relatively resistant but can atrophy in the most severe cases. Alcoholic myopathy may rob an individual of up to 20 to 30% of his entire musculature. This results in muscle weakness leading to difficulties in gait and frequent falls.[3] Between one half to two thirds of all alcohol misusers may suffer from alcoholic myopathy.[4] The exact mechanisms leading to myopathy are not known but they are thought to include malnutrition, reductions in protein synthesis, and altered protein breakdown,[5–7] free radical damage,[8] and concomitant liver disease.[9]

Similar damage can also occur to the heart muscle leading to alcoholic cardiomyopathy. The histological characteristics of alcoholic cardiomyopathy have been characterized in detail and include fibrosis and increased lipid deposits with associated inflammation in some cases. Mitochondrial and sarcoelemmal abnormalities have also been described together with alterations in myofibrillary architecture.[10] Considerable size variation between myofibrils can be seen together with a loss of cross striations, dying cells, vacuolization, and edema.[11,12] These changes result in diastolic dysfunction, atrial fibrillation, myofibrillary disarray and raised cardiac enzyme activities.[13–15] Furthermore, acetaldehyde has been shown to have a direct depressive effect on cardiac contractile function.[16] The etiology of alcoholic cardiomyopathy is at present unclear.

Long-term use of alcohol can lead to brain damage with accompanying cognitive and motor deficits. Imaging techniques have shown enlargement of the ventricles and shrinkage of the brain in humans, especially of the white matter. Animal studies indicate that several areas of the brain are damaged by alcohol, especially the hippocampus and cerebellum.[17] The damage observed includes a reduction in the number of dendritic branches and spines and a loss of neurons.[18–20] In addition, chronic alcohol administration reduces long-term potentiation,[21] a possible mechanism of learning and memory formation. Although the nature of the damage to the brain has been described, relatively little is known about the mechanisms by which alcohol induces brain damage.[22–24] Basic research in the neurosciences suggests that several possible mechanisms including free radicals and excitotoxicity may underlie damage caused by alcohol abuse.

13.3 ETHANOL METABOLISM AND THE GENERATION OF REACTIVE METABOLITES

The primary organ involved in the elimination of ethanol is the liver which carries out enzyme-mediated oxidation of ~90% of the dose at a rate of 10 to 15 g/h.[25] A small amount is metabolized by extrahepatic tissues and the remainder (<10% of load) is excreted as the parent compound in exhaled air and in urinary output.

Since the liver is the main site of metabolism, the enzymes involved in the process in this tissue have been studied in the greatest detail. Hepatocytes, which account for ~85% of the cells in the liver, contain two major systems for the oxidative metabolism of ethanol. The first is located in the cytosol and involves alcohol dehydrogenase.[26–28] Alcohol dehydrogenases comprise a large family of enzymes which are widely distributed in many cell types. Different types of alcohol dehydrogenase have varying affinities for ethanol.[29] The liver contains Class I and Class II alcohol dehydrogenases with the Class I type carrying out the majority of ethanol metabolism at low blood alcohol concentrations. The alcohol dehydrogenase system is not inducible and oxidizes ethanol to acetaldehyde (ethanal) with the concomitant reduction of the cofactor NAD^+ to NADH. If oxidation occurs for a long time, these reducing equivalents alter the redox state ($NADH/NAD^+$) of the liver, leading to major changes in intermediary metabolism.[30] The other main pathway for ethanol oxidation is the microsomal ethanol oxidizing system (MEOS) which is located in the smooth endoplasmic reticulum and is based around the cytochrome P450 termed CYP2E1.[31–34] This enzyme uses molecular oxygen and NADPH to oxidize ethanol to also generate acetaldehyde. This system is inducible but has a lower affinity for ethanol than ADH and only becomes important after several weeks of heavy drinking when it can account for about 70% of ethanol metabolism. As well as producing acetaldehyde there are several other reactive species that are generated by this enzyme due to its "leaky" catalytic cycle. These include α-hydroxyethyl and hydroxyl radicals which are extremely reactive and potentially damaging to the cell. Ironically the metabolism of ethanol produces the much more reactive compound acetaldehyde which then has to be further metabolized before a nonreactive, less toxic metabolite is produced.

The primary product of ethanol oxidation, acetaldehyde, is further oxidized by aldehyde dehydrogenases[26,35-37] situated in the cytosol and mitochondria to produce acetic acid which can then enter intermediary metabolism as acetyl-CoA. These enzymes are also noninducible such that it is possible for ~1 μM acetaldehyde to accumulate in cells during chronic ethanol oxidation.[38]

As well as producing metabolites such as acetaldehyde and α-hydroxyethyl and hydroxyl radicals directly by the action of the enzymes involved, ethanol metabolism also indirectly generates other reactive species by the action of the radicals on cellular components (Figure 13.1) and by the reaction of acetaldehyde with metabolic intermediates. The main target for radical attack is unsaturated fatty acids in lipid bilayers.[39] The radicals react with double bonds in these molecules to produce lipid hydroperoxides (Figure 13.2) which spontaneously break down to generate a series of reactive species including malondialdehyde and 4-hydroxynonenal. These compounds can be thought of as indirect metabolites of ethanol metabolism.

The brain is able to metabolize ethanol to produce acetaldehyde but at a much lower rate than the liver.[40] In rats, the activity of alcohol dehydrogenase in tissues decreases in the following order: liver, intestine, heart, spleen, brain, and skeletal muscle.[41] Analysis of alcohol dehydrogenase activity in bovine brain showed that various regions had differing levels. In decreasing order of activity, the following list of brain areas was generated: cerebellum, white matter of the large hemispheres, grey matter, and subcortex. The overall ethanol metabolizing activity of the brain was calculated to be 1/4000th of that in the liver at physiological pH.[42]

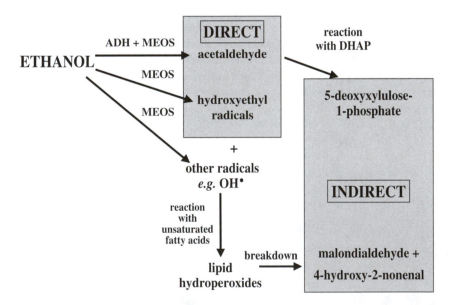

FIGURE 13.1 A scheme showing the production of direct (directly for enzymes metabolizing ethanol) and indirect (generated by other means) metabolites during chronic ethanol oxidation. Abbreviation: ADHs — alcohol dehydrogenase; MEOS — microsomal ethanol oxidizing system; DHAP — dihydroxyacetone phosphate.

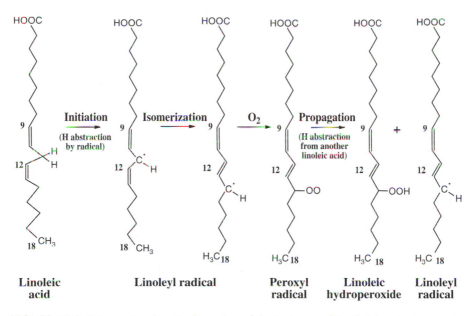

FIGURE 13.2 Scheme showing the formation of the hydroperoxide of oleic acid (an unsaturated fatty acid). The hydroperoxide breaks down to give reactive aldehydes such as malondialdehyde and 4-hydroxy-2-nonenal. The reactions are shown occurring at C-13 but can also occur at C-9.

In human brain the only alcohol dehydrogenase present in significant quantity is the Class III enzyme which has a very low affinity for ethanol[43] and is unlikely to play a major role in ethanol metabolism. This enzyme is widely distributed in the brain including the cortex, subcortex, and cerebellum[44] but is expressed only in small numbers of cells in each area. Class I alcohol dehydrogenase appears absent from the human brain. In fact, enzymes other than alcohol dehydrogenases are used in the oxidation of ethanol in the brain.

It has been known for some time that the brain contains cytochrome P450 enzymes[45] but that they are present in extremely small amounts. The form which metabolizes ethanol in the liver, CYP2E1, was found in the brain[46] in all types of glial cells, nerve cell bodies, terminals, and fibers but maximal activity was found in pyramidal neurons of the frontal cortex and hippocampus, in the bodies of neurons and neuropile of the striatum, in neurons of the substantia nigra, several nuclei, central grey substance, and reticular formation.[47] However, the likely major enzyme that oxidizes ethanol in the brain is one which plays little, if any, part in the liver, namely catalase. Brain catalase can metabolize ethanol in a H_2O_2-dependent manner to produce acetaldehyde.[48] In brain catalase, activity is localized in small cellular organelles and microperoxisomes,[49] and is found uniformly in the cerebellum, medulla, and cerebrum of rats.[50] The highest and lowest activities in small regions of rat brain were found to differ only by twofold.[51] However, histochemical analyses have revealed significant heterogeneity among microregions and discrete cell types.[52] Multiple types of aldehyde dehydrogenase have been detected in the human brain.[53,54]

Ethanol metabolism in other extrahepatic tissues is less well understood. There is some evidence to show that cardiac muscle contains alcohol dehydrogenase,[55] but the activity is extremely low when compared to the liver. It is also believed that catalase may be an important mediator of ethanol metabolism in the heart.[56] Another study showed that cytochrome P450 2E1 mRNA could be detected in all regions of the human heart and the great vessels whereas other P450 mRNA was more regionally expressed.[57] Less is known about alcohol metabolism in skeletal muscle. Cytochrome P450-mediated metabolism appears to occur,[58] with the enzymes probably being located in the sarcoplasmic reticulum.

13.4 REACTIVITY OF ETHANOL METABOLITES WITH PROTEINS

Both the direct and indirect metabolites have been shown to react with macromolecules *in vitro* and also *in vivo*. The best characterized set of reactions are those of acetaldehyde and its interaction with proteins. All of these metabolites can react with other macromolecules such as DNA but only the reactions with proteins will be dealt with in this chapter.

Acetaldehyde is reactive due to the electrophilic nature of the carbonyl carbon and reacts with nucleophilic groups in proteins.[59] The main targets are reactive amino groups such as the α-amino group of the N-terminal amino acid and the ϵ-amino group on the sidechain of internal lysine residues. These readily react with acetaldehyde to produce Schiff bases,[60,61] an unstable form of adduct, which can either break down to regenerate acetaldehyde and a free amino group or can be stabilized by a variety of mechanisms to produce stable adducts (Figure 13.3). In theory, this reaction could occur at any amino group but it is likely that, in the context of a protein, these reactions only occur at those groups which are favorably exposed to the environment and are more reactive than normal amino groups, probably again due to their milieu. If a Schiff base forms on the α-amino group of the N-terminal amino acid, stabilization can occur through cyclization to produce a 2-methyl-imidazolidin-4-one derivative.[62,63] On the other hand if the Schiff base forms on an ϵ-amino group, stabilization can occur through addition across the double bond, either through reduction or nucleophilic addition by a thiol group. Initially it was thought that reduction, which results in the formation of N-ethyllysine, was likely to predominate *in vivo* during chronic ethanol oxidation. However, this hypothesis has recently been under question.[64,65] The adducts formed *in vitro* in the absence of strong reducing agents have been shown to be both chemically[61] and immunologically[64] different from the N-ethylated amino acid derivatives generated in their presence. Proteins lacking free thiol groups and polylysine have been shown to form considerable amounts of adducts when incubated with acetaldehyde even in the absence of reducing agents.[61]

The reaction of acetaldehyde with thiol-containing amino acids and small peptides has been intensively studied *in vitro* at physiological pH and temperature. NMR analysis confirmed that the product with free cysteine or with peptides containing an N-terminal cysteine residue was the expected thiazolidine derivative[66] (Figure

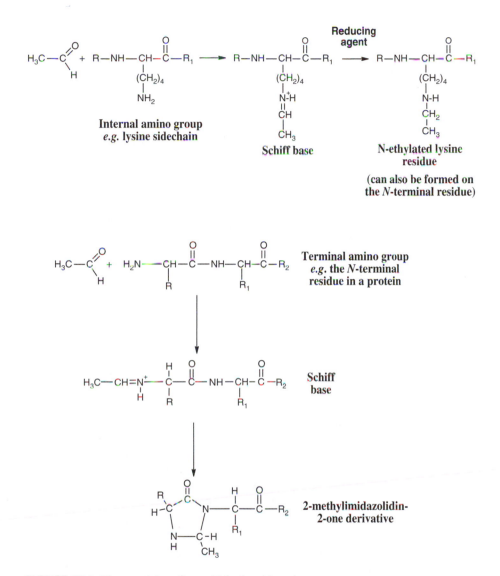

FIGURE 13.3 The reactivity of acetaldehyde with amino groups.

13.4). The reaction was found to be rapid under physiological conditions. However, when acetaldehyde was incubated with peptides containing internal cysteine residues, NMR analysis revealed that the expected hemimercaptal derivative was not formed under these conditions.[66]

Studies have not yet been carried out on the structure of adducts formed by the reaction of exogenously generated hydroxyethyl radicals with amino acids or peptides. However, given their extremely high reactivity, it is expected that they will react with a variety of sites in proteins and other macromolecules.

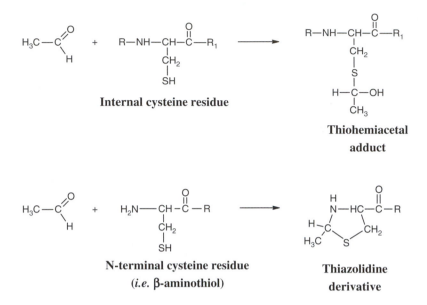

Internal cysteine residue

Thiohemiacetal adduct

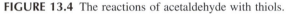

N-terminal cysteine residue
(*i.e.* β-aminothiol)

Thiazolidine derivative

FIGURE 13.4 The reactions of acetaldehyde with thiols.

Acetaldehyde can condense with the glycolytic intermediate dihydroxyacetone phosphate through the action of aldolase to form the sugar 5-deoxyxylulose-1-phosphate.[67] Little is known about the reactivity of this compound with peptides or amino acids except that a stable adduct is formed on incubation with hemoglobin *in vitro*.[68] This adduct is likely to be formed by a series of reactions similar to those of nonenzymic glycation. Initially the deoxyxylulose phosphate forms a Schiff base on an amino group. The Schiff base then undergoes the Amadori rearrangement to finally yield a ketoamine adduct (Figure 13.5). The adduct contains an α-hydrox-yketone group which can react with another amino group through the same reactions to generate crosslinking if the second amino group is on a different peptide.

Malondialdehyde is formed in abnormally large amounts during chronic ethanol oxidation as a result of the breakdown of lipid peroxides formed by radical attack on unsaturated fatty acids in membranes. It is also formed during oxidative stress induced by other agents and because of this its reactivity with macromolecules has been studied in considerable detail. The main form of malondialdehyde in aqueous

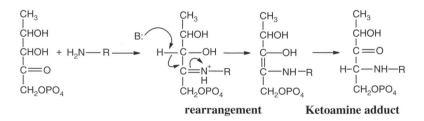

rearrangement   **Ketoamine adduct**

FIGURE 13.5 A likely scheme for adduct formation by 5-deoxyxylulose-1-phosphate.

solution at neutral pH is the enolate anion which is of low reactivity. Thus, in contrast to common belief, malondialdehyde is not a highly reactive compound under physiological conditions.[39] Reactivity increases as pH is lowered when β-hydroxyacrolein becomes the predominant species. This form of malondialdehyde can undergo Michael-type 1,4-addition in a similar manner to other α,β-unsaturated aldehydes such as 4-hydroxy-2-nonenal (another breakdown product of lipid peroxidation). This type of reaction is favored at low pH by resonance stabilization giving a β-substituted acrolein derivative[69] as a product (1:1 adduct). These compounds contain a CC double bond which can further react with another amino acid at low pH to give a 2:1 adduct (Figure 13.6). One study of the reactivity of malondialdehyde with amino acids at pH 4.2 revealed that histidine, tyrosine, tryptophan, and arginine reacted exclusively via their α-amino groups to give 1:1 adducts.[70] Under these conditions formation of 2:1 adduct was not observed, even when amino groups were in large excess. The reaction of cysteine with malondialdehyde generated a product which contained two molecules of cysteine and three molecules of malondialdehyde. Neutral pH did not favor reactivity with amino groups as, at pH 7.0, reactivity with cysteine (thiol and amino groups) could be demonstrated but no reaction with glycine (only an amino group) was seen.[39]

The reaction of malondialdehyde with proteins at neutral pH cannot be totally predicted from the data generated in the preceding studies using amino acids. For example, virtually no reactivity with glutathione (a thiol-containing tripeptide) could be detected at neutral pH but considerable reactivity with bovine serum albumin occurred under the same conditions. However, proteins are generally much more reactive than amino acids at neutral pH. It has been suggested that proteins present amino acids in a more favorable environment such that greater reactivity occurs. It has also been suggested that it is the condensation products of malondialdehyde and not malondialdehyde *per se* that are involved in these reactions. Reaction of malondialdehyde with polylysine lead to three different derivatives of ε-amino groups.[71] About 20% were converted to an unstable aminopropenal adduct, approximately 1% to a dihydropyridine derivative and the remainder to stable crosslinked structures based on amino-imino-propen derivatives. Similar results were obtained by

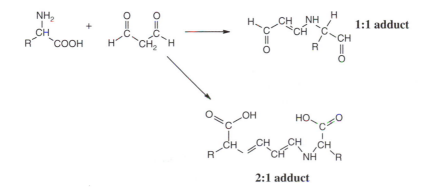

FIGURE 13.6 The reaction of malondialdehyde with amino acids.

incubating bovine serum albumin with malondialdehyde at neutral pH. Under these conditions malondialdehyde was found to modify about 40% of the total ε-amino groups available. The aminopropenal adduct was found on 11 out of the 26 reactive amino groups while the remainder were involved in amino-imino-propen-based crosslinked structures. Only one molecule in twelve carried a single dihydropyridine adduct. Other studies have shown that histidine, tyrosine, arginine, and methionine residues may also be modified to a lesser extent.[72]

4-Hydroxyalkenals such as 4-hydroxy-2-nonenal have three functional groups: namely, an aldehyde group, an hydroxy group, and a carbon–carbon double bond. All three functional groups can participate alone, or in sequence, in reactions with other species. This makes the reactivity of 4-hydroxy-2-nonenal much more complicated than the other metabolites discussed above.[39] The addition of 4-hydroxy-alkenals to cells or tissues results in a rapid loss of thiol groups, suggesting that they are the initial targets of this family of molecules. The initial product is a saturated aldehyde bound to the thiol-containing molecule via a thioether linkage at carbon-3. This can then undergo intramolecular rearrangement to give a five-membered cyclic hemiacetal derivative (Figure 13.7). If an excess of thiol groups is present the initial conjugate can react with another thiol to produce a thiazolidine derivative.[39]

4-Hydroxy-2-nonenal can react with a variety of amino acid residues in proteins. When 5 mM hydroxynonenal is reacted with human apolipoprotein B (M_r 500,000) 2 thiol groups, 45 lysine, 23 serine, 7 histidine, and 51 tyrosine residues are modified.[73] The binding to the lysine residues was reversible, indicating that it was most likely in the form of Schiff bases. Hydroxynonenal can also react with amino groups by nucleophilic Michael addition of the amino group to the carbon–carbon double bond. This can then be stabilized as a cyclic hemiacetal by loss of water. Schiff bases are believed to be minor products in the reaction with amino groups but they can be stabilized by loss of water to form pyrrole derivatives.

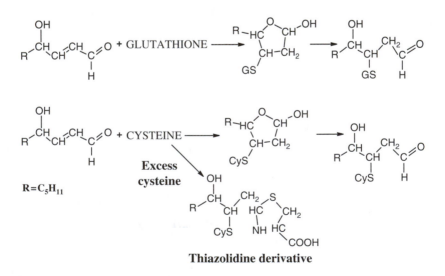

Thiazolidine derivative

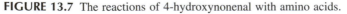

FIGURE 13.7 The reactions of 4-hydroxynonenal with amino acids.

As well as acting alone to produce adducts it is possible for metabolites to react in concert to produce mixed adducts. Recently, Tuma and coworkers have shown that the binding of acetaldehyde is remarkably increased in the presence of malondialdehyde.[74] Incubation of proteins with a mixture of acetaldehyde and malondialdehyde led to the production of two types of adduct, one of which was fluorescent (Figure 13.8). These hybrid adducts were termed malondialdehyde-acetaldehyde (MAA) adducts. They have been identified as 4-methyl-1,4-dihydropyridine-3,5-dicarbaldehyde (MAA 2:1; fluorescent and derived from two molecules of malondialdehyde and one molecule of acetaldehyde)[74] and 2-formyl-3-(alkylamino) butanal (MAA 1:1; nonfluorescent and derived from one molecule of acetaldehyde and one molecule of malondialdehyde),[75] derivatives of protein amino groups. There is now evidence that MAA 1:1 adducts are formed first and then react with malondialdehyde-derived Schiff bases to form the MAA 2:1 adduct.[76]

13.5 FORMATION OF PROTEIN ADDUCTS DURING ETHANOL METABOLISM IN ANIMALS FED ETHANOL AND IN HUMAN ALCOHOLICS

The previous section shows that there is a large body of evidence to demonstrate that direct and indirect metabolites which are generated during ethanol metabolism can react with proteins to produce both stable and unstable modifications. Those studies have been useful in guiding the search for *in vivo* modification by giving us insights into the likely adducts formed and allowing the generation of reagents for their detection.

Initially, I shall concentrate on the evidence for protein modification in the liver, as this organ is responsible for the majority (~90%) of ethanol metabolism and is thus the most likely target for modification by metabolites. I will then discuss the evidence for protein modification in several extrahepatic tissues.

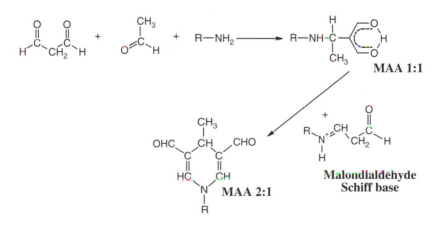

FIGURE 13.8 The reaction of malondialdehyde and acetaldehyde with amino groups to form MAA derivatives.

Initial studies, using cell-free homogenates[60] and liver slices,[77] showed that acetaldehyde generated during ethanol metabolism could react with cellular proteins to form acetaldehyde-protein adducts. In these studies it appeared that unstable adducts, likely to be Schiff bases, were initially formed which became stabilized over time to generate stable adducts. More direct evidence of adduct formation was produced following the generation of polyclonal antisera reactive with proteins modified by acetaldehyde *in vitro*. These reagents were then used in Western blotting and immunohistochemical analyses of liver samples from rodents fed ethanol and from humans consuming ethanol.

All of the early studies using rodents fed ethanol clearly showed that acetaldehyde had reacted with hepatocellular proteins to generate stable adducts but the number and identity of the proteins modified widely differed in each study. Two studies using Western blotting showed that single proteins were modified, namely, CYP2E1 (part of MEOS and responsible for ethanol oxidation in the endoplasmic reticulum)[78] and a 37-kDa cytosolic protein[79–82] later identified as Δ^4-3-ketosteroid-5,-reductase.[83] In contrast, two other studies detected multiple proteins including the 37-kDa protein seen by Lin and colleagues.[84,85] Furthermore, studies using ELISAs demonstrated that cytosolic α-tubulin, glyceraldehyde-3-phosphate dehydrogenase, and calmodulin all carried acetaldehyde-derived modifications[86] and that modified proteins could also be detected in membrane and mitochondrial fractions (Nicholls, R. M., de Jersey, J., Wilce, P. A., and Worrall, S., unpublished observations).

Other studies using immunohistochemistry showed that modified proteins were formed in the cytosol of hepatocytes from human alcoholics.[87] Furthermore, the acetaldehyde-modified epitopes were found to be more intense in the centrilobular regions of the liver,[88,89] the regions associated with the highest levels of ethanol oxidation and the regions most damaged in alcoholic liver disease. Similar studies using ethanol-fed rats also demonstrated a predominantly centrilobular adduct distribution.[90]

Much less work has been carried out on the other metabolites. The α-hydroxyethyl radicals have been shown to be generated by CYP2E1[91–93] and to react with microsomal and other proteins *in vitro*. More recently, hydroxyethyl radical-modified proteins have been detected in the liver and other tissues of ethanol-fed rats[65,94] and human alcoholics.[95] Malondialdehyde and 4-hydroxy-2-nonenal are the major products of oxidative degradation of unsaturated fatty acids as an indirect result of ethanol metabolism. Indeed, elevated levels of malondialdehyde have been detected in humans drinking about 100 g of ethanol per day, with the increase in production seeming to continue for several weeks after cessation of drinking.[96] Malondialdehyde-modified proteins have been detected *in vivo* under a wide range of conditions. For example, hepatic cytosol and plasma from rats with iron overload contained elevated levels of malondialdehyde and hydroxynonenal-derived adducts.[97] In animal models of alcoholic liver disease several researchers have shown that hydroxynonenal- and malondialdehyde-modified epitopes are associated with areas of inflammation and necrosis[98–101] and with iron deposits, probably as a marker of oxidative stress.[102]

Two forms of MAA adduct have been shown to form when acetaldehyde and malondialdehyde react with amino groups *in vitro* but only the MAA 2:1 form has been detected in the livers of rats fed ethanol for extended periods.[65,74,103] There is indirect evidence that the 1:1 adduct was also formed. *In vitro* studies have shown that the MAA 2:1 adduct is formed by the MAA 1:1 adduct reacting with a malondialdehyde Schiff base such that the 1:1 adduct is transferred to the amino carrying the Schiff base.[76] If a tissue contains the 1:1 adduct, then incubation with malondialdehyde should result in an increase in the number of MAA 2:1 adducts. When ethanol-fed rat liver was perfused *in situ* with malondialdehyde, an increase in the amount of the MAA 2:1 adduct was indeed found, whereas similar treatment of control-fed rat livers did not lead to a similar increase. This implies that MAA 1:1 adducts were present in the ethanol-fed rat liver prior to perfusion with malondialdehyde.

More recently, evidence is starting to mount that proteins are also modified by ethanol metabolites in extrahepatic tissues. There is now some evidence for protein modification by ethanol metabolites in the brain. Rats fed ethanol for periods up to 24 months were tested for acetaldehyde adducts in their brain and liver. Only four out of nine ethanol-fed animals exhibited adducts in their brain whereas the majority of animals (seven/nine) had modifications in their livers.[104] Control animals had no such modifications in either tissue. Brain adducts were found in the white matter and some large neurons in layers four and five of the frontal cortex and in the molecular layer of the cerebellum. Mice fed a 5% (v/v) solution of ethanol were shown by immunohistochemistry to have acetaldehyde-modified proteins in the cerebral cortex.[105] Similar modification was observed in rats treated with ethanol for 12 months. In these animals modification occurred in cortical neurons, the granule layer of the dentate gyrus, neurons in the midbrain, and granular cell layers of the cerebellum.[106] Furthermore, unlike the liver, where the major site of modification was often the cytoplasm, modification of brain proteins was apparently confined to the mitochondria.

More recently, ethanol metabolite-modified proteins have been found in cardiac[107] and skeletal muscle[108] of ethanol-fed rats. Rats were pair-fed the ethanol-containing (35% of caloric intake as ethanol) and control (ethanol isocalorically replaced by maltose dextran) forms of the Lieber–DeCarli liquid diet for 6 weeks. This feeding regime causes pathological changes in heart muscle similar to those seen in human alcoholic cardiomyopathy such as a decrease in contractile protein content.[109] Ventricular muscle from ethanol-fed animals showed increased generation of reduced- and unreduced-acetaldehyde and malondialdehyde-acetaldehyde (MAA 2:1) adducts when compared to controls.[107] No increase in malondialdehyde- or α-hydroxyethyl radical-derived protein adducts was seen. This is the only report of protein modification in alcohol-damaged heart muscle and may implicate immune attack or a loss of function due to modification in the pathogenesis of alcoholic cardiomyopathy (see next section). Using the same feeding regime we were also able to demonstrate the elevated production of unreduced acetaldehyde protein adducts in plantaris and soleus muscles of ethanol-fed rats[107] in comparison to pair-fed controls.

Immunohistochemical analysis showed that sarcolemmal and subsarcolemmal regions were the most heavily modified, probably due to acetaldehyde production (i.e., ethanol metabolism) occurring in, or close to, these cellular compartments. While the levels of modification were similar in plantaris (type II fiber-predominant) and soleus (type I fiber-predominant) muscles only the plantaris was affected by ethanol feeding, leading to a decrease in weight. This initial study did not determine whether the same molecular targets were modified in each muscle, so it is presently not clear whether this study implicates acetaldehyde in the etiology of alcoholic skeletal myopathy.

13.6 THE CONSEQUENCES OF PROTEIN MODIFICATION BY ETHANOL METABOLITES

Protein modification can have two major consequences which may occur alone or in combination. Modification may rob a protein of its functionality[110–112] and/or may alter the immunogenicity of the protein such that it becomes a *neoantigen*. In the case of ethanol metabolites there is evidence to show that both of these disparate mechanisms may be occurring.

An important example of the implications of ethanol metabolites binding to cellular components has been provided by studies on the effect of acetaldehyde on microtubular function. It is interesting to note that sulfydryl groups have been implicated in the polymerization of tubulin monomers into microtubules.[113] Given their reactivity with acetaldehyde to form thiazolidine or hemimercaptal derivatives, it was decided to examine whether acetaldehyde could affect tubulin polymerization. Two groups have shown that the addition of acetaldehyde to microtubular proteins had an inhibitory effect on microtubular formation.[114,115] Later studies showed that complete inhibition could be obtained if as little as 5% of the α-tubulin monomers were modified.[116,117]

Two important markers of alcoholic liver damage are liver enlargement and the accumulation of fat. Initially the hepatomegaly was assumed to be due to the fat deposition but more recent studies suggest that fat accounts for only about half of the increase and the remainder is due to an increase in the protein content of liver cells.[118] This increase in protein content appears to be due to an impairment of microtubule-mediated protein secretion.[119,120] The number of microtubules was also found to be decreased in ethanol-affected cells due to an effect of ethanol metabolism on tubulin polymerization to favor the retention of monomers rather than polymerization into microtubules. This effect has been documented in ethanol-fed animals[121] and human alcoholics,[122] and in rat hepatocytes treated with ethanol *in vitro*.[119] Acetaldehyde is known to react with a highly reactive lysine residue in α-tubulin[123] which is only available in the monomeric form and may be important in polymerization. Although it is yet to be fully established, it seems likely that the modification of tubulin by acetaldehyde is responsible for the impairment of protein secretion seen *in vivo* in alcoholic liver disease.

The consequences of this disruption of microtubular function are observable in the accumulation of secretory vesicles and disrupted protein trafficking. The hepatocytes of patients with alcoholic liver disease contain large amounts of cytosolic transferrin, a plasma protein normally secreted by the cell.[120] This accumulation is not seen in cells from patients with nonalcoholic liver disease. Pulse-chase methodology has been used to examine the precise point at which secretion is affected.

Comparison of the incorporation of leucine, glucosamine, fucose, and galactose into secretory proteins by Tuma and colleagues[115,124–126] concluded that ethanol blocked the exit of proteins from the liver by altering processing in the Golgi complex and/or post Golgi compartments of the secretory pathway.

Perturbation of protein trafficking could have many less obvious ramifications for the cell. Vesicular trafficking is responsible, at least in part, for the composition of the plasma membrane by delivering enzymes, receptors, transporters, and structural and cellular recognition proteins. Thus, alterations in vesicular trafficking could have widespread effects on cellular metabolism and functionality by altering the activities of these systems. Interestingly, derangement of receptor-mediated endocytosis is affected much more severely in centrilobular regions of the liver, where alcohol-related injury predominates, than in the periportal regions of the liver.[127] The plasma membrane of ethanol-affected hepatocytes appears very different from that of controls under electron microscopy and appears to have increased lability leading to leakage of alkaline phosphatase.[128,129] Acetaldehyde, but not ethanol *per se*, has been shown to competitively inhibit the membrane-bound enzymes 5′-nucleotidase, Na^+/K^+ ATPase and Mg^{2+} ATPase at high concentrations *in vitro*.[130] Whether this inhibition is significant at physiological concentrations has not been established.

Other proteins accumulating in the liver probably reflect metabolic changes induced by chronic ethanol oxidation. For example, there is a marked increase in the concentration of fatty acid binding protein in ethanol-affected hepatocytes such that it can account for up to 33% of total cellular protein.[131] This accumulation may be a protective response by the hepatocytes so that nonesterified fatty acids do not accumulate and damage the cells by their detergent-like actions.[132]

There is now an extensive body of evidence to show that proteins modified by reactive metabolites are immunogenic, acting as *neoantigens* to elicit an immune response against both the modification (adduct; hapten) and the carrier protein. Research has largely been limited to the detection and characterization of antibodies reactive with the adducts but one group has reported the induction of a cellular response to acetaldehyde-protein adducts.

In 1986 Israel and coworkers[133] were the first to demonstrate the production of antibodies reactive with acetaldehyde-protein adducts in mice chronically fed ethanol. A later study in rats showed that the magnitude of the response was related to the time that the animals were fed ethanol and probably to the cumulative ethanol load.[134] Another study showed that antibodies were generated against at least two broad classes of modification.[135] Similar studies have also shown the generation of antibodies reactive with α-hydroxyethyl radical-,[65,136,137] malondialdehyde-,[65] and 4-hydroxy-2-nonenal-derived epitopes, and against MAA 2:1 adducts.[65,138]

Similarly, many studies have now shown that humans also produce antibodies reactive with epitopes derived from ethanol metabolites. Initial studies concentrated on antibodies reactive with acetaldehyde-containing modifications. Thus, several groups demonstrated antibodies reactive with acetaldehyde-modified proteins before they could show the presence of the modified proteins *per se*.[139–142] These studies used ELISAs to measure serum or plasma reactivity with proteins modified by acetaldehyde *in vitro*, commonly generated under reducing conditions. However, the conditions used to modify the proteins varied greatly, making it likely that different populations of adducts were generated, probably leading to the detection of anti-bodies reactive with different types of adduct. In the rodent experiments mentioned above there was a clear difference between ethanol-fed and control animals, with only ethanol-fed animals exhibiting immunoreactivity with acetaldehyde-modified epitopes. The picture is not so clear in humans as social drinkers (alcohol intake ~50 g per week for males and <30 g for females), patients with nonalcoholic liver disease and alcoholics all exhibited immunoreactivity with the modified proteins.[140] However, more individuals with high immunoreactivity were detected in the alco-holic groups in all of these studies.[139–142]

At present most interest has focused on the reaction of antibodies with modified proteins but it should be noted that these antibodies also react with modified phos-pholipids. Several studies[143,144] have shown that antibodies raised against acetalde-hyde-modified albumin react with acetaldehyde-modified dioleoyl phosphatidyleth-anolamine, presumably because they carry similar adducts on their amino groups. Thus, while modified lipids may be, at least in part, responsible for the generation of such antibodies *in vivo* it is much easier to use modified proteins to detect and measure them.

When antibodies are raised against a modified protein, antibodies are generated which react with the modification but others are also generated which react with the carrier protein alone. Most of the research has concentrated on the antibodies reactive with the adducts. However, an early study[140] showed elevated immunore-activity with unmodified proteins in alcoholics compared to nonalcoholic liver disease and social drinkers. There is also evidence that antibodies are generated against an epitope containing part of the adduct and part of the carrier protein. Koskinas and coworkers[145] demonstrated that 70% of patients with alcoholic hepatitis had antibodies which reacted with a 200-kDa cytosolic protein when it was modified by incubation with acetaldehyde and then treated with a reducing agent. Only 25% of patients with nonalcoholic liver disease and 25% of controls had similar antibodies. The antibodies detected must have some degree of carrier protein specificity since they only detected the 200-kDa protein in a mixture that contained many other modified proteins. However, they did not recognize the protein when it was unmodified, suggesting that the epitope recognized must be largely generated during the modification process. These findings warrant further investigation.

These early studies used ELISAs which were not able to differentiate between the different classes of antibody leading to the measurement of total immunoreac-tivity with the adducts. Later studies used class-specific reagents which enabled IgG, IgA, and IgM reactivity with modified proteins to be determined.[142] One of the rationales behind these further studies was that altered metabolism of immunoglo-bulins was often associated with alcoholism and especially with alcoholic liver disease. For example, (1) serum levels of IgA are elevated in patients with alcoholic liver disease, (2) a "continuous" pattern of perisinusoidal IgA deposition is com-monly seen in the livers of alcoholics, (3) IgA and IgG reactive with liver membranes have been detected in plasma from alcoholics, and (4) circulating immune complexes containing IgA or IgG and ethanol-derived antigens can be found in the blood of alcoholics.[146]

Several studies have now implicated these antibodies in the pathogenesis of alcohol-related liver injury. Initial studies used guinea pigs fed an ethanol-containing diet for 40 d and simultaneously immunized with hemoglobin modified by incubation with acetaldehyde under nonreducing conditions. These animals showed hepatic necrosis with an associated infiltrate of mononuclear cells as well as elevated biochemical markers of liver injury.[147] In contrast, ethanol-fed animals immunized with unmodified hemoglobin only showed steatosis similar to that seen in unimmunized ethanol-fed animals. Animals fed the control diet and immunized with unmodified or modified hemoglobin showed no discernible liver pathology. Extending the period of these treatments to 90 d resulted in producing hepatic fibrosis developing around individual hepatocytes in the terminal hepatic venule areas and portal areas, accompanied by an increase in hepatic hydroxyproline content indicative of increased collagen synthesis.[148] These experiments indicate that immune responses against the adducts may be involved in the generation of inflammation and fibrosis seen in alcoholic liver disease. In a later series of experiments using rats and a similar regime in which they were immunized with autologous liver cytosolic proteins modified by acetaldehyde,[149] my group was able to show that the liver damage could be related to the strength of the antigenic stimulus and to the time of exposure. For example, ethanol-fed rats injected with protein modified by 240 mM acetaldehyde produced major liver damage within 10 weeks whereas those injected with protein modified with 1 mM acetaldehyde required 30 weeks to generate much less damage (Worrall, S., Treloar, W., de Jersey, J., and Wilce, P. A., unpublished observations). The antibodies generated had a similar profile to those seen in human alcoholics.

Evidence for the role of adducts in other tissues is relatively sparse. Acetaldehyde has been shown to bind to actin *in vitro* with the G-form being more reactive than the F-form,[112] implicating it in alcohol-induced muscular dysfunction. Furthermore, acetaldehyde has been shown to alter the contractile properties of cardiomyocytes in culture. These data suggest a role for acetaldehyde in alcoholic cardiomyopathy. There is little direct evidence for the brain, but acetaldehyde has been shown to affect neurotubulin in a manner analogous to liver tubulin.[114]

13.7 THE EFFECT OF NUTRITION ON ALCOHOL-RELATED TISSUE INJURY

Undernutrition/malnutrition has, and continues to be, carefully considered as part of the etiology of alcohol-related tissue injury. Indeed, undernutrition is common in some alcoholics and is a major cause of illness for them. Generally, disturbances in nutrition do not cause pathology similar to that seen in the alcoholic, perhaps with the exception of thiamine deficiency. However, alcohol toxicity can impair nutrition by interfering with absorption, transport, and utilization of essential nutrients.

Alcoholic beverages constitute an appreciable percentage of the total caloric intake (4 to 6%) in Western societies. Ethanol itself can be efficiently used by the body, particularly the liver, as a fuel at intake levels around 45 g/d but the efficiency of utilization may decrease at higher intakes and is likely to be due to the induction of the MEOS which does not produce NADH for ATP synthesis.[150]

Morphological changes in mitochondria may also decrease the efficiency of ATP production. It has been suggested that ethanol has "empty calories" which are lacking in dietary micronutrients and that deficiencies of minerals and vitamins may be important.

Given that the diet of alcoholics is often suboptimal it is not surprising that studies have been carried out to determine if dietary deficiencies play a role in the sequelae of chronic, long-term alcohol abuse. For most of the tissue injury associated with alcoholism there is little evidence to support a role for the diet in their etiology. For example, studies on vitamin D,[151–153] riboflavin, pyridoxine, vitamin B$_{12}$, folate and general nutrition[153–155] have shown that while they are often associated with alcoholism they do not appear to play a role in the pathogenesis of alcoholic cardiomyopathy. Similarly, reductions in muscle and plasma α-tocopherol and selenium concentrations are also associated with alcohol abuse but supplemental α-tocopherol did not prevent acute or chronic muscle injury in rat models of alcoholic myopathy.[156] Paradoxically, muscle antioxidant status seems to be at least partially disturbed by chronic alcoholism, perhaps putting the muscle at greater risk of lipid peroxidation.[157]

There is strong evidence to link thiamine deficiency with Wernicke's encephalopathy, a serious neurological disorder with high morbidity and mortality, encountered in chronic alcoholics and persons with grossly impaired nutritional status. Activities of thiamine-dependent enzymes such as α-ketoglutarate dehydrogenase and transketolase are significantly reduced in affected brains and may be involved in the etiology of the brain injury.[158] Nicotinamide deficiency, leading to alcoholic pellagra encephalopathy, is also seen in alcoholics, albeit at a much lower incidence than Wernicke's encephalopathy.[159]

The rate of malnutrition is relatively modest in alcoholics without liver disease but is much greater in those with alcoholic hepatitis or cirrhosis. Certainly in alcoholic hepatitis some of the reasons for malnutrition are related to the symptoms of the disease *per se* (anorexia, malabsorption, and altered metabolic state) and are probably not underlying causative factors.[160] In other studies where detailed nutritional assessments were made of 250 chronically alcoholic men, the only dietary component which could be positively correlated with cirrhosis and other complications of alcohol abuse was the total lifetime dose of ethanol.[161] Further analysis of this cohort revealed that only 10% had evidence of energy malnutrition and 6% had protein malnutrition while another 6% had both.

One aspect of the diet which does appear to be important in the development of alcoholic liver disease is the dietary intake of fat.[162] Dietary fat appears to be an important factor in the pathogenesis of alcoholic hepatitis and cirrhosis as the degree of fatty infiltration (steatosis) is a risk factor for the development of cirrhosis.[163] One of the principal processes believed to underlie the development of alcoholic liver disease is free radical generation (reactive oxygen species and α-hydroxyethyl radicals) leading to lipid peroxidation. Indeed, lipid peroxidation, as measured by exhaled ethane, correlates with the quantity of ethanol consumed and with the severity of cirrhosis in actively drinking alcoholics[164] and in animals fed ethanol.[100]

In rats fed ethanol, hepatic triacylglycerol accumulates rapidly when the fat content of the diet exceeds 25% of caloric intake.[165] When a low (5%) fat diet is given with ethanol, the animals do not develop steatosis or show evidence of lipid peroxidation, unlike those given 36% of their calories as fat.[166] The animals fed 36% of their calories as fat also show elevated α-hydroxyethyl radical formation.[167]

Although the amount of dietary fat probably plays a role in the development of alcoholic liver disease there is clear evidence that the composition of the fat is also important. Studies on cirrhosis mortality in countries with similar *per capita* alcohol intake show that a high intake of saturated fat is associated with lowered cirrhosis mortality, whereas high unsaturated fat intake is associated with increased mortality from cirrhosis.[168] Potential explanations for these data have been gleaned from animal studies. Use of the Tsukamoto–French intragastric ethanol feeding technique[169] on rats has shown that feeding of ethanol in a high fat diet for 85 to 120 days leads to fatty infiltration, necrosis, polymorphonuclear and mononuclear cell infiltration, stellate cell activation, and fibrosis.[170] In one study where this regimen was used to feed rats with ethanol for 6 months, it was found that inclusion of unsaturated fat (corn oil) lead to severe injury, inclusion of pork fat (lard) lead to less severe injury, and that no injury was seen when beef fat (tallow) was used.[171] The degree of injury was found to correlate with the linolenic acid content of each of the fats used. Furthermore, injury could be generated in the tallow-fed animals if supplemental linolenic acid was added to the diet.[172] This phenomenon may be associated with the induction of CYP2E1 activity.[173] Rats fed fish oil develop even more severe injury than those given corn oil.[174] This is probably because fish oil contains a large percentage of polyunsaturated fatty acids with more than two double bonds making them especially susceptible to lipid peroxidation. This increased injury correlated with elevated CYP2E1 activity and increased lipid peroxidation.[175] However, in these animals liver injury could be reversed if they were placed on a diet rich in saturated fat.[174]

Other studies have shown that ethanol alters the phospholipid composition of membranes, decreasing palmitic and oleic acid content but increasing stearic and arachidonic acids.[176] Administration of soybean lecithin extract containing phosphatidyl choline prevents the development of cirrhosis in ethanol-fed baboons.[177] In these animals phosphatidyl choline appeared to correct the expected changes in membrane composition. This effect may be important in stabilizing the cellular membranes to make them more resistant to lipid peroxidation. This beneficial effect of unsaturated fat is in direct contrast to data from the rat studies where unsaturated fat clearly has deleterious effects.

One aspect of the diet that has not been fully explored is the relationship between dietary deficiencies and the formation of protein-adducts derived from direct and indirect metabolites of ethanol. My group has recently studied the effect of α-tocopherol supplementation on adduct formation in the liver of rats chronically fed ethanol.[178] Supplementary α-tocopherol was found not only to reduce the formation of adducts related to lipid peroxidation such as malondialdehyde- and MAA 2:1 protein adducts and α-hydroxyethyl radicals, as was expected given α-tocopherol's role as a membrane antioxidant, but to also decrease the formation of adducts from the proximal metabolite, acetaldehyde (Figure 13.9).

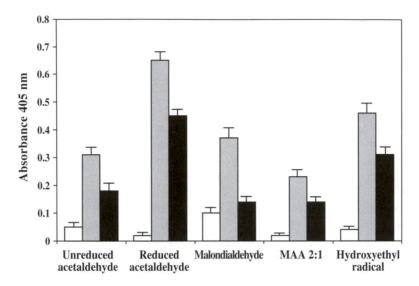

FIGURE 13.9 The effect of α-tocopherol supplementation on adduct formation in ethanol-fed rat liver. Rats were fed control (open bars), ethanol-containing (shaded bars) and ethanol-containing plus supplementary α-tocopherol at 30 mg/kg body weight daily (closed bars) for 4 weeks.

13.8 SUMMARY

There is plenty of evidence that proteins are modified by reactive species produced directly and indirectly during chronic ethanol oxidation. This modification can have deleterious effects causing loss of function or by making the protein a target for immune attack. A recent study on the liver suggests that dietary antioxidants such as α-tocopherol may help to lessen protein modification, thereby decreasing tissue damage.

ACKNOWLEDGMENTS

The author wishes to thank his long-term collaborators Professor John de Jersey and Associate Professor Peter Wilce for their help and guidance over the years. Next I must also thank the many students who have passed through my laboratory, without whom much of this work would not have been carried out. I would also like to thank my international collaborators, Professor Dean Tuma and Professor Geoffrey Thiele (University of Nebraska, Omaha), Associate Professor Victor Preedy (King's College, London), and Onni Niemela (University of Oulu, Finland) for having the courage to work with someone halfway around the world. Finally, I must thank my wife, Linda, and daughters, Elizabeth, Jennifer, and Victoria, for their unstinting support and love.

References

1. Hall, P. M., Pathological spectrum of alcoholic liver disease, in *Alcoholic Liver Disease: Pathology and Pathogenesis*, Hall, P. M., Ed., Edward Arnold, London, 1995, pp. 41.
2. Klassen, L. W., Tuma, D., and Sorrell, M. F., Immune mechanisms of alcohol-induced liver disease, *Hepatology* 22, 355, 1995.
3. Martin, F., Ward, K., Slavin, G., Levi, J., and Peters, T. J., Alcoholic skeletal myopathy, a clinical and pathological study, *Q. J. Med.* 55, 233, 1985.
4. Reilly, M. E., Preedy, V. R., and Peters, T. J., Investigations into the toxic effects of alcohol on skeletal muscle, *Adverse Drug React. Toxicol. Rev.* 14, 117, 1995.
5. Preedy, V. R., Salisbury, J. R., and Peters, T. J., Alcoholic muscle disease: features and mechanisms, *J. Pathol.* 173, 309, 1994.
6. Preedy, V. R., Siddiq, T., Why, H., and Richardson, P. J., The deleterious effects of alcohol on the heart: involvement of protein turnover, *Alcohol Alcohol.* 29, 141, 1994.
7. Preedy, V. R., Peters, T. J., Patel, V. B., and Miell, J. P., Chronic alcoholic myopathy: transcription and translational alterations, *FASEB J.* 8, 1146, 1994.
8. Preedy, V. R., Adachi, J., Asano, M., Koll, M., Mantle, D., Niemela, O., Parkkila, S., Paice, A. G., Peters, T., Rajendram, R., Seitz, H., Ueno, Y., and Worrall, S., Free radicals in alcoholic myopathy: indices of damage and preventive studies, *Free Radic. Biol. Med.* 32, 683, 2002.
9. Marchesini, G., Zoli, M., Angiolini, A., Dondi, C., Bianchi, F. B., and Pisi, E., Muscle protein breakdown in liver cirrhosis and the role of altered carbohydrate metabolism, *Hepatology* 1, 294, 1981.
10. Richardson, P. J., Patel, V. B., and Preedy, V. R., Alcohol and the myocardium, *Novartis Found. Symp.* 216, 35, 1998.
11. Klein, H. and Harmjanz, D., Effect of ethanol infusion on the ultrastructure of human myocardium, *Postgrad. Med. J.* 51, 325, 1975.
12. Hibbs, R. G., Ferrans, V. J., Walsh, J. J., and Burch, G. E., Electron microscopic observations on lysosomes and related cytoplasmic components of normal and pathological cardiac muscle, *Anat. Rec.* 153, 173, 1965.
13. Richardson, P. J., Wodak, A. D., Atkinson, L., Saunders, J. B., and Jewitt, D. E., Relation between alcohol intake, myocardial enzyme activity, and myocardial function in dilated cardiomyopathy. Evidence for the concept of alcohol induced heart muscle disease, *Brit. Heart J.* 56, 165, 1986.
14. Spodick, D. H., Pigott, V. M., and Chirife, R., Preclinical cardiac malfunction in chronic alcoholism. Comparison with matched normal controls and with alcoholic cardiomyopathy, *New Eng. J. Med.* 287, 677, 1972.
15. Wu, C. F., Sudhaker, M., Ghazanfar, J., Ahmed, S. S., and Regan, T. J., Preclinical cardiomyopathy in chronic alcoholics: a sex difference, *Am. Heart J.* 91, 281, 1976.
16. Ren, J. and Brown, R. A., Influence of chronic alcohol ingestion on acetaldehyde-induced depression of rat cardiac contractile function, *Alcohol Alcohol.* 35, 554, 2000.
17. Harper, C. and Kril, J., An introduction to alcohol-induced brain damage and its causes, *Alcohol Alcohol.* (Supplement 2), 237, 1994.
18. Harper, C. and Kril, J., If you drink your brain will shrink. Neuropathological considerations, *Alcohol Alcohol.* (Supplement 1), 375, 1991.
19. Harper, C. and Kril, J., Pathological changes in alcoholic brain shrinkage, *Med. J. Aust.* 144, 3, 1986.
20. Harper, C. and Kril, J., Brain atrophy in chronic alcoholic patients: a quantitative pathological study, *J. Neurol. Neurosurg. Psychiatry* 48, 211, 1985.

21. Ryabinin, A. E., Role of hippocampus in alcohol-induced memory impairment: implications from behavioral and immediate early gene studies, *Psychopharmacology (Berlin)* 139, 34, 1998.

22. Pratt, O. E., Rooprai, H. K., Shaw, G. K., and Thomson, A. D., The genesis of alcoholic brain tissue injury, *Alcohol Alcohol.* 25, 217, 1990.

23. Fadda, F. and Rossetti, Z. L., Chronic ethanol consumption: from neuroadaptation to neurodegeneration, *Prog. Neurobiol.* 56, 385, 1998.

24. Harper, C., The neuropathology of alcohol-specific brain damage, or does alcohol damage the brain? *J. Neuropathol. Exptl. Neurol.* 57, 101, 1998.

25. Lieber, C. S., Ethnic and gender differences in ethanol metabolism, *Alcohol. Clin. Exp. Res.* 24, 417, 2000.

26. Riveros Rosas, H., Julian Sanchez, A., and Pina, E., Enzymology of ethanol and acetaldehyde metabolism in mammals, *Arch. Med. Res.* 28, 453, 1997.

27. Lieber, C. S. and Leo, M. A., Metabolism of ethanol and some associated adverse effects on the liver and the stomach, *Recent Dev. Alcohol.* 14, 7, 1998.

28. Yin, S. J., Han, C. L., Lee, A. I., and Wu, C. W., Human alcohol dehydrogenase family. Functional classification, ethanol/retinol metabolism, and medical implications, *Adv. Exp. Med. Biol.* 463, 265, 1999.

29. Yoshida, A., Hsu, L. C., and Yasunami, M., Genetics of human alcohol-metabolising enzymes, *Prog. Nuc. Acid Res. Mol. Biol.* 40, 255, 1991.

30. Lieber, C. S., Metabolism of ethanol: an update, in *Alcoholic Liver Disease*, Hall, P. M., Ed., Edward Arnold, London, 1995, p. 3.

31. Teschke, R., Hasumura, Y., Joly, J. G., and Lieber, C. S., Microsomal ethanol-oxidizing system (MEOS): purification and properties of a rat liver system free of catalase and alcohol dehydrogenase, *Biochem. Biophys. Res. Commun.* 49, 1187, 1972.

32. Koop, D. R., Morgan, E. T., Tarr, G. E., and Coon, M. J., Purification and characterization of a unique isozyme of cytochrome P-450 from liver microsomes of ethanol-treated rabbits, *J. Biol. Chem.* 257, 8472, 1982.

33. Ryan, D. E., Ramanathan, L., Iida, S., Thomas, P. E., Haniu, M., Shively, J. E., Lieber, C. S., and Levin, W., Characterization of a major form of rat hepatic microsomal cytochrome P-450 induced by isoniazid, *J. Biol. Chem.* 260, 6385, 1985.

34. Wrighton, S. A., Campanile, C., Thomas, P. E., Maines, S. L., Watkins, P. B., Parker, G., Mendez Picon, G., Haniu, M., Shively, J. E., Levin, W. et al., Identification of a human liver cytochrome P-450 homologous to the major isosafrole-inducible cytochrome P-450 in the rat, *Mol. Pharmacol.* 29, 405, 1986.

35. Perozich, J., Nicholas, H., Wang, B. C., Lindahl, R., and Hempel, J., Relationships within the aldehyde dehydrogenase extended family, *Protein Sci.* 8, 137, 1999.

36. Perozich, J., Nicholas, H., Lindahl, R., and Hempel, J., The big book of aldehyde dehydrogenase sequences. An overview of the extended family, *Adv. Exp. Med. Biol.* 463, 1, 1999.

37. Ziegler, T. L. and Vasiliou, V., Aldehyde dehydrogenase gene superfamily. The 1998 update, *Adv. Exp. Med. Biol.* 463, 255, 1999.

38. Irving, M. G., Simpson, S. J., Brooks, W. M., Holmes, R. S., and Dodrell, D. M., Application of the reverse DEPT polarization-transfer pulse sequence to monitor *in vitro* and *in vivo* metabolism of 13C-ethanol by 1H-NMR spectroscopy, *Int. J. Biochem.* 17, 471, 1985.

39. Esterbauer, H., Schaur, R. J., and Zollner, H., Chemistry and biochemistry of 4-hydroxynonenal, malonaldehyde and related aldehydes, *Free Radic. Biol. Med.* 11, 81, 1991.

40. Zimatkin, S. M. and Deitrich, R. A., Ethanol metabolism in the brain, *Addict. Biol.* 2, 387, 1997.

41. Raskin, N. H. and Sokoloff, L., Enzymes catalysing ethanol metabolism in neural and somatic tissues of the rat, *J. Neurochem.* 19, 273, 1972.

42. Chernikevich, I. P., Lomeko, I. E., Yoskoboyev, A. I., and Ostrovsky, Y. M., Evidence on the presence of alcohol dehydrogenase in rat and bovine brain, *Neurokhimia.* 3, 130, 1984.

43. Beisswender, T. V., Holmquist, B., and Vallee, B. L., CADH is the sole form of alcohol dehydrogenase of mammalian brains: implications and inferences, *Proc. Natl. Acad. Sci. U.S.A.* 82, 8369, 1985.

44. Giri, P. R., Linnoila, M., O'Neil, J. B., and Goldman, D., Distribution and possible metabolic role of type III alcohol dehydrogenase in the human brain, *Brain Res.* 481, 131, 1989.

45. Sasame, H. A., Ames, M. M., and Nelson, S. D., Cytochrome P450 and NADPH cytochrome c reductase in rat brain: formation of reactive catechol metabolites, *Biochem. Biophys. Res. Commun.* 78, 919, 1977.

46. Morgan, E. T., Koop, D. R., and Coon, M. J., Catalytic activity of cytochrome P-450 isozyme 3a isolated from liver microsomes of ethanol-treated rabbits. Oxidation of alcohols, *J. Biol. Chem.* 257, 13951, 1982.

47. Hansson, T., Tinberg, N., Ingelman-Sunberg, M., and Kuhler, C., Regional distribution of ethanol-inducible cytochrome P450 IIE1 in the rat central nervous system, *Neuroscience.* 34, 451, 1990.

48. Cohen, G., Sinet, P. M., and Heikkila, R., Ethanol oxidation by rat brain *in vivo*, *Alcohol. Clin. Exp. Res.* 4, 366, 1980.

49. Novikoff, A. B. and Novikoff, P. M., Microperoxisomes, *J. Histochem. Cytochem.* 21, 963, 1973.

50. Gaunt, G. L. and de Duve, C., Subcellular distribution of D-amino acid oxidase and catalase in rat brain, *J. Neurochem.* 26, 749, 1976.

51. Brannan, T. S., Maker, H. S., and Raes, T. P., Regional distribution of catalase in adult rat brain, *J. Neurochem.* 86, 307, 1981.

52. Zimatkin, S. M. and Lindros, K. O., Comparison of catalase and aldehyde dehydrogenase distribution in rat brain: are aminergic neurons affected by acetaldehyde?, *Alcohol. Clin. Exp. Res.* 19, 35 A Abstr. 5.25, 1994.

53. Ryzlak, M. T. and Pietruszko, R., Human brain "high Km" aldehyde dehydrogenase: purification, characterization, and identification as NAD$^+$-dependent succinic semialdehyde dehydrogenase, *Arch. Biochem. Biophys.* 266, 386, 1988.

54. Ryzlak, M. T. and Pietruszko, R., Human brain glyceraldehyde-3-phosphate dehydrogenase, succinic semialdehyde dehydrogenase and aldehyde dehydrogenase isozymes: substrate specificity and sensitivity to disulfiram, *Alcohol. Clin. Exp. Res.* 13, 755, 1989.

55. Nagasawa, H. T. and Alexander, C. S., Ethanol metabolism by the rat heart and alcohol dehydrogenase activity, *Can. J. Biochem.* 54, 539, 1976.

56. Soffia, F. and Penna, M., Ethanol metabolism by rat heart homogenates, *Alcohol* 4, 45, 1987.

57. Thum, T. and Borlak, J., Gene expression in distinct regions of the heart, *Lancet* 355, 979, 2000.

58. Riggs, J. E., Alcohol-associated rhabdomyolisis: ethanol induction of cytochrome P450 may potentiate myotoxicity, *Clin. Neuropharmacol.* 21, 363, 1998.

59. O'Donell, J. P., The reaction of amines with carbonyls; its significance in the nonenzymatic metabolism of xenobiotics, *Drug Metab. Rev.* 13, 1982.

60. Donohue, T. M., Jr., Tuma, D. J., and Sorrell, M. F., Binding of metabolically derived acetaldehyde to hepatic proteins *in vitro*, *Lab. Invest.* 49, 226, 1983.

61. Tuma, D. J., Newman, M. R., Donohue, T. M., Jr., and Sorrell, M. F., Covalent binding of acetaldehyde to proteins: participation of lysine residues, *Alcohol. Clin. Exp. Res.* 11, 579, 1987.

62. Fowles, L. F., Beck, E., Worrall, S., Shanley, B. C., and de Jersey, J., The formation and stability of imidazolidinone adducts from acetaldehyde and model peptides. A kinetic study with implications for protein modification in alcohol abuse, *Biochem. Pharmacol.* 51, 1259, 1996.

63. Sillanaukee, P., Hurme, L., Tuominen, J., Ranta, E., Nikkari, S., and Seppa, K., Structural characterisation of acetaldehyde adducts formed by a synthetic peptide mimicking the N-terminus of the hemoglobin beta-chain under reducing and nonreducing conditions, *Eur. J. Biochem.* 240, 30, 1996.

64. Klassen, L. W., Tuma, D. J., Sorrell, M. F., McDonald, T. L., DeVasure, J. M., and Thiele, G. M., Detection of reduced acetaldehyde protein adducts using a unique monoclonal antibody, *Alcohol. Clin. Exp. Res.* 18, 164, 1994.

65. Worrall, S., de Jersey, J., and Wilce, P. A., Comparison of the formation of proteins modified by direct and indirect ethanol metabolites in the liver and blood of rats fed the Lieber-DeCarli liquid diet., *Alcohol Alcohol.* 35, 164, 2000.

66. Graham, V., Worrall, S., and de Jersey, J., Analysis of adducts formed between acetaldehyde and thiol-containing peptides, in *Proceedings of the Ninth Congress of the International Society for Biomedical Research on Alcoholism*, Copenhagen, Denmark, Williams & Wilkins, Baltimore, MD, 1998, p. 174a.

67. Hoberman, H. D., Synthesis of 5-deoxy-D-xylulose-1-phosphate by human erythrocytes, *Biochem. Biophys. Res. Commun.* 90, 757, 1979.

68. Hoberman, H. D., Adduct formation between hemoglobin and 5-deoxy-D-xylulose-1-phosphate, *Biochem. Biophys. Res. Commun.* 90, 764, 1979.

69. Crawford, D. L., Yu, T. C., and Sinnhuber, R. O., Reaction of malondialdehyde with glycine, *J. Agr. Food Chem.* 14, 182, 1966.

70. Nair, V., Vietti, D. E., and Cooper, C. S., Degenerative chemistry of malondialdehyde. Structure, stereochemistry and kinetics of formation of enaminals from reaction with amino acids, *J. Am. Chem. Soc.* 103, 3030, 1981.

71. Kikugawa, K., Takayanagi, K., and Watanabe, S., Polylysine modified with malondialdehyde, hydroperoxylinoleic acid and monofunctional aldehydes, *Chem. Pharm. Bull.* 33, 5437, 1985.

72. Buttkus, H., Reaction of cysteine and methionine with malondialdehyde, *J. Am. Oil Chem. Soc.* 46, 88, 1966.

73. Jurgens, G., Lang, J., and Esterbauer, H., Modification of human low-density lipoprotein by the lipid peroxidation product 4-hydroxynonenal, *Biochim. Biophys. Acta* 875, 103, 1986.

74. Tuma, D. J., Thiele, G. M., Xu, D., Klassen, L. W., and Sorrell, M. F., Acetaldehyde and malondialdehyde react together to generate distinct protein adducts in the liver during long-term ethanol administration, *Hepatology* 23, 872, 1996.

75. Kearley, M. L., Patel, A., Chien, J., and Tuma, D. J., Observation of a new nonfluorescent malondialdehyde-acetaldehyde-protein adduct by 13C NMR spectroscopy, *Chem. Res. Toxicol.* 12, 100, 1999.

76. Tuma, D. J., Kearley, M. L., Thiele, G. M., Worrall, S., Haver, A., Klassen, L. W., and Sorrell, M. F., Elucidation of reaction scheme describing malondialdehyde-acetaldehyde-protein adduct formation, *Chem. Res Toxicol.* 14, 822, 2001.

77. Medina, V. A., Donohue, T. M., Jr., Sorrell, M. F., and Tuma, D. J., Covalent binding of acetaldehyde to hepatic proteins during ethanol oxidation, *J. Lab. Clin. Med.* 105, 5, 1985.

78. Behrens, U. J., Hoerner, M., Lasker, J. M., and Lieber, C. S., Formation of acetaldehyde adducts with ethanol-inducible P450IIE1 *in vivo*, *Biochem. Biophys. Res. Commun.* 154, 584, 1988.

79. Lin, R. C., Fillenwarth, M. J., Minter, R., and Lumeng, L., Formation of the 37-kDa protein-acetaldehyde adduct in primary cultured rat hepatocytes exposed to alcohol, *Hepatology* 11, 401, 1990.

80. Lin, R. C. and Lumeng, L., Further studies on the 37-kDa liver protein-acetaldehyde adduct that forms in vivo during chronic alcohol ingestion, *Hepatology* 10, 807, 1989.

81. Lin, R. C. and Lumeng, L., Formation of the 37-kDa protein-acetaldehyde adduct in liver during alcohol treatment is dependent on alcohol dehydrogenase activity, *Alcohol. Clin. Exp. Res.* 14, 766, 1990.

82. Lin, R. C. and Lumeng, L., Formation of the 37-kDa liver protein-acetaldehyde adduct *in vivo* and *in vitro*, *Alcohol Alcohol. (Supplement.* 1) 265, 1991.

83. Zhu, Y., Fillenwarth, M. J., Crabb, D., Lumeng, L., and Lin, R. C., Identification of the 37-kDa rat liver protein that forms an acetaldehyde adduct *in vivo* as Δ^4-3-ketosteroid 5 beta-reductase, *Hepatology* 23, 115, 1996.

84. Worrall, S., de Jersey, J., Shanley, B. C., and Wilce, P. A., Detection of stable acetaldehyde-modified proteins in the livers of ethanol-fed rats, *Alcohol Alcohol.* 26, 437, 1991.

85. Yokoyama, H., Ishii, H., Nagata, S., Moriya, S., Ito, T., Kato, S., and Tsuchiya, M., Heterogeneity of hepatic acetaldehyde adducts in guinea-pigs after chronic ethanol administration: an immunohistochemical analysis with monoclonal and polyclonal antibodies against acetaldehyde-modified protein epitopes, *Alcohol Alcohol. (Supplement.* 1a) 91, 1993.

86. Nicholls, R. M., Fowles, L. F., Worrall, S., de Jersey, J., and Wilce, P. A., Distribution and turnover of acetaldehyde-modified proteins in liver and blood of ethanol-fed rats, *Alcohol Alcohol.* 29, 149, 1994.

87. Niemela, O., Juvonen, T., and Parkkila, S., Immunohistochemical demonstration of acetaldehyde-modified epitopes in human liver after alcohol consumption, *J. Clin. Invest.* 87, 1367, 1991.

88. Paradis, V., Scoazec, J. Y., Kollinger, M., Holstege, A., Moreau, A., Feldmann, G., and Bedossa, P., Cellular and subcellular localization of acetaldehyde-protein adducts in liver biopsies from alcoholic patients, *J. Histochem. Cytochem.* 44, 1051, 1996.

89. Holstege, A., Bedossa, P., Poynard, T., Kollinger, M., Chaput, J. C., Houglum, K., and Chojkier, M., Acetaldehyde-modified epitopes in liver biopsy specimens of alcoholic and nonalcoholic patients: localization and association with progression of liver fibrosis, *Hepatology* 19, 367, 1994. [published erratum appears in *Hepatology* 1994 Dec; 20(6): 1664]

90. Lin, R. C., Zhou, F. C., Fillenwarth, M. J., and Lumeng, L., Zonal distribution of protein-acetaldehyde adducts in the liver of rats fed alcohol for long periods, *Hepatology* 18, 864, 1993.

91. Albano, E., Tomasi, A., Goria Gatti, L., and Dianzani, M. U., Spin trapping of free radical species produced during the microsomal metabolism of ethanol, *Chem. Biol. Interact.* 65, 223, 1988.

92. Albano, E., Tomasi, A., and Ingelman-Sundberg, M., Spin trapping of alcohol-derived radicals in microsomes and reconstituted systems by electron spin resonance, *Meths. Enzymol.* 233, 117, 1994.

93. Albano, E., Tomasi, A., Persson, J. O., Terelius, Y., Goria Gatti, L., Ingelman-Sundberg, M., and Dianzani, M. U., Role of ethanol-inducible cytochrome P450 (P450IIE1) in catalysing the free radical activation of aliphatic alcohols, *Biochem. Pharmacol.* 41, 1895, 1991.

94. Iimuro, Y., Bradford, B. U., Gao, W., Kadiiska, M., Mason, R. P., Stefanovic, B., Brenner, D. A., and Thurman, R. G., Detection of alpha-hydroxyethyl free radical adducts in the pancreas after chronic exposure to alcohol in the rat, *Mol. Pharmacol.* 50, 656, 1996.

95. Clot, P., Albano, E., Eliasson, E., Tabone, M., Arico, S., Israel, Y., Moncada, C., and Ingelman-Sundberg, M., Cytochrome P4502E1 hydroxyethyl radical adducts as the major antigen in autoantibody formation among alcoholics, *Gastroenterology* 111, 206, 1996.

96. Clot, P., Tabone, M., Arico, S., and Albano, E., Monitoring oxidative damage in patients with liver cirrhosis and different daily alcohol intake, *Gut* 35, 1637, 1994.

97. Houglum, K., Filip, M., Witztum, J. L., and Chojkier, M., Malondialdehyde and 4-hydroxynonenal protein adducts in plasma and liver of rats with iron overload, *J. Clin. Invest.* 86, 1991, 1990.

98. Kamimura, S., Gaal, K., Britton, R. S., Bacon, B. R., Triadafilopoulos, G., and Tsukamoto, H., Increased 4-hydroxynonenal levels in experimental alcoholic liver disease: association of lipid peroxidation with liver fibrogenesis, *Hepatology* 16, 448, 1992.

99. Li, C. J., Nanji, A. A., Siakotos, A. N., and Lin, R. C., Acetaldehyde-modified and 4-hydroxynonenal-modified proteins in the livers of rats with alcoholic liver disease, *Hepatology* 26, 650, 1997.

100. Niemela, O., Parkkila, S., Yla Herttuala, S., Villanueva, J., Ruebner, B., and Halsted, C. H., Sequential acetaldehyde production, lipid peroxidation, and fibrogenesis in micropig model of alcohol-induced liver disease, *Hepatology* 22, 1208, 1995.

101. Niemela, O., Parkkila, S., Pasanen, M., Iimur, Y., Bradford, B., and Thurman, R. G., Early alcoholic liver injury: formation of protein adducts with acetaldehyde and lipid peroxidation products, and expression of CYP2E1 and CYP3A, *Alcohol. Clin. Exp. Res.* 22, 2118, 1998.

102. Ohhira, M., Ohtake, T., Matsumoto, A., Saito, H., Ikuta, K., Fujimoto, Y., Ono, M., Toyokuni, S., and Kohgo, Y., Immunohistochemical detection of 4-hydroxy-2-nonenal-modified-protein adducts in human alcoholic liver diseases, *Alcohol. Clin. Exp. Res.* 22, 145s, 1998.

103. Xu, D., Thiele, G. M., Kearley, M. L., Haugen, M. D., Klassen, L. W., Sorrell, M. F., and Tuma, D. J., Epitope characterization of malondialdehyde-acetaldehyde adducts using an enzyme-linked immunosorbent assay, *Chem. Res. Toxicol.* 10, 978, 1997.

104. Rintala, J., Jaatinen, P., Parkkila, S., Kiianmaa, K., Hervonen, A., and Niemela, O., Evidence of acetaldehyde-protein adduct formation in rat brain after life-long consumption of ethanol, *Alcohol Alcohol.* 35, 458, 2000.

105. Nakamura, K., Iwahashi, K., Ameno, K., Ijiri, I., Takeuchi, Y., and Suwaki, H., Immunohistochemical study on acetaldehyde adducts in alcohol fed mice, *Alcohol. Clin. Exp. Res.* 24, 93S, 2000.

106. Upadhya, S. C. and Ravindranath, V., Detection and localization of protein-acetaldehyde adducts in rat brain after chronic ethanol treatment, *Alcohol. Clin. Exp. Res.* 26, 856, 2002.

107. Worrall, S., Richardson, P. J., and Preedy, V. R., Experimental heart muscle damage in alcohol feeding is associated with increased amounts of reduced- and unreduced-acetaldehyde and malondialdehyde-acetaldehyde protein adducts, *Addict. Biol.* 5, 421, 2000.

108. Worrall, S., Niemela, O., Parkkila, S., Peters, T. J., and Preedy, V. R., Protein adducts in type I and type II fibre predominant muscles of the ethanol-fed rat: preferential localisation in the sarcolemmal and subsarcolemmal region, *Eur. J. Clin. Invest.* 31, 723, 2001.

109. Preedy, V. R. and Peters, T. J., The acute and chronic effects of ethanol on cardiac muscle protein synthesis in the rat *in vivo*, *Alcohol* 7, 97, 1990.

110. Mauch, T. J., Donohue, T. M., Jr., Zetterman, R. K., Sorrell, M. F., and Tuma, D. J., Covalent binding of acetaldehyde selectively inhibits the catalytic activity of lysine-dependent enzymes, *Hepatology* 6, 263, 1986.

111. Mauch, T. J., Tuma, D. J., and Sorrell, M. F., The binding of acetaldehyde to the active site of ribonuclease: alterations in catalytic activity and effects of phosphate, *Alcohol Alcohol.* 22, 103, 1987.

112. Xu, D. S., Jennett, R. B., Smith, S. L., Sorrell, M. F., and Tuma, D. J., Covalent interactions of acetaldehyde with the actin/microfilament system, *Alcohol Alcohol.* 24, 281, 1989.

113. Luduena, R. F., Roach, M. C., Jordan, M. A., and Murphy, D. B., Different reactivities of brain and erythrocyte tubulins toward a sulfhydryl group-directed reagent that inhibits microtubule assembly, *J. Biol. Chem.* 260, 1257, 1985.

114. McKinnon, G., de Jersey, J., Shanley, B., and Ward, L., The reaction of acetaldehyde with brain microtubular proteins: formation of stable adducts and inhibition of polymerization, *Neurosci. Lett.* 79, 163, 1987.

115. Tuma, D. J., Jennett, R. B., and Sorrell, M. F., The interaction of acetaldehyde with tubulin, *Ann. N.Y. Acad. Sci.* 492, 277, 1987.

116. Smith, S. L., Jennett, R. B., Sorrell, M. F., and Tuma, D. J., Substoichiometric inhibition of microtubule formation by acetaldehyde-tubulin adducts, *Biochem. Pharmacol.* 44, 65, 1992.

117. Smith, S. L., Jennett, R. B., Sorrell, M. F., and Tuma, D. J., Acetaldehyde substoichiometrically inhibits bovine neurotubulin polymerization, *J. Clin. Invest.* 84, 337, 1989.

118. Baraona, E., Leo, M. A., Borowsky, S. A., and Lieber, C. S., Alcoholic hepatomegaly: accumulation of protein in the liver, *Science* 190, 794, 1975.

119. Matsuda, Y., Baraona, E., Salaspuro, M., and Lieber, C. S., Effects of ethanol on liver microtubules and Golgi apparatus. Possible role in altered hepatic secretion of plasma proteins, *Lab. Invest.* 41, 455, 1979.

120. Matsuda, Y., Takase, S., Takada, A., Sato, H., and Yasuhara, M., Comparison of ballooned hepatocytes in alcoholic and non-alcoholic liver injury in rats, *Alcohol* 2, 303, 1985.

121. Matsuda, Y., Takada, A., Kanayama, R., and Takase, S., Changes of hepatic microtubules and secretory proteins in human alcoholic liver disease, *Pharmacol. Biochem. Behav.* 18 Suppl 1, 479, 1983.

122. Baraona, E., Matsuda, Y., Pikkarainen, P., Finkelman, F., and Lieber, C. S., Effects of ethanol on hepatic protein secretion and microtubules. Possible mediation by acetaldehyde, *Curr. Opp. Alcohol.* 8, 421, 1981.

123. Tuma, D. J., Smith, S. L., and Sorrell, M. F., Acetaldehyde and microtubules, *Ann. N.Y. Acad. Sci.* 625, 786, 1991.

124. Tuma, D. J., Zetterman, R. K., and Sorrell, M. F., Inhibition of glycoprotein secretion by ethanol and acetaldehyde in rat liver slices, *Biochem. Pharmacol.* 29, 35, 1980.

125. Sorrell, M. F. and Tuma, D. J., Selective impairment of glycoprotein metabolism by ethanol and acetaldehyde in rat liver slices, *Gastroenterology* 75, 200, 1978.

126. Sorrell, M. F., Nauss, J. M., Donohue, T. M., Jr., and Tuma, D. J., Effects of chronic ethanol administration on hepatic glycoprotein secretion in the rat, *Gastroenterology* 84, 580, 1983.

127. Tuma, D. J., Casey, C. A., and Sorrell, M. F., Effects of ethanol on hepatic protein trafficking: impairment of receptor-mediated endocytosis, *Alcohol Alcohol.* 25, 117, 1990.

128. Yamada, S., Mak, K. M., and Lieber, C. S., Chronic ethanol consumption alters rat liver plasma membranes and potentiates release of alkaline phosphatase, *Gastroenterology* 88, 1799, 1985.

129. Yamada, S., Wilson, J. S., and Lieber, C. S., The effects of ethanol and diet on hepatic and serum gamma-glutamyltranspeptidase activities in rats, *J. Nutr.* 115, 1285, 1985.

130. Gonzalez Calvin, J. L., Saunders, J. B., and Williams, R., Effects of ethanol and acetaldehyde on hepatic plasma membrane ATPases, *Biochem. Pharmacol.* 32, 1723, 1983.

131. Pignon, J. P., Bailey, N. C., Baraona, E., and Lieber, C. S., Fatty acid-binding protein: a major contributor to the ethanol-induced increase in liver cytosolic proteins in the rat, *Hepatology* 7, 865, 1987.

132. Lieber, C. S., Metabolic effects of acetaldehyde, *Biochem. Soc. Trans.* 16, 241, 1988.

133. Israel, Y., Hurwitz, E., Niemela, O., and Arnon, R., Monoclonal and polyclonal antibodies against acetaldehyde-containing epitopes in acetaldehyde-protein adducts, *Proc. Natl. Acad. Sci. U.S.A.* 83, 7923, 1986.

134. Worrall, S., De Jersey, J., Shanley, B. C., and Wilce, P. A., Ethanol induces the production of antibodies to acetaldehyde-modified epitopes in rats, *Alcohol Alcohol.* 24, 217, 1989.

135. Worrall, S., De Jersey, J., Shanley, B. C., and Wilce, P. A., Anti-acetaldehyde adduct antibodies generated by ethanol-fed rats react with reduced and unreduced acetaldehyde-modified proteins, *Alcohol Alcohol.* 29, 43, 1994.

136. Albano, E., Clot, P., Morimoto, M., Tomasi, A., Ingelman-Sundberg, M., and French, S. W., Role of cytochrome P4502E1-dependent formation of hydroxyethyl free radical in the development of liver damage in rats intragastrically fed with ethanol, *Hepatology* 23, 155, 1996.

137. Tsukamoto, H., Horne, W., Kamimura, S., Niemela, O., Parkkila, S., Yla Herttuala, S., and Brittenham, G. M., Experimental liver cirrhosis induced by alcohol and iron, *J. Clin. Invest.* 96, 620, 1995.

138. Xu, D., Thiele, G. M., Beckenhauer, J. L., Klassen, L. W., Sorrell, M. F., and Tuma, D. J., Detection of circulating antibodies to malondialdehyde-acetaldehyde adducts in ethanol-fed rats, *Gastroenterology* 115, 686, 1998.

139. Niemela, O., Klajner, F., Orrego, H., Vidins, E., Blendis, L., and Israel, Y., Antibodies against acetaldehyde-modified protein epitopes in human alcoholics, *Hepatology* 7, 1210, 1987.

140. Worrall, S., De Jersey, J., Shanley, B. C., and Wilce, P. A., Antibodies against acetaldehyde-modified epitopes: presence in alcoholic, non-alcoholic liver disease and control subjects, *Alcohol Alcohol.* 25, 509, 1990.

141. Worrall, S., de Jersey, J., Shanley, B. C., and Wilce, P. A., Antibodies against acetaldehyde-modified epitopes: an elevated IgA response in alcoholics, *Eur. J. Clin. Invest.* 21, 90, 1991.

142. Worrall, S., De Jersey, J., Shanley, B. C., and Wilce, P. A., Alcohol abusers exhibit a higher IgA response to acetaldehyde-modified proteins, *Alcohol Alcohol. (Supplement* 1) 261, 1991.

143. Trudell, J. R., Ardies, C. M., and Anderson, W. R., Cross-reactivity of antibodies raised against acetaldehyde adducts of protein with acetaldehyde adducts of phosphatidyl-ethanolamine: possible role in alcoholic cirrhosis, *Mol. Pharmacol.* 38, 587, 1990.

144. Trudell, J. R., Ardies, C. M., Green, C. E., and Allen, K., Binding of anti-acetaldehyde IgG antibodies to hepatocytes with an acetaldehyde-phosphatidylethanolamine adduct on their surface, *Alcohol. Clin. Exp. Res.* 15, 295, 1991.

145. Koskinas, J., Kenna, J. G., Bird, G. L., Alexander, G. J., and Williams, R., Immunoglobulin A antibody to a 200-kilodalton cytosolic acetaldehyde adduct in alcoholic hepatitis, *Gastroenterology* 103, 1860, 1992.

146. Brown, W. R. and Kloppel, T. M., The liver and IgA: immunological, cell biological and clinical implications., *Hepatology* 9, 763, 1989.

147. Yokoyama, H., Ishii, H., Nagata, S., Kato, S., Kamegaya, K., and Tsuchiya, M., Experimental hepatitis induced by ethanol after immunization with acetaldehyde adducts, *Hepatology* 17, 14, 1993.

148. Yokoyama, H., Nagata, S., Moriya, S., Kato, S., Ito, T., Kamegaya, K., and Ishii, H., Hepatic fibrosis produced in guinea pigs by chronic ethanol administration and immunization with acetaldehyde adducts, *Hepatology* 21, 1438, 1995.

149. Worrall, S., de Jersey, J., and Wilce, P. A., Liver damage in ethanol-fed rats injected with acetaldehyde-modified proteins, *Alcohol Alcohol.* 27 (Suppl. 1) 74, 1992.

150. Mitchell, M. C. and Herlong, H. F., Alcohol and nutrition: caloric value, bioenergetics, and relationship to liver damage, *Ann. Rev. Nutr.* 6, 457, 1986.

151. Wassner, S. J., Li, J. B., Sperduto, A., and Norman, M. E., Vitamin D deficiency, hypocalcemia, and increased skeletal muscle degradation in rats, *J. Clin. Invest.* 72, 102, 1983.

152. Rimaniol, J. M., Authier, F. J., and Chariot, P., Muscle weakness in intensive care patients: initial manifestation of vitamin D deficiency, *Intensive Care Med.* 20, 591, 1994.

153. Hickish, T., Colston, K. W., Bland, J. M., and Maxwell, J. D., Vitamin D deficiency and muscle strength in male alcoholics, *Clin. Sci. (London)* 77, 171, 1989.

154. Duane, P. and Peters, T. J., Nutritional status in alcoholics with and without chronic skeletal muscle myopathy, *Alcohol Alcohol.* 23, 271, 1988.

155. Urbano Marquez, A., Estruch, R., Navarro Lopez, F., Grau, J. M., Mont, L., and Rubin, E., The effects of alcoholism on skeletal and cardiac muscle, *New Eng. J. Med.* 320, 409, 1989.

156. Reilly, M. E., Patel, V. B., Peters, T. J., and Preedy, V. R., *In vivo* rates of skeletal muscle protein synthesis in rats are decreased by acute ethanol treatment but are not ameliorated by supplemental alpha-tocopherol, *J. Nutr.* 130, 3045, 2000.

157. Fernandez Sola, J., Garcia, G., Elena, M., Tobias, E., Sacanella, E., Estruch, R., and Nicolas, J. M., Muscle antioxidant status in chronic alcoholism, *Alcohol. Clin. Exp. Res.* 26, 1858, 2002.

158. Hazell, A. S., Todd, K. G., and Butterworth, R. F., Mechanisms of neuronal death in Wernicke's encephalopathy, *Met. Brain Dis.* 13, 97, 1998.

159. Cook, C. C., Hallwood, P. M., and Thomsom, A. D., B vitamin deficiency and neuropsychiatric syndromes in alcohol misuse, *Alcohol Alcohol.* 33, 317, 1998.

160. Marsano, L. and McClain, C. J., Nutrition and alcoholic liver disease, *J. Parent. Enter. Nutr.* 15, 337, 1991.

161. Estruch, R., Nicolas, J. M., Villegas, E., Junque, A., and Urbano-Marquez, A., Relationship between ethanol-related diseases and nutritional status in chronically alcoholic men, *Alcohol Alcohol.* 28, 543, 1993.

162. Mezey, E., Dietary fat and alcoholic liver disease, *Hepatology* 28, 901, 1998.

163. Sorensen, T. I., Orholm, M., Bentsen, K. D., Hoybye, G., Eghoje, K., and Christoffersen, P., Prospective evaluation of alcohol abuse and alcoholic liver injury in men as predictors of development of cirrhosis, *Lancet* 2, 241, 1984.

164. Letteron, P., Duchatelle, V., Berson, A., Fromenty, B., Fisch, C., Degott, C., Benhamou, J. P., and Pessayre, D., Increased ethane exhalation, an *in vivo* index of lipid peroxidation, in alcohol-abusers, *Gut* 34, 409, 1993.

165. Lieber, C. S. and DeCarli, L. M., Quantitative relationship between amount of dietary fat and severity of alcoholic fatty liver, *Am. J. Clin. Nutr.* 23, 474, 1970.

166. Bloom, R. J. and Westerfeld, W. W., The thiobarbituric acid reaction in relation to fatty livers, *Arch. Biochem. Biophys.* 145, 669, 1971.

167. Reinke, L. A. and McCay, P. B., Spin trapping studies of alcohol-initiated radicals in rat liver: influence of dietary fat, *J. Nutr.* 127, 899s, 1997.

168. Nanji, A. A. and French, S. W., Dietary factors and alcoholic cirrhosis, *Alcohol. Clin. Exp. Res.* 10, 271, 1980.

169. Tsukamoto, H., French, S. W., Benson, N., Delgado, G., Rao, G. A., Larkin, E. C., and Largman, C., Severe and progressive steatosis and focal necrosis in rat liver induced by continuous intragastric infusion of ethanol and low fat diet, *Hepatology* 5, 224, 1985.

170. Tsukamoto, H., Towner, S. J., Ciofalo, L. M., and French, S. W., Ethanol-induced liver fibrosis in rats fed high fat diet, *Hepatology* 6, 814, 1986.

171. Nanji, A. A., Mendenhall, C. L., and French, S. W., Beef fat prevents alcoholic liver disease in the rat, *Alcohol. Clin. Exp. Res.* 13, 15, 1989.

172. Nanji, A. A. and French, S. W., Dietary linoleic acid is required for development of experimentally induced alcoholic liver injury, *Life Sci.* 44, 223, 1989.

173. Morimoto, M., Hagbjork, A. L., Nanji, A. A., Ingelman-Sundberg, M., Lindros, K. O., Fu, P. C., Albano, E., and French, S. W., Role of cytochrome P4502E1 in alcoholic liver disease pathogenesis, *Alcohol* 10, 459, 1993.

174. Nanji, A. A., Yang, E. K., Fogt, F., Sadrzadeh, S. M., and Dannenberg, A. J., Medium chain triglycerides and vitamin E reduce the severity of established experimental alcoholic liver disease, *J. Pharmacol. Exp. Ther.* 277, 1694, 1996.

175. Korourian, S., Hakkak, R., Ronis, M. J., Shelnutt, S. R., Waldron, J., Ingelman-Sundberg, M., and Badger, T. M., Diet and risk of ethanol-induced hepatotoxicity: carbohydrate-fat relationships in rats, *Toxicol. Sci.* 47, 110, 1999.

176. Cunningham, C. C., Sinthusek, G., Spach, P. I., and Leathers, C., Effect of dietary ethanol and cholesterol on metabolic functions of hepatic mitochondria and microsomes from the monkey, *Macaca nemestrina*, *Alcohol. Clin. Exp. Res.* 5, 410, 1981.

177. Lieber, C. S., Robins, S. J., Li, J., DeCarli, L. M., Mak, K. M., Fasulo, J. M., and Leo, M. A., Phosphatidylcholine protects against fibrosis and cirrhosis in the baboon, *Gastroenterology* 106, 152, 1994.

178. Worrall, S., Koll, M., Paice, A., Peters, T., and Preedy, V. R., Tocopherol decreases hepatic protein adduct formation in alcohol-fed rats, *Alcohol. Clin. Exp. Res.* (Supplement 26) 796, 2002.

14 Dietary Arachidonic Acid and Alcohol

Misako Okita, Takayo Sasagawa, and Junko Yokoyama

CONTENTS

14.1 INTRODUCTION

Alcoholic liver injuries such as fatty liver, hepatitis, and fibrosis are frequently observed in patients with a long history of excessive alcohol intake. It is suggested that liver injury due to ethanol may involve the interaction of polyunsaturated fatty acid (PUFA), eicosanoids, and other lipid peroxides.[1–4] Abnormal lipid metabolism is also frequently observed in severe alcoholics. One of the most significant and consistent effects of ethanol on lipid metabolism is the change in the fatty acid composition of phospholipids in liver and other tissues. A common finding in ethanol-treated animals is a decrease in arachidonic acid (20:4 *n*-6) and increased levels of oleic acid (18:1 *n*-9) and linoleic acid (18:2 *n*-6).[5] It has been suggested that the decrease in arachidonic acid induced by ethanol is caused by the reduction in $\Delta 6$ and $\Delta 5$ desaturase activity.[6] On the other hand, increased metabolism of arachidonic acid into epoxides, such as 14,15-epoxy-eicosatrienoic acid (EET), 11,12-EET, and 8,9-EET, was also proposed by French et al.[7] as an important factor in ethanol-induced liver injury. However, they

0-8493-1680-4/04/$0.00+$1.50

suggested that lipid peroxidation by cytochrome P450 (CYP) 2E1 could not totally account for the reduction in arachidonic acid and that the severity of liver pathology correlated negatively with the decrease in arachidonic acid in ethanol-fed rats. In addition, they suggested that reduction of arachidonic acid may be an important mechanism of ethanol-induced liver injury.

To clarify the role of arachidonic acid in liver injury in alcoholic patients, some approaches are presented in the following pages.

14.1.1   ABNORMAL PLASMA FATTY ACID COMPOSITION OBSERVED IN ALCOHOLIC PATIENTS

Malnutrition is often observed in alcoholic patients. We studied the dietary fat intake and the fatty acid composition in plasma phospholipids in two groups of alcoholic patients: eight male patients (48 ± 2 years) with liver injury and seven male patients (57 ± 3 years) without liver injury. In addition, they were compared with 10 healthy male subjects (42 ± 2 years) who did not have habitual alcohol intake. Energy intake from ethanol was 29 ± 16% of total energy intake in the patients with liver injury and 32 ± 14% in the patients without liver injury, and no significant difference was observed. Dietary fat intake in patients with and without liver injury was 34.8 ± 15.2 g/d (13.5 ± 4.9 energy %) and 25.7 ± 16.8 g/d (11.0 ± 6.4 energy %), respectively. As shown in Figure 14.1, significantly low levels of linoleic acid (18:2 n-6), arachidonic acid (20:4 n-6), and docosahexaenoic acid (DHA; 22:6 n-3) in plasma phospholipids were recognized in patients with liver injury compared with controls. In patients without liver injury, significant decreases in linoleic acid and DHA were also recognized. In contrast, saturated fatty acids, palmitic acid (16:0), and stearic acid (18:0), and monounsaturated fatty acid oleic acid (18:1 n-9) were significantly higher in alcoholic patients with liver injury compared with controls. Thus, alcoholic patients, especially those having liver injury, showed low levels of polyunsaturated fatty acids in plasma phospholipids.

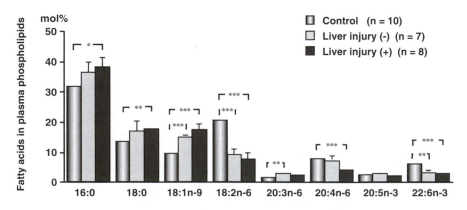

FIGURE 14.1 Fatty acid composition of plasma phospholipids in alcoholic patients with and without liver injury and healthy controls. ***$p < 0.001$, **$p < 0.01$, *$p < 0.05$

Unsaturated fatty acids, linoleic acid, and α-linolenic acid (18:3 *n*-3) are essential for higher animals since they are not synthesized in the body and must be supplied from the diet. Linoleic acid is converted to arachidonic acid via dihomo-γ-linolenic acid (20:3 *n*-6) and α-linolenic acid is also converted to eicosapentaenoic acid (EPA; 20:5 *n*-3) and DHA by desaturation and chain elongation, as shown in Figure 14.2. Although the impaired desaturation step may be a cause for deficiency of arachidonic acid and DHA in alcoholic patients,[6] the very low fat intake in the patients may contribute to the low levels of linoleic acid and arachidonic acid in plasma phospholipids.

14.1.2 DIETARY ARACHIDONIC ACID SUPPLEMENT IN ETHANOL-TREATED RATS

Our previous study of ethanol-treated rats fed with lard[8,9] revealed that arachidonic acid supplement (ethyl ester form, 3% of diet by weight) lowered, but not significantly, the serum alanine aminotransferase (ALT) activity (Figure. 14.3) and, significantly, liver triglyceride content (Figure 14.4). Therefore, arachidonic acid supplement was expected to protect against liver injury induced by ethanol.

To clarify the effect of dietary arachidonic acid supplement on the liver and serum lipids and arachidonate metabolites in ethanol-treated rats, further examinations using arachidonic acid-rich oil (AAoil) was carried out in ethanol-treated rats.[10]

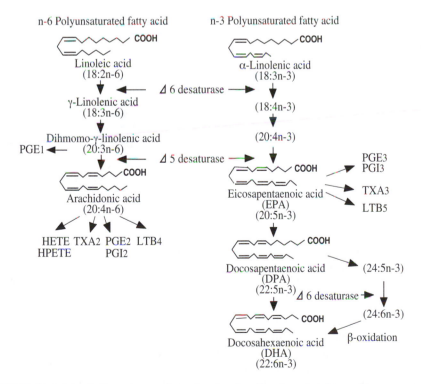

FIGURE 14.2 Metabolic pathways for *n*-6 and *n*-3 polyunsaturated fatty acids.

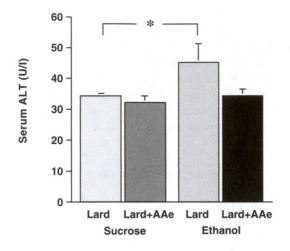

FIGURE 14.3 Serum alanine aminotransferase activities in ethanol-treated rats and control rats fed with 10% lard or 10% lard supplemented with arachidonic acid ethyl-ester (AAe, 3% of total diet) for 14 d. A single daily dose of ethanol (3 g/kg body weight) was administered intragastrically for the experimental feeding period. Control rats were administered isocaloric sucrose instead of ethanol. (n = 6 for each group, $*p < 0.05$).

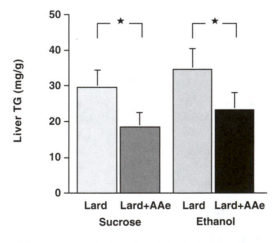

FIGURE 14.4 Liver triglyceride content in ethanol-treated rats and control rats fed with 10% lard or 10% lard supplemented with arachidonic acid ethyl-ester (AAe, 3% of total diet) for 14 d. A single daily dose of ethanol (3 g/kg body weight) was administered intragastrically for the experimental feeding period. Control rats were administered isocaloric sucrose instead of ethanol. (n = 6 for each group, $*p < 0.05$).

Male Sprague-Dawley rats were used and a single daily dose of 3 g/kg body weight of ethanol was administered intragastrically around noon during the 4-week experimental period. Control rats were administered isocaloric sucrose (5 g/kg body weight/d). After 2 weeks of feeding with standard laboratory chow, the rats were separated into two groups and fed two kinds of diet containing 10% lard or 10%

TABLE 14.1
Fatty Acid Composition (Weight %) of Dietary Fats

Fatty acid	Lard	Arachidonic Acid-Rich Oil
Myristic acid (14:0)	1.9	0.3
Palmitic acid (16:0)	25.2	13.5
Palmitoleic acid (16:1)	2.5	0.1
Stearic acid (18:0)	14.6	6.1
Oleic acid (18:1 n-9)	42.0	14.1
Linoleic acid (18:2 n-6)	10.5	23.5
γ-Linolenic acid (18:3 n-6)	0.1	1.9
α-Linolenic acid (18:3 n-3)	0.8	1.8
Arachidic acid (20:0)	0.3	0.7
Gadoleic acid (20:1)	0.9	0.5
Eicosadienoic acid (20:2 n-6)	0.5	0.5
Dihomo-γ-linolenic acid (20:3 n-6)	0.1	3.0
Arachidonic acid (20:4 n-6)	0.2	24.6
Behenic acid (22:0)	0.0	2.0
Docosatetraenoic acid (22:4 n-6)	0.0	0.3
Lignoceric acid (24:0)	0.0	4.1

AAoil (from Tokiwa Chemical Industries Ltd., Osaka) for 2 weeks. Control rats were fed with lard. The fatty acid composition of AAoil and lard tested in the study is shown in Table 14.1.

14.1.2.1 Effect of Arachidonic Acid-Rich Oil on Fatty Acid Composition in Liver Phospholipids

Phospholipids in rat liver tissue are rich in arachidonic acid as shown in Figure 14.5. There were few differences in fatty acid composition between the sucrose–lard (control) and ethanol–lard groups. Comparing with the ethanol–lard group, the ethanol–AAoil group showed significantly higher levels of arachidonic acid (20:4 n-6), docosatetraenoic acid (22:4 n-6) and lignoceric acid (24:0). In contrast, oleic acid (18:1 n-9), linoleic acid (18:2 n-6), and DHA (22:6 n-3) were decreased significantly in the ethanol–AAoil group compared with the ethanol–lard group. Since polyunsaturated fatty acids are esterified in position 2 of glycerol, polyunsaturated fatty acid compensates to esterify in the phospholipids. Therefore, an increase in arachidonic acid may induce decreases in DHA and linoleic acid.

In the phospholipids of red blood cell ghosts of the ethanol–AAoil group (Figure 14.6), significant increases in arachidonic acid (20:4 n-6) and docosatetraenoic acid (22:4 n-6) and decreases in oleic acid (18:1 n-9) and linoleic acid (18:2 n-6) were recognized, compared with the ethanol–lard group, as similar to that in liver phospholipids (Figure 14.4). Few differences were observed in the fatty acid compositions between the control and ethanol–lard groups.

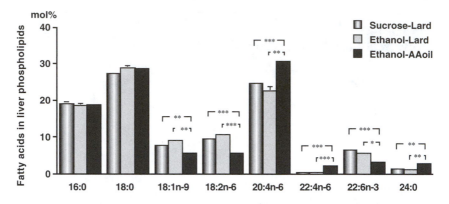

FIGURE 14.5 Fatty acid composition of liver phospholipids in ethanol-treated rats and control rats fed with 10% lard or 10% arachidonic acid-rich oil (AAoil). A single daily dose of ethanol (3 g/kg body weight) was administered intragastrically 2 weeks before and during the 2 weeks of experimental feeding. Control rats were administered isocaloric sucrose instead of ethanol. (n = 6 for each group, ***$p < 0.001$, **$p < 0.01$, *$p < 0.05$)

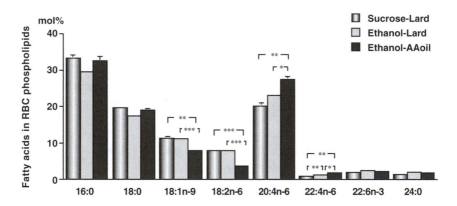

FIGURE 14.6 Fatty acid composition of red blood cell ghosts in ethanol-treated rats and control rats fed with 10% lard or 10% arachidonic acid-rich oil (AAoil). A single daily dose of ethanol (3 g/kg body weight) was administered intragastrically 2 weeks before and during the 2 weeks of experimental feeding. Control rats were administered isocaloric sucrose instead of ethanol. (n = 6 for each group, ***$p < 0.001$, **$p < 0.01$, *$p < 0.05$).

14.1.2.2 Effect of Arachidonic Acid-Rich Oil on Lipid Content in Liver Tissue

A small but not significant decrease in liver triglyceride was observed in the AAoil-fed rats (23.8 ± 5.8 mg/g) compared with the lard-fed rats (27.8 ± 6.7 mg/g) in ethanol-treated rats. In microscopic observation, hepatocytes containing small to large vacuoles were seen in the periportal area in the ethanol–lard group. Compared with the ethanol–lard group, only small vacuoles were seen in the ethanol–AAoil group. These observations may suggest that arachidonic acid-rich oil decreases triglyceride in the liver. However, dietary AAoil did not change the serum triglyceride level. Whelan et al.[11] reported that dietary arachidonic acid (1.1 to 1.5% diet wt/wt) increased circulating triglycerides in hamsters and mice compared with those fed with n-3 polyunsaturated fatty acid or oleic acid enriched diets. Differences in the experimental conditions such as animal species and dietary fat composition may be a reason for the different findings. Mater et al.[12] demonstrated that arachidonic acid suppressed mRNAs encoding fatty acid synthase and S14 chloramphenicol acetyl transferase (CAT) through a prostanoid pathway in 3T3-L1 adipocytes, and they also suggested a different control mechanism from the polyunsaturated fatty acid-mediated suppression of hepatic lipogenic gene expression: the PPAR-mediated pathway.[13]

14.1.2.3 Effect of Arachidonic Acid-Rich Oil on Prostanoid Levels in Plasma and Liver Tissue

Plasma 6-keto-prostaglandin (PG) F1α, a stable metabolite of prostacyclin (PGI$_2$), and thromboxane (TX) B$_2$ levels, liver 6-keto-PGF1α, and leukotriene (LT) B$_4$ contents are shown in Figure 14.7 and Figure 14.8. No significant differences were observed in the plasma 6-keto-PGF1α and TXB$_2$ levels between the sucrose–lard (control) and ethanol–lard groups, though a small decrease was observed in the 6-keto-PGF1α level of the ethanol–lard group. Both plasma 6-keto-PGF1α and TXB$_2$ levels were significantly higher in the AAoil group than in the lard group in ethanol-treated rats. However, the increase in 6-keto-PGF1α in the ethanol–AAoil group was higher than that of TXB$_2$, and the 6-keto-PGF1α/TXB$_2$ ratio in the ethanol–AAoil group was nearly twofold that of the ethanol–lard group.

In the liver tissue of the ethanol–AAoil group, the 6-keto-PGF1α content was more than threefold that of the ethanol–lard group. However, no difference was recognized in LTB$_4$ content between the AAoil and lard groups of ethanol-treated rats. The 6-keto-PGF1α/LTB$_4$ ratio in the ethanol–AAoil group was about threefold that of the ethanol–lard group.

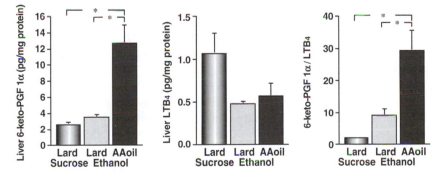

FIGURE 14.7 Plasma 6-keto-PGF1α and TXB$_2$ levels and 6-keto-PGF1α/TXB$_2$ ratio in ethanol-treated rats fed with lard or arachidonic acid-rich oil (AAoil). A single daily dose of ethanol (3 g/kg body weight) was administered intragastrically 2 weeks before and during the 2 weeks of experimental feeding. Control rats were administered isocaloric sucrose instead of ethanol. (n = 6 for each group, ***$p < 0.001$, **$p < 0.01$, *$p < 0.05$).

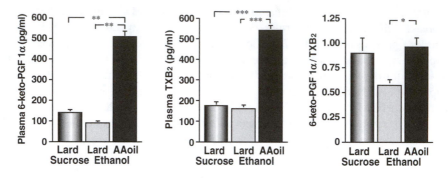

FIGURE 14.8 Liver 6-keto-PGF1α and LTB$_4$ levels and 6-keto-PGF1α/LTB$_4$ ratio in ethanol-treated rats fed with lard or arachidonic acid-rich oil (AAoil). A single daily dose of ethanol (3 g/kg body weight) was administered intragastrically 2 weeks before and during the 2 weeks of experimental feeding. Control rats were administered isocaloric sucrose instead of ethanol. (n = 6 for each group, *$p < 0.05$).

14.1.2.4   Significance of Arachidonate Supplement in Alcoholics

Most tissue has phospholipids in cell membranes, which are characterized by having predominantly polyunsaturated fatty acids such as linoleic acid, arachidonic acid, and eicosapentaenoic acid esterified in position 2. On activation of phospholipase A$_2$, arachidonic acid is normally released and oxidized by both lipoxygenase and cyclooxygenase (COX). This action leads to the instantaneous biosynthesis of various prostaglandins, thromboxanes, or leukotrienes of the 2-type (Figure 14.2). Prostanoids formed in the liver control several functions of hepatocytes, such as glycogenolysis [14] and DNA synthesis.[15] An increased urinary excretion of 6-keto-PGF1α in cirrhotic patients[16] and an elevated level of plasma 6-keto-PGF1α in cirrhotic rats induced by CCl$_4$[17] were reported. From these findings, enhanced synthesis of prostaglandins may be postulated as a possible cause of decreased arachidonic acid content in plasma phospholipids.

In contrast, Wakabayashi et al.[18] observed that COX–2, an inducible form of COX, activity was not affected by ethanol (100 to 400 mM) in RAW macrophages, but the protein expression of COX-2 by lipopolysaccharide (LPS) was significantly increased by ethanol. Therefore, ethanol may suppress utilization of arachidonic acid, resulting in reduction of inducible PG production.

Cell membrane function depends primarily on the fluidity of the lipid matrix of the cell. Polyunsaturated fatty acid content was suggested to play a major role in cell membrane fluidity and integrity.[19] Changes in membrane fluidity in both hepatocyte membranes and erythrocyte membranes have been reported in liver disease.[20,21]

Arachidonic acid is considered a harmful substance if it is consumed in large amounts. However, a human dietary arachidonic acid supplement study, reported by Nelson et al.,[22,23] revealed that dietary arachidonic acid had no deleterious effect on platelet aggregation and plasma lipids. In the study of Nelson et al., a triglyceride produced by algae that contained 50% arachidonic acid (1.5 g arachidonic acid/d) was fed to healthy male subjects for 50 d. Plasma phospholipid and cholesterol ester in the study showed a marked increase in their content of arachidonic acid. A marked increase in the excretion of 11-dehydrothromboxan B_2, a metabolite of TX, and 6-keto-PGF1α was observed after starting the arachidonic acid-rich diet.[24]

The arachidonic acid metabolic cascade consists of COX, lipoxygenases, and CYP. Metabolism by COX generates PGH_2 that rearranges enzymatically or chemically to generate several PGs or TXs.[25] The metabolism by the lipoxygenase generates 5-hydroperoxyeicosatetraenoic acid (5-HPETE), the precursor in the biosynthesis of LTs. In our AAoil study, plasma and liver 6-keto-PGF1α levels and plasma TXB_2 levels were markedly increased, but not liver LTB_4 levels, suggesting selective induction of the COX pathway by dietary AA. A decreased production of a vasodilator prostanoid, PGI_2, enhanced liver injury and portal hypertension.[26] Nanji et al.[27] also recognized reduced PGI_2 production by liver nonparenchymal cells obtained from ethanol treated rats and suggested that decreased PGI_2 production may have contributed to the hepatotoxic effect of ethanol. TXA_2 is the major eicosanoid produced by platelet. TXA_2 is a potent proaggregant and a powerful vasoconstrictor of vascular smooth muscle cells. Nanji et al.[27] suggested the importance of the altered TX: PGI_2 balance in the development of fibrosis and cirrhosis. The present observations showing the increased 6-keto-PGF1α/TXB_2 ratio in the plasma of AAoil-fed rats suggested the usefulness of dietary arachidonic acid for the inhibition of alcoholic liver injury.

LTs may be key mediators in inflammatory liver diseases.[28] Ethanol inhibits the catabolism of LTB_4 in hepatocytes and increases excretion of LTB_4.[29] In the present study, arachidonic acid supplementation did not show any significant increase in LTB_4 in liver tissue of ethanol-treated rats, suggesting no increase in liver synthesis of LTB_4.

14.2 CONCLUSION

Dietary treatment is the basal therapy of liver disease in alcoholics because most patients have some malnutrition. In addition, dietary supplement of arachidonic acid with antioxidative food substances such as vitamin E or C may be expected to protect alcoholic liver injury.

References

1. Nanji, A.A. and French, S.W., Dietary linoleic acid is required for development of experimentally induced alcoholic liver injury, *Life Sci.*, 44, 223, 1989.
2. Okita, M. et al., Fatty acid composition and arachidonate metabolites in the livers of ethanol-treated rats fed an arachidonate-supplemented diet: effect of dietary fat, *J. Nutr. Sci. Vitaminol.*, 44, 745, 1998.
3. Mottaran, E. et al., Lipid peroxidation contributes to immune reactions associated with alcoholic liver disease, *Free Radic. Biol. Med.*, 32, 38, 2002.

4. Hoek, J.B. and Pastorino, J.G., Ethanol, oxidative stress, and cytokine-induced liver cell injury, *Alcohol*, 27, 63, 2002.
5. Nakamura, M.T. et al., Reduced tissue arachidonic acid concentration with chronic ethanol feeding in miniature pigs, *Am. J. Clin. Nutr.*, 56, 467, 1992.
6. Nakamura, M.T. et al., Selective reduction of Δ6 and Δ5 desaturase activities but not Δ9 desaturase in micropigs chronically fed ethanol, *J. Clin. Invest.*, 93, 450, 1994.
7. French, S.W. et al., Lipid peroxidation, CYP2E1 and arachidonic acid metabolism in alcoholic liver disease in rats, *J. Nutr.*, 127, 907S, 1997.
8. Okita, M. et al., Effect of arachidonate on lipid metabolism in ethanol-treated rats fed with lard, *J. Nutr. Sci. Vitaminol.*, 43, 311, 1997.
9. Okita, M. et al., Fatty acid composition and arachidonate metabolites in the livers of ethanol-treated rats fed an arachidonate-supplemented diet: effect of dietary fat, *J. Nutr. Sci. Vitaminol.*, 44, 745, 1997.
10. Okita, M. et al., Effect of arachidonic acid-rich oil on lipids and arachidonate metabolites in ethanol-treated rats, *Prostagl. Leukot. Essent. Fatty Acids*, 64, 273, 2001.
11. Whelan, J. et al., Evidence that dietary arachidonic acid increases circulating triglycerides, *Lipids*, 30, 425, 1995.
12. Mater, M.K. et al., Arachidonic acid inhibits lipogenic gene expression in 3T3-L1 adipocytes through a prostanoid pathway, *J. Lipid Res.*, 39, 1327, 1998.
13. Mater, M.K., Thelen, A.P., and Jump, D.B., Arachidonic acid and PGE2 regulation of hepatic lipogenic gene expression, *J. Lipid Res.*, 40, 1045, 1999.
14. Okumura, T., Sago, K., and Saito, K., Effects of prostaglandins and their analogues on hormone-stimulated glycogenolysis in primary cultures of rat hepatocytes, *Biochem. Biophys. Acta*, 958, 179, 1988.
15. Andreis, P.G., Whitfield, J.F., and Armato, U., Stimulation of DNA synthesis and mitosis of hepatocytes in primary cultures of neonatal rat liver by arachidonic acid and prostaglandins, *Exp. Cell Res.*, 134, 265, 1981.
16. Guarner, C. et al., Systemic prostacyclin in cirrhotic patients, *Gastroenterology*, 102, 303, 1992.
17. Oberti, F. et al., Role of prostacyclin in hemodynamic alterations in conscious rats with extrahepatic or intrahepatic portal hypertension, *Hepatology*, 18, 621, 1993.
18. Wakabayashi, I., Yasui, K., and Negoro, M., Diverse effects of ethanol on the pathway of inducible prostaglandin E2 production in macrophages, *Prostagl. Lipid Mediat.*, 67, 61, 2002.
19. Kakimoto, H. et al., Altered lipid composition and differential changes in activities of membrane-bound enzymes of erythrocytes in hepatic cirrhosis, *Metabolism*, 44, 825, 1995.
20. Schuller, A. et al., The fluidity of liver plasma membranes from patients with different types of liver injury, *Hepatology*, 6, 714, 1986.
21. Owen, J.S. et al., Decreased erythrocyte membrane fluidity and altered lipid composition in human liver disease, *J. Lipid Res.*, 23, 124, 1982.
22. Nelson, G.J. et al., The effect of dietary arachidonic acid on platelet function, platelet fatty acid composition, and blood coagulation in humans, *Lipids*, 32, 421, 1997.
23. Nelson, G.J. et al., The effect of dietary arachidonic acid on plasma lipoprotein distributions, apoproteins, blood lipid levels, and tissue fatty acid composition in humans, *Lipids*, 32, 427, 1997.
24. Ferretti, A. et al., Increased dietary arachidonic acid enhances the synthesis of vasoactive eicosanoids in humans, *Lipids* 32, 435, 1997.
25. Smith, W.L., Garavito, M.R., and Dewitt, D.L., Prostaglandin endoperoxide H synthases (cyclooxygenases)-1 and -2, *J. Biol. Chem.*, 271, 33157, 1996.

26. Lemberg, A. et al., Prostanoid production in endothelial and Kupffer liver cells from monocrotaline intoxicated rats, *Human. Exper. Toxicol.*, 17, 564, 1998.
27. Nanji, A.A., Khwaja, S., and Sadrzadej, S.M.H., Decreased prostacyclin production by liver non-parenchymal cells precedes liver injury in experimental alcoholic liver disease, *Life Sci.*, 54, 455, 1994.
28. Keppler, D. et al., The relation of leukotrienes to liver injury, *Hepatology*, 5, 883, 1985.
29. Uemura, M. et al., Enhanced urinary excretion of cysteinyl leukotrienes in patients with acute alcohol intoxication, *Gastroenterology*, 118, 1140, 2000.

15 Protein Metabolism in Alcohol Misuse and Toxicity

Victor R. Preedy, Michael Koll, Junko Adachi, David Mantle, Vinood B. Patel, and Timothy J. Peters

CONTENTS

0-8493-1680-4/04/$0.00+$1.50
© 2004 by CRC Press LLC

15.1 INTRODUCTION

This review is essentially an update of the article published over a decade ago which was primarily concerned with the effects of alcohol on protein metabolism in the different mammalian tissues such as skeletal muscle, heart, liver, and intestine as well as bone.[1] Since then, there have been considerable advances in our understanding of how these tissues are affected by alcohol at the gross biochemical or molecular levels (for example, see References 2 to 7).

In the present review we focus on skeletal muscle and the whole body metabolism. We also include, where appropriate, studies on heart and liver. Understanding the biochemical mechanisms responsible for the changes in alcoholism is important in developing novel therapeutic strategies, such as administration of hepatic growth factor,[8] catalase,[9] melatonin,[10] glycine,[11] alpha-tocopherol,[12] taurine,[13] s-adenosyl-L-methionine[14] and many other agents. Also, alcohol studies represent a metabolic system in which homeostatic control is disturbed by the presence of a single substance that can be given in precise amounts and the metabolism of the perturbant is largely known. Mechanisms in alcohol-related pathology may thus be applicable to other disease states: for example, the loss of ribosomal RNA and fiber-type specificity of alcoholic myopathy is also identical to other myopathologies, such as those occurring in starvation or diabetes.

The focus on skeletal muscle in this chapter needs to be rationalized. Serious musculoskeletal problems in alcoholism are more common than gastrointestinal and hepatic tissue diseases in alcohol misusers. For example, one study of a cohort of 200 alcohol misusers showed that the prevalence of muscle disease (44%) was nearly five times greater than the incidence of cirrhosis (9%).[15,16] The failure to address alcohol-related research in terms of its prevalence is self-explanatory; while liver failure and/or cirrhosis leads to death, skeletal muscle pathologies are not necessarily life-threatening, though in the long term they lead to impaired morbidity and quality of life measures.

There is a considerable variation in the rates at which proteins are synthesized in the different mammalian organs (Table 15.1). Rates of protein synthesis in skeletal

TABLE 15.1
Average Protein Synthesis Rates in Different Tissues of the Rat

	Fractional Rate of Protein Synthesis (k_s, %/d)	
	Young 100 g Male Rats	Mature 220 g Female Rats
Skeletal muscle	17	5
Brain	ND	12
Heart	20	9
Uterus	ND	34
Kidney	ND	35
Lung	33	22
Skin	64	ND
Spleen	68	38
Bone	90	21
Liver	86	81
Small intestine	119	76

Note: Fractional rates of protein synthesis (k_s) were measured in fed rats with a large flooding dose of [3H]phenylalanine. ND, not determined. Data are mean levels. Skeletal muscle and bone are represented by the gastrocnemius muscle and tibia, respectively. The small intestine pertains to whole segments (mucosa and seromuscular layers combined) of duodenum plus jejunum (young rats) or the entire small bowel (mature rats). Skin protein synthesis is measured in that protein fraction which is soluble in 0.3 mol/l sodium hydroxide. Data compiled from various sources (see References 213 to 216).

muscle are comparatively low (Table 15.1) and by virtue of the fact that muscle is 40% of body weight, this tissue is a major contributor to whole-body metabolism; it accounts for at least a quarter of whole-body protein turnover. In terms of nitrogen economy, the contributions of skeletal muscle are comparable to that of the liver, the gastrointestinal tract, or the combined skin and bone. This implies that changes in skeletal muscle in alcoholism will have major physiological implications for whole-body metabolism. However, despite the prevalence and importance of skeletal muscle, little is known about alcoholic myopathy, compared to the detailed biochemical, genetic, and pathological basis for alcoholic liver disease (for example, see recent articles in this area[17–25]).

15.2 PROTEIN TURNOVER: DEFINITIONS AND COMPONENTS

Protein metabolism has two components, namely *protein synthesis* and *protein breakdown*. Both contribute to "protein turnover" which is defined as the process whereby proteins are continually being synthesized and degraded. At a particular time point, the amount of tissue protein is dependent upon the balance between their respective rates. It follows, therefore, that the rate of protein synthesis will equal the rate of protein degradation only in the steady state, i.e., when the tissue protein content is unaltered. An example of this steady state would be the adult individual or animal where the tissue protein content is generally considered to be constant.[26] This is, of course, a gross simplification, as even in the adult there is an hour-by-hour fluctuation in protein metabolism in response to food, endocrine changes, muscle activity, and other nutritional or physiological factors.[27]

In anabolic phases, such as during growth and development or organ hypertrophy, the synthesis rate will exceed the rate of protein degradation.[28] In the catabolic phase, in contrast, the degradation rate will exceed the rate of protein synthesis. This latter situation can occur in metabolic stress such as ageing, acute injury, or infection,[28-30] or chronic metabolic disturbances such as malnutrition or cancer cachexia.[31] Reductions in tissue protein content also occur in response to alcoholism. This includes alcoholic myopathy,[32] osteopathy,[33] and intestinal atrophy.[34]

There is very little reliable information on the effects of alcohol on protein metabolism in man. Part of the problem relates to the fact that (1) obtaining sufficient human tissue for detailed biochemical analysis is problematical, (2) there are technical problems in routinely measuring protein turnover in humans, and (3) one of the principal determinants of protein turnover is nutritional status, and in human studies this is difficult to control, especially when interventions can perturb nutrient handling or status.[26,28] However, there are some very relevant data on the effects of alcohol on liver protein turnover in humans and these have been reviewed previously.[35] There are also many excellent studies on muscle protein synthesis in humans, although not directly related to alcohol pathology.[36-39] In animal studies, in contrast, protein synthesis rates can be accurately determined in a large number of tissues to allow concomitant analysis of other biochemical variables. The treatment regimens can be designed so that a variety of physiological or regulatory factors can be investigated, such as the use of inhibitors of alcohol metabolism or manipulation of the various endocrine pathways. More importantly, nutritional status or nutrient handling can be strictly controlled.[7] In this review, however, clinical studies have been cited where applicable.

It is often assumed that reductions in tissue protein content occur solely via a fall in the rate of protein synthesis and/or an increase in proteolysis (also termed "breakdown"). However, it is important to emphasize that decreases in tissue protein content arise as a consequence of

1. Increases in both protein synthesis and breakdown, where the increase in protein breakdown is greater than the increase in protein synthesis
2. An increase in the rate of protein breakdown, without alterations in protein synthesis
3. A decrease in the rate of protein synthesis, without alterations in protein breakdown
4. A decrease in both protein synthesis and breakdown, but the decrease in protein synthesis is disproportionately greater than the decrease in protein breakdown
5. A decrease in protein synthesis and an increase in protein breakdown

From the above it is necessary to measure both synthetic and degradative processes in any investigative study into protein metabolism. However, the *in vivo* estimations of rates of protein degradation are not always reliable and a considerable number of assumptions have to be made.[1,40]

15.3 PROTEIN METABOLISM *IN VIVO* AND *IN VITRO*

A variety of techniques have been used to study the effects of alcohol on protein metabolism such as perfused organs (i.e., heart[41]), tissue slices,[42] or isolated cells such as hepatocytes or muscle cells,[43–45] or cocultures of different cells such as hepatocytes and stellate cells.[46] Although useful for dissecting out biochemical events or investigating the role of single substances, results from such experiments must eventually be equated with metabolic events and pathways that occur in the intact animal and ultimately in humans. The failure to reproduce exactly *in vitro* the metabolic conditions occurring in intact organisms has meant that, in general, rates of protein turnover *in vitro* are lower than rates found *in vivo*. In isolated systems, impairment of tissue nutrient supply, membrane damage or disruption, the absence of subcellular organelles necessary for protein trafficking pathways (e.g., Golgi), or lack of external signaling factors (e.g., hormones) may contribute to impairments in protein synthesis. However, if attention is paid to methodological issues, then it is possible to achieve very high rates of protein synthesis in isolated muscle of the same order of magnitude as those occurring *in vivo*.[47–50] Attention to the viability of such *in vitro* preparations are very important. Thus, studies with perfused muscle have shown that *in vitro*, impaired metabolic integrity as reflected by raised lactate or reduced ATP concentrations is associated with impaired rates of protein synthesis.[51] In addition, the composition of the extra-cellular medium for *in vitro* studies has a significant impact on rate of tissue protein synthesis.[48] With these caveats in mind, our subsequent attention has focused largely on *in vivo* observations to overcome these methodological issues, though occasionally we have employed isolated tissue systems to dissect out mechanistic issues, such as whether the increased urinary alanine seen *in vivo* in alcohol-fed rat is due to elevated alanine protein by muscle.

15.4 CLINICAL STUDIES ON THE EFFECTS OF ALCOHOL ON SKELETAL MUSCLE ATROPHY AND PROTEIN SYNTHESIS

Chronic and/or excessive ethanol consumption leads to skeletal muscle myopathy, characterized by a selective reduction in the diameter of Type II skeletal muscle fibers (anaerobic, glycolytic fast-twitch), while Type I (aerobic, oxidative slow-twitch) fibers are only marginally affected[52] (also reviewed in References 53 to 56). The acute form of alcohol-induced muscle damage occurs rarely, and comprises <5% of muscle disorders in alcoholics.

Measurement of urinary creatinine excretion indicates that in chronic alcoholic myopathy, affected subjects lose on average 20% of their whole-body skeletal muscle and in some subjects as much as 30%.[57] In other words, affected subjects have a cachexia similar to that occurring in malignant disease, AIDS, or heart disease. Changes in protein turnover are implicated in the pathogenesis of alcoholic myopathy (that is, changes in either protein synthesis and/or protein breakdown) as skeletal muscle biopsies from patients with alcoholic myopathy have reduced protein content[52,58] that correlates with the degree of fiber atrophy and loss of total ribosomal RNA.[59] Using primed a constant infusion of L[1-^{13}C]-leucine and NaH[13]CO$_3$ it has been shown that chronic alcoholics (>100 g/d, >10 years) exhibit a 40% decline in the fractional rates of skeletal muscle protein synthesis (Table 15.2).[60] Because of these changes, the contribution of skeletal muscle protein synthesis to whole-body protein synthesis falls from approximately 25% to 15% (Table 15.2).[60]

TABLE 15.2
Whole-Body Leucine and Protein Metabolism in Chronic Alcoholics

	Control	Alcoholic	% Change	P
Skeletal Muscle Protein Synthesis				
Fractional rate (%/d)	1.10 ± 0.12	0.66 ± 0.09	−40	<0.001
Percent of whole-body synthesis	27 (Range 23–36)	15 ± 2	−44	<0.001
Whole-Body Leucine Kinetics				
Breakdown (mmol/kg/d)	2.64 ± 0.19	2.32 ± 0.10	−12	NS
Oxidation (mmol/kg/d)	0.43 ± 0.02	0.34 ± 0.04	−21	<0.05
Synthesis (mmol/kg/d)	2.21 ± 0.17	1.98 ± 0.09	−10	NS
Plasma alphaKIC (mol/l)	34 ± 2	30 ± 4	−12	NS
Whole-Body Protein Kinetics				
Breakdown (g/d)	273 ± 28	255 ± 15	−7	NS
Synthesis (g/d)	226 ± 24	218 ± 12	−4	NS

Note: Rates of whole-body and skeletal muscle protein metabolism were measured in six fully-ambulant alcoholics (four males, two females; mean 45 years), and who had a daily alcoholic intake of 100 g or more for over 10 years. Comparisons are made with age- and sex-matched controls. AlphaKIC denotes alphaketoisocaproic acid. All data are mean ± SEM (n = 6). NS, P > 0.05, not significant.

Source: Adapted from Pacy PJ, Preedy VR, Peters TJ, Read M, and Halliday D (1991). The effect of chronic alcohol ingestion on whole body and muscle protein synthesis — a stable isotope study. *Alcohol Alcohol.* 26: 505–513.

15.5 EFFECTS OF ALCOHOL ON MUSCLE PROTEIN BREAKDOWN IN HUMANS

The effects of alcohol on skeletal muscle protein breakdown have also been investigated.[61] Neutral protease activities in skeletal muscle biopsies of myopathic alcoholics are similar to those in biopsies from nonmyopathic alcoholics.[61] However, drawing conclusions from the activity of a single enzyme is somewhat limiting, as there are a considerable number of proteolytic steps involved in the catabolic cascade. Measurement of urinary 3-methylhistidine excretion on the other hand is a suitable way of examining the overall rate of muscle protein degradation *in vivo*.[62–64] When nonskeletal muscle sources of 3-methylhistidine and creatinine are taken into consideration in the analysis (i.e., the Afting correction[65]) myofibrillar protein breakdown rates are shown to be significantly reduced in myopathic alcoholics.[61]

When alcohol or acetaldehyde is added to human muscle, then there are decreases in the activities of a number of proteases such as the cytoplasmic alanyl-, arginyl-, leucyl-, prolyl-, tripeptidyl-aminopeptidase and dipeptidyl aminopeptidase IV as well as the lysosomal cathepsins B, D, H, and L, dipeptidyl aminopeptidase I and II (Table 15.3). However, the metabolic significance of this is difficult to interpret, as very high levels of ethanol or acetaldehyde are needed to show any measurable effect (Table 15.3).[66] There is a wide range of responses, for example, arginyl aminopeptidase decreasing by 90% in response to 170 mM acetaldehyde with no change in cathepsin B activities (Table 15.3). Reductions in protease activities have also been confirmed in rat muscle, albeit for cathepsin D activities which are decreased in muscle homogenates after addition of alcohol and acetaldehyde *in vitro*.[67]

These observations of a reduced rate of protein breakdown in myopathic alcoholics are plausible for the following reason: if fractional rates of skeletal muscle protein synthesis fall by 40%, then the entire skeletal muscle protein mass would be considerably reduced by over 75% in a few years. Such losses of muscle mass will be overtly visible and will undoubtedly lead to death, but these changes do not occur. On the other hand, chronic alcoholics will only lose on average 20% of their muscle/protein mass over 10 years. This implies that there must be some sort of compensatory reaction to account for these gradual losses of skeletal muscle, and this can only be explained by a concomitant decrease in protein degradation when muscle protein synthetic rates are reduced in chronic alcohol toxicity.[1]

15.6 NUTRITIONAL STATUS IN ALCOHOLISM AND ITS RELATIONSHIP TO ALCOHOLIC MYOPATHY IN HUMANS

Nutritional abnormalities in alcohol misusers are very common, arising from either the calorific displacement of nutrients, limitations in financial resources or metabolic deficiencies in nutrient absorption, retention and metabolism, compounded by structural damage at the cellular or gross organ level.[68–72] For example, every single region of the gastrointestinal tract is affected in alcoholism, though not in every individual.[73]

TABLE 15.3
Protease Activities in Human Muscle *In Vitro* in Response to Alcohol and Acetaldehyde

	Effect of Ethanol (% Change)	
	170 mmol/l	1700 mmol/l
Cytoplasmic		
Alanyl aminopeptidase	+1	−10
Arginyl aminopeptidase	+2	−31*
Leucyl aminopeptidase	−20	−58*
Diaminopeptidase IV	0	−48*
Triaminopeptidase	0	−49*
Proline endopeptidase	−11	−63*
Lysosomal		
Diaminopeptidase I	+3	+1
Diaminopeptidase II	0	−42*
Cathepsin B	+5	−58*
Cathepsin H	+6	−56*
Cathepsin L	+1	−12
Cathepsin D	−2	−55*
	Effect of Acetaldehyde (% Change)	
	17 mmol/l	170 mmol/l
Cytoplasmic		
Alanyl aminopeptidase	−63*	−81*
Arginyl aminopeptidase	−72*	−90*
Diaminopeptidase IV	−11	−44*
Triaminopeptidase	−39*	−71*
Proline endopeptidase	−1	−34*
Lysosomal		
Diaminopeptidase I	−39*	−74*
Diaminopeptidase II	−34*	−56*
Cathepsin B	0	+1
Cathepsin H	−64*	−79*
Cathepsin L	−1	−3

Note: Homogenates of human muscle were incubated *in vitro* with alcohol or acetaldehyde *in vitro*. The minus prefix indicates a reduction in mean enzyme activity, where a positive prefix indicates a mean increase. *, $P < 0.05$ in comparison with control preparations without ethanol or acetaldehyde. Leucyl aminopeptidase and cathepsin D activities are only assayed in muscle from alcohol-exposed preparations.

Source: Adapted from Mantle D, Falkous G, Peters TJ, and Preedy VR (1999). Effect of ethanol and acetaldehyde on intracellular protease activities in human liver, brain and muscle tissues *in vitro*. Clin. Chim. Acta 281: 101–108.

It is therefore important to address the issue of whether malnutrition contributes to the muscle wasting in alcoholism.

The liver has a central role in nutritional metabolism and is involved in secondary processing and/or storage of nutritional components or metabolites. Damage to this organ will thus have profound implications for skeletal muscle and consequently whole body protein metabolism.[74,75] For example, the liver is a major site of metabolism for the calciferols where cholecalciferol is converted to 25-hydroxc-holecaliferol. Muscle wasting and/or weakness also arise in vitamin D deficiency.[76,77] However, in the genesis of alcoholic myopathy, vitamin D deficiency is not a contributory factor.[78] There is also a lack of a relationship between riboflavin, pyridoxine, thiamine, vitamin B_{12}, and folate deficiencies with the development of alcoholic myopathy.[57] The activities of serum alkaline ribonuclease, a marker of protein nutrition, are no different in myopathic and nonmyopathic alcoholics.[57] It is erroneous to interpret this as implying that alcoholics are not malnourished, as indeed many of the aforementioned nutrients are markedly impaired in alcohol misusers.[57] For example, deficiencies of one or more of the aforementioned nutrients occur in about 50% of chronic alcoholics. Rather, it is proposed that many of the nutritional deficiencies associated with alcoholism do not play a role in the muscle wasting of alcoholic myopathy.

Presently, the only exception to this conclusion is the observation that in one U.K. study, there was reduced alpha-tocopherol and selenium status in alcoholics with myopathy compared to nonmyopathic alcoholics.[79] The reduced alpha-tocopherol status has, however, not been reproduced in Spanish alcoholics with myopathy.[80] Laboratory animal studies also seem to support the contention that alpha-tocopherol deficiency does not seem to play a role in the genesis of alcohol-induced muscle wasting.

15.7 THE EFFECT OF ALCOHOL ON THE HUMAN LIVER

The effects of alcohol on liver protein metabolism have also been studied using leucine infusions.[2,3,81] Fractional rates of albumin synthesis were measured in non-alcohol misusers in response to wine or water which was administered with food.[81] While meal feeding with water increased albumin synthesis rates, 28 g of ethanol impeded this effect. At a higher dose, 71 g of ethanol decreased albumin synthesis to levels below the pretreatment value.[81] Changes in hepatic protein metabolism may be due to the well-characterized redox changes. In simple terms, ethanol metabolism increases the amount of NADH, thus perturbing the NADH/NAD+ ratio which is also reflected by increased lactate/pyruvate ratios.[82–84] Thus, ethanol administration (as wine) increases the lactate/pyruvate ratio in plasma and is associated with the decreases in albumin synthesis. However, when nicotinamide (a NAD+ donor or precursor) is also administered in alcohol dosing studies to counteract the increased NADH, the increased lactate/pyruvate ratio is ameliorated and the effects of alcohol on albumin synthesis are blunted.[3]

Severe alcoholic liver disease perturbs the biochemical profile of skeletal muscle, reduces its mass, and impairs force generation.[85–87] However, it is important to note that the muscle wasting of alcoholic myopathy is not caused by alcoholic liver disease.[52,78]

There are numerous effects of excessive alcohol on the liver apart from the development of cirrhosis. As mentioned above, the synthesis of albumin is affected by alcohol but there are many other defects that may have profound implications for whole-body metabolism. These abnormalities include possible defects in metal ion transporter proteins such as those pertaining to zinc.[88] Some of these changes in liver may also be related to defective intracellular trafficking or export and endocytosis.[89–91]

15.8 ANIMAL MODELS OF ALCOHOL MISUSE

In our laboratory, we routinely investigate the pathogenesis of alcoholic myopathy using rat models of acute and chronic alcohol exposure. In these studies anatomically distinct skeletal muscles are used to represent the basic fiber types, for example, the soleus representing Type I fibers, whereas the plantaris and gastrocnemius represent the Type II fibers (Table 15.4). The advantage of using the gastrocnemius relates to its relatively large size and is thus amenable for subcellular fractionation or other biochemical procedures. Also, there are distinct biochemical and functional differences between Type I and II fibers, which offer some clues as to the mechanisms involved in the genesis of alcohol-induced muscle disease. For example, Type I fibers have higher concentrations of alpha-tocopherol and other antioxidant defense systems, suggesting that free radicals may be involved in the pathogenesis of alcoholic myopathy.

In acute studies, rats are injected with a bolus of ethanol at a dose of 75 mmol/kg body weight, i.p. Measurements are made up to 24 h later and compared to identically treated control rats injected with saline (0.15 mol/L NaCl). The i.p. route is selected to ensure greater bioavailability of the administered ethanol. Mean blood ethanol levels are 450 mg/100 ml at 20 min, which fall steadily to zero through the following 24 h.[92] In our group, rats are usually sacrificed after 2.5 h treatment in general when ethanol is 200 to 250 mg/100 ml, although both shorter and longer duration studies have been carried out.

In chronic studies, a pair-feeding regimen is employed. Ethanol-treated rats are fed nutritionally complete liquid diets containing all the macro- and micro-nutrients necessary for growth. Ethanol comprises 35% of total dietary intake to ensure high circulating ethanol in the region of 200 to 250 mg/100 ml. Controls are pair-fed the same amount of the same diet in which ethanol is replaced with isocaloric glucose, though some studies have replaced ethanol with isocaloric lipid or protein. This protocol facilitates a direct comparison between glucose and ethanol-fed rats. The pair-feeding protocol is necessary as alcohol feeding in such high concentrations induces anorexia, so appropriate adjustments must be made to the group of animals designated as controls.[93,94] By adopting the pair-feeding regimen, it is possible to exclude the possibility that the metabolic effects observed in alcohol-fed rats may be due to reduced dietary intake or malnutrition and must thus be due to alcohol

TABLE 15.4
Muscles Used in Laboratory Animal Studies and Fiber-Type Differences

(A) Muscles Used

Muscle	Fiber-Type
Soleus	Type I fiber-predominant
Plantaris	Type II fiber-predominant
Gastrocnemius	Type II fiber-predominant

(B) Differences in Red (Type I) and White (Type II) Muscles

Red (Type I)	White (Type II)
High in myoglobin	Low in myoglobin
Slow twitch	Fast twitch
High in slow myosin heavy-chain isoforms	High in fast myosin heavy-chain isoforms
Aerobic	Anaerobic
Oxidative	Glycolytic
Low glycogen	High glycogen
High mitochondria	Few or no mitochondria
High capillary density	Low capillary density
Smaller muscle diameter	Larger muscle diameter
Higher alpha-tocopherol concentrations	Lower alpha-tocopherol concentrations

toxicity which encompass the putative effects of ethanol-related metabolites (for example, acetaldehyde) or ethanol-induced metabolic disturbances (for example, endocrine dysfunction).[93–95] In our group, rats are usually sacrificed after 6 weeks' treatment in general, although both shorter and longer duration studies have been carried out.

15.8.1 EFFECT OF EXPERIMENTAL ALCOHOLISM ON MUSCLE PROTEIN IN THE RAT

In the young male laboratory rat (0.1 kg body weight), chronic ethanol feeding for 6 weeks reduces the weight and protein content of the entire skeletal musculature by one fifth (Table 15.5), which is almost identical to the mean decreases in muscle mass seen in clinical studies.[53–56,95–101] These changes are also accompanied by decreases in the weight of skin, bone, and liver, though the magnitude of these changes depends on whether alcohol feeding commenced in young immature or older mature rats[99] (Table 15.5).

Smaller reductions in muscle protein content are detectable as early as 14 d after the commencement of alcohol feeding using the Lieber–DeCarli protocol[101] and even after 24 h of an acute ethanol dose.[92] An adaptive response in protein metabolism seems to occur as the losses of muscle protein thereafter are less marked.[101] Although mixed muscle protein fractions have been analyzed in the aforementioned studies, there are other specific changes in myopathic muscle, which include significant reductions in myosin, desmin, actin, troponin, nebulin and titin compared to pair-

TABLE 15.5
The Effects of Chronic Ethanol Feeding on Muscle and Body Composition

	Control	Ethanol	% Change	P
Immature Rats				
Body weight (g)	225 ± 3	197 ± 4	−12	<0.001
Carcass (g)	125 ± 2	102 ± 4	−19	<0.001
Bone, tibia (mg)	367 ± 9	340 ± 7	−7	<0.05
Skeletal muscle mass (g)	114 ± 2	92 ± 4	−20	<0.001
Gastrocnemius (mg)	2520 ± 40	1980 ± 50	−21	<0.001
Lung (mg)	1210 ± 110	1040 ± 70	−14	NS
Skin (g)	36 ± 1	29 ± 2	−19	<0.01
Kidney (mg)	872 ± 16	827 ± 19	−5	NS
Liver (g)	9 ± 1	7 ± 1	−17	<0.001
Mature Rats				
Body weight (g)	390 ± 8	361 ± 9	−7	<0.001
Carcass (g)	217 ± 6	194 ± 7	−10	<0.001
Bone, tibia (mg)	608 ± 6	594 ± 12	−2	NS
Skeletal muscle mass (g)	198 ± 5	177 ± 7	−11	<0.01
Gastrocnemius (mg)	4160 ± 80	3940 ± 110	−5	NS
Lung (mg)	1610 ± 130	1500 ± 100	−7	NS
Skin (g)	63 ± 3	55 ± 3	−13	<0.01
Kidney (mg)	1300 ± 40	1210 ± 50	−7	NS
Liver (g)	14 ± 1	13 ± 1	−6	NS

Note: Male Wistar rats of either 0.1 kg (young) or 0.3 kg (mature) body weight were chronically fed with nutritionally complete liquid diets containing 35% of total calories as glucose (controls) or ethanol. All data are mean ± SEM (n = 6–9). NS, $P > 0.05$, not significant.

Source: From Preedy VR and Peters TJ (1988). The effect of chronic ethanol feeding on body and plasma composition and rates of skeletal muscle protein turnover in the rat. *Alcohol Alcohol.* 23: 217–224. With permission.

fed controls.[102,103] Putatively, there are probably other proteins that are also significantly altered and these await elucidation.

Muscles with a predominance of Type II fibers (i.e., plantaris, gastrocnemius) are more susceptible to the detrimental effects of alcohol on protein mass than those muscles containing a predominance of Type I fibers (i.e., soleus). These alcohol-induced lesions are fiber specific, as the diameter of Type II fibers in the Type I fiber-predominant soleus is also preferentially reduced by chronic ethanol feeding.[100] This supports the notion that the metabolic damage is confined to muscle fiber types rather than anatomically located skeletal muscles.[100] The fiber-type specificity of the alcohol-induced damage in the rat model is identical to the situation in humans where the diameter of Type II fibers is preferentially affected in alcoholism[52] (also reviewed in Reference 104). This reaffirms that the rat model of alcohol feeding is suitable for examining the pathogenic mechanisms inherent in the development of alcoholic myopathy.

15.8.2　PROTEIN SYNTHESIS STUDIES IN RAT MODELS OF ALCOHOL TOXICITY

Protein synthesis rates have been measured in alcohol-dosed rats with a flooding dose of [^{3}H] phenylalanine. This is perhaps the gold standard method for measuring protein synthesis in small laboratory animals.[105–107] In these studies, the radiolabeled amino acid is incorporated into protein within 10 min and the amount of radioactivity in the protein is proportional to the rate of protein synthesis. Rates of protein synthesis are measured as a fractional rate, which is the percentage of the tissue protein pool renewed each day, i.e., k_s, %/d.[105–107]

In young rats (0.1 kg body weight), chronic feeding of alcohol for 2 weeks significantly reduces skeletal muscle protein synthesis[108] but less marked reductions that do not achieve significance occur after 6 weeks, which is suggestive of an adaptive response (Table 15.6).[98] Nevertheless, after 2 to 6 weeks of alcohol-feeding in young rats, reductions in muscle protein content occur, particularly in Type II fiber-rich muscle.[98]

In mature rats (0.3 kg body weight), in contrast, there are significant reductions in protein synthesis after 6 weeks of alcohol-feeding (Table 15.6). Although there is no overt loss in muscle protein content of mature rats at 6 weeks, there are measurable decreases at 12 weeks.[109] Reductions in muscle protein synthesis after 3 weeks' ethanol feeding of rats have also been reported by other groups, too.[110] As there is a marked loss in muscle protein and atrophy of Type II fibers in the young rat model of chronic ethanol feeding, we have routinely employed these immature animals in our studies, rather than mature rats.

In acute studies, ethanol dosage decreases k_s in the gastrocnemius muscle (Table 15.6).[111,112] The synthesis rate of the contractile proteins (i.e., myofibrillary fraction) containing the main force generating proteins is also reduced, but synthesis rates in all major fractions, i.e., the cytoplasmic, myofibrillar, and stromal fraction, are affected equally by acute ethanol dosage.[111] However, when the Type II fiber-predominant plantaris is compared with the Type I fiber-predominant soleus, it is apparent that the Type II fiber-predominant muscle shows the greatest change, i.e., decreases in k_s of 30 and 22%, respectively,[111] in Type II and I muscle.

15.8.3　THE FASTING–REFEEDING TRANSITION AND ALCOHOL TOXICITY IN THE RAT

It is possible that some of the effects of alcohol on whole-body protein or nitrogen economy could be due to defects in the fasting–feeding transition. In other words, a defect could lie in the anabolic phase following the ingestion of food. This has been determined in starved rats given food with or without alcohol. Refeeding

TABLE 15.6
Skeletal Muscle Protein Synthesis in Acute and Chronic Ethanol Toxicity Studies

	Acute Effects in Immature Rats (k_s, %/d)			
	Control	Ethanol	% Change	P
Gastrocnemius (fraction)				
sarcoplasmic	18.2 ± 0.6	13.4 ± 1.3	−26	<0.01
myofibrillar	13.8 ± 0.6	10.3 ± 1.0	−26	<0.01
stromal	14.6 ± 0.4	10.3 ± 1.1	−29	<0.01
Soleus	22.5 ± 0.7	17.6 ± 1.1	−22	<0.01
Plantaris	16.9 ± 0.5	11.9 ± 0.6	−30	<0.001
	Chronic Effects in Immature Rats (k_s, %/d)			
Gastrocnemius (fraction)				
sarcoplasmic	8.1 ± 0.2	7.2 ± 0.3	−12	NS
myofibrillar	5.7 ± 0.2	5.1 ± 0.3	−11	NS
stromal	7.2 ± 0.3	6.4 ± 0.3	−11	<0.05
Soleus	11.2 ± 0.5	9.9 ± 0.4	−12	NS
Plantaris	6.9 ± 0.2	6.6 ± 0.2	−6	NS
	Chronic Effects in Mature Rats (k_s,%/d)			
Gastrocnemius (fraction)				
sarcoplasmic	6.2 ± 0.2	5.2 ± 0.2	−16	<0.001
myofibrillar	4.1 ± 0.3	3.2 ± 0.1	−22	<0.05
stromal	5.4 ± 0.2	4.5 ± 0.3	−16	NS
Soleus	9.3 ± 0.8	7.5 ± 0.3	−19	NS
Plantaris	5.2 ± 0.2	4.1 ± 0.3	−21	<0.025

Note: Young (initial body weight 0.1 kg) or mature (initial body weight 0.3 kg) male rats were acutely treated with either saline (controls or ethanol (75 mmol/kg, i.p., 2.5 h) or chronically treated with nutritionally complete liquid diets containing 35% of total calories as glucose (controls) or ethanol. At the end of the studies fractional rates of protein synthesis (k_s) were measured with a large flooding dose of [^{3}H]phenylalanine. All data are mean ± SEM (n = 6 to 9). NS, $P > 0.05$, not significant.

Sources: Data from Preedy VR and Peters TJ (1989). The effect of chronic ethanol ingestion on synthesis and degradation of soluble, contractile and stromal protein fractions of skeletal muscles from immature and mature rats. *Biochem. J.* 259: 261–266; Preedy VR and Peters TJ (1988). The effect of chronic ethanol ingestion on protein metabolism in type-I- and type-II-fibre-rich skeletal muscles of the rat. *Biochem. J.* 254: 631–639; Preedy VR and Peters TJ (1988). Acute effects of ethanol on protein synthesis in different muscles and muscle protein fractions of the rat. *Clin. Sci.* (Colch.) 74: 461–466.

increased muscle k_s, but pretreatment with alcohol prevents this.[7] When the food was given intravenously (i.e., TPN route), there was no effect of alcohol on the increases in muscle k_s seen in the fasting–feeding transition.[7] These results are somewhat similar to those reported by others (see also References 2, 3, and 81) and suggest that impairment of amino acid absorption by alcohol may be significant in blunting the feeding effect.

15.8.4 ALCOHOLIC MUSCLE DISEASE AND CIRRHOSIS IN THE RAT

In our protein synthesis studies in humans and the rat, there is an agreement that alcohol reduces muscle protein synthesis. The notion then that there is an increase in muscle protein turnover in cirrhosis is thus somewhat difficult to explain.[113]

In the rat, we have examined experimental carbon tetrachloride and phenobarbitone-induced cirrhosis to ascertain if liver damage could account for the changes seen in muscle of alcohol-fed rats.[114] These studies showed that there was a confirmed micronodular cirrhosis (loss of normal hepatic architecture, fibrosis, necrosis, etc.) with reduced plasma albumin concentrations and increased alkaline phosphatase and aspartate aminotransferase activities in the cirrhotic group.[114] Despite the fact that cirrhotic rats had been treated for 18 to 20 weeks, there were no significant reductions in either Type I or Type II muscle weights compared to controls.[114] The contents of muscle contractile and noncontractile muscle protein fractions were similarly unaffected by such prolonged treatment.[114] Thus, in a well-characterized model of cirrhosis there were no effects on skeletal muscle, compared with reductions in muscle weight and protein contents after 2 to 12 weeks of chronic alcohol feeding.[114] This should not be interpreted as implying that cirrhosis has no effect on skeletal muscle whatsoever, but rather, consideration should be given to the possibility that longer periods are necessary to elicit muscle-wasting in this condition. Certainly, the data also imply that alcohol acts directly on skeletal muscle to induce wasting and atrophy.

15.8.5 THE ROLE OF APOPTOSIS IN ALCOHOL-EXPOSED SKELETAL MUSCLE IN THE RAT

Reduced muscle mass and decreases in protein turnover may arise as a result of apoptosis. Certainly, the evidence now supports the idea that programmed cell death events are important facets of alcoholic liver disease (for example, see References 115 to 120). However, when we examined apoptosis using DNA fragmentation or the TUNEL (terminal deoxynucleotidyl transferase mediated dUTP nick end labeling) assay, there was no evidence that this cellular process was overtly altered in the muscle of either acutely (2.5 and 6 h) or chronically (6 weeks) alcohol-dosed rats.[121]

15.8.6 EFFECTS OF ALCOHOL ON PROTEIN SYNTHESIS IN THE LIVER OF THE RAT

We have measured protein synthesis in rat muscle at 20-min, 1-, 2.5-, 6-, and 24-h time points after ethanol dosage.[122] In skeletal muscle, there is a progressive fall in k_s between 1 and 24 h (–25 to –69%). These changes can be contrasted with observations in liver where protein and RNA contents and k_s are significantly increased in ethanol-dosed rats relative to saline-injected pair-fed controls at 24 h.[122] Some of the hepatic effects of alcohol may be mediated through defective pathways of transcription (for example, growth factor dysfunction[8]) or translation (initiation or elongation factor dysfunction[4,123]).

The increases in liver protein synthesis *in vivo* in rats dosed with ethanol 24 h previously contrasts with *in vitro* studies showing that ethanol reduces protein synthesis.[124,125] However, there are studies reporting increases in *in vitro* collagen synthesis in response to acetaldehyde.[126–128] This emphasizes the need to employ, where possible, studies in intact animals using appropriate time-course studies.

15.8.7 Effects of Alpha-Tocopherol Supplementation in the Rat

Based on the observation that serum levels of alpha-tocopherol are decreased in alcoholic patients with myopathy, we investigated whether treatment with alpha-tocopherol could ameliorate the ethanol-induced changes in muscle protein synthesis.[129] Young male Wistar rats (90 g body weight) were treated daily with alpha-tocopherol (30 mg/kg body weight) for 5 d and controls were similarly injected with the vehicle alone. However, 5 d of alpha-tocopherol supplementation did not appear beneficial in ameliorating ethanol-induced reductions in protein synthesis.[129] These studies were also extended to 4 weeks of alpha-tocopherol supplementation and similar results were obtained, namely, that neither acute ethanol damage as defined by reductions in protein synthesis nor chronic ethanol-induced muscle damage as defined by decreases in muscle protein content were prevented by such therapeutic treatments.[130] Further, we also showed, in the aforementioned studies, alpha-tocopherol supplementation of control rats increased both protein synthesis and degradation in muscle, resulting in an overall decrease in muscle protein contents.[129,130] In other words, alpha-tocopherol supplementation acted as a prooxidant and induced a myopathy.

15.8.8 Effects of Enzyme Inhibitors with Alcohol Dosage Studies in the Rat

In acute alcohol dosing studies on muscle protein synthesis in the rat, inhibitors of alcohol dehydrogenase (4-methylpyrazole) or aldehyde dehydrogenase (cyanamide) have been employed. In these studies, ethanol by itself reduces muscle k_s by approximately 25%. However, pretreatment of ethanol-dosed rats with 4-methylpyrazole, which inhibits acetaldehyde formation, does not prevent the fall in protein synthesis.[131] More marked effects are observed with cyanamide pretreatment of ethanol-dosed rats, which increases acetaldehyde and also causes striking reductions in muscle k_s by approximately 65%.[131] This suggests that acetaldehyde is a potent protein synthetic perturbant, a supposition supported by the observation that even a small dose of acetaldehyde in the order of 3 mmol/kg body weight reduced k_s by approximately 15% at the end of 2.5 h.[131] These changes can be contrasted with the liver, where acetaldehyde stimulates collagen synthesis.[128] Nevertheless, the data thus suggest that the ethanol-induced inhibition of skeletal muscle protein synthesis may be independently mediated by both ethanol and acetaldehyde.[131]

15.8.9 Myosin Isoforms and Change in mRNA in the Rat

Studies have tested whether experimental alcoholic myopathy occurs as a consequence of changes in myosin heavy-chain mRNA expression. The importance of this relates to the fact that myosin is the principal force generating protein in skeletal muscle, and different muscle types have a characteristic abundance of the specific myosin protein and mRNA isoforms. Myosin consists of two heavy and two light chains, complexed with other myofibrillary proteins such as actin, troponin, and tropomyosin in the muscle sarcomere.[102] Thus, red type aerobic muscles have an abundance of Type I-beta isoform whereas the anaerobic white muscle has an abundance of Type II-a, II-b, II-x informs.[102] In rats fed alcohol for 6 weeks with the Lieber–DeCarli protocol, the contents of total myofibrillary proteins and myosin heavy-chain fraction are reduced in the Type II plantaris.[102] Electrophoretic analysis shows that there are significant reductions in the I-beta, ($P < 0.01$), II-x ($P < 0.05$), and II-b ($P < 0.05$) protein isoforms. Alcohol feeding does not significantly alter the abundance of the myosin heavy-chain II-a protein isoform. However, contrary to expectations, only the mRNA levels of I-beta are reduced in the plantaris ($P < 0.05$) and there are no significant changes in the levels of mRNA encoding the other three fast isoforms of myosin heavy chain.[102] This can be explained by the possibility that there may be either altered proteolysis of myosin heavy chain, perturbations in posttranslational packaging and modifications, or more likely decreases in the translational efficiencies of the fast myosin heavy-chain mRNA in alcoholism.[102]

15.8.10 Other Molecular Events: Translation and Loss of Ribosomal RNA in Muscle in the Rat

Defects in translation may be ascribed to alterations (changes in amount or state of phosphorylation) in one of the many biochemical factors necessary for successful polypeptide formation such as eukaryotic elongation factors (eEF) eEF1A, eEF2, or their binding proteins such as 4E-binding protein −1 (4E-BP1).[7,123,132,133] There are different responses in muscle and liver, as well as differential effects when rats are dosed either acutely or subjected to chronic alcohol feeding.[123,132,133] For example, eEF1A protein decreases after 16 weeks of alcohol feeding, but not at 8 to 12 weeks.[123] More oxidative skeletal muscle, such as the soleus and heart, is particularly resilient to these changes, compared to the anaerobic muscle.[123] In these studies, there were no ethanol-induced reductions in the phosphorylation of eEF2 in skeletal and cardiac muscle, but there were reductions in liver.[123] In acute dosing studies, neither eEF1A nor eEF2 is altered in liver and muscle, yet the phosphorylation states of eEF2 are impaired.[123]

Alcohol feeding also markedly reduces the amount of ribosomal RNA in skeletal muscle[101,134,135] similar to the situation in humans.[59] Most RNA in tissue is ribosomal and effectively corresponds to the amount of protein synthetic machinery. Thus, deficiencies in total and/or ribosomal RNA reduce the potential for protein synthesis.[105] Rat studies have shown that in response to alcohol feeding, total muscle RNA is rapidly decreased compared to pair-fed controls. Using polyclonal antibodies, it has also been shown that losses of ribosomal RNA occur predominantly in the subsarcolemmal region compared to the myofibrillary ribosomes.[135] However, Northern blotting for proteins in the small and large ribosomal subunits shows no change in their mRNA, suggestive of a posttranscriptional regulation. Support for this has been obtained from assays of RNAases in skeletal muscle.[136] In the aforementioned studies, total RNAase, RNAase A, and the specific or "restriction" RNAase T1L were increased in skeletal muscle of ethanol-treated rats.[59,136]

15.8.11 Proteolysis in Rat Muscle and Alcohol Toxicity

We have measured the contribution of proteolysis to the genesis of alcoholic myopathy in a number of ways. When protein breakdown has been measured from the difference between growth and synthesis, the fractional rate of cytoplasmic, myofibrillar, and stromal protein degradation is shown to decrease by approximately 10 to 20%.[96]

An extensive range of proteases, similar to those examined in human muscle, have been investigated in gastrocnemius muscle in response to acute and chronic ethanol dosage but also included proteasomal (chymotrypsin-, trypsin-like, and peptidylglutamyl peptide hydrolase activities) and Ca (2+)-activated (micro- and milli-calpain and calpastatin) activities.[67] Alcohol dosing of young rats for 2.5 h or 4 to 6 weeks has no effect on the activities of any of the muscle enzymes assayed.[67] This lack of effect is not due to the development of tolerance, as the activities of selective enzymes (i.e., cathepsins B and D) are not overtly affected at earlier time points, i.e., 3, 7, 14, 28 d.[67] In contrast to the failure to see changes in the muscle of young immature rats, acute alcohol dosage studies using mature rats show significant reductions in the activities of a number of proteases including the alanyl-, arginyl-, and leucyl-aminopeptidase (cytoplasmic), dipeptidyl aminopeptidase II (lysosomal), and the chymotrypsin- and trypsin-like activities (proteosomal).[67] Overall, this supposes that in mature rats, muscle proteases are more sensitive to acute alcohol dosage.[67]

The measurement of protease activities in muscle homogenates *in vitro* only provides information on the capacity for the tissue to degrade proteins as the aforementioned are measured under artificial conditions. Nevertheless, the above data are contrary to the increased urinary excretion of 3-methylhistidine which is observed in *in vivo* rat models of alcoholism.[137,138] However, the analysis of urinary 3-methylhistidine excretion is subject to some uncertainty as it also can be derived from skin and gastrointestinal tissues, as well as skeletal muscle, and currently there is no corresponding Afting correction factor in rat models. It is also possible that in very severe conditions of experimental alcoholism or when there is a coexisting pathology such as liver disease or infection, increases in muscle proteolysis will occur. Nevertheless, these results overall do not support the contention that alcohol increases muscle proteolysis, which has been confirmed by another group examining radiolabeled amino acid release from muscle *in vitro*.[45]

15.8.12 Proteases in the Liver of Alcohol-Dosed Rats

We have compared the contrasting responses of muscle and liver protease activities 24 h after an acute ethanol bolus.[122] In the liver, there are significant increases in the cytoplasmic proteases (alanyl-, arginyl-, and pyroglutamyl-aminopeptidases and proline-endopeptidase) whereas the activities of the hepatic lysosomal proteases dipeptidyl-aminopeptidase II and cathepsins B, L, and H decrease.[122] The ubiquitin-proteasome pathway of proteolysis is also perturbed in liver of alcohol-fed rats and may play a key role in the pathogenesis of alcoholic liver disease.[139,140]

15.8.13 Changes in Cardiac Protein Synthesis in the Rat

Although moderate alcohol consumption is cardioprotective,[141–144] excessive and prolonged alcohol intake is clearly very damaging.[145–150] There are no studies on the effects of alcohol on human cardiac protein synthesis in response to ethanol so instead, as with skeletal muscle, attention has focused on animals both *in vitro* and *in vivo*. In general, the protein synthesis data on heart are similar to studies on skeletal muscle, though in the former they are less marked (Table 15.7). Thus, acutely, ethanol impairs cardiac protein synthesis *in vivo*[151,152] and time course studies over a day show that the effect is observable at 1 h but not after 20 min. The greatest fall in cardiac protein synthesis occurs 24 h after ethanol dosage and at this point, there is no measurable ethanol in the circulation.[151,152]

TABLE 15.7
Acute Effects of Ethanol with and without ADH and ALDH Inhibitors on Fractional Rates of Ventricular Protein Synthesis in the Rat Heart

Pretreatment (30 min)	Treatment (150 min)	k_s (%/d)	% Change (from saline + saline)	P (vs. saline + saline)
Saline	Saline	24.0 + 0.9		
Saline	Ethanol	18.8 ± 1.2	−22	<0.01
CYN	Saline	24.6 ± 1.5	+3	NS
CYN	Ethanol	4.8 ± 0.8	−80	<0.001
4MP	Saline	23.8 ± 1.7	−1	NS
4MP	Ethanol	18.9 ± 1.5	−21	<0.01

Note: Male Wistar rats were given i.p. injections of either saline, cyanamide (CYN) or 4-methylpyra-zole (4MP) 30 min before i.p. injections of either saline or ethanol. At 150 min after the latter treatments, rates of protein synthesis (k_s) were measured in mixed ventricular homogenates. All data are mean = SEM (n = 4 to 9). NS, $P > 0.05$ not significant.

Source: Adapted from Siddiq T, Richardson PJ, Mitchell WD, Teare J, and Preedy VR (1993). Ethanol-induced inhibition of ventricular protein synthesis *in vivo* and the possible role of acetaldehyde. *Cell Biochem. Funct.* 11: 45–54.

15.9 ALCOHOL AND THE SYNTHESIS OF DIFFERENT CARDIAC REGIONS AND PROTEIN FRACTIONS

As with skeletal muscle, there are different cell types within the heart muscle, and these seem to respond differently to alcohol. The atrial tissue shows a slightly greater decrease in k_s (approximately –30%) when compared to the ventricular regions (approximately –20%) in response to acute ethanol.[153] The imposition of additional metabolic or structural–mechanical stress seems to exacerbate these reductions in protein synthesis.[153,154] Thus the decline in mixed and myofibrillary protein synthesis in heart in response to ethanol is greater in stressed hypertensive animals compared to unstressed normotensive rats.[153,154] This observation has important clinical implications as alcohol misuse is a risk factor of hypertension, and also the reduction in protein synthesis potentially compromises the formation of new myofibrils and contractile elements which are needed for efficient mechanical function.[153,154]

The effects of ethanol on the synthesis rate of ventricular proteins *in vivo* have also been examined using a combination of subcellular fractionation techniques and proteolytic enzyme digestion to release subsarcolemmal and intermyofibrillary mitochondria.[155] In acutely dosed rats, ethanol decreased k_s by –20% ($p < 0.01$) in the mixed fraction and by –25% ($p < 0.05$) in both the subsarcolemmal and intermyofibrillary mitochondrial fractions.[155] The synthesis rates of the nuclear fraction are similarly decreased by acute ethanol dosage (–20%; $p < 0.05$).[155]

15.9.1 USE OF ENZYME INHIBITORS IN ALCOHOL DOSING STUDIES AND EFFECTS ON HEART PROTEIN SYNTHESIS

When ethanol-dosed rats are pretreated with an inhibitor of acetaldehyde dehydrogenase (cyanamide), the fall in protein synthesis is approximately 80% compared to the approximately 15 to 20% depression in k_s seen with alcohol alone (Table 15.7).[156] In these conditions, cardiac ATP content remains unaltered compared to saline or ethanol-injected rats even when ethanol-dosed rats are pretreated with cyanamide.[157] Circulating cardiac troponin-T, a marker of cardiac damage, increases at 2.5 h after an acute dose of alcohol, and this effect is exacerbated with cyanamide pretreatment[158] suggesting that defects in membrane integrity occur in the absence of disturbances in energy-associated nucleotides.

15.9.2 PROPRANOLOL AND ALCOHOLIC HEART MUSCLE DAMAGE

It seems that the mechanism of alcohol-induced heart damage, as reflected by reductions in protein synthesis, is complex. As mentioned above, plasma cardiac troponin-T increases as a consequence of acute alcohol dosage in rats *in vivo*, and pretreatment with propranolol reduces this effect.[158] Propranolol is both a beta-blocker and a xanthine oxidase inhibitor.[158] However, the beta-blockers atenolol and metoprolol are not able to ameliorate the ethanol-induced increases in plasma cardiac troponin-T.[158] In contrast, pretreatment with timolol, another beta-blocker, can ameliorate this effect.[158] This is because propranolol and timolol have similar pharmacological actions compared with atenolol and metoprolol. Moreover, neither allopurinol nor oxypurinol (xanthine oxidase inhibitors) prevent the rise in serum troponin T in these conditions of acute ethanol dosage.[158]

These studies suggest that the increased circulating troponin T is probably due to beta-1 and/or beta-2 adrenergic activation.[158] This would imply that propranolol would also prevent the ethanol-induced decrease in protein synthesis. However, pretreatment of ethanol-dosed rats with propranolol is unable to prevent the decrease in protein synthesis.[159] Indeed, propranolol by itself reduces cardiac protein synthesis, suggesting that the effects of ethanol on cardiac protein synthesis occur independently of beta-receptor activation.[159]

The detailed molecular mechanisms responsible for some of these changes in cardiac protein synthesis due to alcohol have been reported by other groups (see References 123 and 160). These changes include, for example, impairment of 4E-BP1 and p70(S6K) phosphorylation but the reader should refer to these original articles[123,160] and an important review in this area for more details.[5]

15.10 NITROGEN EXCRETION AND WEIGHT LOSS IN HUMANS

Effects of alcohol on the whole body can be assessed in a number of ways, including excretion of urinary compounds, changes in whole-body metabolic dynamics and body composition.[161–163] Subjects on alcohol-feeding regimes for 18 d lose weight when compared to those on iso-caloric control regimes with concomitant increases in urinary excretion of total nitrogen, uric acid, and urea.[163] Other studies have also shown that ethanol enhances urinary nitrogen losses[161,162] although fecal nitrogen is not affected. However, the use of nitrogen balance studies to assess the effects of nutritional interventions has been questioned.[35]

In the 18-d dosing study, urinary creatinine levels did not alter in response to alcohol-feeding, but one patient exhibited a fall in this variable, which is ascribed to reductions in muscle.[163] This subject also displayed the greatest weight loss.[163] However, it is important to mention that ethanol misuse for chronic periods (>100 g/d; >10 years) reduces urinary creatinine excretion by virtue of the fact that muscle mass is lost.[57]

Weight loss because of alcohol ingestion indicates that, at the very least, there is inadequate employment of ethanol-calories or, at the worst, a catabolic effect on one or more organ systems. Naturally, due to the contribution of skeletal muscle to the whole body (40%), suspicion falls on this tissue as being the main target organ of alcohol. It is also important to remember that other tissues such as the gastrointestinal tract,[73,164–171] skin[172–176] and bone[177–179] are also targeted by ethanol, both clinically and experimentally.

An analysis of data from first National Health and Nutrition Examination Survey (HANES I) shows that within the general population, male drinkers (i.e., consuming 56 g of ethanol per day) consume on average 16% more calories than nondrinkers, largely due to the intake of alcoholic calories.[180] In contrast, abstainers have virtually identical body mass (kg/m² or Quetelet's indices), i.e., 26.0 and physical activity levels, i.e., mean 3.2 (arbitrary units), compared to those consuming ethanol

(Quetelet's index of 26.2 and activity scores of 3.2). Female subjects consuming 40 g of ethanol per day have a reduced Quetelet's index.[180,181] These data imply that ethanol ingestion is energetically inefficient. This is consistent with other studies showing either a reduction in body weight with alcohol consumption and/or lack of an increase in body weight when extra calories are consumed as ethanol.[182–184]

It seems that despite the increased calorific intake in the form of ethanol, alcohol drinkers are no more obese than abstainers. Although relatively moderate amounts of alcohol were consumed in the aforementioned studies (for example, see Reference 180), other published material investigating the effects of consuming much higher levels of ethanol (for example, 100 g/d for 10 years or more) have also shown deficits in body weight.[57]

Catabolic effects of alcohol may be due to either (1) the induction of the microsomal ethanol oxidizing system (MEOS) system[185]; (2) inadequate coupling of ATP production,[186,187] or (3) impairment of tissue protein deposition.[1] We believe that the latter is important in the genesis of alcohol-induced weight loss. This is because, in many pathological conditions, the amount of tissue protein in relation to tissue water remains constant. In simple terms the amount of protein per unit wet weight remains constant, i.e., maintaining the relative proportions of the protein-cytoplasmic milieu. A compounded decrease in 1 kg of muscle protein will be associated with an additional loss of 3.75 kg of water. Thus, decrements in tissue protein will hasten disproportionate decreases in tissue weight.[1]

The mechanisms of the alcohol-induced weight losses have been investigated using indirect and direct calorimetric techniques and nasogastric infusions of either control (glucose) or ethanol-containing enteral diets containing various amounts of ethanol (as 30, 40, or 60% of total calories).[188] With such regimens, there were weight losses and elevations in urinary urea nitrogen excretion without thermal energy losses, as determined by both indirect and direct calorimetry. One can conclude that the weight loss seen during ethanol exposure is not related to negative energy balance but may in fact be due to protein, mineral, and fluid loss.[188] Protein loss may be due to increased degradation of muscle proteins, as urinary 3-methyl-histidine excretion is increased.[188] However, as described in the aforementioned sections, such measurements may not be reliable especially without the Afting correction; the apparent contradiction between the aforementioned studies[188] and those of Peters' group[61] may be due to the differences in the period that subjects were exposed to high levels of alcohol. Nevertheless, the authors showed that when they accounted for the energy loses ascribed to urine and breath as well as thermal losses, the fuel value of the diets containing alcohol was 0.95 to 0.99 compared to glucose-containing diets.[188]

15.11 ETHANOL EXCRETION IN HUMAN URINE

It is important to address whether some of the studies in humans are flawed experimentally due to excessive excretion of ethanol in the urine. However, in a well-controlled study where subjects were given 44 g (about 5 to 6 units) ethanol only 0.68 g was recovered in urine which was 1.5% of the administered dose.[189] There are also small losses in breathing, but these concentrations are not thought to contribute significantly to overlay ethanol losses.[190–192]

15.12 WHOLE-BODY PROTEIN TURNOVER IN HUMANS

Whole-body rates of protein turnover have been measured in chronic alcoholic use with primed constant infusion of L[1-13C]-leucine (Table 15.2).[60] Whole-body protein synthesis and breakdown rates also decreased but did not achieve significance: certainly there was no evidence that whole body protein degradation increased in line with traditional thinking (Table 15.2).[60] Whole-body amino acid (leucine) oxidation rates were also significantly reduced in alcoholism (Table 15.2). The significance of these findings relates to the known pathways of leucine catabolism, which is predominantly oxidized in skeletal muscle. However, the alcoholics were not intoxicated with ethanol during the isotopic infusions.

Whole-body protein turnover in abstinent and nonabstinent alcoholic patients with cirrhosis have also been measured using a primed-constant infusion of L-[1-14C] leucine.[193] These studies showed that the flux, oxidation, and nonoxidative disposal of leucine in normal control subjects without metabolic disease and cirrhotic subjects who refrained from continued ethanol consumption were not significantly different, but there was an increase in nonoxidative disposal indicative of whole-body protein synthesis and elevated flux in cirrhotic patients who were drinking, compared to abstinent cirrhotic patients.[193] These results are different from those obtained by our group (Table 15.2),[60] suggesting the need for additional studies in alcoholic myopathy with high prevailing levels of blood ethanol and with varying degrees of liver and muscle disease.[194]

15.13 WHOLE BODY NITROGEN EXCRETION AND PROTEIN TURNOVER IN EXPERIMENTAL ALCOHOLISM

Rat models of alcoholism show similar changes in whole-body protein metabolism.[195–197] These include reduced rates of growth or protein accretion, increases in urinary nitrogen, urea (which is the largest pool of urinary nitrogen), and uric acid excretion (Table 15.8).[195] However, increased urea generation may arise as a consequence of a number of pathways being unregulated, such as flux of ammonia to hepatocytes, carbomyl-phosphate synthetase or ornithine transcarbamoylase activities, and amino acid (i.e., aspartate) availability, as well as liver blood flow. Disturbances in blood flow as a mediating factor in the presentation of ureagenic substrates to the liver can be excluded as this variable appears to be unaltered by chronic alcohol feeding.[198,199]

The urinary excretion of another nitrogenous compound, namely, alanine, is also increased because of alcohol feeding (Table 15.8).[195] This may be due to elevated alanine release by skeletal muscles, a supposition supported by *in vitro* studies. Thus, following 6 weeks of alcohol feeding, mean rate of alanine release from Type II fiber-predominant muscles of rats fed ethanol is 5.8 μmol/g/h, compared to 3.6

TABLE 15.8
Urinary Excretion in the Chronically Treated Alcohol-Fed Rat

	Control	Ethanol	% Change	P
Excretion				
Total nitrogen (mg/d)	137 ± 11	169 ± 12	+23	<0.05
Uric acid (μmol/d)	5.3 ± 0.9	12.1 ± 1.4	+128	<0.01
Urea (mmol/d)	2.1 ± 0.2	3.4 ± 0.2	+62	<0.005
Creatinine (μmol/d)	50 ± 3	46 ± 4	−8	NS
Ethanol (μmol/d)	106 ± 23	1320 ± 100	+92	<0.001
Alanine (μmol/d)	9 ± 1	13 ± 3	+44	<0.025

Note: Data are from chronic ethanol-feeding studies in which young rats were fed a nutritionally complete liquid diet containing either glucose (controls) or ethanol as 35% of total calories. Urine is collected after 6 weeks' treatment.

Source: Data from Preedy VR, Hammond B, Iles RA, Davies SE, Gandy JD, Chalmers RA, and Peters, TJ. (1991). Urinary excretion of nitrogenous and non-nitrogenous compounds in the chronic ethanol-fed rat. *Clin. Sci.* (Colch.) 80: 393–400.

μmol/g/h for corresponding muscles from control animals; $P<0.01$.[200] The mechanism does not appear to be fiber-type specific as similar effects occur in Type I fiber-predominant muscles.[200] This increased alanine production may be due to enhanced synthesis via pyruvate as protein degradation decreases.[200]

Leucine oxidation in response to ethanol has been measured in the laboratory rat *in vivo* and *in vitro* in response to ethanol.[201–203] After 3 weeks' alcohol feeding there is an elevation in whole-body leucine turnover and oxidation.[203] Concomitant changes included a decrease in both muscle and liver protein synthesis.[203] In contrast, it has also been reported that leucine oxidation was unaltered after 4 weeks' treatment with ethanol.[204] These differences may be methodological, such as inclusion of ethanol in drinking water[204] or in nutritional complete liquids diets.[203] It should be emphasized that the changes in protein metabolism are not only related to muscle and liver but also to other tissues such as the intestinal tract[205,206] and skin and bone[173,207–209] (Table 15.9). With reference to the bone, the loss of collagen from this tissue arises as a consequence of reduced rate of protein degradation as the urinary excretion of the specific bone markers pyridinoline and deoxy-pyridinoline actually decrease (Table 15.10).[208,209] This is similar to the directional changes in the degradative pathway of protein in alcohol-exposed skeletal muscle. Urinary hydroxyproline on the other hand increases in alcoholism and may reflect liver collagen metabolism rather than bone (Table 15.10).[208,209]

TABLE 15.9
Acute Effects of Ethanol: A Comparative Study of Liver, Small Intestine, Skin, Bone, and Skeletal Muscle

		Contribution to Whole Body (ks, %/d)			
	Synthesis (%)	Control	Ethanol	% Change	P
Tissue					
Skeletal muscle	20 ± 25	15 ± 1	10 ± 1	−29	<0.001
Small intestine	15 ± 20	119 ± 3	101 ± 8	−18	<0.001
Liver	20 ± 25	86 ± 2	78 ± 4	−10	NS
Skin	15 ± 20	62 ± 2	47 ± 4	−24	<0.001
Bone	5 ± 10	63 ± 2	45 ± 4	−29	<0.001

Note: The effect of an acute dose of ethanol (75 mmol/kg body weight) is examined in 100-g rats.

Sources: Adapted from Preedy VR, Duane P, and Peters TJ (1988). Comparison of the acute effects of ethanol on liver and skeletal muscle protein synthesis in the rat. *Alcohol Alcohol.* 23: 155–162; Preedy VR, Marway JS, Salisbury JR, and Peters TJ (1990). Protein synthesis in bone and skin of the rat are inhibited by ethanol: implications for whole body metabolism. *Alcohol Clin. Exp. Res.* 14: 165–168; McNurlan MA, and Garlick PJ (1980). Contribution of rat liver and gastrointestinal tract to whole-body protein synthesis in the rat. *Biochem. J.* 186: 381–383; Preedy VR and Garlick PJ (1981). Rates of protein synthesis in skin and bone, and their importance in the assessment of protein degradation in the perfused rat hemicorpus. *Biochem. J.* 194: 373–376; Preedy VR, Duane P, and Peters TJ (1988). Acute ethanol dosage reduces the synthesis of smooth muscle contractile proteins in the small intestine of the rat. *Gut* 29: 1244–1248.

15.14 EXCRETION OF ETHANOL IN THE RAT

It is important to address the issue of whether the inefficient utilization of ethanol-derived energy in the rat is due to excretion of ethanol (i.e., unmetabolized component). However, the urinary excretion of ethanol in the rat is 2% of total administered ethanol and thus less than 1% of total energy intake.[195] Alternatively, inefficient peripheral utilization of acetate, perhaps compounded by muscle damage, may account for inefficient utilization of ethanol-derived calories.[210–212] However, we have shown that the initial steps in the conversion of acetate to CO_2 and H_2O via the citric acid cycle is probably unimpaired as 24-h urinary acetate concentrations in glucose-fed controls and ethanol-fed rats are identical and comprise only 0.3% of dietary ethanol.[195]

15.15 CONCLUSIONS

Perturbations in protein metabolism at the whole-body, tissue, and cellular levels occur as a consequence of both acute and chronic alcohol exposures. The etiological

TABLE 15.10
Collagen Degradation in Chronic Alcoholic Rats as Determined by Hydroxyproline, Pyridinoline, and Deoxypyridinoline

	Control	Ethanol	% Change	P
Urinary Excretion (nmol/d/rat)				
Hydroxyproline	4370 ± 460	6130 ± 690	+40	<0.01
Pyridinoline	7.03 ± 0.33	6.06 ± 0.48	−14	<0.05
Deoxy-pyridinoline	7.88 ± 0.45	4.21 ± 0.26	−47	<0.001
Tibia Composition (mg/bone)				
Hydroxyproline	3.27 ± 0.16	2.73 ± 0.10	−17	<0.05
Calcium	43.1 ± 0.9	38.5 ± 1.0	−11	<0.05
Magnesium	0.84 ± 0.04	0.73 ± 0.03	−13	$P = 0.06$*
Phosphate	14.58 ± 1.96	9.57 ± 3.20	−34	$P = 0.06$*

Note: Data are from chronic ethanol-feeding study in which young rats were fed a nutritionally complete liquid diet containing either glucose (controls) or ethanol as 35% of total calories. * indicates that although all pairs demonstrated unidirectional changes, $P = 0.06$.

Sources: Data from Preedy VR, Sherwood RA, Akpoguma CI, and Black D (1991). The urinary excretion of the collagen degradation markers pyridinoline and deoxypyridinoline in an experimental rat model of alcoholic bone disease. *Alcohol Alcohol.* 26: 191–198; Preedy VR, Baldwin DR, Keating JW, and Salisbury JR (1991). Bone collagen, mineral and trace element composition, histomorphometry and urinary hydroxyproline excretion in chronically-treated alcohol-fed rats. *Alcohol Alcohol.* 26: 39–46.

mechanisms involve changes in protein synthesis, perhaps precipitated by acetaldehyde. However, the intervening steps between ethanol and acetaldehyde exposure and changes in protein synthesis are poorly understood, although a number of processes have been proposed.

References

1. Preedy VR, Peters TJ (1992). Protein metabolism in alcoholism. In: Watson RR, Watzl B (Eds.), *Nutrition and Alcohol.* CRC Press, Boca Raton, FL, pp. 143–189.
2. De Feo P, Volpi E, Lucidi P, Cruciani G, Monacchia F, Reboldi G, Santeusanio F, Bolli GB, Brunetti P (1995). Ethanol impairs post-prandial hepatic protein metabolism. *J. Clin. Invest.* 95: 1472–1479.
3. Volpi E, Lucidi P, Cruciani G, Monacchia F, Reboldi G, Brunetti P, Bolli GB, De Feo P (1997). Nicotinamide counteracts alcohol-induced impairment of hepatic protein metabolism in humans. *J. Nutr.* 127: 2199–2204.
4. Lang CH, Frost RA, Kumar V, Wu D, Vary TC (2000). Impaired protein synthesis induced by acute alcohol intoxication is associated with changes in eIF4E in muscle and eIF2B in liver. *Alcohol. Clin. Exp. Res.* 24: 322–331.

5. Lang CH, Kimball SR, Frost RA, Vary TC (2001). Alcohol myopathy: impairment of protein synthesis and translation initiation. *Int. J. Biochem. Cell Biol.* 33: 457–473.

6. Molina PE, McClain C, Valla D, Guidot D, Diehl AM, Lang CH, Neuman M (2002). Molecular pathology and clinical aspects of alcohol-induced tissue injury. *Alcohol. Clin. Exp. Res.* 26: 120–128.

7. Sneddon AA, Koll M, Wallace MC, Jones J, Miell JP, Garlick PJ, Preedy VR (2003). Acute alcohol administration inhibits the refeeding response after starvation in rat skeletal muscle. *Am. J. Physiol. Endocrinol. Metab.* 284: E874–E882.

8. Tahara M, Matsumoto K, Nukiwa T, Nakamura T (1999). Hepatocyte growth factor leads to recovery from alcohol-induced fatty liver in rats. *J. Clin. Invest.* 103: 313–320.

9. Li W, Liu W, Altura BT, Altura BM (2003). Catalase prevents elevation of [Ca^{2+}] induced by alcohol in cultured canine cerebral vascular smooth muscle cells: possible relationship to alcohol-induced stroke and brain pathology. *Brain Res. Bull.* 59: 315–318.

10. Bilici D, Banoglu ZN, Avci B, Ciftcioglu, Bilici S (2002). Melatonin prevents ethanol-induced gastric mucosal damage possibly due to its antioxidant effect. *Dig. Dis. Sci.* 47: 856–861.

11. Iimuro Y, Bradford BU, Forman DT, Thurman RG (1996). Glycine prevents alcohol-induced liver injury by decreasing alcohol in the rat stomach. *Gastroenterology* 110: 1536–1542.

12. Zheng T, Li W, Zhang A, Altura BT, Altura BM (1998). Alpha-tocopherol prevents ethanol-induced elevation of [Ca^{2+}]i in cultured canine cerebral vascular smooth muscle cells. *Neurosci. Lett.* 245: 17–20.

13. Harada H, Kitazaki K, Tsujino T, Watari Y, Iwata S, Nonaka H, Hayashi T, Takeshita T, Morimoto K, Yokoyama M (2000). Oral taurine supplementation prevents the development of ethanol-induced hypertension in rats. *Hypertens. Res.* 23: 277–284.

14. Fernandez-Checa JC, Colell A, Garcia-Ruiz C (2002). S-Adenosyl-L-methionine and mitochondrial reduced glutathione depletion in alcoholic liver disease. *Alcohol* 27: 179–183.

15. Estruch R, Nicolas JM, Villegas E, Junque A, Urbano-Marquez A (1993). Relationship between ethanol-related diseases and nutritional status in chronically alcoholic men. *Alcohol Alcohol.* 28: 543–550.

16. Nicolas JM, Estruch R, Antunez E, Sacanella E, Urbano Marquez A (1993). Nutritional status in chronically alcoholic men from the middle socioeconomic class and its relation to ethanol intake. *Alcohol Alcohol.* 28: 551–558.

17. Brind AM (2001). Genetic predisposition to alcoholic liver disease. *CME J. Gastroenterol. Hepatol. Nutr.* 4: 3–6.

18. Casey CA, Nanji A, Cederbaum AI, Adachi M, Takahashi T (2001). Alcoholic liver disease and apoptosis. *Alcohol. Clin. Exp. Res.* 25: 49S–53S.

19. Albano E (2002). Free radical mechanisms in immune reactions associated with alcoholic liver disease. *Free Radic. Biol. Med.* 32: 110–114.

20. Bailey SM, Cunningham CC (2002). Contribution of mitochondria to oxidative stress associated with alcoholic liver disease. *Free Radic. Biol. Med.* 32: 11–16.

21. Halsted CH, Villanueva JA, Devlin AM (2002). Folate deficiency, methionine metabolism, and alcoholic liver disease. *Alcohol* 27: 169–172.

22. Kwo PY, Crabb DW (2002). Genetics of ethanol metabolism and alcoholic liver disease. In: Sherman DIN, Preedy VR, Watson RR (Eds.), *Ethanol and the Liver: Mechanisms and Management*. Taylor and Francis, London, pp. 95–129.

23. McClain CJ, Hill DB, Song Z, Chawla R, Watson WH, Chen T, Barve S (2002). S-Adenosylmethionine, cytokines, and alcoholic liver disease. *Alcohol* 27: 185–192.

24. McClain CJ, Hill DB, Song Z, Deaciuc I, Barve S (2002). Monocyte activation in alcoholic liver disease. Alcohol 27: 53–61.

25. Wake N (2002). Alcoholic liver disease. *Pharm. Pract.* 12: 62–68.

26. Waterlow JC, Garlick PJ, Millward DJ (1978). *Protein Turnover in Mammalian Tissues and the Whole Body.* North-Holland, Amsterdam.

27. Garlick PJ, Clugston GA, Swick RW, Waterlow JC (1980). Diurnal pattern of protein and energy metabolism in man. *Am. J. Clin. Nutr.* 33: 1983–1986.

28. Waterlow JC (1984). Protein turnover with special reference to man. *Q. J. Exp. Physiol.* 69: 409–438.

29. Jeejeebhoy KN (1985). Energy metabolism in the critically ill. In: Garrow JS, Halliday D (Eds.), *Substrate and Energy Metabolism.* John Libbey, London, pp. 93–101.

30. Ryazanov AG, Nefsky BS (2002). Protein turnover plays a key role in aging. *Mech. Ageing Dev.* 123: 207–213.

31. Morrison WL, Gibson JN, Rennie MJ (1988). Skeletal muscle and whole body protein turnover in cardiac cachexia: influence of branched-chain amino acid administration. *Eur. J. Clin. Invest.* 18: 648–654.

32. Preedy VR, Peters TJ (1990). Alcohol and skeletal muscle disease. *Alcohol Alcohol.* 25: 177–187.

33. Hodges DL, Kumar VN, Redford JB (1986). Effects of alcohol on bone, muscle and nerve. *Am. Fam. Physician* 34: 149–156.

34. Preedy VR, Marway JS, Siddiq T, Ansari FA, Hashim IA, Peters TJ (1993). Gastrointestinal protein turnover and alcohol misuse. *Drug Alcohol Depend.* 34: 1–10.

35. Volpi E (2002). Ethanol and protein turnover. In: Sherman DIN, Preedy VR, Watson RR (Eds.), *Ethanol and the Liver: Mechanisms and Management.* Taylor and Francis, London, pp. 265–296.

36. McNurlan MA, Garlick PJ, Steigbigel RT, Decristofaro KA, Frost RA, Lang CH, Johnson RW, Santasier AM, Cabahug CJ, Fuhrer J, Gelato MC (1997). Responsiveness of muscle protein synthesis to growth hormone administration in HIV-infected individuals declines with severity of disease. *J. Clin. Invest.* 100: 2125–2132.

37. Gamrin L, Berg HE, Essen P, Tesch PA, Hultman E, Garlick PJ, McNurlan, MA, Wernerman J (1998). The effect of unloading on protein synthesis in human skeletal muscle. *Acta Physiol. Scand.* 163: 369–377.

38. Vosswinkel JA, Brathwaite CE, Smith TR, Ferber JM, Casella G, Garlick, PJ (2000). Hyperventilation increases muscle protein synthesis in critically ill trauma patients. *J. Surg. Res.* 91: 61–64.

39. Kleger G-R, Turgay M, Imoberdorf R, McNurlan MA, Garlick PJ, Ballmer PE (2001). Acute metabolic acidosis decreases muscle protein synthesis but not albumin synthesis in humans. *Am. J. Kidney Dis.* 38: 1199–1207.

40. Mantle D, Preedy VR (2002). Adverse and beneficial functions of proteolytic enzymes in skeletal muscle: an overview. *Adverse Drug React. Toxicol. Rev.* 21: 31–49.

41. Schreiber SS, Evans CD, Reff F, Oratz M, Rothschild MA (1984). Prolonged feeding of ethanol to the young growing guinea pig. II. A model to study the effects of severe ischemia on cardiac protein synthesis. *Alcohol. Clin. Exp. Res.* 8: 54–61.

42. Kato S, Murawaki Y, Hirayama C (1985). Effects of ethanol feeding on hepatic collagen synthesis and degradation in rats. *Res. Commun. Chem. Pathol. Pharmacol.* 47: 163–180.

43. Koch F, Koch G (1974). Reversible inhibition of macromolecular synthesis in HeLa cells by ethanol. *Res. Commun. Chem. Pathol. Pharmacol.* 9: 291–298.

44. Harbitz I, Wallin B, Hauge JG, Morland J (1984). Effect of ethanol metabolism on initiation of protein synthesis in rat hepatocytes. *Biochem. Pharmacol.* 33: 3465–3470.

45. Hong-Brown LQ, Frost RA, Lang CH (2001). Alcohol impairs protein synthesis and degradation in cultured skeletal muscle cells. *Alcohol. Clin. Exp. Res.* 25: 1373–1382.

46. Fontana L, Jerez D, Rojas-Valencia L, Solis-Herruzo JA, Greenwel P, Rojkind M (1997). Ethanol induces the expression of alpha 1(I) procollagen mRNA in a co-culture system containing a liver stellate cell-line and freshly isolated hepatocytes. *Biochim. Biophys. Acta* 1362: 135–144.

47. Preedy VR, Garlick PJ (1983). Protein synthesis in skeletal muscle of the perfused rat hemicorpus compared with rates in the intact animal. *Biochem. J.* 214: 433–442.

48. Preedy VR, Smith DM, Kearney NF, Sugden PH (1984). Rates of protein turnover *in vivo* and *in vitro* in ventricular muscle of hearts from fed and starved rats. *Biochem. J.* 222: 395–400.

49. Preedy VR, Smith DM, Kearney NF, Sugden PH (1985). Regional variation and differential sensitivity of rat heart protein synthesis *in vivo* and *in vitro*. *Biochem. J.* 225: 487–492.

50. Preedy VR, Smith DM, Sugden PH (1986). A comparison of rates of protein turnover in rat diaphragm *in vivo* and *in vitro*. *Biochem. J.* 233: 279–282.

51. Preedy VR, Pain VM, Garlick PJ (1984). The metabolic state of muscle in the isolated perfused rat hemicorpus in relation to rates of protein synthesis. *Biochem. J.* 218: 429–440.

52. Martin F, Ward K, Slavin G, Levi J, Peters TJ (1985). Alcoholic skeletal myopathy, a clinical and pathological study. *Q. J. Med.* 55: 233–251.

53. Preedy VR, Ohlendieck K, Adachi J, Koll M, Sneddon A, Hunter R, Rajendram R, Mantle D, Peters TJ (2003). The importance of alcohol induced muscle disease. *J. Muscle Res. Cell Motil.* 24, 55–63.

54. Preedy VR, Adachi J, Asano M, Koll M, Mantle D, Niemela O, Parkkila S, Paice AG, Peters T, Rajendram R, Seitz H, Ueno Y, Worrall S (2002). Free radicals in alcoholic myopathy: indices of damage and preventive studies. *Free Radic. Biol. Med.* 32: 683–687.

55. Preedy VR, Adachi J, Ueno Y, Ahmed S, Mantle D, Mullatti N, Rajendram R, and Peters TJ (2001). Alcoholic skeletal muscle myopathy: definitions, features, contribution of neuropathy, impact and diagnosis. *Eur. J. Neurol.* 8: 677–687.

56. Preedy VR, Peters TJ, Adachi J, Ahmed S, Mantle D, Niemela O, Parkkila S, Worrall S (2001). Pathogenic mechanisms in alcoholic myopathy. In: Agarwal DP, Seitz HK (Eds.), *Alcohol in Health and Disease*. Marcel Dekker, New York, pp. 243–259.

57. Duane P, Peters TJ (1988). Nutritional status in alcoholics with and without chronic skeletal muscle myopathy. *Alcohol Alcohol.* 23: 271–277.

58. Martin FC, Slavin G, Levi AJ, Peters TJ (1984). Investigation of the organelle pathology of skeletal muscle in chronic alcoholism. *J. Clin. Pathol.* 37: 448–454.

59. Wassif WS, Preedy VR, Summers B, Duane P, Leigh N, Peters TJ (1993). The relationship between muscle fiber atrophy factor, plasma carnosinase activities and muscle RNA and protein composition in chronic alcoholic myopathy. *Alcohol Alcohol.* 28: 325–331.

60. Pacy PJ, Preedy VR, Peters TJ, Read M, Halliday D (1991). The effect of chronic alcohol ingestion on whole body and muscle protein synthesis — a stable isotope study. *Alcohol Alcohol.* 26: 505–513.

61. Martin FC, Peters TJ (1985). Assessment *in vitro* and *in vivo* of muscle degradation in chronic skeletal muscle myopathy of alcoholism. *Clin. Sci.* 68: 693–700.

62. Stein TP, Schluter MD (1997). Human skeletal muscle protein breakdown during spaceflight. *Am. J. Physiol.* 272: E688–E695.

63. Wang Z, Deurenberg P, Matthews DE, Heymsfield SB (1998). Urinary 3-methylhistidine excretion: association with total body skeletal muscle mass by computerized axial tomography. *J. Parenter. Enteral Nutr.* 22: 82–86.

64. Nygren J, Thorell A, Brismar K, Wernerman J, McNurlan MA, Garlick PJ, Ljungqvist O (2002). Glucose flux is normalized by compensatory hyperinsulinaemia in growth hormone-induced insulin resistance in healthy subjects, while skeletal muscle protein synthesis remains unchanged. *Clin. Sci.* (Colch.) 102: 457–464.

65. Afting EG, Bernhardt W, Janzen RW, Rothig HJ (1981). Quantitative importance of non-skeletal-muscle N tau-methylhistidine and creatine in human urine. *Biochem. J.* 200: 449–452.

66. Mantle D, Falkous G, Peters TJ, Preedy VR (1999). Effect of ethanol and acetaldehyde on intracellular protease activities in human liver, brain and muscle tissues *in vitro*. *Clin. Chim. Acta* 281: 101–108.

67. Koll M, Ahmed S, Mantle D, Donohue TM, Palmer TN, Simanowski UA, Seitz HK, Peters TJ, Preedy VR (2002). Effect of acute and chronic alcohol treatment and their superimposition on lysosomal, cytoplasmic, and proteosomal protease activities in rat skeletal muscle *in vivo*. *Metabolism* 51: 97–104.

68. Piquet M-A (2002). Nutritional treatment of alcoholism. *Cah. Nutr. Diet.* 37: 136–140.

69. Lieber CS (2000). Hepatic, metabolic, and nutritional disorders of alcoholism: from pathogenesis to therapy. *Crit. Rev. Clin. Lab Sci.* 37: 551–584.

70. Manari AP, Preedy VR, Peters TJ (2000). Nutritional status of harmful drinkers and dependent alcoholics in the UK. *Alcohol. Clin. Exp. Res.* 24, Supplement to issue 5,166A.

71. Nicolas JM, Fernandez-Sola J, Robert J, Antunez E, Cofan M, Cardenal C, Sacanella E, Estruch R, Urbano-Marquez A (2000). High ethanol intake and malnutrition in alcoholic cerebellar shrinkage. *QJM* 93: 449–456.

72. Santolaria F, Perez-Manzano JL, Milena A, Gonzalez-Reimers E, Gomez-Rodriguez MA, Martinez-Riera A, Aleman-Valls MR, Vega-Prieto MJ (2000). Nutritional assessment in alcoholic patients. Its relationship with alcoholic intake, feeding habits, organic complications and social problems. *Drug Alcohol Depend.* 59: 295–304.

73. Preedy VR, Watson RR (1996). *Alcohol and the Gastrointestinal Tract.* CRC Press, Boca Raton, FL.

74. Bunout D (1999). Nutritional and metabolic effects of alcoholism: their relationship with alcoholic liver disease. *Nutrition* 15: 583–589.

75. Diehl AM (2002). Liver disease in alcohol abusers: clinical perspective. *Alcohol* 27: 7–11.

76. Rimaniol JM, Authier FJ, Chariot P (1994). Muscle weakness in intensive care patients: initial manifestation of vitamin D deficiency. *Intensive Care Med.* 20: 591–592.

77. Wassner SJ, Li JB, Sperduto A, Norman ME (1983). Vitamin D deficiency, hypocalcemia, and increased skeletal muscle degradation in rats. *J. Clin. Invest.* 72: 102–112.

78. Hickish T, Colston KW, Bland JM, Maxwell JD (1989). Vitamin D deficiency and muscle strength in male alcoholics. *Clin. Sci.* 77: 171–176.

79. Ward RJ, Peters TJ (1992). The antioxidant status of patients with either alcohol-induced liver damage or myopathy. *Alcohol Alcohol.* 27: 359–365.

80. Fernandez-Sola J, Villegas E, Nicolas JM, Deulofeu R, Antunez E, Sacanella E, Estruch R, Urbano-Marquez A (1998). Serum and muscle levels of alpha-tocopherol, ascorbic acid, and retinol are normal in chronic alcoholic myopathy. *Alcohol. Clin. Exp. Res.* 22: 422–427.

81. Volpi E, Lucidi P, Cruciani G, Monacchia F, Santoni S, Reboldi G, Brunetti P, Bolli GB, De Feo P (1998). Moderate and large doses of ethanol differentially affect hepatic protein metabolism in humans. *J. Nutr.* 128: 198–203.

82. Lieber CS (1993). Biochemical factors in alcoholic liver disease. *Semin. Liver Dis.* 13: 136–153.

83. Lieber CS (1994). Hepatic and metabolic effects of ethanol: pathogenesis and prevention. *Ann. Med.* 26: 325–330.

84. Lieber CS (1997). Role of oxidative stress and antioxidant therapy in alcoholic and nonalcoholic liver diseases. *Adv. Pharmacol.* 38: 601–628.

85. Andersen H, Borre M, Jakobsen J, Andersen PH, Vilstrup H (1998). Decreased muscle strength in patients with alcoholic liver cirrhosis in relation to nutritional status, alcohol abstinence, liver function, and neuropathy. *Hepatology* 27: 1200–1206.

86. Panzak G, Tarter R, Murali S, Switala J, Lu S, Maher B, Van Thiel DH (1998). Isometric muscle strength in alcoholic and nonalcoholic liver-transplantation candidates. *Am. J. Drug Alcohol Abuse* 24: 499–512.

87. Aagaard NK, Andersen H, Vilstrup H, Clausen T, Jakobsen J, Dorup I (2002). Muscle strength, Na,K-pumps, magnesium and potassium in patients with alcoholic liver cirrhosis — relation to spironolactone. *J. Intern. Med.* 252: 56–63.

88. Rocchi E, Borella P, Borghi A, Paolillo F, Pradelli M, Farina F, Casalgrandi G (1994). Zinc and magnesium in liver cirrhosis. *Eur. J. Clin. Invest.* 24: 149–155.

89. Tuma DJ, Casey CA, Sorrell MF (1991). Effects of alcohol on hepatic protein metabolism and trafficking. *Alcohol Alcohol. Suppl.* 1: 297–303.

90. Tuma DJ, Smith SL, Sorrell MF (1991). Acetaldehyde and microtubules. *Ann. N.Y. Acad. Sci.* 625: 786–792.

91. Tuma DJ, Casey CA, Sorrell MF (1991). Chronic ethanol-induced impairments in receptor-mediated endocytosis of insulin in rat hepatocytes. *Alcohol. Clin. Exp. Res.* 15: 808–813.

92. Reilly ME, Mantle D, Richardson PJ, Salisbury J, Jones J, Peters TJ, Preedy VR (1997). Studies on the time-course of ethanol's acute effects on skeletal muscle protein synthesis: comparison with acute changes in proteolytic activity. *Alcohol. Clin. Exp. Res.* 21: 792–798.

93. Lieber CS, DeCarli LM (1986). The feeding of ethanol in liquid diets. *Alcohol. Clin. Exp. Res.* 10: 550–553.

94. Preedy VR, McIntosh A, Bonner AB, Peters TJ (1996). Ethanol dosage regimens in studies of ethanol toxicity: influence of nutrition and surgical interventions. *Addict. Biol.* 1: 255–262.

95. Preedy VR, Duane P, Peters TJ (1988). Biological effects of chronic ethanol consumption: a reappraisal of the Lieber-De Carli liquid-diet model with reference to skeletal muscle. *Alcohol Alcohol.* 23: 151–154.

96. Preedy VR, Peters TJ (1989). The effect of chronic ethanol ingestion on synthesis and degradation of soluble, contractile and stromal protein fractions of skeletal muscles from immature and mature rats. *Biochem. J.* 259: 261–266.

97. Preedy VR, Marway JS, Peters TJ (1989). Use of the Lieber-DeCarli liquid feeding regime with specific reference to the effects of ethanol on rat skeletal muscle RNA. *Alcohol Alcohol.* 24: 439–445.

98. Preedy VR, Peters TJ (1988). The effect of chronic ethanol ingestion on protein metabolism in type-I- and type-II-fibre-rich skeletal muscles of the rat. *Biochem. J.* 254: 631–639.

99. Preedy VR, Peters TJ (1988). The effect of chronic ethanol feeding on body and plasma composition and rates of skeletal muscle protein turnover in the rat. *Alcohol Alcohol.* 23: 217–224.

100. Preedy VR, Bateman CJ, Salisbury JR, Price AB, Peters TJ (1989). Ethanol-induced skeletal muscle myopathy: biochemical and histochemical measurements on type I and type II fibre-rich muscles in the young rat. *Alcohol Alcohol.* 24: 533–539.

101. Marway JS, Preedy VR, Peters TJ (1990). Experimental alcoholic skeletal muscle myopathy is characterised by a rapid and sustained decrease in muscle RNA content. *Alcohol Alcohol.* 25: 401–406.

102. Reilly ME, McKoy G, Mantle D, Peters TJ, Goldspink G, Preedy VR (2000). Protein and mRNA levels of the myosin heavy chain isoforms I[beta], IIa, IIx and IIb in type I and type II fibre-predominant rat skeletal muscles in response to chronic alcohol feeding. *J. Muscle Res. Cell Motil.* 21: 763–773.

103. Hunter R, Neagoe C, Järveläinen HA, Lindros KO, Linke WA, Preedy VR (2003). Alcohol affects the skeletal muscle proteins, titin and nebulin in male and female rats. *J. Nutr.* 133: 1154–1157.

104. Preedy VR, Reilly ME, Peters TJ (1999). A current and retrospective analysis of whether the animal model of alcoholic myopathy is suitable for studying its clinical counterpart. *Addict. Biol.* 4: 241–242.

105. Preedy VR, Why H, Paice AG, Reilly ME, Ansell H, Patel, VB, Richardson PJ (1995). Protein synthesis in the heart *in vivo*, its measurement and pathophysiological alterations. *Int. J. Cardiol.* 50: 95–106.

106. Reeds PJ, Davis TA (1999). Of flux and flooding: the advantages and problems of different isotopic methods for quantifying protein turnover *in vivo*: I. Methods based on the dilution of a tracer. *Curr. Opin. Clin. Nutr. Metab. Care* 2: 23–28.

107. Davis TA, Reeds PJ (2001). Of flux and flooding: the advantages and problems of different isotopic methods for quantifying protein turnover *in vivo*: II. Methods based on the incorporation of a tracer. *Curr. Opin. Clin. Nutr. Metab. Care* 4: 51–56.

108. Bonner AB, Marway JS, Swann M, Preedy VR (1996). Brain nucleic acid composition and fractional rates of protein synthesis in response to chronic ethanol feeding: comparison with skeletal muscle. *Alcohol* 13: 581–587.

109. Ward RJ, Venkatesan S, Swe TN, Preedy VR, Price AB, Peters TJ (1987). An animal model of alcohol-induced myopathy. *Clin. Sci.* 73, Supplement 17: 53–53.

110. Bernal CA, Vazquez JA, Adibi SA (1993). Leucine metabolism during chronic ethanol consumption. *Metabolism* 42: 1084–1086.

111. Preedy VR, Peters TJ (1988). Acute effects of ethanol on protein synthesis in different muscles and muscle protein fractions of the rat. *Clin. Sci.* (Colch.) 74: 461–466.

112. Preedy VR, Duane P, Peters TJ (1988). Comparison of the acute effects of ethanol on liver and skeletal muscle protein synthesis in the rat. *Alcohol Alcohol.* 23: 155–162.

113. Krahenbuhl S, Reichen J (1997). Carnitine metabolism in patients with chronic liver disease. *Hepatology* 25: 148–153.

114. Preedy VR, Gove CD, Panos MZ, Sherwood R, Portmann B, Williams R, Peters TJ (1990). Liver histology, blood biochemistry and RNA, DNA and subcellular protein composition of various skeletal muscles of rats with experimental cirrhosis: implications for alcoholic muscle disease. *Alcohol Alcohol.* 25: 641–649.

115. Mi L-J, Mak KM, Lieber CS (2000). Attenuation of alcohol-induced apoptosis of hepatocytes in rat livers by polyenylphosphatidylcholine (PPC). *Alcohol. Clin. Exp. Res.* 24: 207–212.

116. Casey CA, Nanji A, Cederbaum AI, Adachi M, Takahashi T (2001). Alcoholic liver disease and apoptosis. *Alcohol. Clin. Exp. Res.* 25: 49S–53S.

117. Deaciuc IV, D'Souza NB, Fortunato F, Hill DB, Sarphie TG, McClain CJ (2001). Alcohol-induced sinusoidal endothelial cell dysfunction in the mouse is associated with exacerbated liver apoptosis and can be reversed by caspase inhibition. *Hepatol. Res.* 19: 85–97.

118. Zhou Z, Sun X, Kang YJ (2001). Ethanol-induced apoptosis in mouse liver: Fas- and cytochrome c-mediated caspase-3 activation pathway. *Am. J. Pathol.* 159: 329–338.

119. Cardin R, D'Errico A, Fiorentino M, Cecchetto A, Naccarato R, Farinati F (2002). Hepatocyte proliferation and apoptosis in relation to oxidative damage in alcohol-related liver disease. *Alcohol Alcohol.* 37: 43–48.

120. Neuman MG, Katz GG, Malkiewicz IM, Mathurin P, Tsukamoto H, Adachi M, Ishii H, Colell A, Garcia-Ruiz C, Fernandez-Checa JC, Casey CA (2002). Alcoholic liver injury and apoptosis — synopsis of the symposium held at ESBRA 2001: 8th Congress of the European Society for Biomedical Research on Alcoholism, Paris, September 16, 2001. *Alcohol* 28: 117–128.

121. Paice AG, Hesketh JE, Towner P, Hirako M, Peters TJ, Preedy VR (2003). No change in apoptosis in skeletal muscle exposed acutely or chronically to alcohol. *Addict. Biol.* 8: 97–105.

122. Reilly ME, Salisbury JR, Peters TJ, Preedy VR (2000). Comparative effects of acute ethanol dosage on liver and muscle protein metabolism. *Biochem. Pharmacol.* 60: 1773–1785.

123. Vary TC, Nairn AC, Deiter G, Lang CH (2002). Differential effects of alcohol consumption on eukaryotic elongation factors in heart, skeletal muscle, and liver. *Alcohol. Clin. Exp. Res.* 26: 1794–1802.

124. Girbes T, Susin A, Ayuso MS, Parrilla R (1983). Acute effects of ethanol in the control of protein synthesis in isolated rat liver cells. *Arch. Biochem. Biophys.* 226: 37–49.

125. Girbes T (1986). The acute effects of ethanol on protein synthesis in isolated rat liver cells are pH-dependent. *Biochem. Int.* 12: 313–320.

126. Savolainen ER, Leo MA, Timpl R, Lieber CS (1984). Acetaldehyde and lactate stimulate collagen synthesis of cultured baboon liver myofibroblasts. *Gastroenterology* 87: 777–787.

127. Murawaki Y, Kato S, Hirayama C (1991). Hepatic collagen synthesis in patients with alcoholic and nonalcoholic liver disease. *Gastroenterol. Jpn.* 26: 465–471.

128. Maher JJ, Zia S, Tzagarakis C (1994). Acetaldehyde-induced stimulation of collagen synthesis and gene expression is dependent on conditions of cell culture: studies with rat lipocytes and fibroblasts. *Alcohol. Clin. Exp. Res.* 18: 403–409.

129. Reilly ME, Patel VB, Peters TJ, Preedy VR (2000). *In vivo* rates of skeletal muscle protein synthesis in the rat are decreased by acute ethanol treatment but are not ameliorated by supplemental-tocopherol. *J. Nutr.* 130: 3045–3049.

130. Koll M, Beeso JA, Kelly FJ, Simanowski UA, Seitz HK, Peters TJ, Preedy VR (2003). Chronic alpha-tocopherol supplementation in rats does not ameliorate either chronic or acute alcohol-induced changes in muscle protein metabolism. *Clin. Sci.* (Colch.) 104: 287–294.

131. Preedy VR, Keating JW, Peters TJ (1992). The acute effects of ethanol and acetaldehyde on rates of protein synthesis in type I and type II fibre-rich skeletal muscles of the rat. *Alcohol Alcohol.* 27: 241–251.

132. Lang CH, Wu D, Frost RA, Jefferson LS, Vary TC, Kimball, SR (1999). Chronic alcohol feeding impairs hepatic translation initiation by modulating eIF2 and eIF4E. *Am. J. Physiol.* 277: E805–E814.

133. Ashe MP, Slaven JW, De Long SK, Ibrahimo S, Sachs AB (2001). A novel eIF2B-dependent mechanism of translational control in yeast as a response to fusel alcohols. *EMBO J.* 20: 6464–6474.

134. Paice AG, Reilly ME, Marway JS, Bonner AB, Preedy VR (1995). Compartmentation of total RNA in catabolism: a comparative analysis of skin, bone, skeletal muscle and liver in response to endotoxin and alcohol. *Biochem. Soc. Trans.* 23: 465S.

135. Paice AG (1998). PhD thesis. University of London.

136. Reilly ME, Erylmaz EI, Amir A, Peters TJ, Preedy VR (1998). Skeletal muscle ribonuclease activities in chronically ethanol-treated rats. *Alcohol. Clin. Exp. Res.* 22: 876–883.

137. Tiernan JM, Ward LC (1984). NT-methylhistidine excretion by ethanol-fed rats. *IRCS Med. Sci.* 12: 945–946.

138. Preedy VR, Adachi J, Peters TJ, Worrall S, Parkkila S, Niemela O, Asamo M, Ueno Y, Takeda K, Yamauchi M, Sakamoto K, Takagi M, Nakajima H, Toda G (2001). Recent advances in the pathology of alcoholic myopathy. *Alcohol. Clin. Exp. Res.* 25: 54S–59S.

139. French SW (2000). Mechanisms of alcoholic liver injury. *Can. J. Gastroenterol.* 14: 327–332.

140. French SW, Mayer RJ, Bardag-Gorce F, Ingelman-Sundberg M, Rouach H, Neve E, Higashitsuji H (2001). The ubiquitin-proteasome 26s pathway in liver cell protein turnover: effect of ethanol and drugs. *Alcohol. Clin. Exp. Res.* 25: 225S–229S.

141. Agarwal DP (2002). Cardioprotective effects of light-moderate consumption of alcohol: a review of putative mechanisms. *Alcohol Alcohol.* 37: 409–415.

142. Belleville J (2002). The French paradox: possible involvement of ethanol in the protective effect against cardiovascular diseases. *Nutrition* 18: 173–177.

143. Frishman WH (2002). Alcohol as a cardioprotective agent. *Heart Dis.* 4: 273–275.

144. Wall TL, Carr LG, Ehlers CL (2003). Protective association of genetic variation in alcohol dehydrogenase with alcohol dependence in Native American Mission Indians. *Am. J. Psychiatry* 160: 41–46.

145. Gavazzi A, De Maria R, Parolini M, Porcu M (2000). Alcohol abuse and dilated cardiomyopathy in men. *Am. J. Cardiol.* 85: 1114–1118.

146. Bilora F, Petrobelli F, Boccioletti V, Pomerri F (2002). Treatment of heart failure and ascites with ultrafiltration in patients with intractable alcoholic cardiomyopathy. *Panminerva Med.* 44: 23–25.

147. Dettmeyer R, Reith K, Madea B (2002). Alcoholic cardiomyopathy versus chronic myocarditis — immunohistological investigations with LCA, CD3, CD68 and tenascin. *Forensic Sci. Int.* 126: 57–62.

148. Fernandez-Sola J, Nicolas-Arfelis JM (2002). Gender differences in alcoholic cardiomyopathy. *J. Gend. Specif. Med.* 5: 41–47.

149. Lee WK, Regan TJ (2002). Alcoholic cardiomyopathy: is it dose-dependent? *Prev. Manage. Congest. Heart Failure* 8: 303–306+312.

150. Piano MR (2002). Alcoholic cardiomyopathy: incidence, clinical characteristics, and pathophysiology. *Chest* 121: 1638–1650.

151. Preedy VR, Patel VB, Why HJ, Corbett JM, Dunn MJ, Richardson PJ (1996). Alcohol and the heart: biochemical alterations. *Cardiovasc. Res.* 31: 139–147.

152. Preedy VR, Dunn MJ, Hunter R, Mantle D, Worrall S, Richardson PJ (2002). Alcohol and heart muscle proteins: with special reference to measurement of protein. In: Watson RR, Myers AK (Eds.), *Alcohol and Heart Disease*. Taylor and Francis, London, pp. 197–211.

153. Siddiq T, Richardson PJ, Morton J, Smith B, Sherwood RA, Marway JS, Preedy VR (1993). Rates of protein synthesis in different regions of the normotensive and hypertrophied heart in response to acute alcohol toxicity. *Alcohol Alcohol.* 28: 297–310.

154. Siddiq T, Sandhu G, Richardson PJ, Preedy VR (1997). Effects of acute ethanol on ventricular myofibrillary protein synthesis *in vivo* in normotensive and hypertensive rats. *Addict. Biol.* 2: 87–93.

155. Siddiq T, Salisbury JR, Richardson PJ, Preedy VR (1993). Synthesis of ventricular mitochondrial proteins *in vivo*: effect of acute ethanol toxicity. *Alcohol. Clin. Exp. Res.* 17: 894–899.

156. Siddiq T, Richardson PJ, Mitchell WD, Teare J, Preedy VR (1993). Ethanol-induced inhibition of ventricular protein synthesis *in vivo* and the possible role of acetaldehyde. *Cell Biochem. Funct.* 11: 45–54.

157. Patel VB, Salisbury JR, Rodrigues LM, Griffiths JR, Richardson PJ, Preedy VR (1996). The acute and chronic effects of alcohol upon cardiac nucleotide status. *Addict. Biol.* 1: 171–180.

158. Patel VB, Ajmal R, Sherwood RA, Sullivan A, Richardson PJ, Preedy VR (2001). Cardioprotective effect of propranolol from alcohol-induced heart muscle damage as assessed by plasma cardiac troponin-T. *Alcohol. Clin. Exp. Res.* 25: 882–889.

159. Patel VB, Richardson PJ, Preedy VR (2000). Inability of propranolol to prevent alcohol-induced reductions in cardiac protein synthesis *in vivo*. *Clin. Chim. Acta* 300: 1–12.

160. Vary TC, Lynch CJ, Lang CH (2001). Effects of chronic alcohol consumption on regulation of myocardial protein synthesis. *Am. J. Physiol. Heart Circ. Physiol.* 281: H1242–H1251.

161. Atwater WD, Benedict FG (1902). An experimental inquiry regarding the nutritive value of alcohol. *Mem. Natl. Acad. Sci.* 8: 235–397.

162. Bunout D, Petermann M, Ugarte G, Barrera G, Iturriaga H (1987). Nitrogen economy in alcoholic patients without liver disease. *Metabolism* 36: 651–653.

163. McDonald JT, Margen S (1976). Wine versus ethanol in human nutrition. I. Nitrogen and calorie balance. *Am. J. Clin. Nutr.* 29: 1093–1103.

164. Preedy VR, Peters T (1989). Protein metabolism in the small intestine of the ethanol-fed rat. *Cell Biochem. Funct.* 7: 235–242.

165. Marway JS, Keating JW, Reeves J, Salisbury JR, Preedy, VR (1993). Seromuscular and mucosal protein synthesis in various anatomical regions of the rat gastrointestinal tract and their response to acute ethanol toxicity. *Eur. J. Gastroenterol. Hepatol.* 5: 27–34.

166. Pares X, Farres J (1996). Alcohol and aldehyde dehydrogenases in the gastrointestinal tract. In: Preedy VR, Watson RR (Eds.), *Alcohol and the Gastrointestinal Tract*. CRC Press, Boca Raton, FL, pp. 41–56.

167. Kaur J (2002). Chronic ethanol feeding affects intestinal mucus lipid composition and glycosylation in rats. *Ann. Nutr. Metab.* 46: 38–44.

168. Pronko P, Bardina L, Satanovskaya V, Kuzmich A, Zimatkin S (2002). Effect of chronic alcohol consumption on the ethanol- and acetaldehyde-metabolizing systems in the rat gastrointestinal tract. *Alcohol Alcohol.* 37: 229–235.

169. Roy HK, Gulizia JM, Karolski WJ, Ratashak A, Sorrell MF, Tuma D (2002). Ethanol promotes intestinal tumorigenesis in the MIN mouse. *Cancer Epidemiol. Biomarkers Prev.* 11: 1499–1502.
170. Singer MV (2002). Effect of ethanol and alcoholic beverages on the gastrointestinal tract in humans. *Rom. J. Gastroenterol.* 11: 197–204.
171. Stermer E (2002). Alcohol consumption and the gastrointestinal tract. *Isr. Med. Assoc. J.* 4: 200–202.
172. Laiho K (1998). Myeloperoxidase activity in skin lesions. II. Influence of alcohol and some medicines. *Int. J. Legal Med.* 111: 10–12.
173. Preedy VR, Marway JS, Salisbury JR, Peters TJ (1990). Protein synthesis in bone and skin of the rat are inhibited by ethanol: implications for whole body metabolism. *Alcohol. Clin. Exp. Res.* 14: 165–168.
174. Levine N (2001). Fragile skin. Exposure to the sun makes skin of an alcoholic patient susceptible to traumatic injuries. *Geriatrics* 56: 21.
175. Fung TT, Hunter DJ, Spiegelman D, Colditz GA, Rimm EB, Willett WC (2002). Intake of alcohol and alcoholic beverages and the risk of basal cell carcinoma of the skin. *Cancer Epidemiol. Biomarkers Prev.* 11: 1119–1122.
176. Neuman MG, Haber JA, Malkiewicz IM, Cameron RG, Katz GG, Shear NH (2002). Ethanol signals for apoptosis in cultured skin cells. *Alcohol* 26: 179–190.
177. Hunter DJ, Sambrook PN (2000). Bone loss. Epidemiology of bone loss. *Arthritis Res.* 2: 441–445.
178. Turner RT, Kidder LS, Kennedy A, Evans GL, Sibonga JD (2001). Moderate alcohol consumption suppresses bone turnover in adult female rats. *J. Bone Miner. Res.* 16: 589–594.
179. Nyquist F, Spacing D, Obrant KJ, Bondeson L, Nordsletten L (2002). Effects of alcohol on bone mineral and mechanical properties of bone in male rats. *Alcohol Alcohol.* 37: 21–24.
180. Gruchow HW, Sobocinski KA, Barboriak JJ, Scheller JG (1985). Alcohol consumption, nutrient intake and relative body weight among US adults. *Am. J. Clin. Nutr.* 42: 289–295.
181. Colditz GA, Giovannucci E, Rimm EB, Stampfer MJ, Rosner B, Speizer FE, Gordis E, Willett WC (1991). Alcohol intake in relation to diet and obesity in women and men. *Am. J. Clin. Nutr.* 54: 49–55.
182. Pirola RC, Lieber CS (1972). The energy cost of the metabolism of drugs, including ethanol. *Pharmacology* 7: 185–196.
183. Jones BR, Barrett-Connor E, Criqui MH, Holdbrook MJ (1982). A community study of calorie and nutrient intake in drinkers and nondrinkers of alcohol. *Am. J. Clin. Nutr.* 35: 135–139.
184. Romieu I, Willett WC, Stampfer MJ, Colditz GA, Sampson L, Rosner B, Hennekens CH, Speizer FE (1988). Energy intake and other determinants of relative weight. *Am. J. Clin. Nutr.* 47: 406–412.
185. Pirola RC, Lieber CS (1976). Hypothesis: energy wastage in alcoholism and drug abuse: possible role of hepatic microsomal enzymes. *Am. J. Clin. Nutr.* 29: 90–93.
186. Israel Y, Kalant H, Orrego H, Khanna JM, Videla L, Phillips JM (1975). Experimental alcohol-induced hepatic necrosis: suppression by propylthiouracil. *Proc. Natl. Acad. Sci. U.S.A.* 72: 1137–1141.
187. Blachley JD, Johnson JH, Knochel JP (1985). The harmful effects of ethanol on ion transport and cellular respiration. *Am. J. Med. Sci.* 289: 22–26.
188. Reinus JF, Heymsfield SB, Wiskind R, Casper K, Galambos JT (1989). Ethanol: relative fuel value and metabolic effects *in vivo*. *Metabolism* 38: 125–135.

189. Bendtsen P, Jones AW (1999). Impact of water-induced diuresis on excretion profiles of ethanol, urinary creatinine, and urinary osmolality. *J. Anal. Toxicol.* 23: 565–569.

190. Jones AW, Andersson L (1996). Variability of the blood/breath alcohol ratio in drinking drivers. *J. Forensic Sci.* 41: 916–921.

191. Labianca DA, Simpson G (1996). Statistical analysis of blood- to breath-alcohol ratio data in the logarithm-transformed and non-transformed modes. *Eur. J. Clin. Chem. Clin. Biochem.* 34: 111–117.

192. Jones AW, Norberg A, Hahn RG (1997). Concentration-time profiles of ethanol in arterial and venous blood and end-expired breath during and after intravenous infusion. *J. Forensic Sci.* 42: 1088–1094.

193. Hirsch S, de la Maza MP, Petermann M, Iturriaga H, Ugarte G, Bunout D (1995). Protein turnover in abstinent and non-abstinent patients with alcoholic cirrhosis. *J. Am. Coll. Nutr.* 14: 99–104.

194. Reilly ME, Preedy VR, Peters TJ (1995). Investigations into the toxic effects of alcohol on skeletal muscle. *Adverse Drug React. Toxicol. Rev.* 14: 117–150.

195. Preedy VR, Hammond B, Iles RA, Davies SE, Gandy JD, Chalmers RA, Peters, TJ (1991). Urinary excretion of nitrogenous and non-nitrogenous compounds in the chronic ethanol-fed rat. *Clin. Sci.* (Colch.) 80: 393–400.

196. Rodrigo C, Antezana C, Baraona E (1971). Fat and nitrogen balances in rats with alcohol-induced fatty liver. *J. Nutr.* 101: 1307–1310.

197. Klatskin G (1961). The effect of ethyl alcohol on nitrogen excretion in the rat. *Yale J. Biol. Med.* 34: 124–143.

198. Preedy VR, Nott DM, Yates J, Venkatesan S, Jenkins SA, Peters TJ (1997). Hepatic haemodynamics and reticuloendothelial function in the rat in response to chronic ethanol administration. *Addict. Biol.* 2: 445–454.

199. Preedy VR, Venkatesan S, Peters TJ, Nott DM, Yates J, Jenkins SA (1989). Effect of chronic ethanol ingestion on tissue RNA and blood flow in skeletal muscle with comparative reference to bone and tissues of the gastrointestinal tract of the rat. *Clin. Sci.* (Colch.) 76: 243–247.

200. Cook EB, Adebiyi LA, Preedy VR, Peters TJ, Palmer TN (1992). Chronic effects of ethanol on muscle metabolism in the rat. *Biochim. Biophys. Acta* 1180: 207–214.

201. Ward LC, Carrington LE, Daly R (1985). Ethanol and leucine oxidation-I. Leucine oxidation by the rat *in vivo*. *Int. J. Biochem.* 17: 187–193.

202. Ward LC, Ramm GA, Mason S, Daly R (1985). Ethanol and leucine oxidation — II. Leucine oxidation by rat tissue *in vitro*. *Int. J. Biochem.* 17: 195–201.

203. Bernal CA, Vazquez JA, Adibi SA (1995). Chronic ethanol intake reduces the flux through liver branched-chain keto-acid dehydrogenase. *Metabolism* 44: 1243–1246.

204. Ward LC, Tiernan JM, Fagan C (1985). Ethanol and brain protein synthesis in the rat *in vivo*. *Neurosci. Lett.* 53: 273–278.

205. Marway JS, Miell JP, Jones J, Bonner AB, Preece MA, Hashim I, Preedy, VR (1997). Contractile protein synthesis rates *in vivo* in the rat jejunum: modulating role of adrenalectomy and thyroidectomy on ethanol-induced changes. *Addict. Biol.* 2: 67–79.

206. Marway JS, Preedy VR (1995). The acute effects of ethanol and acetaldehyde on the synthesis of mixed and contractile proteins of the jejunum. *Alcohol Alcohol.* 30: 211–217.

207. Preedy VR, Peters TJ (1992). Effects of chronic ethanol consumption and pair feeding on rates of protein synthesis and nucleic acid composition in rat tibia. *Alcohol Alcohol.* 27: 29–37.

208. Preedy VR, Sherwood RA, Akpoguma CI, Black D (1991). The urinary excretion of the collagen degradation markers pyridinoline and deoxypyridinoline in an experimental rat model of alcoholic bone disease. *Alcohol Alcohol.* 26: 191–198.

209. Preedy VR, Baldwin DR, Keating JW, Salisbury JR (1991). Bone collagen, mineral and trace element composition, histomorphometry and urinary hydroxyproline excretion in chronically treated alcohol-fed rats. *Alcohol Alcohol.* 26: 39–46.

210. Lundquist F, Sestoft L, Damgaard SE, Clausen JP, Trap Jensen J (1973). Utilization of acetate in the human forearm during exercise after ethanol ingestion. *J. Clin. Invest.* 52: 3231–3235.

211. Karlsson N, Fellenius E, Kiessling KH (1975). The metabolism of acetate in the perfused hind-quarter of the rat. *Acta Physiol. Scand.* 93: 391–400.

212. Suokas A, Forsander O, Lindros K (1984). Distribution and utilization of alcohol-derived acetate in the rat. *J. Stud. Alcohol* 45: 381–385.

213. Garlick PJ, McNurlan MA, Preedy VR (1980). A rapid and convenient technique for measuring the rate of protein synthesis in tissues by injection of [3H]phenylalanine. *Biochem. J.* 192: 719–723.

214. Preedy VR, Paska L, Sugden PH, Schofield PS, Sugden MC (1988). The effects of surgical stress and short-term fasting on protein synthesis *in vivo* in diverse tissues of the mature rat. *Biochem. J.* 250: 179–188.

215. Preedy VR, McNurlan MA, Garlick PJ (1983). Protein synthesis in skin and bone of the young rat. *Br. J. Nutr.* 49: 517–523.

216. McNurlan MA, Garlick PJ (1980). Contribution of rat liver and gastrointestinal tract to whole-body protein synthesis in the rat. *Biochem. J.* 186: 381–383.

217. Preedy VR, Garlick PJ (1981). Rates of protein synthesis in skin and bone, and their importance in the assessment of protein degradation in the perfused rat hemicorpus. *Biochem. J.* 194: 373–376.

218. Preedy VR, Duane P, Peters TJ (1988). Acute ethanol dosage reduces the synthesis of smooth muscle contractile proteins in the small intestine of the rat. *Gut* 29: 1244–1248.

Section V

Alcohol and Nutrients

16 Soy Products Affecting Alcohol Absorption and Metabolism

Mitsuyoshi Kano and Fumiyasu Ishikawa

CONTENTS

16.1 INTRODUCTION

Ethanol absorption in the upper gastrointestinal tract is mainly controlled by gastric emptying. Diet components also in the gastrointestinal tract affect the absorption and metabolism. For example, vegetable oils (soybean oil, coconut oil, etc.) not only slow the rate at which gastric ethanol is eliminated but restrain increases of the plasma ethanol concentration.[1] Moreover, sesamin and garlic stimulate ethanol metabolism, especially the clearance of acetaldehyde,[2,3] and are expected to ameliorate alcohol toxicity.

16.1.1 SOY PRODUCTS AND ISOFLAVONES

In Japan five traditional crops (rice, soybean, barnyard grass, foxtail millet, and wheat) are nutritionally important foodstuffs, expressed as *go-koku* (*go* means "five," and *koku* means "cereals and beans" in Japanese). Among these crops, soybean is rich in protein, fat, and carbohydrate, and contributes nutritionally to health as a so-called "field meat." Various types of soy products are available (Figure 16.1): for example, soymilk (soybean extract), tofu (soybean curd from soymilk,), miso (fermented soybean paste), and natto (fermented soybeans with a slimy consistency).

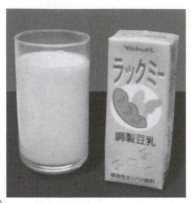

a) Soymilk (soybean extract)

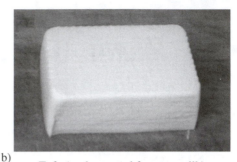

b) Tofu (soybean curd from soymilk)

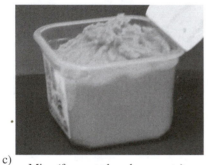

c) Miso (fermented soybean paste)

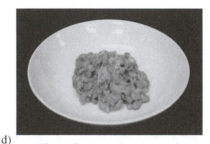

d) Natto (fermented soybean with a slimy consistency)

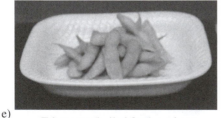

e) Edamame (boiled fresh soybean, popular as a snack with alcohol)

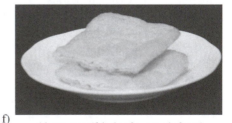

f) Abura-age (fried tofu, pouch form)

FIGURE 16.1 Familiar soy products served in Japan.

Recently, soybean has attracted much attention for its preventive effects on chronic disease such as breast and prostate cancers, hyperlipidemia, atherosclerosis, osteoporosis, and menopausal symptoms.[4–6] Many of these effects would be exerted by soy isoflavones (mainly the glycosides, genistein and daidzein, in soy products) (Figure 16.2). Isoflavones are nonsteroidal phytoestrogenic and antioxidative polyphenolic molecules.[6-8] The effects of isoflavones not derived from soybean on ethanol consumption have been published in some reports, where isoflavones prepared from a crude extract of *Pueraria lobata,* used as a traditional medicine for antiinebriation, suppressed alcohol intake in alcohol-preferring rats.[9,10] The major components (daidzin and daidzein) inhibit mitochondrial low-K_m acetaldehyde dehydrogenase (ALDH)[11] and alcohol dehydrogenase (ADH)[12] *in vitro*, whereas these enzymes are not affected by intragastric or intraperitoneal injection of daidzin.[13,14] Thus, the relationship of isoflavones with alcohol-suppressing performance is yet to be clarified. Furthermore, few reports have been published about the effect of soy on ethanol consumption.

16.1.2 FERMENTED SOYMILK

Soymilk (SM) is a central material for soy products as well as an excellent beverage in itself. We have developed a new soymilk product, fermented soymilk (FSM), by using a probiotic *Bifidobacterium breve* strain Yakult,[15-18] and investigated its physiological functions. SM has almost the glycoside form of isoflavones, which are converted into the aglycone form in FSM. Most of the genistein in FSM is aglycone (Figure 16.3). Isoflavone aglycones are absorbed into blood more rapidly and efficiently than the glycosides.[19,20] This is the case for soymilk products. FSM-fed Sprague–Dawley (SD) rats exhibited a greater increase in the blood concentration of isoflavones than SM-fed rats (Figure 16.4).[21] This difference would be associated with the effect of FSM on lipid metabolism[22-24] and on mammary carcinogenesis.[25] Therefore, ethanol consumption is of possible relevance to the isoflavone form, and probably to the absorbability or availability, too.

16.2 SOYMILK PRODUCTS AND ETHANOL ABSORPTION

Do soymilk products or the difference in the isoflavone form affect ethanol absorption? We investigated the effect of SM and FSM in male SD rats.[26] Overnight-fasted rats were intragastrically given sample beverages in which ethanol (20%) was added to the casein-based control, SM or FSM solutions. The soymilk groups had higher levels of gastric ethanol in the early stages after ethanol injection than the control group; ethanol levels at 3 h were similar in all groups (Figure 16.5). However portal ethanol levels were different between these groups (FSM<SM<control) at early and late stages. Taking into consideration that portal ethanol directly reflects ethanol absorption through the gastrointestinal tract, these findings suggest that FSM components other than those common to SM strongly contribute to ethanol absorption. Because the aortal blood passing the liver reflects hepatic ethanol metabolism as well as absorption, the similar aortal ethanol and acetaldehyde levels with portal ethanol indicates that the FSM effect would be dependent on lowering ethanol absorption or enhancing ethanol metabolism following acute ethanol administration.

Aglycone form

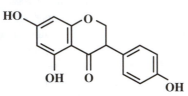

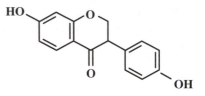

$C_{15}H_{10}O_5$

Genistein

$C_{15}H_{10}O_4$

Daidzein

Glycoside form

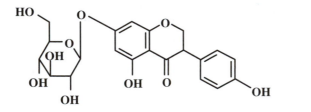

$C_{21}H_{20}O_{10}$

Genistin

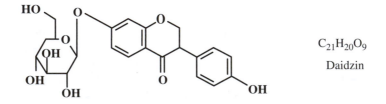

$C_{21}H_{20}O_9$

Daidzin

FIGURE 16.2 Structures of isoflavones, genistein, daidzein, genistin, and daidzin.

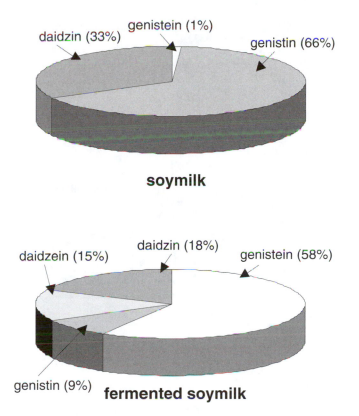

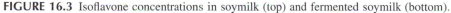

FIGURE 16.3 Isoflavone concentrations in soymilk (top) and fermented soymilk (bottom).

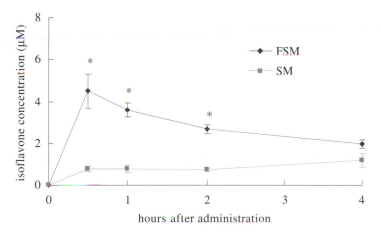

FIGURE 16.4 Time-course change of concentration in plasma after oral administration of soymilk (SM) and fermented soymilk (FSM) (7.5 ml/kg of body weight). Values are means ±SEM of six rats. Asterisk indicates significant difference ($p < 0.05$) from the soymilk value by Tukey's test.

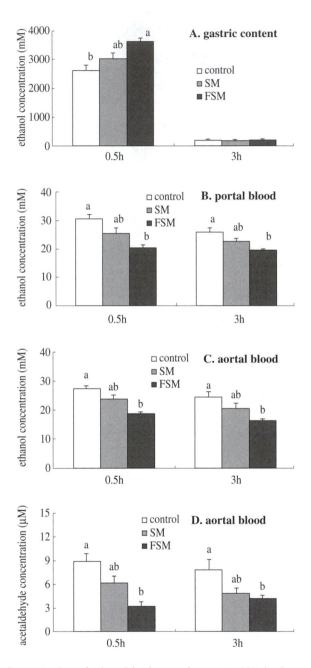

FIGURE 16.5 Concentration of ethanol in the gastric content (A), in the portal blood (B), and in the aortal blood (C); and concentration of acetaldehyde in the aortal blood (D) of rats 0.5 and 3 h after consuming control, soymilk (SM), or fermented soymilk (FSM) solutions containing 20% ethanol. The data represent means ± SEM for eight animals. [ab]Mean values not sharing the same letter above the bars are significantly different at $p < 0.05$ by Tukey's test. (Data from *J. Nutr.,* 132, 238, 2002.)

16.3 SOY ISOFLAVONES AND ETHANOL METABOLISM

Ethanol entering the liver through the portal vein is oxidized into acetaldehyde and, further, to acetate in the hepatocytes. Soy components, especially isoflavones, also flow into the liver through the portal vein. The experiment in the rat hepatocytes cultured with 65 mM ethanol[26] shows that physiological doses of isoflavones (~5 μM) affect ethanol and acetaldehyde metabolism (Figure 16.6). This indicates that the *in vivo* decrease in aortal ethanol and acetaldehyde by FSM would be closely related with the direct effect of soy isoflavones on liver function. Our observations are slightly different from previous reports that isoflavone glucosides, daidzin and genistin, *in vitro* inhibited human ALDH, but not the corresponding aglycones, daidzein, and genistein,[11] and that daidzin suppressed ethanol intake without affecting acetaldehyde metabolism in hamsters.[13]

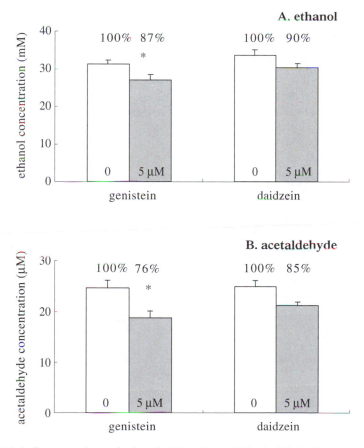

FIGURE 16.6 Concentrations of ethanol (A) and acetaldehyde (B) in the culture filtrates from isolated rat hepatocyte cultures (10^7 cells/10 ml medium) on addition of genistein or daidzein (0 or 5 μM). The data represent the mean ± SEM for six animals. Asterisk indicates significant difference ($p < 0.05$) by Tukey's test.

16.4 SOYMILK PRODUCTS AND ETHANOL METABOLISM

Induction of microsomal ethanol oxidizing system (MEOS) activity and restriction of ALDH activity by ethanol[27] are associated with an accumulation of acetaldehyde and reactive oxygen species upon chronic or high consumption of ethanol. These toxic molecules derived from ethanol are considered to cause cell injury consequently through lipid peroxidation, enzyme inactivation, and DNA damage.[28–30] Glutathione *S*-transferase (GST) participates in detoxification of acetaldehyde through glutathione conjugation,[31] as well as antioxidation of active xenobiotic metabolites and reduction of lipid peroxides.[32] The relationship between soy components and the P450 system is not well understood as yet; genistein acts as a potent inhibitor of CYP1A1 and/or CYP1A2 induced by β-naphthoflavone[33] and soy protein acts as an enhancer of the dexamethasone-induced mRNA expression of hepatic CYP3A2.[34]

In SD rats chronically exposed to ethanol (5%),[26] FSM feeding decreased MEOS activity, probably CYP2E1 (Figure 16.7), but did not affect cytosolic ADH activity. Soymilk products not only enhanced cytosolic GST and mitochondrial low K_m ALDH activities, but restricted hepatic thiobarbituric acid–reactive substances, a putative marker of lipid peroxidation,[35] which was induced by chronic ethanol exposure. These facts suggest that the consumption of soymilk products would contribute to the prevention of ethanol-induced liver injury through enhancement of ethanol metabolism and the antioxidation system. Furthermore, it should be noted

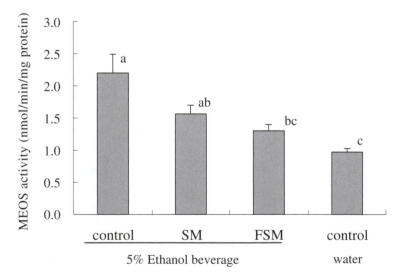

FIGURE 16.7 Microsomal ethanol oxidizing (MEOS) activity in the liver of rats consuming control diet + 5% ethanol (control group), soymilk diet + 5% ethanol (SM group), fermented soymilk diet + 5% ethanol (FSM group) and control diet + water for 24 d. The data represent the mean ± SEM for eight animals. [abc]Mean values not sharing the same letter above the bars are significantly different at $p < 0.05$ by Tukey's test. (Data from *J. Nutr.*, 132, 238, 2002.)

that SM and FSM differed somewhat in their efficacy against ethanol metabolism, as shown by aortal ethanol and acetaldehyde levels after the oral administration of ethanol and in MEOS and GST activities following the chronic exposure. FSM has organic acids (lactic and acetic acids) and probiotic bacteria that accumulate during the fermentation process[36] as well as isoflavone aglycones. It is not clarified whether these components of FSM are directly associated with ethanol consumption.

16.5 CONCLUSION

Soymilk products inhibit ethanol absorption and enhance ethanol metabolism. Isoflavones would be a candidate factor for the metabolism. Reactive metabolites generated in ethanol metabolism would trigger ethanol-induced cell injury, and the antioxidation system would suppress the damage. Soy isoflavones have antioxidative activity, perhaps acting to reinforce the system. These observations indicate that soy would have an unrevealed potential for liver function.

References

1. Tachiyashiki, K. and Imaizumi, K., Effects of vegetable oils and C18-unsaturated fatty acids on plasma ethanol levels and gastric emptying in ethanol-administrated rats, *J. Nutr. Sci. Vitaminol.*, 39, 163, 1993.
2. Yang, Z. et al., Effects of sesamin on ethanol-induced muscle relaxation, *J. Jpn. Soc. Nutr. Food Sci.*, 48, 103, 1995.
3. Kishimoto, R. et al., Combined effects of ethanol and garlic on hepatic ethanol metabolism in mice, *J. Nutr. Sci. Vitaminol.*, 45, 275, 1999.
4. Anderson, J. J. B. et al., Effects of phyto-oestrogens on tissues, *Nutr. Res. Rev.*, 12, 75, 1999.
5. Bingham, S. A. et al., Phyto-oestrogens: where are we now? *Br. J. Nutr.*, 79, 393, 1998.
6. Setchell, K. D. R. and Cassidy, A., Dietary isoflavones: biological effects and relevance to human health, *J. Nutr.*, 129, 758S, 1999.
7. Record, I. R. et al., The antioxidant activity of genistein *in vitro*, *Nutr. Biochem.*, 6, 481, 1995.
8. Robak, J. and Gryglewski, R. J., Flavonoids are scavengers of superoxide anions, *Biochem. Pharmacol.*, 37, 837, 1988.
9. Lin, R. C. et al., Isoflavonoid compounds extracted from *Pueraria lobata* suppress alcohol preference in a pharmacogenetic rat model of alcoholism, *Alcohol. Clin. Exp. Res.*, 20, 659, 1996.
10. Overstreet, D. H. et al., Suppression of alcohol intake after administration of the Chinese herbal medicine, NPI-028, and its derivatives, *Alcohol. Clin. Exp. Res.*, 20, 221, 1996.
11. Keung, W.-M. and Vallee, B. L., Daidzin: a potent, selective inhibitor of human mitochondrial aldehyde dehydrogenase, *Proc. Natl. Acad. Sci. USA*, 90, 1247, 1993.
12. Keung, W.-M., Biochemical studies of a new class of alcohol dehydrogenase inhibitors from Raix puerariae, *Alcohol. Clin. Exp. Res.*, 17, 1254, 1993.
13. Keung, W.-M., Daidzin suppresses ethanol consumption by Syrian golden hamsters without blocking acetaldehyde metabolism, *Pro. Natl. Acad. Sci. USA*, 92, 8990, 1995.

14. Xie, C. I. et al., Daidzin, an antioxidant isoflavonoid, decreases blood alcohol levels and shortens sleep time induced by ethanol intoxication, *Alcohol. Clin. Exp. Res.*, 18, 1443, 1994.
15. Tanaka, R., Probiotics: prospects of use in opportunistic infections, Fuller, R. et al., Eds., Old Herborn University seminar monograph 8, Germany, 1995, 141.
16. Kitajima, H. et al., Early administration of *Bifidobacterium breve* to preterm infants: randomized controlled trial, *Arch. Dis. Child.*, 76, F101, 1997.
17. Tojo, M. et al., The effects of *Bifidobacterium breve* administration on Campylobacter enteritis, *Acta. Paediatr. Jpn.*, 29, 160, 1987.
18. Hotta, M. et al., Clinical effects of Bifidobacterium preparations on pediatric intractable diarrhea, *Keio J. Med.*, 36, 298, 1987.
19. Izumi, T. et al., Soy isoflavone aglycones are absorbed faster and in higher amounts than their glucosides in humans, *J. Nutr.*, 130, 1695, 2000.
20. King, R. A. et al., Absorption and excretion of the soy isoflavone genistein in rats, *J. Nutr.*, 126, 176, 1996.
21. Ishikawa, F., Probiotic foods expected to prevent life-style derived diseases, *Healthist*, 150, 69, 2002. (in Japanese)
22. Kikuchi-Hayakawa et al., Effects of soy milk and Bifidobacterium fermented soy milk on lipid metabolism in aged ovariectomized rats, *Biosci. Biotech. Biochem.*, 62, 1688, 1998.
23. Kikuchi-Hayakawa, H. et al., Effects of soya milk and Bifidobacterium-fermented soya milk on plasma and liver lipids, and faecal steroids in hamsters fed on a cholesterol-free or cholesterol-enriched diet, *Br. J. Nutr.*, 79, 97, 1998.
24. Kikuchi-Hayakawa, H. et al., Effect of soy milk and Bifidobacterium-fermented soy milk on plasma and liver lipids in ovariectomized Syrian hamsters, *J. Nutr. Sci. Vitaminol.*, 46, 105, 2000.
25. Ohta, T. et al., Inhibitory effects of Bifidobacterium-fermented soy milk on 2-amino-1-methyl-6-phenylimidazo [4,5-b] pyridine-induced rat mammary carcinogenesis, with a partial contribution of its component isoflavones, *Carcinogenesis*, 21, 937, 2000.
26. Kano, M. et al., Soymilk products affect ethanol absorption and metabolism in rats during acute and chronic ethanol intake, *J. Nutr.*, 132, 238, 2002.
27. Lebsack, M. E. et al., Effect of chronic ethanol consumption on aldehyde dehydrogenase activity in the baboon, *Biochem. Pharmacol.*, 30, 2273, 1981.
28. Ingelman-Sundberg, M. et al., Ethanol-inducible cytochrome P4502E1: genetic polymorphism, regulation, and possible role in the etiology of alcohol-induced liver disease, *Alcohol*, 10, 447, 1993.
29. Fridovich, I., Oxygen radicals from acetaldehyde, *Free Rad. Biol. Med.*, 7, 557, 1989.
30. Rashba-Step, J. et al., Increased NADPH- and NADH-dependent production of superoxide and hydroxyl radical by microsome after chronic ethanol treatment, *Arch. Biochem. Biophys.*, 300, 401, 1993.
31. Viña, J. et al., Effect of ethanol on glutathione concentration in isolated hepatocytes, *Biochem. J.*, 188, 549, 1980.
32. Tsuchida, S. and Sato, K., Glutathione S-transferase isozymes, *Protein, Nucleic Acid Enzyme* (in Japanese), 33, 1564, 1988.
33. Chae, Y.-H. et al., Effects of synthetic and naturally occurring flavonoids on benzo[a]pyrene metabolism by hepatic microsomes prepared from rats treated with cytochrome P-450 inducers, *Can. Lett.*, 60, 15, 1991.

34. Ronis, M. J. et al., Altered expression and glucocorticoid-inducibility of hepatic CYP3A and CYP2B enzymes in male rats fed diets containing soy protein isolate, *J. Nutr.*, 129, 1958, 1999.
35. Ekström, G. and Ingelman-Sundberg, M., Rat liver microsomal NADPH-supported oxidase activity and lipid peroxidation dependent on ethanol inducible cytochrome P450 (P-450 IIE1), *Biochem. Pharmacol.*, 38, 1313, 1989.
36. Shimakawa, Y. et al., Evaluation of *Bifidobacterium breve* strain Yakult-fermented soymilk as a probiotic food, *Inter. J. Food. Microbio.*, 81, 131, 2003.

17 Alcohol and Retinoid Interaction

Xiang-Dong Wang and Helmut K. Seitz

CONTENTS

17.1 INTRODUCTION

Long-term and excessive alcohol intake induces numerous biochemical and molecular alterations in hepatic tissue, which result in ethanol-related liver disease.[1] Interference with vitamin A metabolism and its nutritional status is one of major alterations caused by alcohol.[2,3] Lower hepatic vitamin A levels have been well documented in alcoholics.[4,5] Several mechanisms have been proposed to explain how ethanol might interfere with retinoid metabolism in the liver (Figure 17.1). Ethanol has been found to lower the level of retinoids (retinyl ester, retinol, and retinoic acid) in the liver through increased catabolism of retinol and retinoic acid into more polar metabolites.[4,6–8] Ethanol has been seen to increase vitamin A mobilization from the liver to other organs, as evidenced by increased vitamin A concentration in extrahepatic tissue after chronic ethanol consumption.[9,10] In addition, ethanol acts as a direct competitive inhibitor of retinol oxidation to retinoic acid in liver and other tissues. These alcohol-induced changes result in decreased hepatic levels of retinol and retinyl esters, which are precursors of retinoic acid, the most active form of vitamin A and a ligand for retinoid receptors. Retinoic acid plays an important

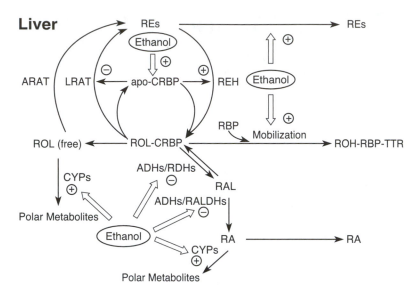

FIGURE 17.1 Simplified schematic illustration of possible interactive metabolic pathways of ethanol effects on hepatic retinoid metabolism (see text for detail). Abbreviations used are: CRBP, cellular retinol-binding protein; RBP, plasma retinol-binding protein; LRAT, lecithin:retinol acyltransferase; ARAT, acyl-CoA-retinol acyltransferase; TTR, transthyretin; ROL, retinol; RAL, retinal; REH, retinyl ester hydrolases; REs, retinyl esters; RDH, retinol dehydrogenase; ADH, alcohol dehydrogenase; ALDH, aldehyde dehydrogenase; RALDH, retinal dehydrogenase; RA, retinoic acid; CYPs, cytochrome P450 enzymes.

role in controlling cell growth, differentiation, and apoptosis and is of potential clinical interest in cancer chemoprevention and treatment.[11] Therefore, interference with the retinoic acid metabolism by ethanol has important impacts on the etiology, prevention, and treatment of alcohol-related disease. In this chapter, recent studies on the ethanol interaction with retinoid homeostasis and signal transduction pathways are discussed.

17.2   ETHANOL ACTS AS A COMPETITIVE INHIBITOR OF RETINOL OXIDATION TO RETINOIC ACID

As a result of earlier reports on ethanol as a competitive inhibitor of retinol oxidation in both liver and other tissues,[12–15] substantial research has been done regarding to the involvement of alcohol dehydrogenases (ADH) as retinol dehydrogenases in retinol oxidation. Han et al.[16] showed that the retinol-oxidizing activity of human class I ADH was 90% inhibited by 5 mM ethanol (blood ethanol levels of 5 to 20 mM are usually reached after social drinking), and the retinol-oxidizing activity of some forms of human class II and III ADH was 60 to 80% inhibited by 20 mM or 50 mM ethanol (only seen in heavy drinking). It has been shown that ethanol inhibits both all-*trans*-retinol and 9-*cis*-retinol oxidation by class IV ADH with K_i values of 6 to 10 mM.[17] Furthermore, Kedishvili et al.[18] showed that the contribution of ADH isozymes to retinoic acid biosynthesis depends on the amount of free retinol in cells, and that physiological levels of ethanol can substantially inhibit the oxidation of retinol by human ADHs. These earlier observations have been substantiated by the demonstration that biosynthesis of retinoic acid following a dose of retinol was reduced by 82% in ADH null mutant mice (*ADH1*[-/-]).[19] This reduction was similar in magnitude to the inhibition in retinoic acid biosynthesis seen in wild-type mice treated with ethanol (87% decrease). Recent study has also shown that the major oxidative metabolite of ethanol, acetaldehyde, inhibits the generation of retinoic acid in human prenatal tissue.[20] In addition, it has been reported that ethanol inhibits the oxidation of retinol into retinoic acid in the human gastric and esophageal mucosa[2] and rat colon mucosa.[21] These studies clearly demonstrate that retinoic acid biosynthesis can be impaired by ethanol, which may contribute the increased risk of developing certain alcohol-related diseases in liver and other tissues, such as cancer, fibrosis, and fetal alcohol syndrome.

17.3 CHRONIC ETHANOL INTAKE INCREASES CATABOLISM OF VITAMIN A AND RETINOIC ACID INTO POLAR METABOLITES

Chronic alcohol intake induces hepatic cytochrome P450 enzymes (CYP), which metabolize numerous compounds and may contribute to ethanol-induced liver disease.[22] Increased catabolism of vitamin A into 4-hydroxy-retinol in the liver has been shown in rats treated with ethanol.[4,6] Many microsomal CYP isozymes such as CYP1A1, CYP2B4, CYP2C3, CYP2C7, CYP2E1, and CYP26 have been found to be involved in retinoid metabolism in rats.[23–26] In a recent study by Liu et al.,[27] treatment of rats with high-dose ethanol led to a significant reduction in hepatic retinol and retinyl ester concentrations, and the occurrence of several polar retinoid metabolites, compared with rats pair-fed with an isocaloric control diet containing the same amount of vitamin A. These results confirm and substantiate data from previous *in vivo* studies.[4,6,7] It is interesting that chlormethiazole, an efficient inhibitor of CYP2E1,[28,29] can prevent this ethanol-enhanced catabolism of retinol and retinoic acid in rats.[8,27] In humans and rats, the main ethanol-induced CYP in the liver is CYP2E1, which plays an important role in the pathogenesis of alcoholic liver disease.[30] Chlormethiazole treatment is associated with significantly reduced formation of oxidative polar metabolites of retinol,[27] consistent with our previous report that CYP2E1 is partially responsible for the catabolism of retinoic acid in hepatic tissue after ethanol treatment.[8] Because the chemical structures of retinol and retinoic acid are very similar, it appears that retinol undergoes CYPs-mediated metabolism similar to that of retinoic acid. The inhibitory effect of chlormethiazole on CYP2E1 may be related to its regulatory effect on CYP2E1 transcription *in vivo* and CYP2E1 catalytic activity *in vitro* mediated by binding to the heme iron of the enzyme.[28,29,31] A recent study also showed that chlormethiazole can inhibit CYP1A and CYP2C at the mRNA level in rat nasal mucosa.[32] Although further investigation of the activity and expression of ethanol-induced CYPs is necessary to determine which other CYPs are involved in the processes, the prevention of reduced retinoid status in the livers of ethanol-fed rats by chlormethiazole treatment indicates that the breakdown of retinoids by microsomal CYP2E1 is key mechanism for the ethanol-enhanced catabolism of retinoids in hepatic tissue after treatment with alcohol.

Since a significant CYP2E1 induction in humans occurs a week following the ingestion of ethanol, and the disappearance of CYP2E1 was found to be significant 3 to 8 d following ethanol withdrawal,[33] it is possible that CYP2E1 enzyme induction in chronic intermittent drinking could continue to be a factor in destroying retinol and retinoic acid, even after alcohol is cleared. This provides a possible explanation for why chronic and excessive alcohol intake is a risk not only for hepatic but also for extra-hepatic cell proliferation and carcinogenesis since it has been reported that CYP2E1 is also present and inducible by alcohol in the esophagus, forestomach, and surface epithelium of the proximal colon.[34] The restoration of vitamin A level by chlormethiazole also provides a possible mechanism for the protective effect of chlormethiazole on ethanol-induced liver injury, as reported recently.[35]

17.4 CHRONIC ETHANOL CONSUMPTION ENHANCES VITAMIN A MOBILIZATION FROM THE LIVER TO OTHER ORGANS

Ethanol increased vitamin A mobilization from the liver to other organs[9,10] although the exact mechanism(s) is still unclear. There are several possible explanations (Figure 17.1). First, it is well known that cellular retinol-binding protein (CRBP) is necessary to maintain normal retinyl ester synthesis and storage.[36] Elevated apo-CRBP (unbound to retinol) has a stimulatory effect on retinyl ester hydrolysis[37] and an inhibitory effect on retinol esterification,[38] particularly in vitamin A deficiency. It has been reported that the expression of CRBP mRNA increased in the liver of ethanol-treated rats[27] and in the fetal snout of rats after alcohol treatment.[39] Therefore, one can hypothesize that elevated apo-CRBP levels in the liver of ethanol-fed rats may stimulate hepatic retinyl ester hydrolase (Figure 17.1). This hypothesis is supported by the findings that the reduction of hepatic retinyl esters in ethanol-fed rats is not due to impairment of retinol esterification[27] and the hydrolysis of retinyl ester can be stimulated by ethanol in rat liver *in vitro*.[40] Since the distribution of retinol between retinol-binding protein (RBP) in plasma and CRBP in cytosol is in equilibrium,[41] retinol produced from ethanol-accelerated hydrolysis of retinyl ester in liver could be transported into peripheral tissue. Another hypothesis is that low levels of retinoic acid in the liver and peripheral tissues due to ethanol may function as "a feedback signal" to regulate hepatic vitamin A metabolism.[42] This concept was supported by our recent demonstration that the restoration of plasma retinoic acid level to normal by chlormethiazole in ethanol-fed rats was correlated with both a reduction in the elevated retinyl palmitate levels in the plasma and an increase in the retinyl palmitate in the liver.[27] It has been demonstrated that retinoic acid treatment increases retinol esterification in the liver of vitamin A-deficient mice and rats.[26] However, the restoration of retinoic acid levels by chlormethiazole treatment did not increase the expression or activity of hepatic lecithin retinal acyltransferase (LRAT) in ethanol-fed rats.[27] This is consistent with our previous observation that retinoic acid treatment did not increase hepatic concentrations of retinyl ester in ethanol-fed rats.[43] It appears that, in the situation of excessive and chronic ethanol consumption, the mechanism of this regulation of retinoic acid is more complicated and involves multiple factors such as enzyme regulation, lipoprotein secretion, and CRBP and RBP function. For example, the restoration of lowered hepatic retinyl palmitate levels and elevated blood levels of retinyl palmitate to normal levels by chlormethiazole treatment in ethanol-fed rats may be due to either blocking the ethanol-induced catabolism of vitamin A or protecting the integrity of the hepatic tissue, which prevents release of retinyl palmitate into the circulation. Clearly, more studies regarding the exact mechanism of ethanol-induced mobilization of hepatic vitamin A are needed.

17.5 CHRONIC AND EXCESSIVE ETHANOL INTAKE INTERFERES WITH RETINOID SIGNAL TRANSDUCTION, RESULTING IN ENHANCED CELL PROLIFERATION AND DYSREGULATED APOPTOSIS

It has been shown that hepatocytes become hyperproliferative after chronic ethanol treatment[43–46] which may contribute to ethanol-induced disease. Recent studies have demonstrated that the restoration of ethanol-lowered retinoic acid levels to normal levels alters hepatocyte proliferation and apoptosis in alcohol-fed rats,[43,46] indicating that retinoids could protect against alcohol-induced diseases. The interaction of ethanol and retinoid signaling may involve several mechanisms (Figure 17.2).

First, retinoid receptors (RARs and RXRs) function as ligand-dependent transcription factors, thereby transcriptionally activating a series of genes with distinct antiproliferative activity and tumor suppressor functions. It has been reported that the expression of the *RARβ* gene, a tumor suppressor, was downregulated by ethanol, even in the presence of retinol,[47] as well as in tumorigenic hepatoma cell lines.[48,49] We have shown that all-*trans*-retinoic acid supplementation in ethanol-fed rats greatly increased the levels of retinoid responsive mitogen-activated kinase phosphatase-1 (MKP-1) in liver tissue.[46] This induction of MKP-1 attenuated the ethanol-induced phosphorylation of Jun N-terminal kinases (JNK) which have been shown to be required for tumorigenesis using a multistep carcinogenesis model in mice lacking the *JNK2* gene.[50] Therefore, the downregulation of specific RARs (e.g., loss or low expression of RARβ as a tumor suppressor) or lack of retinoic acid due to excessive ethanol intake could interfere with retinoid signal transduction, resulting in enhanced cell proliferation, and potentially malignant transformation.[11]

Second, recent evidence has accumulated supporting a role for ethanol in the regulation of activator protein-1 (AP-1, a transcriptionally active dimmer of c-*Jun* and c-*Fos*) gene expression. Antiproliferative and antioncogenic effects of retinoids can be mediated by inhibiting AP-1 activity.[51] Retinoid receptors and the transcription factor AP-1 (Jun/Fos) can interfere with each others' activities.[52] For example, all three RAR subtypes (RARα, β, and γ) could effectively inhibit phorbol ester-induced AP-1 activity in either a retinoic acid-dependent or acid-independent

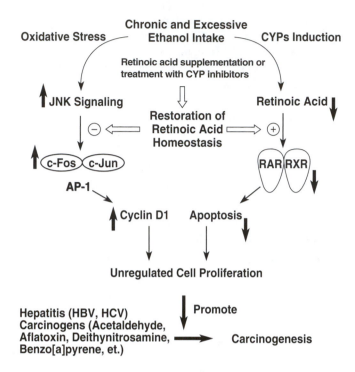

FIGURE 17.2 Simplified schematic illustration of possible interaction of ethanol related to retinoid signal transduction, Jun N-terminal kinases (JNK)-dependent signaling pathway and activator protein-1 (AP-1 [c-*Jun* and c-*Fos*]) nuclear complex on ethanol-promoted carcinogenesis. (Adapted from Wang, X.D. Retinoids and alcohol-related carcinogenesis. *J Nutr* 133, 287S–290S, 2003.)

manner.[53] Recently, we have shown that retinoic acid treatment in ethanol-fed rats dramatically inhibited the ethanol-induced overexpression of c-*Jun*, AP-1 DNA binding activities, the levels of cyclin D1 (an AP-1-dependent player in cell proliferation), and ethanol-induced proliferating cellular nuclear antigen (PCNA)-positive hepatocytes.[43,46] Since the transactivation of AP-1-dependent genes is required for tumor promotion[54] and cyclin D1 plays an important role in tumorigenesis and tumor progression in hepatocellular carcinoma,[55] the identification of c-*Jun* and cyclin D1 as two potential targets of retinoic acid action in ethanol-fed rats indicates that retinoids may play an important role in preventing certain types of ethanol-promoted cancer (Figure 17.2).

Third, retinoids have been implicated in the induction of cell death in many tumor-derived cultured cell systems through retinoid receptors-dependent or receptors-independent mechanisms.[56] Since dysregulated apoptosis contributes to the pathogenesis of a number of human diseases, it is possible that, under certain conditions such as diminished hepatic retinoid signaling due to prolonged alcohol intake, apoptosis may become dysregulated, thereby promoting genomic instability and neoplasia. Recently, we investigated whether hepatocellular apoptosis can be regulated by either ethanol feeding or retinoic acid supplementation. We showed that ethanol feeding in rats for a 1-month period (subacute phase) significantly increased apoptosis; however, after 6 months of ethanol feeding, hepatic apoptosis decreased significantly relative to controls, as assessed by both the Caspase 3 assay as well as the TUNEL method.[46] Interestingly, retinoic acid supplementation increased apoptosis by fourfold in ethanol-fed rats, as compared with ethanol treatment alone.[46] Although the mechanism is not well defined, these data indicate that induction of apoptosis by retinoic acid plays an important role in preventing ethanol-promoted carcinogenesis by eliminating cells with unrepairable alterations in the genome or killing neoplastic cells.

17.6 SUMMARY

Understanding the metabolic and molecular details behind the altered homeostasis of retinoids (retinyl esters, retinol, and retinoic acid) by ethanol may yield insights into pathophysiological processes in human disease. The restoration of retinoic acid homeostasis with either retinoic acid or an inhibitor of retinoic acid catabolism suppresses alcohol-induced cell hyperproliferation and restores alcohol-dysregulated apoptosis, thereby reducing the risk of alcohol-related disease in the liver as well as in peripheral organs. The mechanism of retinoic acid action may involve induction of tumor suppressors, a "cross talk" with other signaling pathways activated by alcohol, inhibition of AP-1 (c-*Jun* and c-*Fos*) activity and induction of apoptosis. A deeper understanding of the molecular mechanism(s) involved is needed before pursuing retinoids in the prevention and treatment of alcohol-related disease.

ACKNOWLEDGMENT

This work was supported by NIH/NIAAA Grant R01AA12628.

References

1. Lieber, C.S. and Leo, M.A. Metabolism of ethanol and some associated adverse effects on the liver and the stomach. *Recent Dev Alcohol* 14, 7–40, 1998.
2. Crabb, D.W. et al. Alcohol and retinoids. *Alcohol Clin Exp Res* 25, 207S–217S, 2001.
3. Wang, X.-D. Retinoids and alcoholic liver disease. In: Agarwal, D.P. and Seitz, H.K. Eds. *Alcohol in Health and Disease*. pp. 427–452. New York: Marcel Dekker, 2001.
4. Leo, M.A. and Lieber, C.S. Hepatic vitamin A depletion in alcoholic liver injury. *N Engl J Med* 307, 597–601, 1982.
5. Hautekeete, M.L. et al. Hepatic stellate cells and liver retinoid content in alcoholic liver disease in humans. *Alcohol Clin Exp Res* 22, 494–500, 1998.
6. Sato, M. and Lieber, C.S. Increased metabolism of retinoic acid after chronic ethanol consumption in rat liver microsomes. *Arch Biochem Biophys* 213, 557–564, 1982.
7. Wang, X.D. et al. Chronic alcohol intake reduces retinoic acid concentration and enhances AP-1 (c-*Jun* and c-*Fos*) expression in rat liver. *Hepatology* 28, 744–750, 1998.
8. Liu, C. et al. Ethanol enhances retinoic acid metabolism into polar metabolites in rat liver via induction of cytochrome P4502E1. *Gastroenterology* 120, 179–189, 2001.

9. Leo, M.A., Kim, C., and Lieber, C.S. Increased vitamin A in esophagus and other extrahepatic tissues after chronic ethanol consumption in the rat. *Alcohol Clin Exp Res* 10, 487–492, 1986.

10. Mobarhan, S. et al. Age-related effects of chronic ethanol intake on vitamin A status in Fisher 344 rats. *J Nutr* 121, 510–517, 1991.

11. Lippman, S.M. and Lotan, R. Advances in the development of retinoids as chemopreventive agents. *J Nutr* 130, 479S–482S, 2000.

12. Mezey, E. and Holt, P.R. The inhibitory effect of ethanol on retinol oxidation by human liver and cattle retina. *Exp Mol Pathol* 15, 148–156, 1971.

13. Julia, P., Farres, J., and Pares, X. Ocular alcohol dehydrogenase in the rat: regional distribution and kinetics of the ADH-1 isoenzyme with retinol and retinal. *Exp Eye Res* 42, 305–314, 1986.

14. Yang, Z.N. et al. Catalytic efficiency of human alcohol dehydrogenases for retinol oxidation and retinal reduction. *Alcohol Clin Exp Res* 18, 587–591, 1994.

15. Boleda, M.D. et al. Physiological substrates for rat alcohol dehydrogenase classes: aldehydes of lipid peroxidation, omega-hydroxyfatty acids, and retinoids. *Arch Biochem Biophys* 307, 85–90, 1993.

16. Han, C.L. et al. Contribution to first-pass metabolism of ethanol and inhibition by ethanol for retinol oxidation in human alcohol dehydrogenase family — implications for etiology of fetal alcohol syndrome and alcohol-related diseases. *Eur J Biochem* 254, 25–31, 1998.

17. Allali-Hassani, A. et al. Retinoids, omega-hydroxyfatty acids and cytotoxic aldehydes as physiological substrates, and H2-receptor antagonists as pharmacological inhibitors, of human class IV alcohol dehydrogenase. *FEBS Lett* 426, 362–366, 1998.

18. Kedishvili, N.Y. et al. Effect of cellular retinol-binding protein on retinol oxidation by human class IV retinol/alcohol dehydrogenase and inhibition by ethanol. *Biochem Biophys Res Commun* 249, 191–196, 1998.

19. Molotkov, A. and Duester, G. Retinol/ethanol drug interaction during acute alcohol intoxication in mice involves inhibition of retinol metabolism to retinoic acid by alcohol dehydrogenase. *J Biol Chem* 277, 22553–22557, 2002.

20. Khalighi, M. et al. Inhibition of human prenatal biosynthesis of all-*trans*-retinoic acid by ethanol, ethanol metabolites, and products of lipid peroxidation reactions: a possible role for CYP2E1. *Biochem Pharmacol* 57, 811–821, 1999.

21. Parlesak, A. et al. Inhibition of retinol oxidation by ethanol in the rat liver and colon. *Gut* 47, 825–831, 2000.

22. Lieber, C.S. Mechanisms of ethanol–drug–nutrition interactions. *J Toxicol Clin Toxicol* 32, 631–681, 1994.

23. Raner, G.M., Vaz, A.D., and Coon, M.J. Metabolism of all-*trans*, 9-*cis*, and 13-*cis* isomers of retinal by purified isozymes of microsomal cytochrome P450 and mechanism-based inhibition of retinoid oxidation by citral. *Mol Pharmacol* 49, 515–522, 1996.

24. Roberts, E.S., Vaz, A.D., and Coon, M.J. Role of isozymes of rabbit microsomal cytochrome P-450 in the metabolism of retinoic acid, retinol, and retinal. *Mol Pharmacol* 41, 427–433, 1992.

25. Tomita, S. et al. Identification of a microsomal retinoic acid synthase as a microsomal cytochrome P-450-linked monooxygenase system. *Int J Biochem* 25, 1775–1784, 1993.

26. Zolfaghari, R. and Ross, A.C. Lecithin: retinol acyltransferase from mouse and rat liver. CDNA cloning and liver-specific regulation by dietary vitamin A and retinoic acid. *J Lipid Res* 41, 2024–2034, 2000.

27. Liu, C. et al. Chlormethiazole treatment prevents reduced hepatic vitamin A levels in ethanol-fed rats. *Alcohol Clin Exp Res* 26, 1703–1709, 2002.

28. Gebhardt, A.C. et al. Chlormethiazole inhibition of cytochrome P450 2E1 as assessed by chlorzoxazone hydroxylation in humans. *Hepatology* 26, 957–961, 1997.

29. Hu, Y. et al. Chlormethiazole as an efficient inhibitor of cytochrome P450 2E1 expression in rat liver. *J Pharmacol Exp Ther* 269, 1286–1291, 1994.

30. Lieber, C.S. Cytochrome P-4502E1: its physiological and pathological role. *Physiol Rev* 77, 517–544, 1997.

31. Simi, A. and Ingelman-Sundberg, M. Post-translational inhibition of cytochrome P-450 2E1 expression by chlomethiazole in Fao hepatoma cells. *J Pharmacol Exp Ther* 289, 847–852, 1999.

32. Longo, V. et al. Effect of starvation and chlormethiazole on cytochrome P450s of rat nasal mucosa. *Biochem Pharmacol* 59, 1425–1432, 2000.

33. Oneta, C.M. et al. Dynamics of cytochrome P4502E1 activity in man: induction by ethanol and disappearance during withdrawal phase. *J Hepatol* 36, 47–52, 2002.

34. Shimizu, M. et al. Immunohistochemical localization of ethanol-inducible P450IIE1 in the rat alimentary tract. *Gastroenterology* 99, 1044–1053, 1990.

35. Gouillon, Z. et al. Inhibition of ethanol-induced liver disease in the intragastric feeding rat model by chlormethiazole. *Proc Soc Exp Biol Med* 224, 302–308, 2000.

36. Napoli, J.L. Biochemical pathways of retinoid transport, metabolism, and signal transduction. *Clin Immunol Immunopathol* 80, S52–62, 1996.

37. Boerman, M.H. and Napoli, J.L. Cholate-independent retinyl ester hydrolysis. Stimulation by Apo-cellular retinol-binding protein. *J Biol Chem* 266, 22273–22278, 1991.

38. Herr, F.M. and Ong, D.E. Differential interaction of lecithin-retinol acyltransferase with cellular retinol binding proteins. *Biochemistry* 31, 6748–6755, 1992.

39. Zachman, R.D. and Grummer, M.A. Prenatal ethanol consumption increases retinol and cellular retinol-binding protein expression in the rat fetal snout. *Biol Neonate* 80, 152–157, 2001.

40. Friedman, H. et al. *In vitro* stimulation of rat liver retinyl ester hydrolase by ethanol. *Arch Biochem Biophys* 269, 69–74, 1989.

41. Noy, N. and Blaner, W.S. Interactions of retinol with binding proteins: studies with rat cellular retinol-binding protein and with rat retinol-binding protein. *Biochemistry* 30, 6380–6386, 1991.

42. Ross, A.C., Zolfaghari, R., and Weisz, J. Vitamin A: recent advances in the biotransformation, transport, and metabolism of retinoids. *Curr Opin Gastroenterol* 17, 184–192, 2001.

43. Chung, J. et al. Restoration of retinoic acid concentration suppresses ethanol-enhanced c-Jun expression and hepatocyte proliferation in rat liver. *Carcinogenesis* 22, 1213–1219, 2001.

44. Baroni, G.S. et al. Chronic ethanol feeding increases apoptosis and cell proliferation in rat liver. *J Hepatol* 20, 508–513, 1994.

45. Halsted, C.H. et al. Ethanol feeding of micropigs alters methionine metabolism and increases hepatocellular apoptosis and proliferation. *Hepatology* 23, 497–505, 1996.

46. Chung, J. et al. Retinoic acid inhibits hepatic Jun N-terminal kinase-dependent signaling pathway in ethanol-fed rats. *Oncogene* 21, 1539–1547, 2002.

47. Grummer, M.A. and Zachman, R.D. Interaction of ethanol with retinol and retinoic acid in RAR beta and GAP-43 expression. *Neurotoxicol Teratol* 22, 829–836, 2000.

48. Li, C. and Wan, Y.J. Differentiation and antiproliferation effects of retinoic acid receptor beta in hepatoma cells. *Cancer Lett* 124, 205–211, 1998.

49. Wan, Y.J., Cai, Y., and Magee, T.R. Retinoic acid differentially regulates retinoic acid receptor-mediated pathways in the Hep3B cell line. *Exp Cell Res* 238, 241–247, 1998.

50. Chen, N. et al. Suppression of skin tumorigenesis in c-Jun NH(2)-terminal kinase-2-deficient mice. *Cancer Res* 61, 3908–3912, 2001.

51. Altucci, L. and Gronemeyer, H. The promise of retinoids to fight against cancer. *Nat Rev Cancer* 1, 181–193, 2001.

52. Gottlicher, M., Heck, S., and Herrlich, P. Transcriptional cross-talk, the second mode of steroid hormone receptor action. *J Mol Med* 76, 480–489, 1998.

53. Lin, F. et al. Unique anti-activator protein-1 activity of retinoic acid receptor beta. *Cancer Res* 60, 3271–3280, 2000.

54. Young, M.R. et al. Transgenic mice demonstrate AP-1 (activator protein-1) transactivation is required for tumor promotion. *Proc Natl Acad Sci USA* 96, 9827–9832, 1999.

55. Uto, H. et al. Transduction of antisense cyclin D1 using two-step gene transfer inhibits the growth of rat hepatoma cells. *Cancer Res* 61, 4779–4783, 2001.

56. Simoni, D. and Tolomeo, M. Retinoids, apoptosis and cancer. *Curr Pharm Des* 7, 1823–1837, 2001.

57. Wang, X.D. Retinoids and alcohol-related carcinogenesis. *J Nutr* 133, 287S–290S, 2003.

18 Plasma Lipids, Lipoproteins, and Alcohol

William V. Rumpler, David J. Baer, and Beverly A. Clevidence

CONTENTS

18.1 INTRODUCTION

18.1.1 ALCOHOL CONSUMPTION AND CARDIOVASCULAR DISEASE RISK

In 1974 Klatsky et al.[1,2] reported a clear relationship between alcohol consumption and decreased risk of heart attack after taking into consideration smoking habits. Two decades later, Maclure[3] in a meta-analysis of cohort studies demonstrated a reduced risk of myocardial infarction (MI) in individuals consuming 2 to 3 drinks per day, when compared to nondrinkers. This reduction in risk of MI has been observed in high-risk populations such as diabetics,[4] older individuals, individuals with ischemic left-ventricular dysfunction,[5] or individuals with prior year MI.[6]

In addition to reduced risk of MI, light or moderate alcohol consumption may be protective against stroke. Reynolds et al.[7] reported that light to moderate alcohol consumption was associated with a decrease in overall risk of stroke. Risk of ischemic stroke, the major type of stroke, decreased but there was an increasing incidence of hemorrhagic stroke with increased alcohol consumption. Reduced risk of total and ischemic stroke was observed with alcohol consumption in male physicians[8] although greater than one drink per day did not increase the observed benefit.

The reduced risk of coronary heart disease (CHD) observed with light to moderate alcohol consumption has been attributed to a number of physiological changes. Alcohol consumption affects blood lipid and lipoprotein concentrations, platelet function, fibrinolytic activity, and vascular wall inflammatory responsiveness. Klatsky[2] recently identified reductions in inflammation, blood clotting, and stress as possible contributors to the reduction in risk associated with CHD. However, most studies identify improvements in blood lipid profile as accounting for more than half of the reduction in risk of CHD.[9]

18.1.2 Blood Lipids and CHD

Current thinking on the etiology of CHD suggests that accumulation of low-density lipoprotein particles in the arterial wall and their subsequent oxidation precipitates an inflammatory reaction and subsequent immune response. The infiltration of arterial walls by macrophages and the formation of foam cells ultimately result in plaque formation. In the most common scenario for heart attack, a plaque in a coronary artery ruptures, triggering thrombus formation and occlusion of the artery. Blood lipid and lipoprotein concentrations play a central role in the progression of CHD and are strong indicators of future risk for development of the disease. Thus, much of the work over the last two decades regarding CHD risk has focused on the various lipoproteins and how to change, through lifestyle or drug intervention, their concentrations or ratios.

Lipoproteins are broadly classified by particle size and sedimentation behavior in an ultracentrifuge. The most common categories are (from least to most dense) chylomicrons, very-low density lipoprotein (VLDL), low-density lipoprotein (LDL), and high-density lipoprotein (HDL). Viewed simplistically, these categories of lipoproteins perform different functions in the transport of triglycerides and cholesterol. Chylomicrons are principally involved in the transport of triglycerides and cholesterol from the intestine to the liver. VLDL, which is high in triglyceride, and LDL, which is high in cholesterol, transport lipid to peripheral tissues. HDL serves to transport cholesterol from peripheral tissues to the liver where it can be processed for excretion.

Elevated concentrations of LDL cholesterol (LDL-C) and decreased concentrations of HDL cholesterol (HDL-C) have consistently been shown to be risk factors for CHD.[10–13] Intervention studies suggest that a 25% reduction in LDL-C concentration results in greater than 30% reduction in CHD.[14,15] In the Lipid Research Clinics Coronary Primary Prevention Trial[16] a 35% reduction in LDL-C, induced by a cholesterol-lowering drug, reduced the incidence of CHD by half when compared to controls. HDL–C concentrations have also been shown to be a strong predictor of CHD.[17,18] Concentrations of HDL–C in the lowest quintile of prospective studies have been associated with a three-[19] and a fourfold[20] increase in risk of CHD.

It has been estimated that an increase in HDL–C of 1.0 mg/dl is associated with a 2% reduction in risk of CHD in men and 3% in women.[11]

In addition to the cholesterol content, the particle size and specific apoprotein content of LDL and HDL have been related to cardiovascular risk. There is a clear inverse relationship between LDL particle size and increased risk for ischemic heart disease.[21] A similar relationship has been observed between HDL particle size and cardiovascular disease risk[22] but may be dependent on the apoprotein content. Gotto[23] describes HDL lipid–protein complex as being comprised of two major classes based on density. The HDL_2 is larger and less dense than the HDL_3 particle. HDL_2 is generally thought to be more protective against CVD than is HDL_3.[19,24]

Another approach, subfractioning HDL based on apoprotein content, characterizes HDL as those that contain apo A-I but not apo A-II (LpA-I) and those that contain apo A-I and A-II (LpA-I: A-II). Although HDL_2 is richer in LpA-I and HDL_3 is richer in LpA-I: A-II, the apo A-defined and density-defined particles are not identical. The apo A-defined approach gained attention when Barbaras et al.[25] reported that the HDL subfraction containing predominantly apo A-I was involved in the movement of cholesterol out of cultured adipocytes. More recently, CHD patients have been reported to have lower amounts of LpA-I[26–29] or proportions[29]of LpA-I to LpA-I:A-II relative to controls.

Lipoprotein (a) [Lp(a)] is a highly atherogenic lipoprotein comprised of a glycoprotein, apolipoprotein (a) that is attached to LDL. Lp(a) levels are thought to be under genetic control[30] and not readily altered by diet.[31]

18.2 ALCOHOL AND BLOOD LIPIDS

18.2.1 TOTAL BLOOD LIPID CONCENTRATIONS

A number of population-based studies have revealed a significant relationship between alcohol consumption and changes in blood lipids and lipoproteins.[12,32–37] In one of the first reports to examine the relationship between alcohol consumption and blood lipid concentrations Ostrander et al.[38] reported significantly higher triglyceride concentrations in men who drank regularly. Their observation of higher circulating triglycerides has been a consistent finding in subsequent studies with high concentrations of alcohol consumption, but an alcohol intake below 60 to 80 g/d[39] may not elevate plasma triglyceride. In studies where both diet and alcohol were controlled for 2 months, Clevidence et al.[40] did not observe a change in triglyceride concentrations in premenopausal women who consumed two drinks per day, and Rumpler et al.[41] did not observe an effect of alcohol on triglyceride concentrations in a mixed population of pre- and postmenopausal women who consumed one drink per day. However, in postmenopausal women Baer et al.[42] reported a significant decrease in triglyceride with consumption of one and two drinks per day. In addition, they reported that the greatest response was in individuals with the highest level of triglycerides. In some uncontrolled diet studies, triglyceride concentrations increased after alcohol consumption.[43] On the other hand, a stratified random sample of English women aged 25 to 69 years who consumed moderate amounts of alcohol (1 to 20 g/d) had lower plasma triglyceride concentrations than did nondrinkers in a cross-sectional study of the population.[44] There are also gender differences in the response of triglyceride to alcohol. In a comparison of drinkers and nondrinkers, higher triglyceride concentrations were observed in men but not women and only for men with high levels of alcohol consumption.[36]

The effect on circulating cholesterol concentrations has been less consistent with some studies reporting higher concentrations in drinkers[45,46] and other studies reporting no effect.[47,48] Ostrander et al.[38] reported elevated cholesterol concentrations in drinking men under 50 years of age but no difference in men over 50. Srivastava et al.,[39] in a review, suggested that some of the inconsistency seen in the response of cholesterol to alcohol consumption might be related to the fat level in the diet. They observed that individuals consuming a high fat diet might be more sensitive to the effects of alcohol on blood lipids.

18.2.2 LDL–CHOLESTEROL

Prospective studies have examined the relationship between lipoprotein concentrations, alcohol consumption, and CHD. The association between LDL and drinking has been inconsistent with some studies showing no effect[49,50] and others reporting a reduction of LDL–C.[51,52] The few clinical trials in which alcohol intake was controlled have generally, but not always,[53,54] found a decrease in LDL–C concentrations due to alcohol consumption in men,[55,56] premenopausal women,[40] and postmenopausal women.[41,42]

The reduction in LDL–C is not necessarily accompanied by a reduction in the amount of apoprotein B (apo B), the primary protein in LDL. In a study[53] with both obese and lean men, alcohol consumption increased apo B concentrations and decreased LDL–C concentrations in the lean men but not the obese. Furthermore, an alcohol-induced reduction in LDL–C level was not accompanied by a reduction in the apo B level in a group of premenopausal women.[40] Since the amount of apo B is proportional to the number of LDL particles, the reduction in LDL–C may be a function of each LDL particle carrying less cholesterol and not a reduction in total number of particles.

The effect of moderate intake of alcohol on Lp(a) concentration has been reported for few studies. Alcohol intake did not alter the Lp(a) concentration of healthy subjects in studies that controlled alcohol intake at 30 mg/d for 2 months[57] and at 60 mg/d for 3 weeks.[58] However, variable results have been reported for alcohol-dependent subjects. Lp(a) concentration has been reported to both increase[59,60] and decrease[61] following abstinence for 3 to 4 weeks. In patients with untreated essential hypertension,[62] self-reported alcohol consumption was inversely and dose dependently related to Lp(a) concentrations.

18.2.3 HDL–CHOLESTEROL

At least half of the reduced risk in CHD associated with alcohol consumption has been attributed to changes in circulating concentrations of HDL–C and HDL subfractions.[9] Observational studies of large populations have shown that regular consumers of alcohol have higher circulating concentrations of HDL–C than do those who abstain from alcohol,[63–65] and these higher HDL–C concentrations are associated with lower CVD risk. Clinical trials have confirmed the effect of alcohol consumption on circulating HDL–C concentrations in men[66,67] and pre-[40] and postmenopausal[42] women. However, there does seem to be some gender difference in the response to alcohol consumption.[36,37] Women may be more sensitive to the effect of alcohol on HDL–C. At least two studies have reported more pronounced HDL–C changes in women than in men with consumption of one drink per day or less.[36,68]

Not only is there a consistent effect of alcohol consumption on HDL-C concentrations, there appears be a dose–response relationship between the two. A significant positive linear relationship between alcohol intake, ranging from 13 to 51 g/d, and an increase in HDL–C concentration was observed in a mixed population of 14 subjects by De Oliveira et al.[56] Baer et al.[42] reported HDL–C concentrations of 54, 55, and 57 mg/dl with alcohol intakes of 0, 15, and 30 g/d in postmenopausal women.

Although the effect of alcohol on HDL–C has been shown consistently, the effect on HDL subfractions is not entirely clear. Alcohol-induced increases in HDL_2 and HDL_3 have been reported in premenopausal women consuming 30 g alcohol/d,[40] in men consuming 60 g alcohol/d,[58] and in men and women who reported regular alcohol consumption.[49] A dose-dependent response was observed by Valimaki et al.[67] HDL_2 increased when men consumed approximately two drinks per day and both HDL_2 and HDL_3 increased when alcohol consumption was increased to five drinks per day. Recent studies observed higher concentrations of HDL_3 but not HDL_2 as alcohol consumption increased up to 40 g alcohol/d[50] or 160 g alcohol/d.[69]

Alcohol modulates apo A-defined particles, most typically increasing LpA-I[55] or LpA-I:A-II[27,33] or both.[40,58] Only a couple of studies have assessed apo A-defined particles while controlling the alcohol intake of subjects. In these, alcohol consumption in the range of 30 to 60 g/d increases both LpA-I and LpA-I:A-II.[40,58] It has been suggested,[56] based on fractional catabolic rates and transport rates of apo A-I and II, that HDL–C levels increase in response to moderate alcohol consumption as a result of increased production of the lipoprotein rather than decreased removal from circulation.

18.2.4 INTERACTION WITH MENOPAUSE

A woman's risk of CHD increases after menopause, whether the hormonal change is natural or artificially induced. For example, the incidence of coronary artery disease in women increases after bilateral oophorectomy[70] or early natural menopause.[71] The risk of CHD has been linked to decreases in endogenous estrogens after cessation of menses.[72] One possibility is that the increase in plasma LDL–C that occurs with and before[73] menopause is associated with the increase in risk of CHD. Even more so than a lowered LDL–C concentration, high HDL–C is an important predictor of a decreased risk of coronary artery disease in women.[17,18] Alcohol has been shown to decrease the risk of CHD in middle-aged women[12,74] and affects both LDL–C and HDL–C metabolism in premenopausal women[40] and postmenopausal women.[12]

Studies conducted in our laboratory suggest that the effects of alcohol on plasma LDL–C and HDL–C of postmenopausal women are generally consistent with the effects observed in premenopausal women.[40–42] However, it appears that the magnitude of the response to alcohol is less in postmenopausal women than in premenopausal women. In premenopausal women who consumed 30 g alcohol/d, the LDL–C concentration was 8% lower than observed after consumption of a controlled diet with no alcohol.[40] In postmenopausal women who ate a diet of similar composition, the LDL–C concentration was 5% lower with the consumption of an equivalent amount of alcohol.[42] Similarly, the HDL–C concentration increased by 10% in premenopausal women who consumed 30 g alcohol/d compared with a 5% increase in postmenopausal women. Thus, although the pattern of change for LDL–C and HDL–C was similar, alcohol may not modulate plasma lipoproteins in postmenopausal women to the same degree as in premenopausal women consuming similar diets and amounts of alcohol.

In postmenopausal women[42] the increase in HDL_2 cholesterol accounted for the increase in HDL–C in response to alcohol consumption. However, in premenopausal women there was a proportional increase in HDL_2 and HDL_3 fractions.[40] The magnitude of the effect of alcohol on apolipoprotein concentrations may also be less pronounced in postmenopausal women than in premenopausal women. In response to drinking 30 g alcohol/d, apo A-I increased by 8% in premenopausal women[40] but only 3% in postmenopausal women.[42] When Rumpler et al.[41] fed the equivalent of one drink per day to women (mixed population of pre- and postmenopausal women with and without hormone replacement), the apo A-I concentration increased by only 2%, which was not a significant change compared with the value after the control diet. Similarly, in postmenopausal women who consumed one drink per day, the apo A-I concentration increased by <1% (also not a significant change relative to the value after the control diet). Thus, it appears that 15 g alcohol/d may not be sufficient to elicit a change in apo A-I concentrations, and the change in apo A-I concentrations after 30 g alcohol/d may not be as great in postmenopausal women as in premenopausal women. Alcohol-related changes in apo A-II concentrations have not been observed in postmenopausal women but have been observed in premenopausal women. The nonsignificant 3% increase in the apo A-II concentration in the postmenopausal women consuming 30 g alcohol/d is not as large as the significant (4%) increase observed in premenopausal women. Changes in apo A-I and apo A-II concentrations also suggest that apo A-I is more responsive to alcohol than is apo A-II.

In contrast with the similar directional effects of alcohol on LDL–C and HDL–C seen in premenopausal and postmenopausal women, our data suggest that the effect of alcohol on fasting triglyceride concentrations may differ by menopause status. We have shown that triglyceride concentrations decrease in postmenopausal women[42] but are not altered in premenopausal women[40] in response to alcohol intake. The reasons for the discrepancies in triglyceride metabolism between premenopausal and postmenopausal women are not clear, but the data suggest that changes associated with menopause may mediate the triglyceride response to alcohol. In premenopausal women, alcohol increased circulating estrogens.[75] However, this increase was not observed in postmenopausal women in another study.[76] The triglyceride concentration-lowering effect of alcohol observed in postmenopausal women may be masked in premenopausal women by the alcohol mediated increase in estrogens and consequent increase in triglyceride concentrations.[77–79]

18.2.5 BEVERAGE TYPE, DRINKING PATTERN, AND AMOUNT

Within the last 20 years, the observation that alcohol lowered CVD risk has gained popular awareness as the "French paradox." The French paradox is based on the observation that regions in France with known high concentrations of fat intake (a strong risk factor for heart disease) have a lower rate of heart disease than other countries with similar characteristics.[80] This reduction in risk has been attributed to the regular consumption of wine.[2]

However, in a review of 25 studies, Rimm[81] found that the association between alcohol and lower risk of CHD was consistent across beverage type. Recent data from the U.S. Males Health Professional Study (USMHPS) support the similarity of response across beverage type.[82] Frequency and the regularity of alcohol drinking were associated with lower risk of CHD more so than either the type of beverage or consumption with meals. Beer and liquor, the alcoholic beverage types most widely consumed by the study population, were more strongly associated with the reduction in risk observed in their study than other beverage types. The authors suggest that this observation supports their previous hypothesis that associations of reduction in risk of CVD with certain beverage types is more a function of the regional differences in the predominant type of beverage consumed by the population[83] than the direct association with the beverage type. There have been no clinical intervention studies that have examined the impact of beverage type on circulating blood lipids and lipoproteins. The lack of impact of beverage type in reducing CVD risk suggests that any effect of beverage type will be small. It should be noted, however, that some alcoholic beverages, in particular, red wine, contain polyphenols that are under study for possible cardioprotective effects.

There is a substantial body of information that suggests that regular frequent consumption of light to moderate amounts of alcohol provides some protective effect from CHD. The amount and pattern of consumption which defines light to moderate drinking has not been consistent across studies but is generally confined to two drinks per day or less. One of the early meta-analyses of 42 prospective studies suggested that a maximum reduction in CHD risk was achieved at less than one drink per day.[3] However, a recent meta-analysis of 28 cohort studies[84] suggests a maximum reduction in relative risk of CHD of 15% in women and 23% in men with alcohol consumption of 10 g/d in women and 25 g/d in men. This translates into slightly less than one drink (12 g alcohol per drink) for women and two drinks per day for men. However, consumption below 52 g/d in women and 114 g/d in men still provided some protection from CHD in this analysis.

The role of drinking patterns in the risk of CHD is not entirely resolved. Most prospective studies are unable to discriminate drinking patterns beyond the broad categories of occasional, light to moderate, and heavy. Gruchow et al.[85] categorized regular drinkers by either a consistent or variable intake pattern. These authors found that variable intake pattern provided little increase in HDL–C concentrations. This observation was supported by Taskinen et al.[86] who showed that consumption of high concentrations of alcohol over a weekend had little impact on HDL–C concentrations. In one of the few controlled studies of drinking patterns, the blood lipid concentrations were measured in men consuming similar amounts of alcohol per week with either a weekend or daily drinking pattern.[54] Alcohol consumption was restricted for 4 weeks (by consumption of low alcohol beer). The men then returned to their normal drinking habit for 4 weeks. Changes in HDL–C, LDL–C, and apo A-I and II, in response to the two drinking patterns, were similar in both groups of drinkers and consistent with those associated with alcohol consumption. In a review, Puddey et al.[87] suggest that a pattern of drinking may have little impact on blood lipid responses to alcohol but for other aspects of CHD, such as coagulation and fibrinolysis, risk may be markedly affected by drinking pattern.

18.2.6 INTERACTION WITH DIETARY FAT CONCENTRATION

According to a number of studies utilizing a variety of methodologies, a reduction in the risk of CVD can be achieved by the consumption of a diet lower in fat than currently consumed by the American population.[91] This reduction in risk of CVD is generally accepted to be a consequence of a decrease in circulating concentrations of LDL cholesterol. However, in controlled feeding studies low fat diets reduce both LDL–C and HDL–C concentrations but may not lead to an improvement in the ratio of LDL–C to HDL–C.[41,88]

In a recent study, Rumpler et al.[41] found a significant interaction of fat concentration (38% vs. 20% of energy from fat) in the diet with changes in blood lipids associated with alcohol consumption (one drink per day). Women consuming the lower-fat diet had lower concentrations of plasma cholesterol as well as LDL–C and HDL–C than those consuming the higher-fat diet. This resulted in no significant change in the LDL–C to HDL–C ratio. The plasma lipid response to consumption of alcohol in conjunction with the higher-fat diet was also as expected. LDL–C concentrations were decreased and HDL–C concentrations were increased by alcohol consumption. However, when the data were separated by dietary fat treatment there was little or no effect of alcohol consumption on the blood lipid variables measured in those subjects consuming the lower-fat diet. The significant effects of alcohol treatments occurred in subjects that consumed the higher-fat diet. In subjects consuming the higher-fat diet, consumption of alcohol decreased plasma cholesterol by 6% and LDL–C by 11%. These lower concentrations were similar to those produced by the lower-fat diet with or without alcohol consumption. HDL–C, in particular HDL_2, increased in response to alcohol consumption when subjects consumed the higher-fat diet in conjunction with alcohol. The response to alcohol when the women consumed the higher-fat diet was similar in direction and magnitude to those differences reported between drinkers and nondrinkers in population-based studies.[35,38] This was expected since the higher-fat diet used in this study is similar in fat concentration to the "typical diet" consumed by free-living individuals in the U.S. The lack of response to alcohol consumption in individuals consuming a low fat diet complicates further the interpretation of studies on alcohol consumption in which diet composition is not controlled.

18.3 SUMMARY

Interpretation of the existing literature on the effects of alcohol on lipids and lipo-proteins is hampered by the wide variability in study designs and populations studied. Most of the data collected on the relationship between alcohol intake and blood lipid concentrations is from cross-sectional or longitudinal surveys. These studies provide much qualitative data but often are confounded with cultural and lifestyle changes that coincide with differences in alcohol intake. For example, in the Health Professionals Follow-Up Study (HPFUS)[32,89] those individuals who consumed the highest concentrations of total fats and saturated fats also consumed the lowest concentrations of alcohol, fruits, vegetables, and dietary fiber. The clustering of dietary habits, as observed in the HPFUS study, would indicate that the assessment of alcohol-induced changes in population studies is difficult due to changes in a number of other dietary variables.

In addition, these studies do not lend themselves well for quantifying amounts of alcohol consumed and developing dose–response relationships. Of the few studies that have controlled alcohol intake, most fail to control known factors that influence lipids and lipoproteins, particularly diet composition. In many alcohol intervention studies, the subjects are free-living with no dietary restrictions. Clearly, dietary fat, fatty acids, carbohydrates, and other components have a significant influence on circulating cholesterol and triglyceride concentrations. Also, the very short intervention periods may be insufficient, as in many studies of alcohol intake, to observe a change in steady-state cholesterol concentrations.[90] All these factors contribute to the inconsistencies observed in the response to alcohol.

However, after three decades of research on the relationship between alcohol and blood lipids a fairly clear picture has emerged. Moderate alcohol consumption may have little impact on circulating triglyceride concentration in individuals with triglyceride concentration in the normal range, but clearly lowers LDL–C and raises HDL–C concentrations. There is still some question whether there is an effect of alcohol consumption on apo B concentration. If there is an effect it seems to be small. Changes in subfractions of HDL are due to increases in both apo A-I and II and appear to be alcohol-dose dependent. The increase in HDL–C and decrease in LDL–C are consistent with the observed decrease in risk of CHD. Although alcohol consumption has been shown to affect other risk factors for CHD, it is clear much of the reduction in risk of CHD is a consequence of the effect on blood lipids.

From a public health standpoint, the data from a variety of studies suggest that even low concentrations of alcohol consumption can improve the lipoprotein profile of individuals consuming the high fat diet typical in the U.S. However, most of the beneficial effects of alcohol consumption on blood lipids can be achieved by a low fat diet alone and little additional benefit is garnered by the inclusion of alcohol in the diet. This observation could simplify the choice to drink or not by individuals at high risk for diseases, such as breast cancer, for which alcohol consumption may be a risk factor.

References

1. Klatsky, A. L., Friedman, G. D., and Siegelaub, A. B., Alcohol consumption before myocardial infarction. Results from the Kaiser-Permanente epidemiologic study of myocardial infarction, *Ann Intern Med* 81 (3), 294–301, 1974.
2. Klatsky, A. L., Drink to your health? *Sci Am* 288 (2), 74–81, 2003.
3. Maclure, M., Demonstration of deductive meta-analysis: ethanol intake and risk of myocardial infarction, *Epidemiol Rev* 15 (2), 328–51, 1993.
4. Valmadrid, C. T., Klein, R., Moss, S. E., Klein, B. E., and Cruickshanks, K. J., Alcohol intake and the risk of coronary heart disease mortality in persons with older-onset diabetes mellitus, *JAMA* 282 (3), 239–46, 1999.
5. Cooper, H. A., Exner, D. V., and Domanski, M. J., Light-to-moderate alcohol consumption and prognosis in patients with left ventricular systolic dysfunction, *J Am Coll Cardiol* 35 (7), 1753–9, 2000.
6. Mukamal, K. J., Maclure, M., Muller, J. E., Sherwood, J. B., and Mittleman, M. A., Prior alcohol consumption and mortality following acute myocardial infarction, *JAMA* 285 (15), 1965–70, 2001.
7. Reynolds, K., Lewis, L. B., Nolen, J. D., Kinney, G. L., Sathya, B., and He, J., Alcohol consumption and risk of stroke: a meta-analysis, *JAMA* 289 (5), 579–88, 2003.
8. Berger, K., Ajani, U. A., Kase, C. S., Gaziano, J. M., Buring, J. E., Glynn, R. J., and Hennekens, C. H., Light-to-moderate alcohol consumption and risk of stroke among U.S. male physicians, *N Engl J Med* 341 (21), 1557–64, 1999.
9. Langer, R. D., Criqui, M. H., and Reed, D. M., Lipoproteins and blood pressure as biological pathways for effect of moderate alcohol consumption on coronary heart disease, *Circulation* 85 (3), 910–5, 1992.
10. Campos, H., Genest, J. J., Jr., Blijlevens, E., McNamara, J. R., Jenner, J. L., Ordovas, J. M., Wilson, P. W., and Schaefer, E. J., Low density lipoprotein particle size and coronary artery disease, *Arterioscler Thromb* 12 (2), 187–95, 1992.
11. Gordon, D. J., Probstfield, J. L., Garrison, R. J., Neaton, J. D., Castelli, W. P., Knoke, J. D., Jacobs, D. R., Jr., Bangdiwala, S., and Tyroler, H. A., High-density lipoprotein cholesterol and cardiovascular disease. Four prospective American studies, *Circulation* 79 (1), 8–15, 1989.
12. Stampfer, M. J., Colditz, G. A., Willett, W. C., Speizer, F. E., and Hennekens, C. H., A prospective study of moderate alcohol consumption and the risk of coronary disease and stroke in women, *N Engl J Med* 319 (5), 267–73, 1988.
13. Manninen, V., Elo, M. O., Frick, M. H., Haapa, K., Heinonen, O. P., Heinsalmi, P., Helo, P., Huttunen, J. K., Kaitaniemi, P., Koskinen, P. et al., Lipid alterations and decline in the incidence of coronary heart disease in the Helsinki Heart Study, *JAMA* 260 (5), 641–51, 1988.
14. Shepherd, J., A tale of two trials: the West of Scotland Coronary Prevention Study and the Texas Coronary Atherosclerosis Prevention Study, *Atherosclerosis* 139 (2), 223–9, 1998.
15. Gotto, A. M., Jr., Insights on treating an over-the-counter-type subgroup: data from the Air Force/Texas Coronary Atherosclerosis Prevention Study Population, *Am J Cardiol* 85 (12A), 8E–14E, 2000.
16. The Lipid Research Clinics Coronary Primary Prevention Trial results. II. The relationship of reduction in incidence of coronary heart disease to cholesterol lowering, *JAMA* 251 (3), 365–74, 1984.
17. Crouse, J. R., III, Gender, lipoproteins, diet, and cardiovascular risk. Sauce for the goose may not be sauce for the gander, *Lancet* 1 (8633), 318–20, 1989.

18. Bass, K. M., Newschaffer, C. J., Klag, M. J., and Bush, T. L., Plasma lipoprotein levels as predictors of cardiovascular death in women, *Arch Intern Med* 153 (19), 2209–16, 1993.

19. Salonen, J. T., Salonen, R., Seppanen, K., Rauramaa, R., and Tuomilehto, J., HDL, HDL2, and HDL3 subfractions, and the risk of acute myocardial infarction. A prospective population study in eastern Finnish men, *Circulation* 84 (1), 129–39, 1991.

20. Wilson, P. W., Abbott, R. D., and Castelli, W. P., High density lipoprotein cholesterol and mortality. The Framingham Heart Study, *Arteriosclerosis* 8 (6), 737–41, 1988.

21. Lamarche, B., Tchernof, A., Mauriege, P., Cantin, B., Dagenais, G. R., Lupien, P. J., and Despres, J. P., Fasting insulin and apolipoprotein B levels and low-density lipoprotein particle size as risk factors for ischemic heart disease, *JAMA* 279 (24), 1955–61, 1998.

22. Freedman, D. S., Otvos, J. D., Jeyarajah, E. J., Barboriak, J. J., Anderson, A. J., and Walker, J. A., Relation of lipoprotein subclasses as measured by proton nuclear magnetic resonance spectroscopy to coronary artery disease, *Arterioscler Thromb Vasc Biol* 18 (7), 1046–53, 1998.

23. Gotto, A. M., Jr., Low high-density lipoprotein cholesterol as a risk factor in coronary heart disease: a working group report, *Circulation* 103 (17), 2213–8, 2001.

24. Miller, N. E., Hammett, F., Saltissi, S., Rao, S., van Zeller, H., Coltart, J., and Lewis, B., Relation of angiographically defined coronary artery disease to plasma lipoprotein subfractions and apolipoproteins, *Br Med J (Clin Res Ed)* 282 (6278), 1741–4, 1981.

25. Barbaras, R., Puchois, P., Fruchart, J. C., and Ailhaud, G., Cholesterol efflux from cultured adipose cells is mediated by LpAI particles but not by LpAI:AII particles, *Biochem Biophys Res Commun* 142 (1), 63–9, 1987.

26. Cheung, M. C., Brown, B. G., Wolf, A. C., and Albers, J. J., Altered particle size distribution of apolipoprotein A-I-containing lipoproteins in subjects with coronary artery disease, *J Lipid Res* 32 (3), 383–94, 1991.

27. Puchois, P., Ghalim, N., Zylberberg, G., Fievet, P., Demarquilly, C., and Fruchart, J. C., Effect of alcohol intake on human apolipoprotein A-I-containing lipoprotein subfractions, *Arch Intern Med* 150 (8), 1638–41, 1990.

28. Genest, J. J., Jr., Bard, J. M., Fruchart, J. C., Ordovas, J. M., Wilson, P. F., and Schaefer, E. J., Plasma apolipoprotein A-I, A-II, B, E and C-III containing particles in men with premature coronary artery disease, *Atherosclerosis* 90 (2–3), 149–57, 1991.

29. Asztalos, B. F., Roheim, P. S., Milani, R. L., Lefevre, M., McNamara, J. R., Horvath, K. V., and Schaefer, E. J., Distribution of ApoA-I-containing HDL subpopulations in patients with coronary heart disease, *Arterioscler Thromb Vasc Biol* 20 (12), 2670–6, 2000.

30. Boerwinkle, E., Leffert, C. C., Lin, J., Lackner, C., Chiesa, G., and Hobbs, H. H., Apolipoprotein(a) gene accounts for greater than 90% of the variation in plasma lipoprotein(a) concentrations, *J Clin Invest* 90 (1), 52–60, 1992.

31. Lippel, K., Gianturco, S., Fogelman, A., Nestel, P., Grundy, S. M., Fisher, W., Chait, A., Albers, J., and Roheim, P. S., Lipoprotein heterogeneity workshop. *Arteriosclerosis* 7, 315–323, 1987.

32. Ascherio, A., Hennekens, C., Willett, W. C., Sacks, F., Rosner, B., Manson, J., Witteman, J., and Stampfer, M. J., Prospective study of nutritional factors, blood pressure, and hypertension among U.S. women, *Hypertension* 27 (5), 1065–72, 1996.

33. Branchi, A., Rovellini, A., Tomella, C., Sciariada, L., Torri, A., Molgora, M., and Sommariva, D., Association of alcohol consumption with HDL subpopulations defined by apolipoprotein A-I and apolipoprotein A-II content, *Eur J Clin Nutr* 51 (6), 362–5, 1997.

34. Ettinger, W. H., Wahl, P. W., Kuller, L. H., Bush, T. L., Tracy, R. P., Manolio, T. A., Borhani, N. O., Wong, N. D., and O'Leary, D. H., Lipoprotein lipids in older people. Results from the Cardiovascular Health Study. The CHS Collaborative Research Group, *Circulation* 86 (3), 858–69, 1992.

35. Hegsted, D. M. and Ausman, L. M., Diet, alcohol and coronary heart disease in men, *J Nutr* 118 (10), 1184–9, 1988.

36. Taylor, K. G., Carter, T. J., Valente, A. J., Wright, A. D., Smith, J. H., and Matthews, K. A., Sex differences in the relationships between obesity, alcohol consumption and cigarette smoking and serum lipid and apolipoprotein concentrations in a normal population, *Atherosclerosis* 38 (1–2), 11–8, 1981.

37. Weidner, G., Connor, S. L., Chesney, M. A., Burns, J. W., Connor, W. E., Matarazzo, J. D., and Mendell, N. R., Sex differences in high density lipoprotein cholesterol among low-level alcohol consumers, *Circulation* 83 (1), 176–80, 1991.

38. Ostrander, L. D., Jr., Lamphiear, D. E., Block, W. D., Johnson, B. C., Ravenscroft, C., and Epstein, F. H., Relationship of serum lipid concentrations to alcohol consumption, *Arch Intern Med* 134 (3), 451–6, 1974.

39. Srivastava, L. M., Vasisht, S., Agarwal, D. P., and Goedde, H. W., Relation between alcohol intake, lipoproteins and coronary heart disease: the interest continues, *Alcohol Alcohol* 29 (1), 11–24, 1994.

40. Clevidence, B. A., Reichman, M. E., Judd, J. T., Muesing, R. A., Schatzkin, A., Schaefer, E. J., Li, Z., Jenner, J., Brown, C. C., Sunkin, M. et al., Effects of alcohol consumption on lipoproteins of premenopausal women. A controlled diet study, *Arterioscler Thromb Vasc Biol* 15 (2), 179–84, 1995.

41. Rumpler, W. V., Clevidence, B. A., Muesing, R. A., and Rhodes, D. G., Changes in women's plasma lipid and lipoprotein concentrations due to moderate consumption of alcohol are affected by dietary fat level, *J Nutr* 129 (9), 1713–7, 1999.

42. Baer, D. J., Judd, J. T., Clevidence, B. A., Muesing, R. A., Campbell, W. S., Brown, E. D., and Taylor, P. R., Moderate alcohol consumption lowers risk factors for cardiovascular disease in postmenopausal women fed a controlled diet, *Am J Clin Nutr* 75 (3), 593–9, 2002.

43. Nishiwaki, M., Ishikawa, T., Ito, T., Shige, H., Tomiyasu, K., Nakajima, K., Kondo, K., Hashimoto, H., Saitoh, K., Manabe, M. et al., Effects of alcohol on lipoprotein lipase, hepatic lipase, cholesteryl ester transfer protein, and lecithin:cholesterol acyltransferase in high-density lipoprotein cholesterol elevation, *Atherosclerosis* 111 (1), 99–109, 1994.

44. Razay, G., Heaton, K. W., Bolton, C. H., and Hughes, A. O., Alcohol consumption and its relation to cardiovascular risk factors in British women, *BMJ* 304 (6819), 80–3, 1992.

45. Barboriak, J. J., Alcohol, lipids and heart disease, *Alcohol* 1 (4), 341–5, 1984.

46. Cushman, P., Jr., Barboriak, J., and Kalbfleisch, J., Alcohol: high density lipoproteins, apolipoproteins, *Alcohol Clin Exp Res* 10 (2), 154–7, 1986.

47. Avogaro, P. and Cazzolato, G., Changes in the composition and physico-chemical characteristics of serum lipoproteins during ethanol-induced lipaemia in alcoholic subjects, *Metabolism* 24 (11), 1231–42, 1975.

48. Burr, M. L., Fehily, A. M., Butland, B. K., Bolton, C. H., and Eastham, R. D., Alcohol and high-density-lipoprotein cholesterol: a randomized controlled trial, *Br J Nutr* 56 (1), 81–6, 1986.

49. Gaziano, J. M., Buring, J. E., Breslow, J. L., Goldhaber, S. Z., Rosner, B., VanDenburgh, M., Willett, W., and Hennekens, C. H., Moderate alcohol intake, increased levels of high-density lipoprotein and its subfractions, and decreased risk of myocardial infarction, *N Engl J Med* 329 (25), 1829–34, 1993.

50. Sillanaukee, P., Koivula, T., Jokela, H., Pitkajarvi, T., and Seppa, K., Alcohol consumption and its relation to lipid-based cardiovascular risk factors among middle-aged women: the role of HDL(3) cholesterol, *Atherosclerosis* 152 (2), 503–10, 2000.

51. Criqui, M. H., Cowan, L. D., Tyroler, H. A., Bangdiwala, S., Heiss, G., Wallace, R. B., and Cohn, R., Lipoproteins as mediators for the effects of alcohol consumption and cigarette smoking on cardiovascular mortality: results form the Lipid Research Clinics Follow-up Study, *Am J Epidemiol* 126 (4), 629–37, 1987.

52. Castelli, W. P., Doyle, J. T., Gordon, T., Hames, C. G., Hjortland, M. C., Hulley, S. B., Kagan, A., and Zukel, W. J., Alcohol and blood lipids. The cooperative lipoprotein phenotyping study, *Lancet* 2 (8030), 153–5, 1977.

53. Glueck, C. J., Hogg, E., Allen, C., and Gartside, P. S., Effects of alcohol ingestion on lipids and lipoproteins in normal men: isocaloric metabolic studies, *Am J Clin Nutr* 33 (11), 2287–93, 1980.

54. Rakic, V., Puddey, I. B., Burke, V., Dimmitt, S. B., and Beilin, L. J., Influence of pattern of alcohol intake on blood pressure in regular drinkers: a controlled trial, *J Hypertens* 16 (2), 165–74, 1998.

55. Hagiage, M., Marti, C., Rigaud, D., Senault, C., Fumeron, F., Apfelbaum, M., and Girard-Globa, A., Effect of a moderate alcohol intake on the lipoproteins of normotriglyceridemic obese subjects compared with normoponderal controls, *Metabolism* 41 (8), 856–61, 1992.

56. De Oliveira, E. S. E. R., Foster, D., McGee Harper, M., Seidman, C. E., Smith, J. D., Breslow, J. L., and Brinton, E. A., Alcohol consumption raises HDL cholesterol levels by increasing the transport rate of apolipoproteins A-I and A-II, *Circulation* 102 (19), 2347–52, 2000.

57. Clevidence, B. A., Taylor, P. R., Campbell, W. S., and Judd, J. T., Lean and heavy women may not use energy from alcohol with equal efficiency, *J Nutr* 125 (10), 2536–40, 1995.

58. Valimaki, M., Laitinen, K., Ylikahri, R., Ehnholm, C., Jauhiainen, M., Bard, J. M., Fruchart, J. C., and Taskinen, M. R., The effect of moderate alcohol intake on serum apolipoprotein A-I-containing lipoproteins and lipoprotein (a), *Metabolism* 40 (11), 1168–72, 1991.

59. Huang, C. M., Elin, R. J., Ruddel, M., Schmitz, J., and Linnoila, M., The effect of alcohol withdrawal on serum concentrations of Lp(a), apolipoproteins A-1 and B, and lipids, *Alcohol Clin Exp Res* 16 (5), 895–8, 1992.

60. Delarue, J., Husson, M., Schellenberg, F., Tichet, J., Vol, S., Couet, C., and Lamisse, F., Serum lipoprotein(a) [Lp(a)] in alcoholic men: effect of withdrawal, *Alcohol* 13 (3), 309–14, 1996.

61. Budzynski, J., Klopocka, M., Swiatkowski, M., Pulkowski, G., and Ziolkowski, M., Lipoprotein(a) in alcohol-dependent male patients during a six-month abstinence period, *Alcohol Alcohol* 38 (2), 157–62, 2003.

62. Catena, C., Novello, M., Dotto, L., De Marchi, S., and Sechi, L. A., Serum lipoprotein(a) concentrations and alcohol consumption in hypertension: possible relevance for cardiovascular damage, *J Hypertens* 21 (2), 281–8, 2003.

63. Jackson, R., Scragg, R., and Beaglehole, R., Alcohol consumption and risk of coronary heart disease, *BMJ* 303 (6796), 211–6, 1991.

64. Paunio, M., Virtamo, J., Gref, C. G., and Heinonen, O. P., Serum high density lipoprotein cholesterol, alcohol, and coronary mortality in male smokers, *BMJ* 312 (7040), 1200–3, 1996.

65. Hein, H. O., Suadicani, P., and Gyntelberg, F., Alcohol consumption, serum low density lipoprotein cholesterol concentration, and risk of ischaemic heart disease: six year follow up in the Copenhagen male study, *BMJ* 312 (7033), 736–41, 1996.

66. Belfrage, P., Berg, B., Hagerstrand, I., Nilsson-Ehle, P., Tornqvist, H., and Wiebe, T., Alterations of lipid metabolism in healthy volunteers during long-term ethanol intake, *Eur J Clin Invest* 7 (2), 127–31, 1977.

67. Valimaki, M., Taskinen, M. R., Ylikahri, R., Roine, R., Kuusi, T., and Nikkila, E. A., Comparison of the effects of two different doses of alcohol on serum lipoproteins, HDL-subfractions and apolipoproteins A-I and A-II: a controlled study, *Eur J Clin Invest* 18 (5), 472–80, 1988.

68. Taskinen, M. R., Nikkila, E. A., Valimaki, M., Sane, T., Kuusi, T., Kesaniemi, A., and Ylikahri, R., Alcohol-induced changes in serum lipoproteins and in their metabolism, *Am Heart J* 113 (2 Pt 2), 458–64, 1987.

69. Gardner, C. D., Tribble, D. L., Young, D. R., Ahn, D., and Fortmann, S. P., Associations of HDL, HDL(2), and HDL(3) cholesterol and apolipoproteins A-I and B with lifestyle factors in healthy women and men: the Stanford Five City Project, *Prev Med* 31 (4), 346–56, 2000.

70. Rosenberg, L., Hennekens, C. H., Rosner, B., Belanger, C., Rothman, K. J., and Speizer, F. E., Early menopause and the risk of myocardial infarction, *Am J Obstet Gynecol* 139 (1), 47–51, 1981.

71. van der Schouw, Y. T., van der Graaf, Y., Steyerberg, E. W., Eijkemans, J. C., and Banga, J. D., Age at menopause as a risk factor for cardiovascular mortality, *Lancet* 347 (9003), 714–8, 1996.

72 Colditz, G. A., Willett, W. C., Stampfer, M. J., Rosner, B., Speizer, F. E., and Hennekens, C. H., Menopause and the risk of coronary heart disease in women, *N Engl J Med* 316 (18), 1105–10, 1987.

73. Akahoshi, M., Soda, M., Nakashima, E., Shimaoka, K., Seto, S., and Yano, K., Effects of menopause on trends of serum cholesterol, blood pressure, and body mass index, *Circulation* 94 (1), 61–6, 1996.

74. Nanchahal, K., Ashton, W. D., and Wood, D. A., Alcohol consumption, metabolic cardiovascular risk factors and hypertension in women, *Int J Epidemiol* 29 (1), 57–64, 2000.

75. Reichman, M. E., Judd, J. T., Longcope, C., Schatzkin, A., Clevidence, B. A., Nair, P. P., Campbell, W. S., and Taylor, P. R., Effects of alcohol consumption on plasma and urinary hormone concentrations in premenopausal women, *J Natl Cancer Inst* 85 (9), 722–7, 1993.

76. Dorgan, J. F., Baer, D. J., Albert, P. S., Judd, J. T., Brown, E. D., Corle, D. K., Campbell, W. S., Hartman, T. J., Tejpar, A. A., Clevidence, B. A., Giffen, C. A., Chandler, D. W., Stanczyk, F. Z., and Taylor, P. R., Serum hormones and the alcohol–breast cancer association in postmenopausal women, *J Natl Cancer Inst* 93 (9), 710–5, 2001.

77. Schaefer, E. J., Foster, D. M., Zech, L. A., Lindgren, F. T., Brewer, H. B., Jr., and Levy, R. I., The effects of estrogen administration on plasma lipoprotein metabolism in premenopausal females, *J Clin Endocrinol Metab* 57 (2), 262–7, 1983.

78. Kuhl, H., Marz, W., Jung-Hoffmann, C., Weber, J., Siekmeier, R., and Gross, W., Effect on lipid metabolism of a biphasic desogestrel-containing oral contraceptive: divergent changes in apolipoprotein B and E and transitory decrease in Lp(a) levels, *Contraception* 47 (1), 69–83, 1993.

79. Taves, E. H. and Wolfe, B. M., Estradiol is a potent inhibitor of the hypotriglyceri-demic effect of levonorgestrel in female rats, *Lipids* 24 (7), 669–72, 1989.

80. Criqui, M. H. and Ringel, B. L., Does diet or alcohol explain the French paradox? *Lancet* 344 (8939–8940), 1719–23, 1994.

81. Rimm, E., Alcohol and coronary heart disease: can we learn more? *Epidemiology* 12 (4), 380–2, 2001.

82. Mukamal, K. J., Conigrave, K. M., Mittleman, M. A., Camargo, C. A., Jr., Stampfer, M. J., Willett, W. C., and Rimm, E. B., Roles of drinking pattern and type of alcohol consumed in coronary heart disease in men, *N Engl J Med* 348 (2), 109–18, 2003.

83. Rimm, E. B., Alcohol consumption and coronary heart disease: good habits may be more important than just good wine [see comments], *Am J Epidemiol* 143 (11), 1094–8; discussion 1099, 1996.

84. Corrao, G., Rubbiati, L., Bagnardi, V., Zambon, A., and Poikolainen, K., Alcohol and coronary heart disease: a meta-analysis, *Addiction* 95 (10), 1505–23, 2000.

85. Gruchow, H. W., Hoffmann, R. G., Anderson, A. J., and Barboriak, J. J., Effects of drinking patterns on the relationship between alcohol and coronary occlusion, *Atherosclerosis* 43 (2–3), 393–404, 1982.

86. Taskinen, M. R., Valimaki, M., Nikkila, E. A., Kuusi, T., and Ylikahri, R., Sequence of alcohol-induced initial changes in plasma lipoproteins (VLDL and HDL) and lipolytic enzymes in humans, *Metabolism* 34 (2), 112–9, 1985.

87. Puddey, I. B., Rakic, V., Dimmitt, S. B., and Beilin, L. J., Influence of pattern of drinking on cardiovascular disease and cardiovascular risk factors — a review, *Addiction* 94 (5), 649–63, 1999.

88. Clevidence, B. A., Judd, J. T., Schatzkin, A., Muesing, R. A., Campbell, W. S., Brown, C. C., and Taylor, P. R., Plasma lipid and lipoprotein concentrations of men consuming a low-fat, high-fiber diet, *Am J Clin Nutr* 55 (3), 689–94, 1992.

89. Ascherio, A., Rimm, E. B., Giovannucci, E. L., Spiegelman, D., Stampfer, M., and Willett, W. C., Dietary fat and risk of coronary heart disease in men: cohort follow up study in the United States, *BMJ* 313 (7049), 84–90, 1996.

90. Kris-Etherton, P. M. and Dietschy, J., Design criteria for studies examining individual fatty acid effects on cardiovascular disease risk factors: human and animal studies, *Am J Clin Nutr* 65 (5 Suppl), 1590S–1596S, 1997.

91. National Research Council (U.S.) Committee on Diet and Health. Diet and health: implications for reducing chronic disease risk. Washington, D.C.: National Academy Press, 1989.

19 Alcohol-Induced Membrane Lipid Peroxidation

Robert R. Miller, Jr.

CONTENTS

19.1 INTRODUCTION

The effects of ethanol (EtOH) on membrane fatty acid composition have been intensely studied and reviewed.[1–4] EtOH-induced reductions in long-chain, polyunsaturated fatty acid (PUFA) levels were reported in adult brain[3–9] and in adult retina.[9] EtOH-induced reductions in membrane PUFA levels were also reported in adult liver[10–12] and adult erythrocytes.[13] In adult liver membranes, reduced levels of long-chain polyunsaturated membrane fatty acids (PUFAs) correlated with alcohol-induced liver damage[14,15] and decreased levels of long-chain PUFAs were reported during necrosis and apoptosis.[16–19]

These EtOH-induced changes in membrane fatty acid composition may partially explain EtOH-induced changes in membrane fluidity.[4,20–22] In many systems, EtOH-induced increases in membrane fluidity have been observed in membranes isolated from EtOH-intolerant animals. Meanwhile, membranes isolated from EtOH-tolerant animals resist the fluidizing effects of EtOH. These observations led to an interesting hypothesis by Hagai Rottenberg and colleagues[23–25] who speculated that EtOH-induced increases in membrane fluidity are damaging while the ability to resist EtOH-induced increases in membrane fluidity in EtOH-tolerant animals is a component of EtOH-tolerance. In EtOH-dependency, EtOH may be required to fluidize overly nonfluid and nonfunctional membranes into near normal levels of membrane fluidity and may be required to reestablish normal membrane functionality.

19.1.1 MEMBRANE FLUIDITY

Membrane fluidity can be influenced by four different biochemical configurations. These four biochemical configurations include the degree of membrane hydration, membrane cholesterol levels, the ratio of cylindrical-shaped phospholipids/triangular-shaped phospholipids (phosphatidylcholine/phosphatidylethanolamine), and membrane fatty acid composition. A highly hydrated membrane is less fluid than a dehydrated membrane because water molecules can form hydrogen bonds with the phosphates of adjacent phospholipids. Dehydration of a membrane increases molecular motion and increases membrane fluidity.[26] Cholesterol decreases the molecular motion of phospholipids by insertion into the hydrophobic regions of membranes and forming a hydrogen bond with an adjacent phospholipid through the hydroxyl group on the cholesterol molecule. Membranes rich in cylindrical-shaped phospholipids such as phosphatidylcholine form membrane bilayers with high packing orders. Meanwhile, membranes rich in triangular-shaped phospholipids such as phosphatidylethanolamine fall out of their bilayer configurations and adopt hexagonal$_{II}$ micelles and have large spaces between the hexagonal$_{II}$ micelles.[1,4,22,27,28] Membranes rich in saturated long-chain fatty acids are less fluid and more gel-like because of the higher melting points of long-chain fatty acids. Meanwhile, short-chain saturated fatty acids are more fluid and are more liquid-like because of their lower melting points. Membranes rich in saturated fatty acids are less fluid because of the high packing order that is created by closely spaced phospholipids. Meanwhile, membranes rich in unsaturated fatty acids are more fluid because of the low packing order that is created by the presence of *cis*-bonds in the fatty acids of adjacent phospholipids.[1,4,22,27–29]

19.1.2 EtOH-INDUCED REDUCTIONS IN MEMBRANE PUFAS IN DEVELOPING SYSTEMS

While EtOH-induced changes in membrane fatty acid composition have been intensely studied in adult tissues, only a few studies have been directed at developing systems. EtOH-induced decreases in the levels of brain membrane docosahexaenoic acid (22:6, *n*-3 and 22:6, *n*-6) have been reported in fetal guinea-pigs[30] and in neonatal mice at 32 d postconception.[31] In developing chick embryos, EtOH-induced decreases in the levels of brain oleic acid (18:1, *n*-9), linoleic acid (18:2, *n*-6), linolenic acid (18:3, *n*-6), and arachidonic acid (20:4, *n*-6) were observed at 18 d of development within microsomal membranes (stage 44; see Reference 32). These EtOH-induced decreases in long-chain, unsaturated fatty acids correlated with decreased neuron densities in the cerebral hemispheres and optic lobes with correlation coefficients ranging from 0.44 [$F = (1, 32)$ 7.84; $p \leq 0.009$] to 0.59 [$F = (1, 32)$ 17.38; $p \leq 0.0002$].[33] EtOH-induced decreases in long-chain PUFAs within embryonic chick brains also correlated with EtOH-induced decreases in brain mass, increased levels of brain lipid hydroperoxides, and decreased activity by the membrane-bound enzyme acetylcholine esterase (AChE; EC 3.1.1.7).[34] Thus, EtOH-induced decreased in brain long-chain PUFAs correlate with EtOH-induced changes in brain morphology and physiology.

It has recently been demonstrated that a single dose of either EtOH or nicotine at 0 d of incubation induced decreased levels of brain membrane long-chain PUFAs, increased levels of brain lipid hydroperoxides, and reduced brain AChE activities in the brains of stage 44 (18 d of incubation), stage 45 (20 d of incubation), and 2-day-old neonatal chicks.[35] While a single dose of either EtOH or nicotine promoted decreased levels of brain membrane PUFAs, the dual treatment of EtOH and nicotine failed to promote decreased levels of long-chain PUFAs in either a compensatory or synergistic manner. Embryonic exposure to either EtOH or nicotine promoted reduced levels of unsaturated/saturated brain membrane fatty acids and increased levels of brain lipid hydroperoxides when experimental groups were compared to controls. However, these values were unchanged in EtOH- and nicotine-treated chicks as compared to either EtOH-treated or nicotine-treated chicks.[35] These observations are in conflict with the findings of Ashakumary and Vijayammal[36,37] who reported an additive effect by EtOH and nicotine on lipid peroxidation in adult rats.

19.2 MECHANISM(S) UNDERLYING ETOH-INDUCED REDUCTIONS IN PUFAs

In 1992, Ronald C. Reitz presented a wonderful review article that attempted to explain the underlying mechanism of EtOH-induced reductions in long-chain PUFAs.[2] Reitz stated that the most consistent finding in the literature at that time was an increase in linoleic acid (18:2) and a decrease in arachidonic acid (20:4).[38–46]

Because *in vitro* studies in rats[47–49] demonstrated EtOH-induced inhibition of Δ-5 and Δ-6 desaturases, Reitz[2] suggested that EtOH-induced reductions in long-chain PUFAs and EtOH-induced increases in shorter, less unsaturated fatty acids were caused by changes in *de novo* synthesis. Through EtOH-induced inhibition of Δ-5 and Δ-6 desaturases, cells may not be able to convert dietary linoleic acid (18:2) or dietary linolenic acid (18:3) into either arachidonic acid (20:4), docosapentaenoic acid (22:5), or docosahexaeneoic acid (22:6) (Figure 19.1).

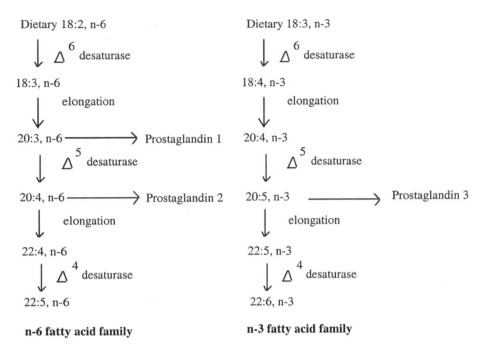

n-6 fatty acid family   **n-3 fatty acid family**

FIGURE 19.1 The role of desaturases in the *de novo* synthesis of long-chain PUFAs.

While EtOH-induced inhibition of Δ-5 and Δ-6 desaturases may explain EtOH-induced reductions in long-chain PUFAs in many biological systems, it does not appear to fully explain the phenomenon in all biological systems. Pawlosky and Salam[9] reported that chronic EtOH exposure in adult cats promoted reduced levels of docosahexaeneoic acid (22:6, *n-3*) in brain and retina membranes. Meanwhile, a compensatory increase in the levels of docosapentaenoic acid (22:5, *n-6*) was observed in feline brain and retina membranes, This change in the ratio of 22:6, *n-3*/22:5, *n-6* is associated with a loss of nervous system function. An EtOH-induced inhibition of Δ-5 and Δ-6 desaturases could explain the EtOH-induced decrease in 22:6, *n-3* that Pawlosky and Salam observed[9] (Figure 19.1). However, an EtOH-induced increase in (22:5, *n-6*) levels would require an EtOH-induced stimulation of the Δ-6, Δ-5, and Δ-4 desaturases used in the elongation and desaturation of *n-6* fatty acids (Figure 19.1). Thus, an EtOH-induced inhibition of Δ-5 and Δ-6 desaturases is either not universal in all biological systems, or EtOH selectively inhibits only some Δ-5 and Δ-6 desaturases. The Δ-5 and Δ-6 desaturases that are used in the elongation and desaturation of *n-3* fatty acids may be inhibited, while EtOH may stimulate the Δ-5 and Δ-6 desaturases used in the elongation and desaturation of *n-6* fatty acids.

EtOH-induced inhibition of Δ-5 and Δ-6 desaturases would promote decreased levels of arachidonic acid (20:4), docosapentaenoic acid (22:5), and docosahexaeneoic acid (22:6), and increased levels of linoleic acid (18:2) and linolenic acid (18:3).[2] However, in developing chicks, a single dosage of EtOH at 0 d of incubation promoted decreased levels of linoleic acid (18:2, *n-6*), linolenic acid (18:3, *n-3*), arachidonic acid (20:4, *n*-6), and docosahexaeneoic acid (22:6, *n*-3) in the membranes of embryonic chick brains at 18 d of incubation (stage 44; see Reference 32).[34,35] In later stages of embryonic development, a single dosage of EtOH at 0 d of embryonic incubation promoted decreased levels of linoleic acid (18:2, *n*-6), linolenic acid (18:3, *n*-3), arachidonic acid (20:4, *n*-6), docosapentaenoic acid (22:5, *n*-3), and docosahexaeneoic acid (22:6, *n*-3) in the membranes of embryonic chick brains at 20 d of incubation (stage 45; see Reference 32). This same trend was observed in the brains of 2-d-old neonatal chicks after embryonic exposure to EtOH.[35] Meanwhile, EtOH-induced increases in the levels of myristic acid (14:0) were observed in brain membranes at 18 d of incubation (stage 44), 20 d of incubation (stage 45), and 2-d-old neonatal chicks.[34,35] This trend has also been observed at earlier stages of development in the brain membranes of chick embryos at 11 d of incubation (stage 37; see Reference 32).[50] These developmental stages in chicks are analogous to the second and third trimesters of mammalian development. This universal decrease in linoleic acid (18:2, *n*-6), linolenic acid (18:3, *n*-3), arachidonic acid (20:4, *n*-6), and docosahexaeneoic acid (22:6, *n*-3) levels in developing chick brains indicates that an additional mechanism may exist which works along side EtOH-induced inhibition of Δ-5 and Δ-6 desaturases.

19.2.1 LIPID PEROXIDATION

A second mechanism has emerged that explains EtOH-induced decreases in long-chain PUFAs and EtOH-induced increases in shorter-chain fatty acids. This mechanism is lipid peroxidation through the Fenton reaction (Figure 19.2). Iron and other transition metals such as copper can act as Fenton reagents. As Fe^{+2} is oxidized to Fe^{+3}, reactive oxygen radicals (2 O–) and hydroxyl radicals (OH–) can be synthesized as O_2 and OH– ions absorb electrons.[51–53] These oxygen and hydroxyl radicals can attack the unsaturation sites of membrane PUFAs and cleave the long-chain PUFAs into short-chain, saturated fatty acids and a variety of short-chain alcohols. The appearance of short-chain membrane fatty acids can promote increased membrane fluidity, necrosis, and apoptosis.[16,17,54,55]

Lipid peroxidation is dependent on the formation of oxygen and hydroxyl radicals that catalyze the formation of lipid peroxides, lipid hydroperoxides, conjugated lipid dienes, and thiobarbituric acid-reactive substances (TBARs) (Figure 19.2). TBAR assays measure breakdown products from all lipid hydroperoxides including malondialdehyde. EtOH-induced increases in lipid peroxides, lipid hydroperoxides, and conjugated lipid dienes have been observed. Some of these lipid peroxidation products, such as 4-hydroxynonenal, are also involved in EtOH-induced mitochondrial damage.[56]

The synthesis of EtOH-induced oxygen radicals, lipid peroxidation, and mitochondrial malfunction has been demonstrated in adult rat brain,[57,58] neuronal cell cultures,[59] and glial cell cultures.[60,61] Chronic EtOH exposure has induced oxidative stress in adult rat cerebellum,[62] and chronic EtOH exposure induced oxygen radical formation and protein peroxidation in the central and peripheral nervous system of adult rats.[63,64] In embryonic chick brains, EtOH exposure induced the formation of

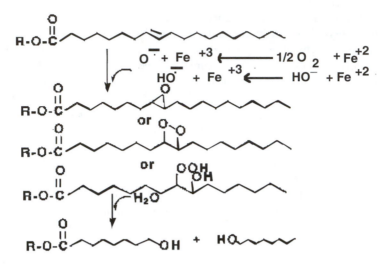

FIGURE 19.2 Lipid peroxidation via the Fenton reaction.

lipid hydroperoxides and EtOH-induced increases in lipid hydroperoxide levels correlated with the loss of membrane PUFAs.[34,35,50]

The early work of Di Luzio and Hartman[65] and Comporti et al.[66] demonstrated that a large single dosage of EtOH promoted increased lipid peroxide levels in adult rat liver and they suggested that lipid peroxidation contributes to the pathogenesis of EtOH-induced fatty infiltration of the liver. Hepatic microsomes isolated from adult rats exhibited EtOH-induced increases in the levels of oxygen radicals, hydroxyl radicals, H_2O_2, and enhanced lipid peroxidation.[67–73] In addition, the oxidation of EtOH to the reactive 1-hydroxyethyl radical has been reported in adult rat liver[74,75] and adult heart.[74]

19.2.2 ANTIOXIDANT ENZYMES AND THE PRODUCTION OF HYDROXYL RADICALS FROM H_2O_2

The removal of oxygen radicals is catalyzed by superoxide dismutase (SOD; EC 1.15.1.1). SOD removes oxygen radicals by forming hydrogen peroxide (H_2O_2) and water. Because H_2O_2 can form hydroxyl radicals through the Haber–Weiss reaction,[76] H_2O_2 must be removed by either catalase (CATAL; E.C. 1.11.1.6) or selenium-dependent and selenium-independent isozymes of GSH-Px. CATAL and GSH-Px enzymes convert H_2O_2 to molecular H_2O and O_2. During this reaction, GSH-Px isozymes bond two molecules of glutathione (GSH) to one another through a disulfide bond and thus form the GSSH dimer. Collectively, SOD, CATAL, and GSH-Px isozymes serve as antioxidant enzymes.

Any Fe^{+2}-containing enzyme or any enzyme that produces H_2O_2 can potentially generate hydroxyl radicals (HO-·). This is especially true if the newly produced H_2O_2 cannot be converted to H_2O and O_2 by either catalase or glutathione peroxidase. As

H_2O_2 levels increase, H_2O_2 can decompose into HO- by use of the Haber–Weiss reaction.[76]

$$H_2O_2 + Fe^{+2} \rightarrow OH^- + HO^\bullet + Fe^{+3} \qquad \text{Fenton reaction}$$

$$+ Fe^{+3} + O_2^\bullet \rightarrow Fe^{+2} + O_2 \qquad \text{Reduction of the ferric ion}$$

$$H_2O_2 + O_2^\bullet \xrightarrow[\text{catalyst}]{Fe^{+2}} OH^- + HO^\bullet + O_2 \quad \text{Haber – Weiss reaction}$$

19.2.3 KUPFFER CELLS AND EtOH-INDUCED LIVER DAMAGE

EtOH-induced oxidative stress and EtOH-induced liver parthenogenesis employ Kupffer cells. Kupffer cells are resident macrophages of the liver, and inhibition of Kupffer cells partially attenuates EtOH-induced free radical formation and EtOH-induced liver damage.[77,78] Free radical products have been demonstrated in rats fed a high fat diet rich in unsaturated fatty acids and these free radical products were associated with EtOH-induced liver damage.[10,11,74,79] Since macrophages (Kupffer cells) are Fe^{+2}-containing cells and kill through oxidative bursts, it is not surprising to find that the destruction of Kupffer cells by chronic administration of $GdCl_3$ decreased the formation of EtOH-induced free radicals by approximately 50% in the livers of adult rats fed an EtOH-containing, high-fat diet.[78] In this study, the destruction of hepatic Kupffer cells also decreased the severity of EtOH-induced pathogenesis as measured by the histological examination of hepatic tissue.[78] Adachi et al.[77] previously demonstrated that chronic exposure of rats to $GdCl_3$ decreased serum levels of aspartate aminotransferase (AST) in $GdCl_3$- and EtOH-treated adult rats as compared to EtOH-treated adult rats. Since hepatic cells have high levels of AST, this study[77] implied that the destruction of Kupffer cells partially attenuated EtOH-induced liver damage. Considerable evidence has arisen in supporting the role of Kupffer cells in mediating EtOH-induced peroxidation and EtOH-induced liver damage, and the role of Kupffer cells in mediating alcohol-induced liver damage has recently been reviewed.[80]

19.2.4 VITAMIN E ATTENUATES EtOH-INDUCED DAMAGE

Vitamin E (tocopherol) slows the propagation of hydroxyl radicals (HO-).[81,82] As a fat-soluble vitamin, vitamin E is found in extremely low concentrations within membranes and can quench membrane lipid peroxidation.[83,84] This is accomplished by the donation of H^+ form phenolic hydroxyl groups of vitamin E molecules and the extraction of an electron from either oxygen or hydroxyl radicals, resulting in the formation of α-tocopheroxyl radicals, tocopherol quinines, and tocopherol dimers. Because membrane levels of α-tocopherol are very low, the regeneration of α-tocopherol from the α-tocopheroxyl radical is accomplished by the reduction of cytoplasmic ascorbate.[85]

EtOH-induced cerebrovascular spasms, the rupturing of micro-vessels, micro-hemorrhaging, and intracranial hemorrhages have been reported in adult mammals,[86–89] and EtOH-induced cerebral vascular damage may utilize oxidative stress.

Altura and Gebrewold[90] reported that the chronic treatment of exogenous α-tocopherol (1.25 to 5 mg/d for 14 d), a known antioxidant, attenuated EtOH-induced cerebral vascular damage in adult rats. Altura and Gebrewold[90] delivered exogenous α-tocopherol to adult rats for 2 weeks by the subcutaneous injection of α-tocopherol-containing pellets. Since the mass of the rats ranged from 125 to 135 g, this exogenous treatment of α-tocopherol ranged from 21.5 μmol/kg/d to 92.87 μmol/kg/d. Vitamin E (tocopherol) slows the propagation of hydroxyl radical damage.[81,82] This is accomplished by the donation of H^+ from phenolic hydroxyl groups of vitamin E molecules and the extraction of an electron from oxygen and hydroxyl radicals resulting in the formation of tocopherol quinines or tocopherol dimers. Thus, Altura and Gebrewold[90] attenuated the EtOH-induced destruction of endothelial cells of blood vessels and they hypothesized that the EtOH-induced destruction of endothelial cells utilized membrane lipid peroxidation.

EtOH-induced cerebrovascular spasms are also associated with a very rapid decrease in serum Mg^{+2}.[84,88,89,91,92] Since Mg^{+2} is a known antagonist to Ca^{+2} uptake, the EtOH-induced cerebrovascular spasms may involve Ca^{+2} stimulation. Recently, Li et al.[93,94] demonstrated that exogenous α-tocopherol ameliorated the EtOH-induced reductions in Mg^{+2} levels in cultured canine cerebral vascular smooth muscle. Thus, EtOH-induced lipid peroxidation may disrupt Ca^{+2}/Mg^{+2} transport from the circulatory system into cerebral vascular smooth muscle cells.

Zhang et al.[95] have studied the influence of EtOH, acute Fe^{+2} overload, and exogenous α-tocopherol on lipid peroxidation in rat testes. Acute Fe^{+2} and EtOH overload was obtained by the intraperitoneal injection of iron-dextran (500 mg/kg) with and without EtOH (50 mmol/kg). After 18 h of treatment, a significant increase in total iron levels was observed in testis. Total testis iron levels were 6.8 times greater than control values in iron-treated rats and 9.1 times greater in iron and EtOH-treated rats as compared to controls. As testicular iron levels increased, lipid peroxidation products, as measured by TBARs (2-thiobarbituric acid–reactive substances), increased as α-tocopherol levels decreased within the rat testis. As testicular EtOH levels increased, lipid peroxidation products, as measured by TBARs, increased as α-tocopherol levels decreased within the rat testis. The supplementation of exogenous α-tocopherol may be necessary during EtOH intoxication because EtOH-induced depletion of endogenous α-tocopherol levels has previously been reported in rat liver[96] and human liver.[97] In adult rats, exogenous α-tocopherol is able to enter the brain and liver. Bondy et al.[98] administered a daily intraperitoneal injection of α-tocopherol succinate (200 mg/kg/d; 376.83 μmol/kg/d) for 15 d before EtOH ingestion. Endogenous levels of α-tocopherol increased in the brains and livers of α-tocopherol-treated and α-tocopherol- and EtOH-treated rats as compared to untreated animals. While exogenous α-tocopherol treatments promoted elevated endogenous α-tocopherol levels in both brains and livers, the increase was more pronounced in the liver, and the levels of reactive oxygen species were diminished in hepatic cells after α-tocopherol treatment in the presence or absence of EtOH. The levels of reactive oxygen species in the cerebral cortex of the brain were unaffected by α-tocopherol.[98]

While exogenous α-tocopherol can serve as an antioxidant, low to moderate concentrations of exogenous α-tocopherol must be used. Bondy et al.[98] reported that when rats received high concentrations of α-tocopherol succinate (200 mg/kg/d; 376.83 μmol/kg/d) for 15 d prior to either water or EtOH ingestion, fibrosis of the liver and peritoneal cavities containing ascites fluid was observed. In addition, the high concentrations of exogenous α-tocopherol promoted increased hepatic protease activities. This suggested that the high, chronic dosage of exogenous α-tocopherol (376.83 μmol/kg/d) used in this study was hepatotoxic. The authors cited that exogenous α-tocopherol could occasionally enhance oxidative events because the catabolic products of vitamin E, such as the α-tocopheroxyl radical, can have pro-oxidant activities.[99,100] Bondy et al.[98] suggested that low to moderate concentrations of exogenous α-tocopherol is an antioxidant, while high concentrations may serve as a pro-oxidant. Bondy et al.[98] also reported that the administration of exogenous α-tocopherol promoted higher levels of glutathione (GSH) in both brain and liver while EtOH treatment depressed glutathione (GSH) levels in both tissues. Glutathione (GSH) serves as a substrate for the antioxidant enzyme glutathione peroxidase (GSH-Px; EC 1.11.1.9).

EtOH-induced peroxidation has been demonstrated in embryos. In a very clever *in vitro* study by Kotch et al.,[101] EtOH-induced teratogenesis was studied in gestational day 8 mouse embryos that were exposed to EtOH for 6 h in whole embryo cultures. Embryonic EtOH exposure promoted increased levels of superoxide anions, increased rates of lipid peroxidation, and excessive cell death. However, in the presence of the antioxidant enzyme superoxide dimutase (SOD; EC 1.15.1.1), the EtOH-induced increased levels of reactive oxygen species, the EtOH-induced increased levels of lipid peroxidation metabolites, and EtOH-induced cell-death were attenuated.

Miller et al.[34] demonstrated EtOH-induced membrane lipid peroxidation in chick embryos. At 0 d of development, fertile chicken eggs were injected with a single dose of either saline, EtOH (6.05 mmol/kg), EtOH and α-tocopherol (6.05 mmol EtOH/kg and 2.5 μmol α-tocopherol/kg), or EtOH and γ-tocopherol (6.05 mmol EtOH/kg and 2.5 μmol γ-tocopherol/kg). At 18 d of development (stage 44, see Reference 32), EtOH-induced reductions in brain membrane long-chain, unsaturated fatty acids were observed with EtOH-induced increases in brain membrane short-chain, saturated fatty acids. EtOH-induced decreases in the levels of brain membrane oleic acid (18:1, *n*-9), linoleic (18:2, *n*-6), linolenic (18:3, *n*-3), arachidonic (20:4, *n*-6), and docosahexaenoic acid (22:6, *n*-3) were observed, and EtOH-induced increases in the levels of brain membrane lauric acid (12:0) and myristic acid (14:0) were observed. These EtOH-induced decreases in long-chain unsaturated fatty acids correlated with EtOH-induced reductions in brain mass, EtOH-induced reductions in brain acetylcholine esterase activities (AChE; EC 3.1.1.7), and EtOH-induced increases in brain lipid hydroperoxide levels. Exposure to either α-tocopherol or γ-tocopherol attenuated EtOH-induced changes in brain fatty acid composition, brain mass, AChE activities, and lipid hydroperoxide levels. Thus, the exogenous use of an antioxidant ameliorated EtOH-induced brain membrane lipid peroxidation in an embryonic system.

We have recently studied the effects of exogenous EtOH, EtOH and α-tocopherol, and EtOH and γ-tocopherol treatments on endogenous vitamin E levels in embryonic chick brains and livers. This was accomplished by injecting fertile chicken eggs with a single dose of saline, EtOH (6.05 mmol/kg), EtOH and α-tocopherol (6.05 mmol EtOH/kg and 2.5 μmol α-tocopherol/kg), or EtOH and γ-tocopherol (6.05 mmol EtOH/kg and 2.5 μmol γ-tocopherol/kg) at 0 days of development. At 18 d of development (stage 44; see Reference 32), embryonic chick brains and livers were removed and lipids and lipid-soluble materials were extracted. Fat-soluble vitamins were separated by high-pressure liquid chromatography with a fluorescence detector. A Prevail C18 HPLC column (5 μm, 150 mm × 4.6 mm) (Alltech Associates, Deerfield, IL) was used with a mobile phase of acetonitrile–methanol (75:25, v/v) at a flow rate of 1.5 ml/min. The excitation wavelength of the fluorescence detector was 295 nm and the emission wavelength was 330 nm. In this study, a single dose of EtOH (6.05 mmol/kg) promoted decreased levels of endogenous α-tocopherol in both brains and livers at 18 d of development as compared to controls (Figure 19.3). Meanwhile, exposure to EtOH and α-tocopherol (6.05 mmol EtOH/kg and 2.5 μmol α-tocopherol/kg) caused endogenous levels of α-tocopherol to return to near normal levels in embryonic brains and livers (Figure 19.3). Thus exposure to exogenous α-tocopherol attenuated EtOH-induced reductions in endogenous vitamin E levels within an embryonic system.

19.2.5 CAN MELATONIN ATTENUATE EtOH-INDUCED DAMAGE?

There are many antioxidants other than vitamin E. Consequently, there has been a recent interest in testing whether or not other antioxidants attenuate EtOH-induced damage. Melatonin is one such antioxidant. Melatonin (*N*-acetyl-5-methoxytratamine) is an indole that is produced in the pineal gland. Besides involvement in circadian rhythms, the immune system, and endocrine system,[102,103] melatonin has been demonstrated as an antioxidant in neural, hepatic, and pulmonary tissues.[104–107]

Melatonin can attack hydroxyl radicals and superoxide anions. The resulting complexes are then excreted.[107–109] Melatonin can also stimulate the activity of the antioxidant enzyme GSH-Px in adult brain[110] and melatonin pretreatment attenuated bleomycin-induced increases in lipid peroxidation products in adult rat pulmonary tissues.[111]

Exogenous melatonin has been shown to attenuate EtOH-induced reductions in total glutathione levels (GSH), EtOH-induced reductions in glutathione reductase (GSSH Rd) activities, and EtOH-induced invasion of macrophages into adult rat gastric mucosa.[112] Recently, 4-d-old neonatal rats were given exogenous EtOH (97.68 mmol/kg/d), melatonin (43.1 μmol/kg/d), or EtOH and melatonin (97.68 mmol EtOH/kg/d and 43.1 μmol melatonin/kg/d) for 5 d prior to the histological staining of Purkinje cells within the vermis of the cerebellum.[113] EtOH-induced decreases in Purkinje neuron densities were observed in the vermis and lobule I of the cerebellum as compared to controls. However, exogenous melatonin failed to affect Purkinje neuron densities in the cerebellum. Exogenous melatonin failed to ameliorate EtOH-induced reductions in neonatal Purkinje neuron densities in the cerebellum.[113] Thus, the efficacy of exogenous melatonin in attenuating EtOH-induced damage is still in question.

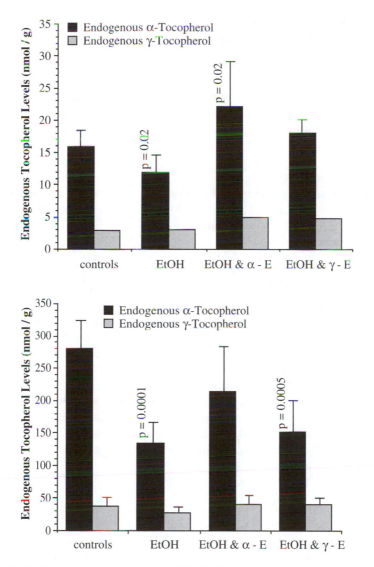

FIGURE 19.3 The effect of exogenous EtOH, EtOH and α-tocopherol, and EtOH and γ-tocopherol on endogenous vitamin E levels in brains and livers isolated from stage 44 chick embryos. At 0 d of development, fertile chicken eggs were injected with a single dose of either saline, EtOH (6.05 mmol/kg), EtOH and α-tocopherol (6.05 mmol EtOH/kg and 2.5 µmol α-tocopherol/kg), or EtOH and γ-tocopherol (6.05 mmol EtOH/kg and 2.5 µmol γ-tocopherol/kg). At 18 d of development (stage 44, see Reference 32), brain and liver tissue was removed and lipid soluble material extracted. Fat-soluble vitamins were separated by HPLC with a fluorescence detector (Thermo-Finnegan, Austin, TX). A Prevail C18 column (5 µm, 150 mm × 4.6 mm) (Alltech Associates, Deerfield, IL) was used with a mobile phase of acetonitrile-methanol (75: 25, v/v) at a flow rate of 1.5 ml/min. The excitation wavelength of the fluorescence detector was 295 nm and the emission wavelength was 330 nm.

19.2.6 ANTIOXIDANTS IN RED AND WHITE WINE CAN ATTENUATE EtOH-INDUCED DAMAGE

Red and white wines contain a number of polyphenolic antioxidants and polyphenols that are not only antioxidants but appear to alleviate EtOH-induced damage. These antioxidants include *trans*-resveratrol, catechin, and a number of anthocyanins. While *trans*-resveratrol, catechin, and anthocyanins are found in both white wines and red wines, their concentrations are generally higher in red wines. In red wines, *trans*-resveratrol levels are approximately 1.0 mg/l (0.1 to 2.3 mg/l) while their concentrations in white wines are only 0.22 mg/l (0.003 to 2.0 mg/l). In red wines, catechin levels are approximately 89 mg/l (27 to 191 mg/l) while their concentrations in white wines are only 17.3 mg/l (3 to 35 mg/l). In red wines, anthocyanin levels are approximately 281 mg/l (20 to 500 mg/l) while only trace amounts are found in white wines.[114] While white wines have lower levels of these antioxidants as compared to red wines, Cui et al.[115] recently reported that some white wines scavenge both superoxide anions and hydroxyl radicals in postischemic rat hearts. Sato et al.[116] demonstrated EtOH induced oxidative stress and the induction of HSP-70 (heat shock protein — 70,000 Da) in adult rat hearts. Meanwhile feeding adult rats red wine extracts or polyphenolic antioxidants with EtOH improved postischemic recovery by triggering a signal-transduction cascade by reducing proapoptotic transcription factors such as JNK-1 and c-Jun, and attenuating cell death.[116]

In 1991, the CBS television show, 60 *Minutes*, presented epidemiological observations that are now known as the "French paradox." While the French diet is typically rich in saturated fats, the incidence of atherosclerosis and other cardiovascular diseases is lower in France as compared to other countries. This decrease in atherosclerosis and other cardiovascular diseases correlated with wine consumption.[117] Since the positive effects of moderate wine consumption have recently been reviewed,[114,118-120] only recent observations will be presented.

19.2.6.1 CYP2E1 Involvement

It has long been known that chronic EtOH exposure increases the activity of cytochrome P-450 2E1 (CYP2E1) in a wide variety of cell types and at a variety of developmental time periods.[18,54,55,121-128] CYP2E1 is a Fe^{+2}-containing microsomal isozyme in the cytochrome p450 family that is not only induced by EtOH but also catalyzes the metabolism of EtOH. CYP2E1 and alcohol dehydrogenase catalyze the conversion of EtOH to acetaldehyde which in turn is oxidized to acetate through the use of aldehyde dehydrogenase and CYP2E1.[129-131] Besides metabolizing EtOH, CYP2E1 is a leaky enzyme that metabolizes a large number of nonpolar compounds to more polar metabolites that are easier to excrete.[125]

19.2.6.2 Attenuating EtOH-Induced Damage by Inhibiting CYP2E1

Because CYP2E1 as well as other CYP isozymes contains Fe^{+2}, CYP2E1 has been implicated in the production of oxygen radicals, hydroxyl radicals, and hydroxyethyl radicals, and EtOH-induced increases in CYP2E1 activities correlate with EtOH-induced toxicity.[74,122-124,132] Morimoto et al.[18,54,55] have reported that adult rats fed known CYP2E1 inhibitors (either diallyl sulfide or phenethyl isothiocyanate) had an attenuation of EtOH-induced increases in CYP2E1 mRNA levels, EtOH-induced reductions of long-chain membrane PUFAs, and EtOH-induced liver damage. Miller et al.[34] reported that embryonic exposure to the CYP2E1 inhibitor diallyl sulfide (DAS) attenuated EtOH-induced reductions in the levels of brain membrane long-chain PUFAs in embryonic chick brains. However in this last paper, DAS appears to have some teratogenic effects because DAS-induced reductions in embryonic brain mass were observed.[34] In regards to the antioxidant capabilities of red wine, Orellana et al.[133] demonstrated that chronic consumption of either red wine or red wine extracts decreased hepatic CYP2E1 activities while EtOH alone promoted elevated CYP2E1 activities.

While EtOH-induced induction of CYP2E1 has been linked to the generation of oxygen radicals, hydroxyl radicals, hydroxyethyl radicals, and subsequent lipid peroxidation,[18,54,55,74,122–124,131] EtOH-induced lipid peroxidation may also occur in CYP2E1-free cellular environments. Kono et al.[134,135] recently reported the production of CYP2E1 knockout mice (CYP2E1$^{-/-}$). EtOH-induced liver steatosis, EtOH-induced increases in reactive oxygen species (radicals), and EtOH-induced necrosis were reported in CYP2E1 $^{+/+}$, CYP2E1 $^{+/-}$, and CYP2E1$^{-/-}$ mice. However, there were insignificant differences when comparing EtOH-induced damage in CYP2E1 $^{+/+}$ mice to CYP2E1$^{-/-}$ (CYP2E1 knockout) mice. In response, Cederbaum et al.[136] recently reported the establishment of HepG2 cell lines that overexpress CYP2E1. Addition of EtOH or an unsaturated fatty acid such as arachidonic acid or iron supplementation promoted apoptosis and elevated lipid peroxidation. The inclusion of antioxidants and CYP2E1 inhibitors attenuated EtOH-induced, arachidonic acid-induced, and Fe^{+2}-induced apoptosis and lipid peroxidation in HepG2 cell lines.[133] The apparent conflict between the work of Kono et al.[134,135] and Cederbaum et al.[136] may be the result of EtOH-induced production of reactive oxygen and hydroxyl radicals through other Fe^{+2}-containing proteins other than CYP2E1.

19.2.7 GREEN TEA EXTRACTS MAY ATTENUATE EtOH-INDUCED DAMAGE

The polyphenols and flavonoids found in wine can attenuate EtOH toxicity.[114,118,119] However, polyphenols and flavonoids are also found in other dietary substances, and it is not surprising that other dietary substances have been reported to attenuate EtOH-induced peroxidation. Polyphenolic extracts of green tea, composed primarily of epigallocatechin gallate, protect against EtOH-induced liver damage. Arteel et al.[137] fed rats high-fat diets with and without ethanol (10 to 14 g/kg/d), with and without green tea (300 mg/kg/d) for a period of 4 weeks. EtOH-induced increases in serum alanine transaminase (ALT) were observed which indicated hepatic trauma. Inclusion of green tea significantly reduced the EtOH-induced increase in serum ALT activity.[137] In a similar paper, Skrzydlewska et al.[138] reported EtOH-induced damage in rats by monitoring EtOH-induced increases in serum lipid peroxidation products (malondialdehyde and 4-hydroxynonenal) and EtOH-induced increases in serum proteases (cathepsin G and elastase). While the inclusion of green tea failed to affect EtOH-induced increases in serum protease activities, it attenuated EtOH-induced increases in serum lipid peroxidation products (malondialdehyde and 4-hydroxynonenal).[138]

EtOH-induced increases in serum lipid peroxidation products and EtOH-induced decreases in hepatic superoxide dimutase (SOD; EC 1.15.1.1), hepatic catalase (CATAL; EC 1.11.1.6), hepatic glutathione peroxidase (GSH-Px 1.11.1.9), and reduced hepatic glutathione (GSH) levels have been observed.[139,140] Skrzydlewska et al.[140] have also reported EtOH induced decreases in the levels of ascorbic acid, vitamin A, vitamin E, and beta-carotene. The inclusion of green tea attenuated these EtOH-induced markers of lipid peroxidation.[140]

19.3   REACTIVE OXYGEN SPECIES AND IRON OVERLOAD

CYP2E1, as well as other CYP isozymes, contains Fe^{+2}, and CYP2E1 has been implicated in the production of oxygen radicals, hydroxyl radicals, and hydroxyethyl radicals. EtOH-induced increases in CYP2E1 activities have been observed and correlated with EtOH-induced toxicity.[75,122–124,132] However recent discrepancies in regards to the importance of CYP2E1[134–136] indicate that the production of reactive oxygen species (oxygen radicals and hydroxyl radicals) can be accomplished by other means.

EtOH-induced cytotoxicity is associated with elevated levels of iron (Fe^{+2}). In one out of three chronic alcoholics, increased levels of hepatic iron were seen,[141,142] and ethanol-induced increases in nontransferrin-bound iron levels were reported in the serum of chronic alcoholics.[143] De Lorgeril et al.[144] reported that EtOH ingestion promoted elevated levels of serum iron and ferritin in humans, and they reported significant Spearman's rank order correlation coefficients between EtOH ingestion and the levels of serum iron (r = 0.21; $p \leq 0.0001$) and ferritin (r = 0.23; $p \leq 0.0001$). Although the storage protein ferritin itself does not produce hydroxyl radicals via the Fenton reaction,[145] iron released from ferritin can produce hydroxyl radicals.[146,147] In patients suffering from alcohol-induced liver damage, excess hepatic iron accumulation was observed with an upregulation of liver transferrin receptor expression as compared to patients with normal liver pathology.[148]

In laboratory animals, the effects of EtOH on iron levels have been inconsistent. In adult rats, chronic EtOH exposure promoted increased plasma Fe^{+2} levels. However, EtOH failed to alter Fe^{+2} levels in the cerebral cortex and the liver, and EtOH-induced decreases in Fe^{+2} levels were seen in the cerebellum.[149] Meanwhile, in adult rats, chronic EtOH treatments promoted cirrhosis of the liver and increased levels of hepatic iron.[150]

In order to study the effects of exogenous EtOH and/or Fe^{+2} on membrane lipid peroxidation, exogenous EtOH, $FeCl_2$, $FeCl_2$ and EtOH, NaCl, and NaCl and EtOH were injected into fertile chicken eggs.[50] Controls were either shams or injected with saline. The experimental groups were as follows.

Experimental Treatments	Concentrations
EtOH	3.025 mmol EtOH/kg
$FeCl_2$	3.003 µmol $FeCl_2$/kg
$FeCl_2$ and EtOH	3.003 µmol $FeCl_2$/kg and
	3.025 mmol EtOH/kg
NaCl	6.006 µmol NaCl/kg
NaCl and EtOH	6.006 µmol NaCl/kg and
	3.025 mmol EtOH/kg

The Fe^{+2} dosage used in this study was selected because many pregnant women consume iron supplements that range from 15 mg/d to 240 mg/d.[151,152] If maternal weight ranges from 130 to 200 lbs, a daily dosage of 15 mg of Fe^{+2} would range from 2.96 μmol/kg/d to 4.56 μmol/kg/d. Thus, Miller et al.[50] selected a dosage of 3.003 μmol $FeCl_2$/kg per egg. These injections were made at 0 d or 0 to 2 d of development and tissue removed at 11 d of embryonic development. Embryonic exposure to exogenous EtOH and/or Fe^{+2} promoted decreased brain mass, decreased levels of brain membrane PUFAS, elevated levels of brain lipid hydroperoxides, and elevated levels of Fe^{+2} within embryonic brain and liver. These alterations were more severe in triple-injected embryos (E0-2/E11) as compared to single-injected embryos (E0/E11). While exogenous treatments of either EtOH and/or $FeCl_2$ promoted increased levels of endogenous brain Fe^{+2}, the effects were not additive. These observations are consistent with the hypothesis that embryonic exposure to exogenous EtOH and/or Fe^{+2} promotes brain membrane lipid peroxidation.

19.4 REACTIVE OXYGEN SPECIES AND XANTHINE OXIDASE

One enzyme of interest in the production of oxygen radicals is xanthine oxidase (XO; EC 1.2.3.2). Xanthine oxidase consists of two dissociable subunits where each subunit contains a molybdenum atom, one FAD^+ molecule, and two Fe^{+2}/S_2 complexes.[153] Xanthine oxidase and xanthine dehydrogenase (EC 1.2.1.37) catalyzes the conversion of hypoxanthine to xanthine during purine catabolism. Normally, XDH would be the preferred enzyme in converting hypoxanthine to xanthine.

$$\text{Hypoxanthine} + H_2O + NAD^+ \xrightarrow[\text{dehydrogenase}]{\text{xanthine}} \text{Xanthine} + NADH + H^+$$

$$\text{Hypoxanthine} + H_2O + 2O_2 \xrightarrow[\text{oxidase}]{\text{xanthine}} \text{Xanthine} + O_2^{\bullet} + H_2O_2$$

However, during EtOH metabolism, NAD^+ levels decrease because of the actions of alcohol dehydrogenase (ADH; EC 1.1.1.1) and aldehyde dehydrogenase (ALDH; EC 1.2.1.3).[154,155] As ADH converts ethanol to acetaldehyde, NADH is synthesized from NAD^+. As ALDH converts acetaldehyde to acetate, NADH is synthesized from NAD^+, and thus intercellular levels of NAD^+ decline. As intercellular levels of NAD^+ decline, xanthine dehydrogenase is no longer the favored enzyme over xanthine oxidase and as xanthine oxidase activity increases, the levels of hydroxyl radicals increase.[153,156]

Younes and Strubelt[156] argued that during EtOH metabolism, depletion of the NAD^+ pool would slow XDH activity and allow XO to produce H_2O_2, and the subsequent H_2O_2 decomposition would generate hydroxyl radicals. In support of this hypothesis, Younes and Strubelt reported EtOH-induced liver damage in perfused adult rats as monitored by increases in serum glutamate-pyruvate transaminase [GPT; also known as alanine transaminase (ALT)].[156] As EtOH-induced liver hypoxia was monitored, Kreb's cycle activity slowed and the levels of serum lactate and pyruvate increased as serum GSH levels decreased. Since allopurinol is a known inhibitor of XO, Younes and Strubelt administered allopurinol (100 mg/l) to the EtOH-containing (3 g/l) perfusion medium and reported an attenuation of EtOH-induced changes in hepatic activities. This paper suggested that XO mediates EtOH-induced liver damage.[156]

Recent work in adult rats indicates that the conversion of ethanol to acetaldehyde and the formation of 1-hydroxyethyl free radicals can also be catalyzed by XDH, and by XO.[157,158] The administration of the XDH and XO inhibitor, allopurinol, reduced the transformation of ethanol to acetaldehyde and reduced the levels of 1-hydroxyethyl free radicals.[157,158] Kono et al. reported that exogenous allopurinol had no effect of urine ethanol levels in rat. However, exogenous allopurinol significantly blunted EtOH-induced increases in serum aspartate aminotransferase and ALT levels. Thus, inhibition of XO attenuated EtOH-induced liver damage in adult rats.[159] Wright et al.[160] reported that the EtOH-induced formation of reactive oxygen species and the levels of reactive oxygen species correlate to EtOH-induced increases in XO activities in alcohol-induced breast cancer. Thus, ethanol metabolism is linked to xanthine oxidase activity.

EtOH-induced increase in xanthine oxidase activity can also mediate EtOH-induced increases in serum Fe^{+2}, and EtOH-induced increases in serum Fe^{+2} levels have been reported.[141–144] In adults, dietary Fe^{+2} is absorbed through the small intestine and bound to transferrin, and the uptake of Fe^{+2} by transferrin is mediated by XO.[161] While XO activity is found in all tissues, it is highest within the liver and small intestine. In the small intestine, the generation of oxygen radicals, largely by XO, can catalyze the release of Fe^{+2} from ferritin.[146,162] Ferritin released Fe^{+2} ions can produce more hydroxyl radicals,[146,147] and the hydroxyl radicals can not only produce lipid peroxidation, as discussed in this paper, but can also promote the peroxidation of DNA.[124] Thus, EtOH-induced mobilization of iron and the production of oxygen radicals and hydroxyl radicals by xanthine oxidase can enhance ETOH-induced cellular damage.

ACKNOWLEDGMENTS

This author is indebted to a large number of students who have worked in my lab and, thereby, contributed to this manuscript. The most recent group of students includes Dan Coughlin, Sabrina Fraser-Thomson, Betsy Noe, Beth Olson, Amanda Palenick, and Emily Voorhees. I am also indebted to the entire Hillsdale College community.

References

1. Geer, B.W., Miller, R. R., Jr., Heinstra, P.W.H. (1991) Genetic and dietary control of alcohol degradation in *Drosophila*: role in cell damage. In: R. R. Watson (Ed.), *Drug and Alcohol Abuse Reviews, Vol. 2: Liver Pathology and Alcohol*. Humana Press, Totowa, NJ, pp. 325–373.

2. Reitz, R .C. (1992) Effects of dietary fatty acids and alcohol on fatty acid composition in cellular membranes. In: R. R. Watson, B. Watzl (Eds.), *Nutrition and Alcohol.* CRC Pess, Boca Raton, FL, pp. 191–204.

3. Salam, N., Jr., Ward G. (1993) The effects of ethanol on polyunsaturated fatty acid composition. In: C. Alling, I. Diamond, S. W. Leslie, G.Y. Sun, W. Gibson Wood (Eds.), *Alcohol, Cell Membranes and Signal Transduction in Brain.* Plenum Press, New York, pp. 55–62.

4. Sun, G.Y., Sun, A.Y. (1985) Ethanol and membrane lipids. *Alcohol. Clin. Exp.* Res. 9: 164–180.

5. Aloia, R. C., Paxton, J. Daviau, J. S., Van Gelb, O., Mlekusch, W., Truppe, W., Meyer, J.A., Braver, F.S. (1985) Effect of chronic alcohol consumption on rat brain microsome lipid composition, membrane fluidity, and Na⁺-K⁺-ATPase activity. *Life Sci.* 36: 1003–1010.

6. Beauge, F. J. (1993) Relevant effects of dietary polyunsaturated fatty acids on synaptic membrane responses to ethanol and chronic ethanol intoxication. In: C. Alling, I. Diamond, S. W. Leslie, G. Y. Sun, W. Gibson Wood (Eds.), *Alcohol, Cell Membranes, and Signal Transduction in Brain*, Plenum Press, New York, pp. 47–54.

7. Lesch, P., Schmidt, E., Schmidt, F. W. (1973) Effects of chronic alcohol abuse on the fatty acid composition of major lipids in the human brain. *Z. Klin. Chem. Klin. Biochem.* 11: 159–166.

8. Littleton, J. M. (1990) Effects of ethanol on membranes and their associated functions. In: K. E. Crowe, R.D. Batt (Eds.) *Human Metabolism of Alcohol, Vol. 3.* CRC Press, Boca Raton, FL, pp. 161–173.

9. Pawlosky, R. J., Salam, N. Jr. (1995) Ethanol exposure causes a decrease in docosa-hexaenoic acid and an increase in docosapentaenoic acid in feline brain and retinas. *Am. J. Clin. Nutr.* 61: 1284–1289.

10. Nanji, A. A., French, S.W. (1989) Dietary linoleic acid is required for development of experimental alcoholic liver disease. *Life Sci.* 44: 223–227.

11. Nanji, A. A., Mendenhall, C. L., French, S.W. (1989) Beef fat prevents alcoholic liver disease in rat. *Alcohol. Clin. Exp. Res.* 13: 15–19.

12. Nanji, A. A., Zhao, S., Lamb, R. G., Sadrzadeh, S. M. H., Dannenberg, A. J., Waxman, D. J. (1993) Changes in microsomal phospholipases and arachidonic acid in experimental alcoholic liver injury: relationship to levels of cytochrome p450 2E1 induction and conjugated dienes formation. *Alcohol. Clin. Exp. Res.* 17: 598–603.

13. Shiraishi, K., Matsuzaki, S., Iyakura, M., Ishida, H. (1996) Abnormality in membrane fatty acid composition of cells measured in erythrocytes in alcoholic liver disease. *Alcohol. Clin. Exp. Res.* 20: 56A–59A.

14. Nanji, A.A., Zhao, S., Hossein, S.M., Sadrzadeh, S.M.H. (1994) Liver microsomal fatty acid composition in ethanol-fed rats: effects of dietary fats and relationship to liver injury. *Alcohol. Clin. Exp. Res.* 18: 1024–1028.

15. Nanji, A.A., Zhao, S., Hossein, S.M., Sadrzadeh, S.M.H., Dannenberg, A.J., Waxman, D.J. (1994) Markedly enhanced cytochrome p450 2E1 induction and lipid peroxida-tion is associated with severe liver injury in fish-oil-ethanol-fed rats. *Alcohol. Clin. Exp. Res.* 18: 1280–1994.

16. Bondy S. C., Marwah, S. (1995) Stimulation of synaptosomal free radical production by fatty acids: relation to estrification and to degree of unsaturation. *FEBS Lett.* 375: 53–55.

17. Chen, Q., Galleano, M., Cederbaum, A. I. (1997) Cytotoxicity and apoptosis produced by arachidonic acid in Hep G2 cells over-expressing human cytochrome p450 2E1. *J. Biol. Chem.* 272: 14532–14541.

18. Morimoto, M., Zern, M.A., Hagbjork, A-L., Ingelman-Sundberg, M, French, S.W. (1994) Fish oil, alcohol, and liver pathology: role of cytochrome P450 2E1. *Proc. Soc. Exp. Biol. Med.* 207: 197–205.

19. Porter, N. A., Mills, K.A., Caldwell S.E. (1995) Mechanisms of free radical oxidation of unsaturated lipids. *Lipids* 30: 277–290.

20. Chin, J.H., Goldstein, D.B. (1977) Drug tolerance in biomembranes: a spin label study of the effects of ethanol. *Science* 196: 684–85.

21. Miller R.R., Jr., Dare, A.O., Moore, M.L., Kooser, R.G., Geer, B.W. (1993) Long-chain fatty acids and ethanol affect the properties of membranes in *Drosophila melanogaster* larvae. *Biochem. Genet.* 31: 113–31.

22. Tarashi, T.F., Rubin, E. (1985) Biology of disease: effects of ethanol on the chemical and structural properties of biologic membranes. *Lab. Invest.* 52: 120–131.

23. Waring, A.J., Rottenberg, H., Ohnishi, T., Rubin, E. (1981) Membranes and phospholipids of liver mitochondria from chronic alcoholic rats are resistant o membrane disordering by alcohol. *Proc. Natl. Acad. Sci. U.S.A.* 78: 2582–2586.

24. Rottenberg, H. (1987) Partition of ethanol and other amphiphilic compounds modulated by chronic alcoholism. *Ann. N.Y. Acad. Sci.* 492: 112–124.

25. Rottenberg, H. (1991) Liver cell membrane adaptation to chronic alcohol consumption. In: R.R. Watson (Ed.), *Drug and Alcohol Abuse Reviews, Vol. 2: Liver Pathology and Alcohol.* Humana Press, Totowa, NJ, pp. 91–115.

26. Ho, C., Slater, S.J., Stubbs, C.D. (1995) Hydration and order in lipid bilayers. *Biochemistry* 34: 6188–6195.

27. Cullis, P.R., de Kruijff, B. (1979) Lipid polymorphism and the functional roles of lipids in biological membranes. *Biochim. Biophys. Acta* 559: 399–420.

28. Tilcock, C.P.S., Cullis, P.R. (1987) Lipid polymorphism. *Ann. N.Y. Acad. Sci.* 492: 88–101.

29. Jain, M. (1972) *The Biomolecular Membrane.* Van Nostrand, New York, pp. 1–51.

30. Burdge, G. C., Postle A. D. (1995) Effect of maternal ethanol consumption during pregnancy on the phospholipid molecular species composition of fetal guinea-pig brain, liver, and plasma. *Biochim. Biophys. Acta* 1256: 346–352.

31. Wainwright, P.E., Huang, Y.-S., Simmons, V., Mills, D.E., Ward, R.P., Ward, G.R. Winfeld, D., McCutcheon, D. (1990) Effects of prenatal ethanol and long-chain n-3 fatty acid supplementation of development in mice. 2. Fatty acid composition of brain membrane phospholipids. *Alcohol. Clin. Exp. Res.* 14: 413–420.

32. Hamburger, V., Hamilton H. L. (1951) A series of normal stages in the development of the chick embryo. *J. Morphol.* 88: 49–92.

33. Miller, R.R., Jr., Taylor, C.L., Spidle, D.L., Ugolini, A.M., Nothdorf, R.A. (1996) Ethanol-induced decreases in membrane long-chain unsaturated fatty acids correlate with impaired chick brain development. *Comp. Biochem. Physiol.,* 115B: 465–474.

34. Miller, R.R., Jr., Slathar. J.R., Luvisotto, M.L. (2000) α-tocopherol and γ-tocopherol attenuate ethanol-induced changes in membrane fatty acid composition in embryonic chick brains. *Teratology* 62: 26–35.

35. Miller, R.R., Jr., Heckel, C.D., Koss, W.J., Montague, S.L., Greenman, A.L. (2001) Ethanol-induced and nicotine-induced membrane changes in embryonic chick brains. *Comp. Biochem. Physiol.* 130C: 163–178.

36. Ashakumary, L., Vijayammal, P.L. (1993) Additive effect of alcohol and nicotine on lipid metabolism in rats. *Indian J. Exp. Biol.* 31: 270–274.

37. Ashakumary, L., Vijayammal, P.L. (1996) Additive effect of alcohol and nicotine on lipid peroxidation and antioxidant defense mechanism in rats. *J. App. Toxicol.* 16: 305–308.

38. Turchetto, E., Ottani, V., Zanetti, P., Weiss, H. (1968) Hepatic fatty acids after ethanol ingestion. *Nutr. Diet. Basal.* 10: 224–228.

39. French, S.W., Ihrig, T.J., Morin, R.T. (1970) Lipid composition of RBC ghost, liver mitochondria and microsomes of ethanol-fed rats. *Q. J. Stud. Alcohol* 31: 801–809.

40. French, S.W., Ihrig, T.J., Shaw, G.P., Tanaka, T.T., Norum, M.L. (1971) The effect of ethanol on the fatty acid composition of hepatic microsomes and inner and outer membranes. *Res. Commun. Chem. Pathol. Pharmacol.* 2: 561–585.

41. Thompson J.A., Reitz, R.C. (1978) Effects of ethanol ingestion and dietary fat levels on mitochondrial lipids in male and female rats. *Lipids* 13: 540–550.

42. Roa, G.A., Goheen, S.C., Manix, M., Larkin, E.C. (1980) Enhanced ratio of linoleic acid to arachidonic acid in erythrocyte phosphatidylcholine in rats withdrawal from ethanol. *Toxicol. Lett.* 7: 37–40.

43. Foudin, L., Sun, G.Y., Sun, A.Y. (1986) Changes in lipid composition of rat heart mitochondria after chronic ethanol administration. *Alcohol. Clin. Exp. Res.* 10: 606–609.

44. Ellingson, J.S., Jones, N., Taraschi, T.F., Rubin, E. (1991) The effect of chronic ethanol administration on the fatty acid composition of phosphatidylinositol in rat liver microsomes as determined by gas chromatography and 1-H-NMR. *Biochim. Biophys. Acta* 1062: 199–205.

45. Rouach, H., Clement, M., Orfanelli, M.-T., Janvier, B., Nordmann, R. (1984) Fatty acid composition of rat liver mitochondrial phospholipids during ethanol inhalation. *Biochim. Biophys. Acta* 795: 125–129.

46. Reitz, R.C., Helsabeck, E., Mason, D.P. (1973) Effects of chronic alcohol ingestion on the fatty acid composition of the heart. *Lipids* 8: 80–84.

47. Nervi, A.M., Peluffo, R.O., Brenner, R.R. (1980) Effect of ethanol administration on fatty acid desaturation. *Lipids* 15: 263–268.

48. Reitz, R.C. (1982) Relationship of the acyl-CoA desaturases to certain membrane fatty acid changes induced by ethanol consumption. *Proc. West. Pharmacol. Soc.* 27: 247–249.

49. Wang, D.L., Reitz, R.C. (1983) Ethanol ingestion and polyunsaturated fatty acids: effects on the acyl-CoA desaturases. *Alcohol. Clin. Exp. Res.* 7: 220–226.

50. Miller, R.R., Jr., Coughlin, D.J, Fraser-Thomson, E.S., Noe, E.C., Palanick, A., Voorhees, E.B. (2003) Ethanol- and Fe^{+2}-induced membrane lipid oxidation is not additive in developing chick brains. *Comp. Biochem. Physiol.* 134C: 267–279.

51. Van Albert, B.C. (1990) Oxygen toxicity: role of hydrogen peroxide and iron. In: I. Emeritt (Ed.), *Anti-oxidants in Therapy and Preventive Medicine*. Plenum Press, New York, pp. 235–246.

52. Lalonde, C., Picard, L., Campbell, C., Demling, R. (1994) Lung and systemic oxidant and anti-oxidant activity after graded smoke exposure in the rat. *Circ. Shock* 42: 7–13.

53. Benzie, I.E.F. (1996) Lipid peroxidation: a review of causes, consequences, measurement, and dietary influences. *Int. J. Food Sci. Nutr.* 47: 233–261.

54. Morimoto, M., Reitz, R. C., Morin, R. J., Nguyen, K., Ingelman-Sundberg, M., French S. W. (1995a) Cytochrome P450 2E1 inhibitors partially ameliorate the changes in fatty acid composition induced in rats by chronic administration of ethanol and high fat diets. *J. Nutr.* 125: 2953–2964.

55. Morimoto, M., Hagbjork, A.-L., Wan, Y.-J., Y., Fu, P.C., Clot, P., Albano, E., Ingelman-Sundberg, M., French, S.W. (1995b) Modulation of experimental alcohol-induced liver disease by cytochrome P450 2E1 inhibitors. *Hepatology* 21: 1610–1617.

56. Chen, J., Schenker, S., Henderson, G.I. (2002) 4-hydroxynonenal detoxification by mitochondrial glutathione S-transferase is compromised by short-term ethanol consumption in rats. *Alcohol. Clin. Exp. Res.* 26: 1252–1258.

57. Bondy, S.C., Guo, S.X. (1995) Regional selectivity in ethanol-induced pro-oxidant events within the brain. *Biochem. Pharmacol.* 49: 69–72.

58. Montoliu, C., Valles, S., Renau-Piqueras, J., Guerri, C. (1994) Ethanol-induced oxygen radical formation and lipid peroxidation in rat brain: effects of alcohol consumption. *J. Neurochem.* 63: 1855–1862.

59. Sun, A.Y., Chen, Y.M., James-Kracke, M., Wixom, P., Cheng, Y. (1997) Ethanol-induced cells death by lipid peroxidation in PC 12 cells. *Neurochemistry* 22: 1187–1192.

60. Gonthier, B., Eysseric, H., Soubeyran, A. Daveloose, D., Saxod, R., Barret, L. (1997) Free radical production after exposure of astrocytes and astrocytic C6 glioma cells to ethanol. Preliminary results. *Free Radic. Res.* 27: 645–656.

61. Montoliu, C., Sauncho-tello, M., Azorin, I., Burgal, M., Valles, S., Renau-Piqueras, J., Guerri, C. (1995) Ethanol increases cytochrome P4502E1 and induces oxidative stress in astrocytes. *J. Neurochem.* 65: 2561–2570.

62. Rouach, H., Houze, P., Gentil., M., Orfanelli, M.T., Nordmann, R. (1997) Changes in some pro-and antioxidants defense system in rat brain subcellular fractions. *Neurotoxicology* 20: 977–987.

63. Calabrese, V., Renis, M., Calderone, A., Russo, A., Reale, S., Barcellona, M.L., Rizza, V. (1998a) Stress proteins and SH-groups in oxidant-induced cellular injury after chronic administration of ethanol in rat. *Free Radic. Biol. Med.* 24: 1159–1167.

64. Calabrese, V., Randazzo, G., Ragusa, N., Rizza, V. (1998b) Long-term ethanol administration enhances age-dependent modulation of redox status in central and peripheral organs of rat: protection by metadoxine. *Drugs. Exp. Clin. Res.* 24: 85–91.

65. Di Luzio, N.R., Hartman, A.D. (1967) Role of lipid peroxidation in the pathogenesis of the ethanol-induced fatty liver. *Fed. Proc.* 26: 1436–1442.

66. Comporti. M., Hartman, A., Di Luzio, N.R. (1967) Effect of *in vivo* and *in vitro* ethanol administration on liver peroxidation. *Lab. Invest.* 16: 616–624,

67. Boveris, A., Fraga, C.G., Varsavsky, A.I., Koch, O.R. (1983) Increased chemiluminescence and superoxide production in the liver of chronically ethanol-fed rats. *Arch. Biochem. Biophys.* 227: 534–541.

68. Dicker, E., Cederbaum, A.I. (1988) Increased oxygen radical-dependent inactivation of metabolic enzymes by liver microsomes after chronic ethanol consumption. *FASEB J.* 2: 2901–2906.

69. Ekstrom, G., Ingelman-Sundberg, M. (1989) Rat liver microsomal NADPH-supported oxidase activity and lipid peroxidation on ethanol-inducible cytochrome P450 (P-450 IIE1). *Biochem. Pharmacol.* 38: 1313–1318.

70. Ekstrom, G., Cronholm, T., Ingelman-Sundberg, M. (1986) Mechanisms of lipid peroxidation dependent upon cytochrome P-450 LM2. *Biochem. J.* 233: 755–761.

71. Puntarulo, S., Cederbaum, A.I. (1988a) Increased NADPH-dependent chemiluminescence by microsomes after chronic ethanol consumption. *Arch. Biochem. Biophys.* 266: 435–445.

72. Puntarulo, S., Cederbaum, A.I. (1988b) Effect of oxygen radical concentration on microsome oxidation of ethanol production of oxygen radicals. *Biochem. J.* 251: 787–794.

73. Rashba-Step, J., Turro, N., Cederbaum, A.I. (1993) Increased NADPH- and NADH-dependent production of superoxide and hydroxyl radicals by microsomes after chronic ethanol treatment. *Arch. Biochem. Biophys.* 300: 401–408.

74. Reinke, L. A., Lai, E.K., DuBose, C.M., McCay, P.B. (1987) Reactive free radical generation in the heart and liver of ethanol-fed rats: correlation with *in vitro* radical formation. *Proc. Natl. Acad. Sci. U.S.A.* 84: 9223–9227.

75. Albano, E., Tomasi, A., Persson. J.-O., Terelius, Y., Goria-Gatti, L., Ingelman-Sundberg, M., Dianzani, M.U. (1991) Role of ethanol-inducible cytochrome P450 (P450IIE1) in catalyzing the free radical activation of aliphatic alcohols. *Biochem. Pharmacol.* 41: 1895–1902.

76. Nordmann, R., Ribiere, C., Rouach, H. (1987) Involvement of iron and iron-catalyzed free radical production in ethanol metabolism and toxicity. *Enzyme* 37: 57–69.

77. Adachi, Y., Bradford, B.U., Wenshi, G., Bojes, H.K., Thurman, R.G. (1994) Inactivation of Kupffer cells prevents early alcohol-induced liver injury. *Hepatology* 20: 453–460.

78. Knecht, K.T., Adachi, Y., Bradford, B.U., Iimuro, Y., Kadiiska, M., Qun-Hui, X., Thurman, R.G. (1995) Free radical adducts in the bile of rats treated chronically with intragastric alcohol: inhibition by destruction of Kupffer cells. *Mol. Pharmacol.* 47: 1028–1034.

79. Knecht, K.T., Bradford, B.U., Mason, R.P., Thurman, G. (1990) *In vivo* formation of a free radical metabolite of ethanol. *Mol. Pharmacol.* 38: 26–30.

80. Wheeler, M.D., Kono, H., Yin, M., Nakagami, M., Uesugi, T., Arteel, G.E., Gabelle, E., Rusyn, I., Yamashina, S., Froh, M., Adachi, Y., Iimuro, Y., Bradford, B.U., Smutney, O.M., Connor, H.D., Mason, R.P., Goyert, S.M., Peters, J.M., Gonzalez, F.J., Samulski, R.J., Thurman, R.G. (2001) The role of Kupffer cell oxidant production in early ethanol-induced liver disease. *Free Radic. Biol. Med.* 31: 1544–1549.

81. Halliwel, B. (1996) Antioxidants in human health and disease. *Annu. Rev. Nutr.* 16: 33–50.

82. Thomas, J.A. (1994) Oxidative stress, oxidant defense, and dietary constituents. In: M.E. Shils, J.A. Olson, M. Shike (Eds.), *Modern Nutrition in Health and Disease*, 8th ed. Lea and Febiger, Malvern, PA, pp. 501–512.

83. Niki, E., Chemistry and biochemistry of vitamin E and coenzyme Q as antioxidant, in *Free Radicals and Antioxidants in Nutrition*, Corogiu, F., Banni, S., Dessi, M.A., and Rice-Evans, C., Eds., Richelieu Press, London, 1993, 13.

84. Packer, L., Kagan, V.E., Vitamin E: the antioxidant harvesting center of membranes and lipoproteins, in *Vitamin E in Health and Disease*, Packer, L., Fuchs, J., Eds., Marcel Dekker, New York, 1993, 179.

85. Packer, L., Slater, T.F., and Wilsson, R.L., Direct observation of a free radical interaction between vitamin E and vitamin C, *Nature* 278, 737, 1979.

86. Altura, B.M., Altura, B.T. (1984) Alcohol, the cerebral circulation, and strokes. *Alcohol* 1: 325–331.

87. Camargo, C.A., Jr. (1989) Moderate alcohol consumption and stroke: the epidemiologic evidence. *Stroke* 20: 1611–1626.

88. Donahue, R.P., Abbott, R.D., Reed, D.M., Yano, K. (1986) Alcohol and hemorrhagic stroke. *J. Am. Med. Assoc.* 225: 2311–2314.

89. Mullins, P.G.M., Vink, R. (1995) Chronic alcohol exposure decreases brain intracellular free magnesium concentration in rats. *Neuro Report* 6: 1633–1636.

90. Altura, B.M., Gebrewold, A. (1996) α-Tocopherol attenuates alcohol-induced cerebral vascular damage in rats: possible role of anti-oxidants in alcohol brain pathology and stroke. *Neurosci. Lett.* 220: 207–210.

91. Altura, B.M., Altura, B.T (1994) Role of magnesium and calcium in alcohol-induced hypertension and strokes as probed by *in vivo* television microscopy, digital image microscopy, optical spectroscopy, ^{31}P-NMR spectroscopy, and a unique magnesium ion-selective electrode. *Alcohol. Clin. Exp. Res.* 18: 1057–1068.

92. Altura, B.M., Gebrewold, A., Altura, B.T., Gupta, R.K. (1995) Role of brain [Mg^{2+}] in alcohol-induced hemorrhagic stroke in a rat model: a ^{31}P-NMR *in vivo* study. *Alcohol* 12: 131–136.

93. Li, W., Zheng, T., Alura, B.T., Altura, B.M. (2001) Antioxidants prevent depletion of [Mg^{2+}] induced by alcohol in cultured canine cerebral vascular smooth muscle cells: possible relationship to alcohol-induced stroke. *Brain Res. Bull.* 55: 475–478.

94. Li, W., Zheng, T., Alura, B.T., Altura, B.M. (2001) Antioxidants prevent ethanol-induced contractions of canine cerebral vascular muscle: relationship to alcohol-induced brain injury. *Neurosci. Lett.* 30: 91–94.

95. Zhang, X., Liu, Q., Ha, J. (1998) Protection of vitamin E against testis lipid peroxidation induced by iron and ethanol. *Wei sheng yan jiu (J. Hygiene Res.)* 27: 184–186.

96. Hagen, B.F., Bjoerneboe, A., Bjoerneboe, G.E.A., Drevon, C.A. (1989) Effect of chronic ethanol consumption on the content of α-tocopherol in subcellular fractions of rat liver. *Alcohol. Clin. Exp. Res.* 13: 246–251.

97. Bell, H., Bjoerneboe, A., Eidsvoll, B., Norum, K.R., Raknerund, N., Try, K., Thomassen, Y., Drevon, C.A. Reduced concentrations of hepatic α-tocopherol in patients with alcoholic liver cirrhosis. *Alcohol Alcohol.* 27, 39, 1992.

98. Bondy, S.C., Guo, S.X., Adams, J.D. (1996) Prevention of ethanol-induced changes in reactive oxygen parameters by α-tocopherol. *Alcohol Alcohol.* 31: 403–410.

99. Maiorino, M., Zamburlini, A., Roveri, A., Ursini, F. (1993) Prooxidant role of vitamin E in copper induced lipid peroxidation. *FEBS Lett.* 33: 174–176.

100. Iwatsuki, M., Niki, E., Stone, D., Darley-Usmar, V., Drevon, C.A. (1995) Alpha-tocopherol-mediated peroxidation in the copper (II) and metmyoglobin induced oxidation of human low density lipoprotein: the influence of lipid hydroperoxides. *FEBS Lett.* 360: 271–276.

101. Kotch L.E., Chen, S.-Y., Sulik, K.K. (1995) Ethanol-induced teratogenesis: free radical damage as a possible mechanism. *Teratology* 52:128–136.

102. Maestroni, G.J.M. (1993) The immunoneuroendocrine role of melatonin. *J. Pineal. Res.* 14: 1–10.

103. Reiter, R.J. (1993) The melatonin rhythm: both a clock and a calendar. *Experientia* 49: 654–664.

104. Lipartiti, M., Franceschini, D., Zanoni, R., Gusella, M., Giusti, P., Cagnoli, C.M., Kharlamov, E., Manev, H. (1996) Neuroprotective effects of melatonin. *Adv. Exp. Med. Biol.* 398: 315–321.

105. Mansouri, A., Demeilliers, C., Amsellem, S., Pessayre, D., Fromenty, B. (2001) Acute ethanol administration oxidatively damages and depletes mitochondrial DNA in mouse liver, brain, heart, and skeletal muscles: protective effects of antioxidants. *J. Pharmacol. Exp. Ther.* 298: 737–743.

106. Melchiorri, D., Reiter, R.J., Attia, A.M., Masayuki, H., Burgos, A., Nistico, G. (1995) Potent protective effect of melatonin on *in vivo* paraquat-induced oxidative damage in rats. *Life Sci.* 56: 83–89.

107. Reiter, R.J. (1996) The indoleamine melatonin as a free radical scavenger, electron donor, an antioxidant. *Adv. Exp. Med. Biol.* 398: 307–313.
108. Reiter, R.J., Tan, D.X., Poeggler, B., Chen, L.D., Manchester, L.C. (1994) Melatonin as a free radical scavenger: implications for aging and age-related diseases. *Ann. N.Y. Acad. Sci.* 719: 1–12.
109. Tan, D.X., Chen, L.D., Poeggler, B., Manchester, L.C., Reiter, R.J. (1993) Melatonin: a potent endogenous hydroxyl scavenger. *Endocr. J.* 1: 57.
110. Barlow-Walden L.R., Reiter, R.J., Abe, M., Pablos, M.,Menedez-Pelaez, A., Chen, L.D., Poeggeler, B. (1995) Melatonin stimulates brain glutathione peroxidase activity. *Neurochem. Int.* 26: 497–502.
111. Arslan, S.O., Zerin, M., Vural, H., Coskun, A. (2002) The effect of melatonin on bleomycin-induced pulmonary fibrosis in rats. *J. Pineal. Res.* 32: 21–25.
112. Bilici, D., Suleyman, H., Banoglu, Z.N., Kiziltunc, A., Avci, B., Ciftcioglu, Bilici, S. (2002) Melatonin prevents ethanol-induced gastric mucosal damage possibly due to its antioxidant activity. *Dig. Dis. Sci.* 47: 856–861.
113. Edwards, R.B., Manzana, E.J.P., Chen, W.-J.A. (2002) Melatonin (an antioxidant) does not ameliorate alcohol-induced Purkinje cell loss in the developing cerebellum. *Alcohol. Clin. Exp. Res.* 26: 1003–1009.
114. German, J.B., Walsem, R.L. (2000) The health benefits of wine. *Annu. Rev. Nutr.* 20: 561–593.
115. Cui, J., Tosaki, A., Cordis, G.A., Bertelli, A.A., Bertelli, A., Maulik, N., Das, D.K. (2002) Cardioprotective abilities of white wine. *Ann. N.Y. Acad. Sci.* 957: 308–316.
116. Sato, M., Maulik, N., Das, D.K. (2002) Cardioprotection with alcohol: role of both alcohol and polyphenolic antioxidants. *Ann. N.Y. Acad. Sci.* 957: 122–135.
117. Renaud S., de Lorgeril, M. (1992) Wine, alcohol, platelets, and the French Paradox of coronary heart disease. *Lancet* 339: 1523–1526.
118. Parks, D.A., Booyse, F.M. (2002) Cardiovascular protection by alcohol and polyphenols: role of nitric oxide. *Ann. N.Y. Acad. Sci.* 957: 115–121.
119. Rodrigo, R., Rivera, G. (2002) Renal damage mediated by oxidative stress: a hypothesis of protective effects of red wine. *Free Radic. Biol. Med.* 33: 409–422.
120. Sun, A.Y., Simonyi, A., Sun, G. Y. (2002) The "French paradox" and beyond: neuroprotective effects of polyphenols. *Free Radic. Bio. Med.* 32: 314–318.
121. Boutelet-Bochan, H., Huang, Y., Juchau, M.R. (1997) Expression of CYP 2E1 during embryogenesis and fetogenesis in human cephalic tissues: implications for the fetal alcohol syndrome. *Biochem. Biophys. Res. Commun.* 238: 443–447.
122. Cederbaum, A.I. (1989) Introduction: role of lipid peroxidation and oxidative stress in alcohol toxicity. *Free Radic. Biol. Med.* 7: 559–567.
123. Cederbaum, A.I. (1989) Oxygen radical generation by microsomes: role of iron and implications for alcohol metabolism and toxicity. *Free Radic. Biol. Med.* 7: 559–567.
124. Kukielka, E., Dicker, E., Cederbaum, A.J. (1994) Increased production of reactive oxygen species by rat liver mitochondria after chronic ethanol treatment. *Arch. Biochem. Biophys.* 309: 377–386.
125. Lieber, C.S. (1999) Microsomal ethanol-oxidizing system (MEOS): the first 30 years (1968–1998)-a review. *Alcohol. Clin. Exp. Res.* 23: 991–1007.
126. Oesterheld, J.R. (1998) A review of developmental aspects of cytochrome P450. *J. Chil Adolesc. Psychopharmacol.* 8: 161–174.
127. Rasheed, A., Hines, R.N., McCarver-May, D.G. (1997) Variation in induction of human placental CYP 2E1: possible role in susceptibility to fetal alcohol syndrome? *Toxicol. App. Pharmacol.* 144: 396–400.

128. Yoo, M., Ryu, H.-M., Shin, S.-W., Yun, C.-H., Lee, S.-C., Ji, Y.-M., You, K.-H. (1997) Identification of cytochrome P450 2E1 in rat brain. *Biochem. Biophys. Res. Commun.* 231: 254–256.

129. Burnell, J.C., Li, T.K., Bosron, W.Y. (1989) Purification and steady-state kinetic characterization of human liver β3β3 alcohol dehydrogenase. *Biochemistry* 28: 6810–6815.

130. Lieber, C.S., DeCarli, L.M. (1968) Ethanol oxidation by hepatic microsomes: adaptive increase after ethanol feeding. *Science* 162: 917–918.

131. Terelius, Y., Norsten-Hoog, C., Cronholm, T., Ingelman-Sundberg, M. (1991) Acetaldehyde as a substrate for ethanol-inducible cytochrome P450 (CYP2E1). *Biochem. Biophys. Res. Commun.* 179: 689–694.

132. Albano, E., Clot, P., Morimoto, M., Tomasi, A., Ingelman-sundberg, M., French, S.W. (1996) Role of cytochrome P450 2E1-dependent formation of hydroxyethyl free radical in development of liver damage in rats intragastrically fed with ethanol. *Hepatology* 23: 155–163.

133. Orellana, M., Varela, N., Guajardo, V., Araya, J., Rodrigo, R. (2002) Modulation of rat liver cytochrome P450 activity by prolonged red wine consumption. *Comp. Biochem. Physiol.* 131C: 161–166.

134. Kono, H., Bradford, B.U., Yin, M., Sulik, K.K., Koop, D.R., Peters, J.M., Gonzalez, F.J., McDonald, T., Dikalova, A., Kadiiska, M.B., Mason, R.P., Thurman, R.P. (1999) CYP2E1 is not involved in early alcohol-induced liver injury. *Am. J. Physiol.* 277: G1259–G1267.

135. Kono, H., Bradford, B.U., Rusyn, I., Fujii, H., Matsumoto, Y., Yin, M., Thurman, R.G. (2000) Development of an intragastric entral model in the mouse: studies of alcohol-induced liver disease using knockout technology. *J. Hepatobiliary Pancreat. Surg.* 7: 395–400.

136. Cederbaum, A.I., Wu, D., Mari, M., Bai, J. (2001) CYP2E1-dependent toxicity and oxidative stress in HepG2 cells. *Free Radic. Biol. Med.* 31: 1539–1543.

137. Arteel, G.E., Uesugi, T., Bevan, L.N., Gabelle. E., Wheeler, M.D., McKim, S.E., Thurman, R.G. (2002) Green tea extract protects against early alcohol-induced liver injury in rats. *Biol. Chem.* 383: 663–670.

138. Skrzydlewska E., Roszkowska, A., Makiela, M., Skrzydlewska, Z. (2001) The influence of green tea on the activity of proteases and their inhibitors in plasma of rats after ethanol treatment. *Rocz. Akad. Med. Bialymst. (Roczniki Akademii Medycznej w Bialymstoku)* 46: 240–250.

139. Polavarapu, R., Spitz, D.R., Sim, J.E., Follanssbee, M.H., Oberly, L.W., Rahemtulla, A., Nanji, A.A. (1998) Increased lipid peroxidation and impaired antioxidant enzyme function is associated with pathological liver injury in experimental alcohol liver disease in rats fed diets high in corn oil and fish oil. *Hepatology* 27: 1317–1323.

140. Skrzydlewska, E., Ostrowska, J., Stankiewicz, A., Fabiszewski, R. (2002) Green tea as a potent antioxidant in alcohol intoxication. *Addict. Biol.* 7: 307–314.

141. Chapman, R.W., Morgan, M.Y., Laulicht, M., Hoffbrand, V., Sherlock, S. (1982) Hepatic iron stores and markers of iron overload in alcoholics and patients with idiopathic hemochromatosis. *Dig. Dis. Sci.* 27: 909–916.

142. Potter, B.J. (1991) Alcohol and hepatic iron homeostasis. In: R.R. Watson (Ed.), *Liver Pathology and Alcohol*. Humana Press, Totowa, NJ, pp. 1–60.

143. De Feo, T.M., Fargion, S., Duca, L., Cesana, B.M., Boncinelli, L., Lozza, P., Cappelini, M.D., Fiorelli, G. (2001) Non-transferrin-bound iron in alcohol abusers. *Alcohol. Clin. Exp. Res.* 25: 1494–1499.

144. De Lorgeril, M., Salen, P., Boucher, F., de Leiris, J., Paillard, F. (2001) Effect of wine ethanol on serum iron and ferritin levels in patients with coronary heart disease. *Nutr. Metab. Cardiovasc. Dis.* 11: 176–180.

145. Maguire, J.J., Kellog, E.W., Packer, L. (1982) Protection against free radical formation by protein bound iron. *Toxicol. Lett.* 14: 27–34.

146. Biemond, P., Swaak, A.J.G., Beindorff, C.M., Koster, J.F. (1986) Superoxide-dependent and -independent mechanisms of iron mobilization from ferritin by xanthine oxidase. Implications for oxygen-free-radical-induced tissue destruction during ischaemia and inflammation. *Biochem. J.* 239: 169–173.

147. Carlin, G., Djursater, R. (1984) Xanthine oxidase induced depolymerization of hyaluronic acid in the presence of ferritin. *FEBS Lett.* 177: 27–30.

148. Suzuki, Y., Saito, H., Suzuki, M., Hosoki, Y., Sakurai, S., Fujimoto, Y., Kohgo, Y. (2002) Up-regulation of transferrin receptor expression in hepatocytes by habitual alcohol drinking is implicated in hepatic iron overload in alcoholic liver disease. *Alcohol. Clin. Exp. Res.* 26: 26S–31S.

149. Xia, J., Simonyl, A., Sun, G.Y. (1999) Chronic ethanol and iron administration on iron content, neuronal nitric oxide synthetase, and superoxide dimutase in rat cerebellum. *Alcohol. Clin. Exp. Res.* 23, 702–707.

150. Powell, L.W. (1966) Normal human iron storage and its relation to ethanol consumption. *Australian Ann. Med.* 15: 110–115.

151. Beard, J., Dawson, H. (1994) Iron. In: B. O'Dell, R. Sunde (Eds.), *Handbook of Nutritionally Essential Mineral Elements*. Marcel Dekker, New York.

152. Guthrie, H., Picciano, M.F. (1995) Micronutrient minerals. In: *Human Nutrition*. Mosby, St. Louis, MO, pp. 333–380.

153. Soranno, T.M., Sultatos, L.G. (1991) Biochemical properties and physiological functions of xanthine dehydrogenase and xanthine oxidase. In: R.R. Watson (Ed.), *Drug and Alcohol Abuse Reviews: Liver Pathology and Alcohol*. Humana Press, Totowa, NJ, pp. 427–440.

154. Crow, K.E., Hardman, M.J. (1989) Regulation of rates of ethanol metabolism. In: K.E. Crow, R.D. Batt (Eds.), *Human Metabolism of Alcohol, Vol. II, Regulation, Enzymology, and Metabolites of Ethanol*. CRC Press, Boca Raton, FL, pp. 3–15.

155. Thurman, R.G., Glassman, E.B., Handler, J.A., Forman, D.T. (1989) The swift increase in alcohol metabolism (SIAM): a commentary on the regulation of alcohol metabolism in mammals. In: K.E. Crow, R.D. Battt (Eds.), *Human Metabolism of Alcohol, Vol. II*: Regulation, Enzymology, and Metabolites of Ethanol. CRC Press, Boca Raton, FL, pp. 17–30.

156. Younes, M., Strubelt, O. (1987) Enhancement of hypoxic liver damage by ethanol: involvement of xanthine oxidase and the role of glycolysis. *Biochem. Pharmacol.* 36: 2973–2977.

157. Castro, G.D., Delgado de Layno, A.M., Costantini, M.H., Castro, J.A. (2001) Cytosolic xanthine oxidoreductase mediated bioactivation of ethanol to acetaldehyde and free radicals in rat breast tissue. Its potential role in alcohol-promoted mammary cancer. *Toxicology* 160: 11–18.

158. Castro, G.D., Delgado de Layno, A.M., Costantini, M.H., Castro, J.A. (2001) Rat ventral prostate xanthin oxidase bioactivation of ethanol to acetaldehyde and 1-hydroxyethyl free radicals: analysis of its potential role in heavy alcohol drinking tumor-promoting effects. *Teratog. Carcinog. Mutagen* 21: 109–119.

159. Kono, H., Rusyn, I., Bradford, B.U., Connor, H.D., Mason, R.P., Thurman, R.G. (2000) Allopurinol prevents early alcohol-induced liver injury in rats. *J. Pharmacol. Exp. Ther.* 293: 296–303.

160. Wright, R.M., McManaman, J.L. Repine, J.E. (1999) Alcohol-induced breast cancer: a proposed mechanism. *Free Radic. Biol. Med.* 26: 348–354.
161. Topham, R.C., Walker, M.C., Calisch, M.P., Williams, R.W. (1982) Evidence for the participation of intestinal xanthine oxidase in the mucosal processing of iron. *Biochemistry* 21: 4529–4535.
162. Bolann, B.J., Ulvik, R.J. (1987) Release of iron from ferritin by xanthine oxidase. *Biochem. J.* 243: 55–59.

20 Alcohol, Overweight, and Obesity

S. Goya Wannamethee and A.G. Shaper

CONTENTS

20.1 INTRODUCTION

In many developed countries the average alcohol intake among those who drink is about 10 to 30 g/d or 3 to 9% of the total energy intake,[1] and the efficiency of alcohol for the maintenance of metabolizable energy is the same as for carbohydrate.[2] Alcohol suppresses the oxidation of fat, favoring fat storage, and can serve as a precursor for fat synthesis.[3,4] Moderate alcohol consumers usually add alcohol to their daily energy intake rather than substituting it for food, thus increasing energy balance.[4] On the basis of this it would seem surprising if alcohol did not contribute directly to body weight. However, the relationship between alcohol consumption and body weight "remains an enigma to nutritionists and in many instances para-doxical."[5] The epidemiological evidence is inconsistent, with numerous studies suggesting absent or positive associations in men and strong inverse relationships in women.[1,4,6,7] A comprehensive review of representative studies of the relationship between alcohol intake and body weight found remarkable inconsistency between studies which is explained to some degree by confounding factors.[4] Another recent review concludes that "there is no consensus on the relationship between moderate alcohol intake and body weight,"[1] and the issue of whether or not alcohol calories "count" has been the topic of recent editorials.[5] Most epidemiological studies of this issue have been cross-sectional in nature. There have been relatively few prospective studies of the relation between alcohol and weight gain. The aim of this chapter is to review the epidemiological evidence in population studies for alcohol as a risk factor for overweight and obesity with particular focus on prospective studies.

20.2 EPIDEMIOLOGICAL EVIDENCE

While laboratory studies on energy and nutrient balances show that alcohol is a nutrient that is efficiently utilized by the body and that alcohol calories do count, the epidemiological evidence is conflicting.[1,3,4] In several reviews of studies of the alcohol and obesity relation, most of which are cross-sectional in nature, the association between alcohol intake and body weight has been inconsistent and has varied between men and women.[1,4,6,7] In men, the association between alcohol and body weight has been found to be almost equally positive or nonexistent but in women the majority of cross-sectional studies report an inverse relationship.[1,4,6–9]

20.3 CONFOUNDING AND BIAS

It has been suggested that the inconsistencies between studies may be caused by incomplete control for confounding, by heterogeneity of study populations regarding alcohol consumption, by socioeconomic factors and lifestyle characteristics, or by differences in other lifestyle characteristics among drinkers which may offset the additional energy from alcohol.[3,4] Much of the inconsistency in the evidence relating to the relationship between alcohol intake and body weight has arisen from the confounding effects of cigarette smoking, as smoking is associated consistently with lower body weight than observed in nonsmokers.[10] An early report using cross-sectional data from the British Regional Heart Study (BRHS), a prospective study of 7735 middle-aged men, showed that current smokers (light and moderate/heavy) had a lower mean BMI than nonsmokers (never and ex-smokers) at almost every level of alcohol intake.[11] The strongest influence of alcohol on body weight was seen in nonsmokers. Among moderate/heavy smokers, alcohol consumption had virtually no influence on BMI, reflecting the stronger influence of smoking on body weight.[11] In a later prospective analysis from the BRHS on heavy drinking and weight gain, the increased risk of weight gain associated with heavy drinking was most apparent in never smokers.[12] The strength of the association between alcohol and body weight or weight gain in any population may be conditioned by the prevalence and intensity of smoking in that population.

20.4 PROSPECTIVE STUDIES

Cross-sectional analyses are limited in assessing cause and effect. The patterns of higher obesity rates in nondrinkers compared to drinkers commonly seen in women may reflect a history of dieting or current dieting to lose weight. The higher BMI levels in nondrinkers may in part be due to self-selection bias. Women who are more prone to weight gain for reasons other than alcohol may abstain from drinking because of their belief that alcohol causes weight gain.

There have been relatively few prospective studies of the relation between alcohol intake and weight gain in men and women, and the findings have been inconsistent.[12–23] Table 20.1 summarizes the main findings from prospective studies on alcohol and weight change and adiposity.[12–23] Early data from the Framingham study showed that after 20 years' follow-up, men who were drinkers at baseline weighed more than nondrinkers. Both men and women who took up drinking or increased their alcohol intake during follow-up experienced weight gain.[13] In a study of over 12,000 adult Finns, heavier drinking (>75 g/week) was associated with increased prevalence of obesity and with a significantly increased risk of >5 kg weight gain in men compared to nondrinkers.[14] In women, an inverse relationship was seen between prevalence of obesity and alcohol intake but in prospective analyses risk of weight gain $\geq$ 5 kg increased at higher levels of drinking (> 10 g/d). Nondrinkers and lighter drinkers showed similar risk.[14] In a study of over 2000 Chinese adults, alcohol consumption was associated with significant weight gain in men while in women only a small but positive association was seen.[15] Strong evidence supporting the effects of alcohol on obesity and weight gain comes from the British Regional Heart Study. The prevalence of men with high BMI ($\geq$ 28 kg/m^2) tended to increase with increasing alcohol intake[12] (Figure 20.1) An examination of the association between changes in alcohol intake and body weight over 5 years showed stable heavy drinkers ($\geq$ 30 g/d) and new heavy drinkers to have the greatest weight gain and the highest prevalence of obesity[12] (Figure 20.1). Light and moderate drinkers showed no increased risk in weight gain compared to nondrinkers. These positive findings in heavier drinkers have been confirmed in recent prospective analyses carried out in a U.S. cohort of over 40,000 female nurses aged 29 to 42 years at baseline in 1989 (Nurses II Health Study). An inverse relationship was seen between alcohol and BMI in cross-sectional analyses, but in prospective analyses, light to moderate drinkers (up to 30 g/d) had a significantly lower risk of weight gain (>5 kg) over 8 years than nondrinkers; heavy drinkers ($\geq$ 30 g/d/3 UK units/d) had the highest risk of weight gain (>5 kg) (Wannamethee et al., personal communication). In a recent prospective study of alcohol and subsequent high waist to-hip ratio in the Copenhagen City Heart Study, a positive linear relationship was seen between alcohol intake and high WHR measured 10 years later in both men and women.[16] Men drinking more than 28 beverages/week showed significant increased risk of high WHR compared to those drinking 1 to 6 beverages/week. These prospective data supported the concept of alcohol as a risk factor for obesity. However, weak positive or no association has been reported between alcohol and weight change and weight gain in five prospective studies from the U.S.A.[17–21] In these studies, data by levels of alcohol consumption were not presented and the average intake in these populations is not known. By contrast in the Nurses I Health Study of women aged 30 to 55 years at baseline in 1976, an inverse correlation was observed between alcohol (g/d) and subsequent weight gain.[22] In the NHANES I study of over 7000 men and women aged 25 to 74 years, female drinkers were significantly less likely to gain weight than nondrinkers during the 10 year follow-up even after adjustment for a wide range of confounders.[23] In men, a small but nonsignificant inverse relationship was seen. The progressive inverse pattern seen in the heavier drinkers in the NHANES study particularly in women may in part be due to the small number

TABLE 20.1
Prospective Studies on the Association between Alcohol and Weight Gain and Adiposity

Study Population	Subjects	Weight Index	Alcohol Categories	Main Findings
Framingham Study (1983)[13]	5209 men and women, age 29–62	20-year weight change	ozs/month	Men and women increasing alcohol intake had greater weight gain than those decreasing alcohol intake ($p < 0.01$)
Nurses I Health Study. (1990)[22]	31,940 nonsmoking women age 30–55	8-year weight gain	g/d (continuous variable)	Inverse association
Social Insurance Institution Finland (1991)[14]	12,669 adult Finns. age 30–64	5-year weight gain (≥5kg)	None, 1–300 g/month >300 g/month	Men/women drinking >300 g/month showed increased weight gain compared to nondrinkers Adjusted OR of weight gain 1.4 (1.1–1.6) in men and 1.3 (0.9–1.9) in women
Healthy Worker Project (1993)[17]	1639 male and 1913 female employees	2-year change in body weight	Alcohol frequency/week (continuous variable)	No association in men or women
NHANES I Study (1994)[23]	7230 U.S. adults age 25–74	10-year weight gain (≥10kg)	None, <12 dr/year, 1 dr/week, 1–7 dr/week, 1–1.9 dr/d, ≥2dr/d	Significant inverse relationship in women; small nonsignificant inverse relationship in men The adjusted relative odds of weight gain in men drinking >2 dr/d compared to nondrinkers was 0.9 (0.5, 1.6) in men and 0.5 (0.3–1.0) in women
Male Firefighters (1996)[18]	438 male fire service personnel, aged 20–58	7-year weight gain (≥ 5 lbs)	Alcoholic beverages/week (continuous variable)	No association seen between alcohol and weight gain
American Cancer Society (1997)[19]	79,236 adults	10-year weight gain	Frequency of alcohol consumption None, <5 d/week, ≥ 5 d/week.	No association was seen between frequency of alcohol intake and waist gain in men or women
Pound of Prevention Study (2000)[20]	826 women, 218 men age 20–45	3-year weight gain (≥5lb)	% energy from alcohol (continuous variable)	No association between alcohol and weight gain in men or women

Study (reference)	Sample	Outcome measure	Alcohol measure	Results
Male athletes (2000)[21]	1143 men, age 36–88	10-year weight change	Alcohol g/week (continuous variable)	No significant association seen between alcohol and weight change
Chinese adults (2001)[15]	2488 adults 20–45 years	8-year weight gain (>5 kg)	Alcohol in past year (yes/month)	Male drinkers showed significant increase in odds of large weight gain in men (OR = 1.55, 1.01–2.33) compared to nondrinkers. Smaller but positive association in women (OR = 1.08, 0.68–1.71)
British Regional Heart Study (2003)[12]	7608 men, age 40–59 with no history of diabetes	5-year weight gain (≥4% body weight)	Non/occasional, light to moderate, heavy (≥3 dr/d), new heavy drinkers	Compared to stable nonoccasional drinkers over 5 years, those who remained heavy drinkers showed significant increase in risk of weight gain (OR = 1.29, 1.10–1.51) Those who increased their intake and became heavy drinkers also showed increased risk (OR = 1.45, 1.09–1.92)
Copenhagen City Heart Study (2003)[16]	2916 men and 3970 women, age 20–83	High waist–hip ratio (WHR) (>102 cm for men; >88 cm for women) After 10 years	Beverage/week <1, 1–7, 7–14, 14–28, ≥28	Compared to those drinking <1 dr/week, the odds ratio of having a high WHR in men drinking >28 beverages/week was 1.65 95% CI 1.07–2.55 and in women the corresponding odds ratio was 2.16 (0.86–5.14)

Note: dr = drink, d = day/s.

of men and women who drank more than two drinks a day, the level at which alcohol appeared to have an effect on increased weight gain. It was concluded that alcohol was not a risk factor for obesity.[23] It appears likely that higher levels on a regular basis are required to have an effect on body weight. Intervention studies are inconclusive.[24] Cordain et al. reported that the addition of 35 g/d of wine to the daily energy requirements during a period of 6 weeks does not affect body weight and or energy metabolism.[24] This is consistent with the findings in the BRHS and Nurses II Health Study in which up to 30 g (3 UK units) was not associated with weight gain. Overall, prospective data support the conclusion that heavier alcohol intake contributes directly to body weight and the prevalence of obesity, as one might expect if the energy derived from alcohol consumption was added to the usual dietary calorie intake.

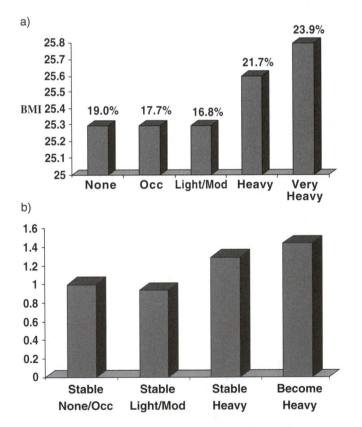

FIGURE 20.1 (a) Alcohol intake and age-adjusted mean BMI (kg/m²) and percentage of men with high BMI (≥28 kg/m²) in 7608 men aged 40 to 59. (b) Adjusted relative odds of 5-year weight gain (≥4% body weight) in 6832 men with data on weight change and no history of diabetes. Relative odds adjusted for age, social class, physical activity, and cigarette smoking. Occ = occasional (<1/week), Light/Mod (1–20 units/week), Heavy (21–42 units/week), Very Heavy (>42 units/week). [1 UK unit = 10 g alcohol].

20.4.1 ALCOHOL AND BODY FAT DISTRIBUTION

Evidence from a number of studies suggests that in drinkers, fat is preferentially deposited in the abdominal area.[4] In contrast to the cross-sectional relationship between alcohol and body weight many cross-sectional studies have reported positive associations between alcohol and WHR in men and women. Studies in Switzerland have found a significant relationship between the frequency of alcohol consumption and WHR.[25] In the French MONICA study, alcohol consumption was positively associated with WHR, independently of BMI, in both men and women.[26] Positive associations have also been reported in American men and women,[27] and Italian women,[28] as well as in Japanese men.[29] Prospective studies are few. As mentioned earlier, in the Copenhagen City Heart Study alcohol was positively associated with increased WHR measured 10 years later in both men and women.[16] The mechanisms are not clearly established but endocrine changes reflected by increased cortisol secretion appear to be involved.[30,31]

20.5 TYPE OF ALCOHOL AND OBESITY

It has been suggested that the type of alcohol consumed might explain the discrepant results in studies of alcohol and body weight. The common belief is that drinking beer promotes abdominal fat distribution and that wine in contrast has no effect and may even have beneficial effects on metabolism.[26,32] The relationships reported between type of drink and body weight and obesity have been unequivocal. Some studies have reported differing effects of type of beverage on body weight and obesity rates while others have not.[8,9,12,16,26,27] In the Nurses I Health Study and the Health Professionals Follow-Up Study, the lack of relationship between alcohol intake and BMI was similar for men who drank only wine and those who drank only beer.[8] In a study of some 3500 French men and women aged 35 to 64 years drawn from three distinct geographic areas of France (MONICA centers), wine was the main source of alcohol (67% of intake). Wine and beer consumption were positively and strongly associated with WHR in women but only poorly associated with WHR in men.[26] In the Spanish national survey[9] there appeared to be a positive association between wine intake and the prevalence of obesity in women and between spirit intake and obesity in men. No significant trends of association were observed for beer or wine in men or for beer or spirits in women. In a U.S. study of 12,000 men and women aged 45 to 64 years, the WHRs of those consuming more than six beer drinks/week were significantly greater than in than nondrinkers, while those drinking more than six wine drinks/week were significantly smaller (than nondrinkers). The findings were regarded as supporting the popular concept of the "beer belly."[27] In the Japanese study of male self-defense officials, abdominal obesity was associated with shochu ethanol (Japanese spirits) but not with other types of alcohol.[29] In the British Regional Heart Study, mean BMI increased with increasing alcohol intake from light to moderate to heavy, irrespective of type of drink, although men who reported spirit drinking tended to be heavier than beer and wine drinkers.[12] Prospective studies on the effects of alcohol on weight gain and adiposity by type of drink are sparse. The Copenhagen City Heart Study reported high consumption of beer and spirits to be associated with increased waist circumference whereas moderate to high wine consumption was associated with lower WHR.[16] The differences in findings between studies may be associated with unrecorded differences in lifestyle or differences in nutritional characteristics among wine, spirit, and beer drinkers.

20.5.1 MECHANISMS

There is a considerable literature on the influence of alcohol on fat storage and metabolism.[4,33] In a comprehensive review of the effects of alcohol on energy metabolism and body weight regulation, Suter and colleagues point out that alcohol cannot be stored in the body and appears to have priority in metabolism.[4] This takes place at the expense of other metabolic pathways including the suppression of lipid oxidation which appears to be a critical factor in the development of a positive energy balance.[2] Even in healthy young men, low-dose alcohol consumption results in hepatic production of acetate and release into the plasma, with consequent inhibition of lipolysis in peripheral tissues by 53% and decrease in whole-body lipid oxidation by 73%.[33,34] Suter and colleagues also note the significant positive relationship between alcohol and fat intakes and the lack of inhibitory effect of moderate alcohol intake on daily energy and fat intake. It has been suggested that alcohol consumers on a high fat diet may experience weight gain more easily than an alcohol consumer with a lower dietary fat intake due to the metabolic effects of alcohol on suppressing fat oxidation rate leading to a positive fat balance.[33] These findings are of considerable relevance in view of the observation that alcohol intake, especially when accompanied by a high fat diet, favors truncal obesity, particularly in women.[35]

Although alcohol appears to be added to the diet, light and moderate drinkers have often been shown to have significantly lower body weight and weight gain than nondrinkers.[1,4,6,7,22,23] This lower weight gain in light and moderate drinkers may be due to residual confounding or it may reflect a true physiological effect of alcohol on increased basal energy expenditure and inefficient energy utilization.[4,36] In a carefully controlled isoenergenic dietary study, Pirola and Lieber[36] suggested that alcohol was not as effective as carbohydrate or fat in causing weight gain. However, this was carried out in a hospital-based group of heavy alcohol consumers and the result may not be generalized to the general population. It has further been suggested that alcohol enhances weight gain in obese subjects, but not in lean subjects.[37,38] In a recent study of 37 healthy premenopausal women aged 21 to 40 years, heavier subjects (mean BMI 25.2 kg/m^2) required fewer calories to maintain body weight when consuming alcohol than leaner women (mean BMI 22.6 kg/m^2). It was suggested that heavier women utilize alcohol more efficiently than lean women.[38] If these finding are confirmed, the examination of data on women's response to alcohol may require stratification by BMI, body weight, or WHR for proper interpretation.

20.6 CONCLUSION

While metabolic studies indicate fairly unequivocally that alcohol consumption even in moderate amounts contributes to weight gain,[4] the epidemiological evidence on the relationship between alcohol intake and body weight based on cross-sectional studies is conflicting. This may not be surprising, given the heterogeneity of the groups studied, the problems of assessing true alcohol intake in men and in women, and the wide range of variables affecting energy balance, such as overall diet, physical activity, and ill health and selection bias. Findings from more recent prospective population studies suggest that light to moderate drinking is not associated with weight gain but that heavier levels (≥3 drinks/d; ≥30 g alcohol/d) contribute to weight gain and obesity in men and women. Overall evidence from prospective studies supports the concept that alcohol is a risk factor for obesity, as one might expect if the energy derived from alcohol consumption was added to the usual dietary calorie intake.

References

1. Westerterp KR, Prentice AM, Jequier E. Alcohol and body weight. In: McDonald I (Ed.), *Health Issues Related to Alcohol Consumption* (2nd ed.). ILSI Europe, Brussels 1999, pp. 103–123.
2. Rumpler WV, Rhodes DG, Baer DJ, Conway JM, Seale JL. Energy value of moderate alcohol consumption by humans. *Am J Clin Nutr* 1996; 64: 108–114.
3. Prentice AM. Alcohol and obesity. *Int J Obesity* 1995; 19: Suppl. 5 S44–S50.
4. Suter PM, Hasler E, Vetter W. Effects of alcohol on energy metabolism and body weight regulation: is alcohol a risk factor for obesity? *Nutr Rev* 1997; 55: 157–171.
5. Jequier E. Alcohol intake and body weight: a paradox. *Am J Clin Nutr* 1999; 69: 173–174.
6. McDonald I, Debry G, Westerterp K. Alcohol and overweight. In: Verschuren PM (Ed.). *Health Issues Related to Alcohol Consumption*. ILSI Europe, Brussels, 1993, pp. 263–279.
7. Hellerstedt WL, Jeffery RW, Murray DM. The association between alcohol intake and the general population. Reviews and commentary. *Am J Epidemiol* 1990; 132: 594–611.
8. Colditz GA, Giovannucci E, Rimm EB, Stampfer MJ, Rosner B, Speizer FE, Gordis E, Willett WC. Alcohol in relation to diet and obesity in women and men. *Am J Clin Nutr* 1991; 54: 49–55.
9. Gutierrez-Fisac JL, Rodriguez-Artalejo F, Rodriguez-Blas C, del Rey-Calero J. Alcohol consumption and obesity in the adult population of Spain. *J Epidemiol Community Health* 1995; 49: 108–109.
10. U.S. Department of Health and Human Services. The health consequences of smoking: nicotine addiction. A report of the Surgeon General, Washington D.C. U.S. GPO 1988 (DHHS Pub.No. [CDC] 88–8406.
11. Wannamethee G, Shaper AG. Blood lipids: the relationship with alcohol intake, smoking, and body weight. *J Epidemiol Community Health* 1992; 46: 197–202.
12. Wannamethee SG, Shaper AG. Alcohol, body weight and weight gain in middle-aged men. *Am J Clin Nutr* 2003; 77: 1312–1317.

13. Gordon T, Kannell WB. Drinking and its relation to smoking, blood pressure, blood lipids and uric acid: the Framingham study. *Arch Int Med* 1983; 143: 1366–1374.

14. Rissanen AM, Heliovaara M, Knekt P, Reunanen A, Aromaa A. Determinants of weight gain and overweight in adult Finns. *Eur J Clin Nutr* 1991; 45: 419–430.

15. Bell AC, Ge K, Popkin BM. Weight gain and its predictor in Chinese adults. *Int J Obesity* 2001; 25: 1079–1086.

16. Vadstrup ES, Petersen L, Sorensen TIA, Gronbaek M. Waist circumference in relation to history of amount and type of alcohol: results from the Copenhagen City Heart Study. *Int J Obesity* 2003; 27: 238–246.

17. French SA, Jeffery RW, Forster JL, McGovern PG, Kelder SH, Baxter JE. Predictors of weight change over two years among a population of working adults: the Healthy Worker Project. *Int J Obesity* 1993; 18: 145–154.

18. Gerace TA, George VA. Predictors of weight increases over 7 years in fire fighters and paramedics. *Prev Med* 1996; 25: 593–600.

19. Kahn H, Tatham LM, Rodriguez C, Eugenia E, Thun MJ, Clark CW. Stable behaviours associated with adults's 10-year change in body mass index and likelihood of gain at the waist. *Am J Public Health* 1997; 87: 747–754.

20. Sherwood NE, Jeffery RW, French SA, Hannan PJ, Murray DM. Predictors of weight gain in the Pound of Prevention Study. *Int J Obesity* 2000; 24: 395–403.

21. Fogelholm M, Kujala U, Kaprio J, Sarna S. Predictors of weight change in middle-aged and old men. *Obes Res* 2000; 8: 367–373.

22. Colditz GA, Willett WC, Stampfer MJ, London SJ, Segal MR, Speizer F. Patterns of weight change and their relation to diet in a cohort of healthy women. *Am J Clin Nutr* 1990; 51: 1100–1105.

23. Liu S, Serdula MK, Williamson DF, Mokdad AH, Byers T. A prospective study of alcohol intake and change in body weight among U.S. adults. *Am J Epidemiol* 1994; 140: 912–920.

24. Cordain L, Bryan ED, Melby CL, Smith MJ. Influence of moderate daily wine consumption on body weight regulation and metabolism in healthy free-living males. *J Amer Coll Nutr* 1997; 16: 134–139.

25. Suter PM, Maire R, Vetter W. Alcohol consumption: a risk factor for abdominal fat accumulation in men. *Addiction Biol* 1997; 2: 101–103.

26. Dallongeville J, Marecaux N, Ducimetiere P, Ferrieres J, Arveiler D, Bingham A, Ruidavets JB, Simon C, Amouyel P. Influence of alcohol consumption and various beverages on waist girth and waist-to-hip ratio in a sample of French men and women. *Int J Obesity Relat Metab Disord* 1998; 22: 1178–1183.

27. Duncan BB, Chambless LE, Schmidt MI, Folsom AR, Szklo M, Crouse JR III, Carpenter MA. Association of the waist-to-hip ratio is different with wine than with beer or hard liquor consumption. Atherosclerosis risk in communities study investigators. *Am J Epidemiol* 1995; 142: 1034–1038.

28. Armellini F, Zamboni M, Frigo L, Mandragona R, Robbi R, Micciolo R et al. Alcohol consumption, smoking habits and body fat distribution in Italian men and women aged 20–60 years. *Eur J Clin Nutr* 1993; 47: 52–60.

29. Sakurai Y, Umeda T, Shinchi K, Honjo S, Wakabayashi K, Todoroki I et al. Relation of total and beverage-specific alcohol intake to body mass index and waist-to-hip ratio: a study of self-defense officials in Japan. *Eur J Epidemiol* 1997; 13: 893–898.

30. Zakhari S. Alcohol and the endocrine system. Research Monograph No. 23. Bethesda, MD. National Institutes of Health, National Institute on Alcohol Abuse and Alcoholism (NIH-NIAAA) 1993; pp. 411.

31. Kissebah A, Krakower GR. Regional adiposity and morbidity. *Physiol Rev* 1994; 74: 761–811.

32. Gronbaek M., Deiss A, Sorensen TIA, Becker U, Schnohr P, Jensen G. Mortality associated with moderate intakes of wine beer or spirits. *BMJ* 1995; 310: 1165–1169.

33. Suter PM, Schutz Y, Jequier E. The effect of ethanol on fat storage in healthy subjects. *N Engl J Med* 1992; 326: 983–987.

34. Siler SQ, Neese RA, Hellerstein MK. *De novo* lipogenesis, lipid kinetics and whole-lipid balances in humans after acute alcohol consumption. *Am J Clin Nutr* 1999; 70: 928–936.

35. Feinman L, Lieber CS. Ethanol and lipid metabolism. *Am J Clin Nutr* 1999; 70: 791–792.

36. Pirola RC and Lieber CS. The energy cost of the metabolism of drugs, including ethanol. *Pharmacology* 1972; 7: 185–196.

37. Crouse JR, Grundy SM: Effects of alcohol on plasma lipoproteins and cholesterol and triglyceride metabolism in man. *J Lipid Res* 1984; 25: 486–496.

38. Clevidence BA, Taylor PR, Campbell WS, Judd JT. Lean and heavy women may not use energy from alcohol with equal efficiency. *J Nutr* 1995; 125: 2536–2540.

21 Alcohol Use during Lactation: Effects on the Mother and the Breastfeeding Infant

Julie A. Mennella

CONTENTS

21.1 INTRODUCTION

There is a growing recognition of the importance of cultural differences, as well as commonalities, in the use of alcohol for medicinal purposes.[1,2] Of particular interest is its use by women during lactation since alcohol was, and continues to be, believed by many to possess galactogenic (milk-producing) properties.[3,4] Although some physicians during the 19th century counseled lactating women to abstain from alcohol because it was believed that the most frequent source of acquired alcoholism was exposure to alcohol in mother's milk, others argued that drinking spirits could enhance a woman's appetite and stimulate milk production which, in turn, would strengthen the breastfed infant.[5,6] This latter folklore was so well ingrained in American tradition that, back in 1895, a major U.S. brewery produced a low-alcoholic beer known as Malt-Nutrine™ that was sold exclusively in drugstores and prescribed by physicians as a tonic for pregnant and lactating women as well as a nutritional beverage for children.[7] Its production was halted during the Prohibition because it contained more than 0.5% alcohol.

0-8493-1680-4/04/$0.00+$1.50
© 2004 by CRC Press LLC

That the belief in alcoholic beverages as galactagogues continues to be ingrained in current-day medical practice is evident from a recent study on lactating women living in the Delaware Valley.[4] According to 25% of these women, a health professional encouraged them to drink alcohol; approximately half of the women reported receiving no advice at all, whereas the remainder were advised to refrain from drinking. Of particular interest is the finding that approximately one quarter of the women who were discouraged from drinking alcohol while they were pregnant reported that their health professionals actually encouraged them to drink once they began lactating. The advice ranged from the recommendation that drinking small quantities of alcohol shortly before nursing will facilitate the letdown and production of milk, to the belief that by drinking such milk, the infant will relax, become less colicky, and obtain warmth (see also References 8 to 11). Interestingly, the type of alcoholic beverage believed to possess galactogenic properties appears to be, in part, culturally driven. For example, women in Mexico are encouraged to drink as much as two liters of *pulque*, a low alcoholic beverage made of the fermented juice of a local fruit, *Agave atrovirens*, daily during both pregnancy and lactation[12]; Indochinese women in California drink wine steeped with herbs,[10] whereas the magic elixir in Argentina[13] and Germany[8] is malt beer.

It is important to note that the claims that alcohol benefits the lactating mother and her infant are not accompanied by any controlled scientific evidence. In this chapter, we explore the scientific literature, albeit limited, on the transfer of alcohol to mothers' milk and the effects that maternal alcohol consumption has on maternal health and infant nutrition and behavior. As will be discussed, this research suggests that, contrary to the folklore, the recommendation for a nursing mother to drink a glass of beer or wine shortly before nursing actually may be counterproductive.

21.2 THE LACTATING MOTHER

The notion that a woman can optimize the quality and quantity of her milk to meet the needs of the infant through her own diet and psychological well-being is ingrained in the traditional wisdom of many cultures. The following discussion focuses on the science that investigates the folklore that alcohol ingestion benefits lactating women. Specifically, we discuss the effects of ethanol ingestion on ethanol pharmacokinetics, lactational performance and hormonal profile, as well as changes in the sensory properties of their milk.

21.2.1 ETHANOL PHARMACOKINETICS AND MILK FLAVOR

Research conducted at the turn of the 20th century, and then again almost a century later, revealed that the ethanol content in human milk, which is almost identical to that detected in a woman's blood, peaked one hour after ingestion and declined thereafter.[14-18] The amount of alcohol in mother's milk presented to the infant is a minute fraction of that consumed by the mother (generally less than 2% of the maternal dose). As shown in Figure 21.1, the presence of ethanol in the milk produced a significant change in the flavor of the milk which paralleled the changes in its ethanol content,[3,17,18] a finding which is similar to that reported for a variety of foods and beverages consumed by the lactating mother.[19]

Whether the lactational state alters ethanol pharmacokinetics is still unresolved. To our knowledge, there is only one published study in which only five women were tested in the fed state.[20] Here they reported that the average time to reach maximal blood ethanol levels was significantly longer (1 h) in lactating women when compared to nonlactating controls (0.5 h), a finding consistent with animal model studies.[21,22] That the change in ethanol metabolism is due, in part, to liver hypertrophy during lactation is suggested by a study in lactating rats in which the faster ethanol elimination was not evident when the disappearance rates were expressed per gram of liver.[22] Additional research is needed to further explore whether the dynamic physiological changes that occur during lactation influence the pharmacokinetic processes of the absorption, distribution, and elimination of a wide variety of drugs including ethanol.[23,24]

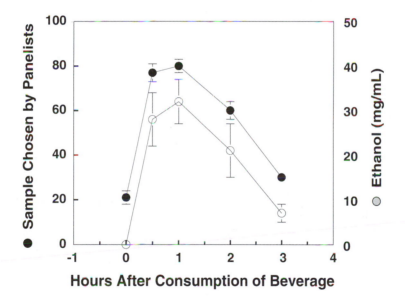

FIGURE 21.1 The ethanol content of milk samples (open circles) and the percentage of time panelists chose milk samples (closed circles) obtained at baseline (0) and 30 min, 1, 2, and 3 h after the mothers consumed a 0.3 g/kg dose of alcohol in orange juice or an equal volume of orange juice alone (see inset). Using a forced-choice paradigm, the panelists were presented individually with each set of milk samples and asked to indicate which of the paired smelled "stronger" or more like alcohol. A value of 50% would be expected if there were no difference in the odor of the samples and hence the panelists responded at random. Values below 50% for the samples collected at base line and after 3 h are a consequence of these samples' being paired with a stronger-smelling sample (e.g., one collected 30 min or 1 or 2 h after alcohol consumption). The bars indicate standard errors. To convert values for ethanol to millimoles per liter, multiply by 0.2171. (From Mennella, J.A. and Beauchamp, G.K. The transfer of alcohol to human milk: effects on flavor and the infant's behavior. *N. Engl. J. Med.*, 325, 8, 1991. With permission.)

21.2.2 LACTATIONAL PERFORMANCE

Because women are often advised to drink alcohol shortly before they nurse their babies to promote milk production, an experimental study was conducted to determine whether milk production is indeed enhanced during the immediate hours following maternal alcohol consumption. Contrary to the lore, but consistent with research in animal models,[25–28] women produced a significant decrease in milk yield within the immediate hours after they consumed an alcoholic beverage (0.3 g/kg dose of alcohol), compared to when they consumed a nonalcoholic beverage.[29] There were no changes in the milk's caloric content.

Research on the effects of ethanol consumption on milk composition in animal models is limited to a few studies that revealed that chronic ethanol consumption by lactating rat dams during both pregnancy and lactation resulted in a reduction of milk production and the milk produced was higher in lipid and lower in lactose content, when compared to the milk of control rat dams.[28] Because there was no alteration in its protein or water content, the milk of ethanol-exposed rats had a higher energy content owing to the greater energetic value of lipids compared to proteins and lactose. This increase in milk lipid content may be due to the increased rate of lipogenesis of the mammary gland following ethanol treatment.[30] Future research is needed to determine whether this alteration in milk composition was a direct consequence of ethanol intake or malnutrition and whether ethanol intake, in the long term, has similar effects on milk composition or yield in humans.

21.2.3 HORMONAL MILIEU

The production, secretion, and ejection of milk are the result of highly synchronized endocrine and neuroendocrine processes, which are governed, in part, by the frequency and intensity of the infant's sucking. This multistage process is controlled by several hormones, the most important of which are prolactin and oxytocin. The amount of oxytocin released is positively correlated with the amount of milk transferred from mother to baby[31] and may be involved in maternal behaviors and mother–infant bonding.[32] Prolactin also increases transiently in response to the suckling stimulus and is important for the secretory transformation of the mammary gland epithelium. No clear temporal correlation exists between plasma prolactin levels and milk yield of a particular breastfeed in humans, although prolactin appears to be essential for the maintenance of lactation in the longer term.[33]

Prolactin. Research on the effects of ethanol consumption on prolactin secretion is limited to studies that yielded conflicting results and, perhaps more important, focused *not* on lactating women, but on normal men and nonlactating women.[34–44] The majority of the research studies revealed that ethanol consumption increases plasma prolactin. In striking contrast to the finding that prolactin increases following ethanol consumption in humans, the majority of the animal model studies of Subramanian and colleagues revealed that ethanol administration decreased suckling-induced prolactin.[25,26,45] However, closer examination of their most recent study, which extended the observation period, actually demonstrated significant suckling-induced increases in prolactin following ethanol administration. This latter study led authors to conclude that "oxytocin, rather that prolactin may be the primary avenue by which alcohol induces growth retardation during lactation."[46]

Oxytocin. The study of ethanol's effect on milk ejection dates back to the late 1960s when ethanol was used in medical practices to treat premature labor. Complete or partial blockage of the milk-ejection reflex, as assessed by either intra-mammary pressure[47,48] or uterine contraction[49] recordings (an indirect measure of oxytocin), was observed in peripartum women. Recent studies that used RIA methods to measure oxytocin demonstrated that suckling-induced oxytocin levels are attenuated following ethanol consumption in *nonlactating* women[36] and lactating rats.[50]

Because there is a positive correlation between oxytocin and milk ejection/volume in humans, we hypothesized that the hormonal mechanisms underlying the depression in milk production following maternal ethanol consumption is that ethanol decreases suckling-induced plasma oxytocin. This hypothesis is also supported by the finding that infants sucked significantly more during the first minutes of all feeds that occurred during the immediate hours following maternal ethanol consumption.[17] We suggest that such changes in the patterning of suckling may reflect a difficulty in obtaining milk from the breast, since infants suck at faster rates when milk flow is lower.[51] Research is presently underway in our laboratory to determine the effects of acute alcohol consumption on the hormonal milieu of the lactating woman.

21.3   THE BREASTFEEDING INFANT

Because the amount of ethanol transmitted to human milk is a minute fraction of that consumed by the mother,[14–18] occasional exposure is often considered insignificant[11,40,52,53] and consequently many authorities, such as the Committee on Drugs of the American Academy of Pediatrics (AAP)[54] regard ethanol as a "drug usually permissible with breastfeeding" except in such rare cases of intoxication when the lactating mothers drank quite heavily[55,56] or when infants were inadvertently fed large amounts of alcohol in a bottle.[57] However, research conducted during the past decade strongly suggests that exposure to ethanol via mothers' milk affects breastfed infants in several important ways.

21.3.1   NUTRITION

Contrary to this lore that ethanol is a galactagogue, but consistent with research in other animals,[25–28] human infants consumed approximately 23% *less* milk during the 4 h that follow their mothers' drinking of an alcoholic beverage.[17,18] The dosage of alcohol used in these studies (0.3 g/kg body weight of mother) was chosen because it represents approximately the amount of alcohol in a can of beer or glass of wine for the average-sized woman. The diminished intake at the breast was not due to infants feeding for shorter periods of time following maternal ethanol consumption since there was no significant difference in the number of feedings. Nor was it due to infants rejecting the altered flavor in their mother's milk, which also resulted from maternal ethanol consumption.[58] Rather, as was discussed previously, maternal ethanol consumption significantly reduced the amount of milk produced by the mother without altering its caloric content.[29]

Although the infants consumed less milk following their mothers' consumption of alcoholic relative to nonalcoholic beverages, the mothers were apparently unaware of this difference.[17] Because milk intake and the rate of synthesis of human milk varies from feed to feed,[59] a difference of this small magnitude may be difficult for women to perceive.[60] Moreover, breastfed infants often determine the pace and duration of the feeding[61] and regulate the amount of milk they ingest, as shown by the finding that milk usually can be expressed from the mother's breasts after a feeding.[59] Perhaps one reason why the folklore that alcohol is a galactagogue has persisted for centuries is because the breastfeeding mother, unlike the bottle-feeding caretaker who often feeds in response to the amount of formula remaining in the bottle,[61] does not have an immediate means of assessing whether her infant consumes more milk in the short term, making her particularly vulnerable to such lore.

Because breastfed infants are clearly capable of regulating milk intake, we hypothesized they would compensate for the diminished intake that occurs following exposure to ethanol in mothers' milk if their mothers then refrained from drinking alcohol. This was indeed the case. As shown in the left panel of Figure 21.2, the compensation occurred within the 8 to 12 h following exposure and was due, in part, to the increased number of breastfeedings that occurred during this time period.[62] Perhaps one reason for the persistence of the folklore that occasional drinking by the nursing mother enhances breastfeeding is because the infants feed more later to compensate for the ethanol-induced deficits in their mothers' milk production. The effects are subtle and remarkably similar to the changes in active sleep that follow exposure to ethanol in mothers' milk.[17,63,64]

21.3.2 THE BEHAVIORAL STATE OF THE INFANT

Much of the scientific information regarding alcohol's effect during lactation has been limited to occasional case histories.[55–57] However, recent studies have begun to systematically explore the effects of maternal consumption of acute doses of alcohol on the flavor of human milk and the behavior of breastfed infants in the short term.[17,18,62–64] Contrary to the lore that contends that drinking ethanol shortly before breastfeeding relaxes and sedates the infant, experimental studies revealed that infants whose mothers drank little during both pregnancy and lactation slept for significantly shorter periods of time during the immediate hours following the consumption of ethanol in their mothers' milk when compared to mothers' milk alone.[63,64] This reduction was due, in part, to shortening in the amount of time that infants spent in active sleep, a finding consistent with that observed in the near-term fetuses[65] of nonalcoholic adults[66,67] and other animals.[68] Similar to that reported above for compensation of milk deficits and as shown in Figure 21.2, infants then compensated for this reduction in active sleep during the 20.5 h following ethanol exposure during which their mothers refrained from drinking alcohol.[64] Taken together with the findings on milk compensation, these data highlight the infants' resiliency in modulating behaviors in response to acute ethanol exposure. Whether ethanol consumption by lactating women disrupts other aspects of maternal–infant interaction is an important area for future research.

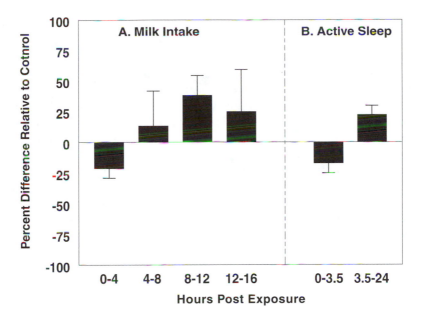

FIGURE 21.2 Mean percentage difference in the amount of milk consumed at the breast (left panel A) and the amount of time the infants spent in active sleep (right panel B) during the hours following their consumption of mothers' milk with alcohol when compared to mother's milk alone. For milk intake, the time intervals are 0–4, 4–8, 8–12, and 12–16 h post consumption, whereas for active sleep the time intervals are 0–3.5 and 3.5–24 h postconsumption.

To our knowledge, the one epidemiological study of 400 breastfed infants and their mothers suggested that such exposure can also affect the infant in the long term.[69] Gross motor development at one year of age, as assessed by the Bayley Psychomotor Index, was slightly but significantly altered in infants who were exposed regularly (at least daily) to ethanol in their mothers' milk. There were no significant differences in the motor and mental development of infants whose mothers drank less than one drink per day when compared with either infants whose mothers did not drink at all or those who were formula fed. This association between maternal drinking and motor development persisted even after controlling for more than 100 potentially confounding variables, including heavy maternal use of tobacco, marijuana, and caffeine.[69–71]

Little and colleagues[69] hypothesized that either the developing brain may be exquisitely sensitive to small quantities of alcohol, or that, following repeated exposure, the alcohol accumulates in the infant because it is metabolized or excreted more slowly than in adults.[72] Research on other animals has demonstrated permanent neuronal cell loss in the cerebellum of rats exposed to continuous low blood alcohol levels during the brain growth spurt.[73] Moreover, chronic exposure to alcohol during periods of cellular proliferations, migration and final maturation can result in extensive damage to the brain which, in turn, can affect motor development and behavior.[74,75]

21.3.3 EARLY SENSORY LEARNING

Research on humans and animal models has focused on the ontogeny of responsiveness to the sensory qualities of alcohol in humans in an attempt to identify some of the developmental, experiential, and cultural factors that contribute to an individual's hedonic responses to alcohol. Because of the olfactory system's intense and immediate access to the neurological substrates underlying emotion,[76] such investigations on the hedonic responses to sensory stimuli may provide a window into children's emotional responses and reveal information about contextual effects of learning and the role of early experience on the development of preferences and aversions. Moreover, the early state of maturity and plasticity of the chemical senses favors its involvement in the adaptive responses to the challenges of normal or atypical development.

During the past decade, animal model studies have elegantly revealed that early experiences with the smell and taste of alcohol can affect later responsiveness to the drug. Learning occurs when the young animal experiences alcohol in amniotic fluid,[77–80] mother's milk,[81–83] and as an ambient odor,[84,85] when the drug is intra-orally infused,[86] and even during acute stages of intoxication when perception is probably mediated by nonmetabolic routes of elimination such as respiration, or salivation, or both.[87]

Consistent with these findings in animal models, recent experimental studies in humans suggest that pre- and postnatal experiences with odors and flavors, including ethanol, bias the infants' behaviors and preferences during infancy and childhood. Not only can newborns discriminate full-strength homologous alcohols (ethanol to decanol) in much the same way as the perceived intensity of these alcohols decreased as the chain length increased for adults,[88] but they retain information about ethanol when experienced in amniotic fluid[89] mother's milk,[90] and/or the home.[91] Using a nonassociative learning paradigm (e.g., habituation), it was revealed that day-old infants born to frequent drinkers exhibited heightened reactivity (as assessed by head and facial activity) towards ethanol odor when compared to newborns of infrequent drinkers; the response did not generalize to other odors such as citral,[89] thus suggesting that the effects were not due to a generalized hyperreactivity to odors in general.

Experiences with ethanol odors can continue to impact upon infants' behaviors throughout the first years of life. When breastfed infants (6 to 13 months) were exposed to toys that were identical in appearance but differed in their characteristic scent (e.g., vanilla-scented, ethanol-scented, or no scent), we found that those infants who had more exposure to ethanol, as inferred from questionnaires about maternal and paternal alcoholism and alcohol intake, behaved differently in the presence of an ethanol-scented toy when compared with less exposed infants.[90] Of the four behaviors monitored in the study (mouthing, looking, manipulating the toy, and vocalizing), this differential response was manifested in mouthing the ethanol-scented toy more. This finding might be anticipated based on animal model studies that indicated that pups that were exposed to the flavor of ethanol in milk increased their mouthing rates to the odor of ethanol and were more willing to ingest ethanol-flavored solutions.[83] Whether mouthing the ethanol-odorized toy more reflects their familiarity with the flavor of ethanol which, in turn, leads to a greater willingness to accept ethanol-flavored substances remains to be investigated. Nevertheless, these data provide circumstantial evidence that prior ethanol exposure in humans alters the willingness of infants to orally explore toys scented with this odor. Moreover, this learning appears to be keenly selective, as it allows for the discrimination of closely related aromas, vanilla and ethanol.

That early experiences can also result in the generation of aversive memories about alcohol was evident in a study on older children who were between the ages of 3 and 6 years.[91] Here the children's hedonic response to the odor of alcohol was related to the emotional context in which parents experience alcohol and the parents' frequency of drinking. That is, children of a parent or parents who drank alcohol to change their state of mind or reduce dysphoric feelings (hereafter referred to as "escape drinking") were significantly more likely to judge the odor of beer as unpleasant when compared to similarly aged children whose parents did not drink to escape (see Figure 21.3). This difference between the groups was odor specific. That is, the children in the two groups were similar in their preference for the bubble gum and rejection of the pyridine odors. These findings concur with previous

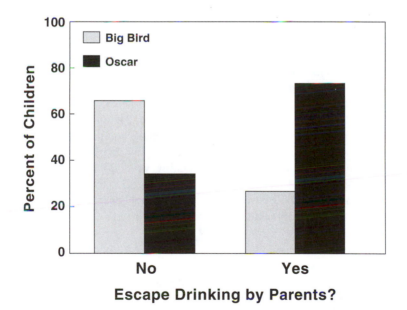

FIGURE 21.3 The percentage of children in each group who rated the odor of beer as good or bad. Children were told that if they liked the smell inside the bottle, then they should give it to a stuffed toy of Big Bird (a likeable, well-known television character puppet), but if they did not like the smell, they should give it to another well-known puppet, Oscar the Grouch, "so that he can throw it in his trash can." One group of children lived in a household in which one or both parents drank alcohol to change their state of mind, or reduce dysphoric feelings, or both ("escape drinkers"), whereas the parents of the children in the other group did not drink to escape. (From Mennella, J.A. and Garcia, P.L. The child's hedonic response to the smell of alcohol: effects of parental drinking habits. *Alcohol. Clin. Exp. Res.*, 24, 1167, 2000. With permission.)

studies on elementary school-aged children of alcoholic parents[92] and are consistent with animal model studies that demonstrate that pups exposed to an intoxicated mother develop aversive memories towards the odor of alcohol.[93,94]

Early childhood represents a critical period for the development of expectancies about, and the affective disposition toward alcohol, which may impact on alcohol use during adolescence.[95,96] The research in both humans and animal models suggests that at least some of the early learning about alcohol is based on sensory experiences and clearly anchor sit to children's experiences at home and the frequency and the emotional context in which their parents experience alcohol. These data support the hypothesis that associative learning in the context of emotionally salient conditions is a powerful mechanism by which odors acquire personal significance and that the emotional context in which children experience an odor can influence subsequent behaviors. Whether the emotional response to the scent of alcohol conditioned during early childhood persists or can explain behaviors during later childhood and adolescence is not known.

21.4 CONCLUDING REMARKS

Although there has been considerable research on the effects of prenatal alcohol exposure, the scientific information on the long-term effects of postnatal exposure to alcohol on the infants' behavioral state is quite limited. Nevertheless, recent findings on acute alcohol use during lactation in humans and animal models have consistently found that alcohol consumption by nursing mothers results in a decrease in milk production and a reduction in milk intake by their infants in the short term as well as the formation of alcohol-related memories. The mechanisms underlying this reduction in intake, and the long-term effects on the composition of milk remain to be elucidated. We emphasize that the scientific data described here do not imply that occasional alcohol consumption by lactating women would decrease overall milk intake or negatively affect their infants' development in the long term. However, until more is known, the folklore that claims that alcohol benefits the lactating mother and the breastfeeding infant should be carefully evaluated.

References

1. Marshall, M., Ames, G.M., and Bennett, L.A. Anthropological perspectives on alcohol and drugs at the turn of the millennium. *Soc. Sci. Med.*, 53, 153, 2001.
2. Hunt, G., Barker J.C. Socio-cultural anthropology and alcohol and drug research: towards a unified theory. *Soc. Sci. Med.*, 53, 165, 2001.
3. Mennella, J.A. The transfer of alcohol to human milk: sensory implications and effects on mother–infant interaction. In: Hannigan, J.H., Spear, N., Spear, L., and Goodlett, C.R. (Eds.). *Alcohol and Alcoholism: Brain and Development.* Lawrence Erlbaum Associates, NJ, 177, 1999.
4. Mennella, J.A. Alcohol and lactation: the folklore versus the science. In: Auerbach, K.G. (Ed.). *Current Issues in Clinical Lactation.* Jones and Bartlett, Boston, MA, pp. 3–10, 2002.
5. Robinovitch, L.G. Infantile alcoholism. *Q. J. Inebriety*, 25, 231, 1903.

6. Routh, C.H.F. *Infant Feeding and its Influence on Life*. New York: William Wood, 1879.

7. Krebs, R. *Making Friends Is Our Business — 100 Years of Anheuser-Busch*. A-B, Inc., St. Louis, MO, 1953.

8. Walter, M. The folklore of breastfeeding. *Bull. N.Y. Acad. of Med.*, 51, 870, 1975.

9. Riordan, J. *A Practical Guide to Breastfeeding*. C. V. Mosby, St. Louis, MO, 1983, 64.

10. Fishman, C., Evans, R., and Jenks, E. Warm bodies, cool milk: conflicts in post-partum food choice for Indochinese women in California. *Soc. Sci. Med.*, 26, 1125, 1988.

11. Lawrence, R.A. *Breastfeeding: A Guide for the Medical Profession*, 3rd ed. C. V. Mosby, St. Louis, MO, 1989.

12. Flores-Heurta, S. et al. Effects of ethanol consumption during pregnancy and lactation on the outcome and postnatal group of the offspring. *Ann. Nutr. Metab.*, 36, 121, 1992.

13. Pepino, M.Y. and Mennella, J.A. Advice given to pregnant and lactating women in Argentina: a pilot study. *Alcohol. Clini. Exp. Res.*, 26, A419, 2002.

14. Nicloux, M. Sur le passage de l'alcool ingéré dans le lait chez la femme. *Comptes Rendus de la Societe de Biologie*, Paris, 6, 982,1899. [Concerning the passage of ingested alcohol into the milk of women.]

15. Kesäniemi, Y.I. Ethanol and acetaldehyde in the milk and peripheral blood of lactating women after ethanol administration. *J. Obstet. Gynaecol. Br. Commonw.*, 81, 84, 1974.

16. Lawton, M.E. Alcohol in breast milk. *Aust. J. Obstet. Gynaecol.*, 25, 71, 1985.

17. Mennella, J.A. and Beauchamp, G.K. The transfer of alcohol to human milk: effects on flavor and the infant's behavior. *N. Engl. J. Med.*, 325, 8, 1991.

18. Mennella, J.A. and Beauchamp, G.K. Beer, breast-feeding and folklore. *Dev. Psychobiol.*, 26, 459, 1993.

19. Mennella, J.A., and Beauchamp, G.K. Early flavor experiences: research update. *Nutr. Rev.*, 56, 205, 1998.

20. Da-Silva, V.A. et al. Ethanol pharmacokinetics in lactating women. *Braz. J. Med. Biol. Res.*, 26, 1097, 1993.

21. Da-Silva, V.A., McLean, A.E.M., and Beales, D. Ethanol elimination by rats as a function of reproductive state, gender and nutritional status. *Braz. J. Med. Biol. Res.*, 29, 651, 1996.

22. Abel, E.L., Greizerstein, H.B., and Siemens, A.J. Influence of lactation on rate of disappearance of ethanol in the rat. *Neurobehav. Toxicol.*, 1, 185, 1979.

23. Gordon, B.H.J. et al. Exaggerated acetaldehyde response after ethanol administration during pregnancy and lactation. *Alcohol. Clin. Exp. Res.*, 9, 17, 1985.

24. Briggs, G.G., Freeman, R.K., and Yaffe, S.J. *A Reference Guide to Fetal and Neonatal Risk: Drugs in Pregnancy and Lactation*, 4th ed., Williams and Wilkins, Philadelphia, 1994.

25. Subramanian, M.G. and Abel, E.L. Alcohol inhibits suckling-induced prolactin release and milk yield. *Alcohol*, 5, 95, 1988.

26. Subramanian, M.G., Chen, X., and Bergeski, B.A. Pattern and duration of the inhibitory effect of alcohol administered acutely on suckling-induced prolactin in lactating rats. *Alcohol. Clin. Exp. Res.*, 14, 771, 1990.

27. Swiatek, K.R., Dombrowski G.J., Jr., and Chao, K.-L. The inefficient transfer of maternally fed alcohol to nursing rats. *Alcohol*, 3, 169, 1986.

28. Vilaró, S., Viñas, O., Remesar, X., and Herrera, E. Effects of chronic ethanol consumption on lactational performance in the rat: mammary gland and milk composition and pups' growth and metabolism. *Pharmacol. Biochem. Behav.*, 27, 333, 1987.

29. Mennella, J.A. Short-term effects of maternal alcohol consumption on lactational performance. *Alcohol. Clin. Exp. Res.*, 22, 1389, 1998.

30. Tavares-do-Carmo, M. and Nascimento-Curi, C.M. Effect of ethanol during lactation on the metabolism of dams and on pup development. *Braz. J. Med. Biol. Res.*, 23, 1161, 1990.

31. Chatterton, R.T. et al. Relation of plasma oxytocin and prolactin to milk production in mothers of preterm infants: influence of stress. *J. Clin. Endocrinol. Metab.*, 85, 3661, 2000.

32. Carter, C.S. and Altemus, M. Integrative functions in lactational hormones in social behavior and stress management. *Ann. N. Y. Acad. Sci.*, 807, 164, 1996.

33. Cox, D.B., Owens, R.A., and Hartmann, P.E. Blood and milk prolactin and the rate of milk synthesis in women. *Exp. Physiol.*, 81, 1007, 1996.

34. Becker, U., Gluud, C., Bennett, P., Micic, S. et al. Effect of alcohol and glucose infusion on pituitary-gonadal hormones in normal females. *Drug Alcohol Depend.*, 22, 141, 1988.

35. Carlson, H.E., Wasser, H.L., and Reidelberger, R.D. Beer-induced prolactin secretion: a clinical and laboratory study of the role of salsolinol. *J. Clin. Endocrinol. Metab.*, 60, 673, 1985.

36. Coira, V., Alboni, A., Gramellini, D. et al. Inhibition by ethanol of the oxytocin response to breast stimulation in normal women and the role of endogenous opioids. *Acta Endocrinol.*, 126, 213, 1992.

37. De Rosa, G., Corsello, S.M., Ruffilli, M. et al. Prolactin secretion after beer. *Lancet*, ii, 934, 1981.

38. Earll, J.M. et al. Effect of ethyl alcohol on ionic calcium and prolactin in man. *Avia. Space Environ. Med.*, 47, 808, 1976.

39. Ellingboe, J. et al. Effect of acute alcohol ingestion on integrated plasma prolactin levels in normal men. *Pharm. Biochem. Behav.*, 12, 297, 1980.

40. Grossman, E.R. Beer, breast-feeding and the wisdom of old wives. *JAMA*, 259, 1016, 1987.

41. Mendelson, J.H., Mello, N.K., and Ellingboe, J.J. Acute alcohol intake and pituitary gonadal hormones in normal human females. *J. Pharmacol Exp. Ther.*, 218, 23, 1981.

42. Soyka, M., Görig, E., and Naber, D. Serum prolactin increase induced by ethanol: a dose-dependent effect not related to stress. *Psychoneuroendocrinology*, 16, 441, 1991.

43. Teoh, S.K. et al. Alcohol effects on hCG-stimulation gonadal hormones in women. *J. Pharmacol. Exp. Ther.*, 254, 407, 1990.

44. Volpi, R. et al. Endogenous opioid mediation of the inhibitory effect of ethanol on the prolactin response to breast stimulation in normal women. *Life Sci.*, 54, 739, 1994.

45. Subramanian. M.G. Inhibitory effect of alcohol on the established suckling-induced prolactin surge in lactating rats. *Proc. Soc. Exp. Biol. Med.*, 198, 579, 1991.

46. Heil, S.H. and Subramanian, M.G. Chronic alcohol exposure and lactation: extended observations. *Alcohol*, 21, 127, 2000.

47. Cobo, E. Effect of different doses of ethanol on the milk-ejecting reflex in lactating women. *Am. J. Obstet. Gynecol.*, 115, 817, 1973.

48. Cobo, E. and Quintero, C.A. Milk-ejecting and antidiuretic activities under neurohypophyseal inhibition with alcohol and water overload. *Am. J. Obstet. Gynecol.*, 105, 877, 1969.

49. Wagner, G. and Fuchs, A.-R. Effect of ethanol on uterine activity during suckling in post-partum women. *Acta Endocrinol.*, 58, 133, 1968.

50. Subramanian, M.G. Alcohol inhibits suckling-induced oxytocin release in the lactating rat. *Alcohol*, 19, 51, 1999.

51. Bowen-Jones, A., Thompson, C., and Drewett, R.F. Milk flow and sucking rates during breast-feeding. *Dev. Med. Child. Neurol.*, 24, 626, 1982.
52. Auerbach, K.G. et al. Beer and the breast-feeding mom. *JAMA*, 258, 2126, 1987.
53. Berlin C.M., Jr. Drugs and chemicals: exposure of the nursing mother. *Clin. Pharmacol.*, 36, 1089, 1989.
54. American Academy of Pediatrics: Committee on Drugs. The transfer of drugs and other chemicals into human milk. *Pediatrics*, 108, 776, 2001.
55. Bisdom, C.J.W. Alcohol — en nicotinevergiftifing bij zuigelingen. *Maandschr Kindergeneesk*, 6, 332, 1937.
56. Binkiewicz, A., Robinson, M. J., and Senior, B. Pseudo-Cushing syndrome caused by alcohol in breast milk. *J. Pediatr.*, 93, 965, 1978.
57. Yamagishi, M., and Iwasaki, T. Acute alcohol intoxication in a two-month-old baby. *J. UOEH*, 9, 53, 1987.
58. Mennella J.A. The human infants' suckling responses to the flavor of alcohol in mother's milk. *Alcohol. Clin. Exp. Res.*, 21, 581, 1997.
59. Daley, S.E.J. et al. The determination of short-term breast volume changes and the rate of synthesis of human milk using computerized breast measurement. *Exp. Physiol.*, 77, 79, 1992.
60. Auerbach, K.G. Breastfeeding fallacies: their relationship to understanding lactation. *Birth*, 17, 44, 1990.
61. Wright, P. Learning experiences in feeding behavior during infancy. *J. Psychosom. Res.*, 32, 613, 1988.
62. Mennella, J.A. Regulation of milk intake following exposure to alcohol in mothers' milk. *Alcohol. Clin. Exp. Res.*, 25, 590, 2001.
63. Mennella, J.A. and Gerrish, C.J. Effects of exposure to alcohol in mother's milk on infant sleep. *Pediatrics*, 101, e21, 1998.
64. Mennella, J.A. and Garcia-Gomez, P.L. Sleep disturbances following acute exposure to alcohol in mothers' milk. *Alcohol*, 25, 153, 2001.
65. Mulder, E.J.H. et al. Acute maternal alcohol consumption disrupts behavioral state organization in the near-term fetus. *Pediatr. Res.*, 44, 774, 1998.
66. Rundell, O.H. et al. Alcohol and sleep in young adults. *Psychopharmacologia (Berlin)*, 26, 201, 1972.
67. Williams, D.L., MacLean, A.W., and Cairns, J. Dose-response effects of ethanol on the sleep of young women. *J. Stud. Alcohol.*, 44, 515, 1983.
68. Mendelson, W.B. and Hill, S.Y. Effects of the acute administration of ethanol on the sleep of the rat: a dose-response study. *Pharmacol. Biochem. Behav.*, 8, 723, 1978.
69. Little, R.E. et al. Maternal alcohol use during breast-feeding and infant mental and motor development at one year. *N. Engl. J. ed.*, 321, 425, 1989.
70. Little, R.E. Maternal use of alcohol and breast-fed infants — reply. *N. Engl. J. Med.*, 322, 339, 1990.
71. Little, R.E., Lambert, M.D., and Worthington-Roberts, B. Drinking and smoking at 3 months postpartum by lactation history. *Paediatr. Perinat. Epidemiol.*, 4, 290, 1990.
72. Manning, G.J. Drug metabolism in the newborn. *Fed. Proc.*, 44, 2302, 1985.
73. Napper, R.M.A. and West, J.R. Permanent neuronal cell loss in the cerebellum of rats exposure to continuous low blood alcohol levels during the brain growth spurt: a stereological investigation. *J. Com. Neurol.*, 362, 283, 1995.
74. Clarren, S.K., Astley, S.J., and Bowden, D.M. Physical anomalies and developmental delays in nonhuman primate infants exposed to weekly doses of ethanol during gestation. *Teratology*, 37, 561, 1988.

75. Barr, H.M. et al. Prenatal exposure to alcohol, caffeine, tobacco, and aspirin: effects on fine and gross motor performance in 4-year-old children. *Dev. Psychol.*, 26, 339, 1990.

76. Cahill, L. et al. The amygdala and emotional memory. *Nature*, 377, 295, 1995.

77. Chotro, M.G. and Molina, J.C. Acute ethanol contamination of the amniotic fluid during gestational day 21: postnatal changes in alcohol responsiveness in rats. *Dev. Psychobiol.*, 23, 535, 1990.

78. Abate, P. et al. Neonatal activation of alcohol-related prenatal memories: impact on the first suckling responses. *Alcohol. Clin. Exp. Res.*, 26, 1512, 2002.

79. Abate, P., Spear, N.E., and Molina, J.C. Fetal and infantile alcohol-mediated associative learning in the rat. *Alcohol. Clin. Exp. Res.*, 25, 989–98, 2001.

80. Domínguez, H.D., Chotro, M.G., and Molina, J.C. Alcohol in the amniotic fluid prior to cesarean delivery: effects of subsequent exposure to the drug's odor upon alcohol responsiveness. *Behav. Neural Biol.*, 60, 129, 1993.

81. Pepino, M.Y. et al. Infant rats respond differently to alcohol during nursing from an alcohol-intoxicated dam. *Alcohol,* 18, 189, 1999.

82. Phillips, D.S. and Stainbrook, G.L. Effects of early alcohol exposure upon adult learning ability and taste preferences. *Physiol. Psychol.*, 4, 473, 1976.

83. Hunt, P.S. et al. Enhanced ethanol intake in preweanling rats following exposure to ethanol in a nursing context. *Dev. Psychobiol.*, 26, 133, 1993.

84. Molina, J.C., Serwatka, J., and Spear, N.E. Changes in alcohol intake resulting from prior experiences with alcohol odor in young rats. *Pharm. Biochem. Behav.*, 21, 387, 1984.

85. Molina, J.C. et al. Differential ethanol olfactory experiences affect ethanol ingestion in preweanlings but not in older rats. *Behav. Neural Biol.*, 44, 90, 1985.

86. Molina, J.C., Hoffmann, H., and Spear, N.E. Conditioning of aversion to alcohol orosensory cues in 5- and 10-day-old rats: subsequent reduction in alcohol ingestion. *Dev. Psychobiol.*, 19, 175, 1986.

87. Molina, J.C., Chotro, M.G., and Spear, N.E. Early (preweanling) recognition of alcohol's orosensory cues resulting from acute ethanol intoxication. *Behav. Neural Biol.*, 51, 307, 1989.

88. Rovee, C.K. Psychophysical scaling of olfactory response to aliphatic alcohols in human neonates. *J. Exp. Child. Psychol.*, 7, 245, 1969.

89. Faas, A. et al. Differential responsiveness to alcohol odor in human neonates: effects of maternal consumption during gestation. *Alcohol,* 22, 7, 2000.

90. Mennella, J.A. and Beauchamp, G.K. The infant's response to scented toys: effects of exposure. *Chem. Senses*, 2, 11, 1998.

91. Mennella, J.A. and Garcia, P.L. The child's hedonic response to the smell of alcohol: effects of parental drinking habits. *Alcohol. Clin. Exp. Res.*, 24, 1167, 2000.

92. Noll, R.B., Zucker, R.A., and Greenberg, G.S. Identification of alcohol by smell among preschoolers: evidence for early socialization about drugs occurring in the home. *Child Dev.*, 61, 1520, 1990.

93. Molina, J.C. et al. The infant rat learns about alcohol through interaction with an intoxicated mother. *Alcohol. Clin. Exp. Res.*, 24, 428, 2000.

94. Pepino, M.Y., Spear, N.E., and Molina J.C. Nursing experiences with an alcohol-intoxicated rat dam counteract appetitive conditioned responses toward alcohol. *Alcohol. Clin. Exp. Res.*, 25, 18, 2001.

95. Miller, P.M., Smith, G.T., and Goldman, M.S. Emergence of alcohol expectancies in childhood: a possible critical period. *J. Stud. Alcohol*, 31, 343, 1990.

96. Wiers, R.W., Gunning, W.B., and Sergeant, J.A. Do young children of alcoholics hold more positive or negative alcohol-related expectancies than controls? *Alcohol. Clin. Exp. Res.*, 22, 1855, 1998.

22 Alcohol, Acetaldehyde, and Digestive Tract Cancer

Mikko P. Salaspuro

CONTENTS

393

22.1 INTRODUCTION

Excessive alcohol consumption is one of the strongest risk factors for upper digestive tract cancers.[1] In addition, there is increasing evidence that heavy drinking may increase cancer risk also in other parts of the gastrointestinal tract. The exact mechanism of ethanol-associated cancers has remained obscure since ethanol itself is not a carcinogen.[2] In contrast to alcohol, the first metabolite of ethanol oxidation, acetaldehyde, has multiple carcinogenic effects according to cell culture and animal studies.[3] On the other hand, alcohol abuse has also been associated with several indirect tumor-promoting effects. These may include for instance malnourishment, increased exposure to other carcinogens, increased production of free radicals, and local effects of strong alcoholic beverages.[4,5]

After its oral intake, alcohol is at first absorbed to the portal blood from the stomach and upper part of the small intestine. Thereafter, it is rapidly transported by blood circulation to other organs including the digestive tract. Finally, ethanol is evenly distributed to the water phase of all organs. After the distribution phase, ethanol levels in saliva, tears, and urine, as well as in the contents of the terminal ileum and large intestine, are equal to those of the blood and the liver.[6–8] Although the main organ for ethanol oxidation is the liver, there is increasing evidence that alcohol is not merely an innocent bystander in the digestive tract. Ethanol can be oxidized to acetaldehyde by many microbes representing normal gut flora, and also by salivary glands and mucous membranes. However, as compared to the liver, the detoxification of acetaldehyde by either microbes or mucous membranes is limited. This results after ingestion of alcoholic beverages in strikingly high local concentrations of carcinogenic acetaldehyde throughout the whole gastrointestinal tract.

In the past 10 years a great deal of work has been done to characterize those factors that regulate the concentration of acetaldehyde in various parts of the GI tract.[9–11] Those environmental and hereditary factors that are associated with increased risk of digestive tract cancers appeared to be also factors that increase the local concentrations of carcinogenic acetaldehyde in human saliva. These include for instance smoking, heavy drinking, poor oral hygiene, and a hereditary deficiency of acetaldehyde metabolizing enzyme, aldehyde dehydrogenase (ALDH2). The combined evidence derived from these epidemiological and biochemical studies opens a new microbiological approach to the pathogenesis of digestive tract cancer and may have an influence on future preventive strategies.

22.2 EPIDEMIOLOGY

22.2.1 CANCER OF THE OROPHARYNX AND ESOPHAGUS

An association between heavy drinking and esophageal cancer was recognized already at the beginning of the 19th century.[12] A massive body of epidemiological evidence later on accumulated to show that excessive alcohol consumption is a strong risk factor for upper digestive tract cancer.[1,2] It has been estimated that 25 to 68% of upper GI tract cancers are attributable to alcohol and that up to 80% of these tumors can be prevented by abstaining from alcohol and smoking.[13] Poor oral

TABLE 22.1
Relative Risks of Oral and Esophageal Cancer by Drinking Habit

Drinks/d	Type of Cancer	
	Oral	Esophageal
0	1.0	1.0
1 or less	0.7	1.3
2–3	1.4	2.2
4–5	3.1	4.8
6+	6.2	5.8

Data from Boffeta, P. and Garfinkel, L., Alcohol drinking and mortality among men enrolled in an American Cancer Society prospective study, *Epidemiology*, 1, 342, 1990.

hygiene, nutritional deficiencies, and human papilloma virus are other independent risk factors of these cancers.[13]

22.2.1.1 Upper Digestive Tract Cancer Risk Is Dose-Dependent

Most epidemiological cohort and case-control studies adjusted for smoking show a dose-dependent effect of alcohol. According to American Cancer Society's cohort study on one million subjects, the relative risk of oral cancer was 6.2 and that of esophageal cancer 5.8 among those having six or more drinks per day (Table 22.1).[14] A similar dose-dependent relationship has been demonstrated in case control studies comprising nonsmokers.[15–17] Alcohol consumption exceeding 1.5 bottles of wine daily results in males in about a 100-fold risk of esophageal cancer (Table 22.2).[17]

22.2.1.2 Carcinogenic Effect of Alcohol and Smoking Is Synergistic

Strong evidence suggests that alcohol and smoking have a greater relative effect together than alone. This is clearly illustrated by a case-control study on 598 men with squamous cell carcinoma of the mouth and pharynx (Table 22.3).[18] Confirming results have been obtained in France, where much larger quantities of alcohol are consumed. Individuals drinking more than 1.5 bottles of wine and smoking 10 to 30 cigarettes daily have about a 150-fold risk of esophageal cancer (Table 22.4).[19] Moderate cigarette smoking without drinking and moderate drinking without smoking have a slight or negligible effect on esophageal cancer risk. However, simultaneous exposure to the same moderate amounts increases the risk 12- to 19-fold in men and women, respectively.[20]

22.2.1.3 ALDH2 Deficiency Enhances Cancer Risk

The association between heavy drinking and the risk of digestive tract cancers is particularly prominent in individuals who have a genetically deficient ability to detoxify acetaldehyde. Mitochondrial class II aldehyde dehydrogenase (ALDH2) is responsible for the main part of acetaldehyde oxidation.[21] The ALDH2*2 is a result

TABLE 22.2
Relative Risk of Esophageal Cancer in Relation to Alcohol Consumption among Nonsmokers

Alcohol Consumption, g/d	Relative Risk	
	Males	Females
0–49	1.0	1.0
41–80	3.8	5.6
81–120	10.2	11.9
>121	101.0	

Data from Tuyns, A.G., Oesophageal cancer in non-smoking drinkers and in non-drinking smokers, *Int. J. Cancer*, 32, 443, 1983.

TABLE 22.3
Relative Risk of Oral and Pharyngeal Cancer by Level of Smoking and Drinking

Drinking, ml/d	Smoking, Cigarette Equivalents/d			
	0–10	>20	20–39	yli 40
0	1.0	1.5	1.4	2.4
< 12	1.4	1.7	3.2	3.3
12–44	1.6	4.4	4.5	8.2
>45	2.3	4.1	9.6	15.5

Data from Rothman, K. and Keller R., The effect of joint exposure of alcohol and tobacco on risk of cancer of the mouth and pharynx, *J. Chron. Dis.*, 25, 711, 1972.

TABLE 22.4
Relative Risk of Esophageal Cancer by Level of Smoking and Drinking

Drinking, g/d	Smoking, g/d		
	0–10	10–30	yli 30
0–40	1.0	3.9	7.8
40–80	7.3	8.6	33.6
80–120	11.7	13.1	87.0
>120	49.7	78.7	149.1

Data from Tuyns, A.J., Pequignot, G., and Jensen, O.M., Les cancers de l'oesophage an Ille-et-Villaine en fonction des niveaux de consommation d'alcool et de tabac, Des risques qui se multiplient, *Bull. Cancer*, 64, 45, 1977.

of a single point mutation in chromosome six coding the normal ALDH2*1 allele. Individuals homozygous for the mutated ALDH2*2 allele lack ALDH2 activity, whereas heterozygous individuals with the ALDH2*1/*2 genotype have 30 to 50% of the activity of ALDH2*1 homozygotes.[22] Some Asian populations show high frequencies of the ALDH2*2 allele, e.g., about 50% of the Japanese are ALDH2-deficient, while it is extremely rare in Caucasian populations.[23]

Because of elevated blood acetaldehyde levels, ALDH2-deficient subjects receive after alcohol ingestion unpleasant symptoms such as flushing of the face and body, tachycardia, drop in blood pressure, headache, and nausea.[24] Because of these adverse reactions totally ALDH2-deficient subjects are protected against alcoholism.[25] However, heterozygotic subjects may become heavy drinkers, or even alcoholics.[26] Many recent epidemiological studies have shown that the risk of alcohol related digestive tract cancers is markedly increased in Asian heavy drinkers with deficient ALDH2 enzyme as compared to those heavy drinkers with the normal enzyme (Table 22.5).[27,28]

22.2.1.4 Cancer Risk among Those with High Activity ADH Enzyme

The most important enzymes in ethanol elimination and acetaldehyde formation in humans are class I alcohol dehydrogenases (ADHs), which are expressed by three genes, ADH1, ADH2, and ADH3. Three different allelic forms have been found for ADH2 and two for *ADH3*.[29] Alleles ADH2*2 and ADH3*1 encode the most active enzymatic forms, e.g., individuals having ADH3*1/*1 genotype metabolize ethanol to acetaldehyde 2.5 times faster than individuals with other ADH3 genotypes. ADH2*2/*2 genotypes metabolize ethanol even 40 times faster than individuals with the ADH2*1/*1 genotype.

An enhanced risk of upper digestive tract cancers has been associated with the rapidly metabolizing ADH3 genotype in some studies.[30,31] However, this association

TABLE 22.5
Relative Risk (Odds Ratios) of Digestive Tract Cancers among Japanese Alcoholics after Adjustment for Confounders among ALDH2-Deficient Subjects as Compared to Those with the Normal ALDH2-Enzyme

Type of Cancer	Odds Ratios
Oropharyngolaryngeal	11.1
Esophageal	12.5
Stomach	3.5
Colon	3.4
Esophageal cancer concomitant with oropharyngolaryngeal and/or stomach cancer	54.2

Data from Yokoyama, A. et al., Alcohol-related cancers and aldehyde dehydrogenase-2 in Japanese alcoholics, *Carcinogenesis*, 19, 1383, 1998.

could not be confirmed in two other studies.[32,33] The two negative studies used hospital patients as controls and included less heavy drinkers than the positive studies. These differences in study design may explain the controversy. It can be concluded that the present epidemiological data support an association between *ADH3*1* and increased upper GI tract cancer risk, but further population-based studies with a larger number of subjects are still needed.

22.2.1.5   Cancer Risk in Relation to the Type of Alcoholic Beverage and Nutrition

Some studies have attempted to determine whether different types of alcoholic beverages are associated with different risks of upper digestive tract cancers. Unfortunately, most studies lack accurate data on types of alcoholic beverages or are based on a single center, so that the beverage associated most strongly with cancer risk is the one most frequently used.

In France, the highest incidence of esophageal cancer has been reported in the West (Calvados, Normandy), especially among rural populations.[34] Consumption of hot Calvados (a dry apple brandy) appeared to explain about two thirds of the interregional and urban/rural differences in incidence, whereas total alcohol consumption explained less than 1/5.[35] Our preliminary studies indicate that Calvados may contain as a congener up to 100 times higher concentrations of carcinogenic acetaldehyde than other alcoholic beverages (unpublished observation). So far, it has been generally believed that possible congeners play a minor role in the pathogenesis of upper digestive tract cancers.

Already in 1957 cancer of hypopharynx was related to iron deficiency and the Plummer–Winson syndrome.[36] Furthermore, some indirect evidence suggests that the risk from exposure to many carcinogenic agents may be reduced by regular consumption of fruit and green vegetables.[13] Nutritional deficiencies have also been proposed to play a major role in the high incidence of esophageal cancer in some parts of Asia.[37]

22.2.2   Cancer of the Stomach

The epidemiological data concerning the association between alcohol consumption and stomach cancer are controversial. The general conclusion derived from 18 cohort and 40 case-control studies is that alcohol could have an etiological role in stomach cancer, albeit minor and unproven.[1,2,38] In some case-control studies the relative risk caused by heavy drinking has ranged from 1.5 to 1.7. However, a relative risk up to 3.5 has been reported among the Japanese,[27,39] who frequently have a genetically determined deficiency to detoxify acetaldehyde.[23]

22.2.3   Cancer of the Large Intestine

The association between alcohol consumption and cancer of the large intestine has also been long debated. Controversial epidemiological studies based on at least 15 cohort and 18 case-control studies have been published.[1,2] It can be concluded that there is some evidence suggesting that excessive drinking leads to a relative risk of

1.1 with regard to colon cancer, and that the risk for rectal cancer is somewhat larger.[40,41] According to a recent WHO consensus statement, epidemiological data indicate that the consumption of alcoholic beverages, even at low intake, results in an increased risk of colorectal adenomas and cancer.[42] The association seems to be more consistent for beer and rectal cancer. Furthermore, there is some evidence suggesting that the relative risk of alcohol-related colorectal cancers is higher among Japanese[43] and especially among those with a genetic deficiency to detoxify acetaldehyde.[27,28]

22.3 PATHOGENESIS

22.3.1 LOCAL AND SYSTEMIC EFFECTS OF ALCOHOL

Ethanol itself is not carcinogenic. However, it may have tumor-promoting local or systemic effects. The risk of oropharyngeal cancer is increased both in men and women who regularly use mouthwashes with a high alcohol content.[44] Alcohol concentration of more than 20% may have local injurious effects on mucous membranes.[45] This may lead to accelerated cell division and regeneration and could explain why chronic alcohol intake is frequently associated with hyperproliferation, which might subsequently trigger replication errors during DNA synthesis.[46]

Ethanol has been postulated to act as a solvent that might enhance the penetration of carcinogenic substances from either tobacco smoke or food into the mucous membranes.[47] This mechanism could be particularly relevant in case of ethanol-induced injuries in cell membranes. Moreover, chronic alcohol abuse may lead to the atrophy of parotid glands and reduced saliva flow.[48] These mechanisms could result in higher local concentration and prolonged contact times of potential carcinogens.

Heavy drinking may impair esophageal motility and enhance gastroesophageal reflux leading to esophagitis and Barrett's esophagus[49] that is a well known precancerous lesion for the adenocarcinoma of the distal esophagus.

Alcohol abuse may enhance digestive tract cancer risk also by indirect nutritional or direct metabolic means. Chronic alcoholism is frequently associated with malnutrition. This may lead to decreased intake of cancer-protective fruits, vegetables, trace elements such as zinc and selenium, and vitamins such as folic acid, riboflavin, retinol, ascorbic acid, and alpha-tocopherol.[50] By another systemic mechanism, heavy drinking may induce cytochrome P-450-dependent metabolic pathways which have been suggested to lead to the activation of procarcinogens to carcinogens.[51] On the other hand, the inhibition of cytochrome P-450-dependent mechanisms may impair the detoxification of carcinogenic compounds to less toxic metabolic products.[4]

22.3.2 ACETALDEHYDE

After its oral intake alcohol is absorbed to the portal blood from the stomach and upper part of the small intestine. Thereafter it is rapidly transported by blood circulation to other organs including the digestive tract. Due to its water solubility, ethanol levels in saliva and in the contents of large intestine are equal to those of the blood and the liver.[7] In the saliva and large bowel ethanol can be oxidized to acetaldehyde by many microbes representing normal gut flora, and also by salivary glands and mucous membranes.[9–11] However, as compared to the liver the detoxification of acetaldehyde by either microbes or mucous membranes is limited. This results in strikingly high local concentrations of carcinogenic acetaldehyde throughout the whole gastrointestinal tract.[9–11]

22.3.2.1   Acetaldehyde as a Carcinogen

Acetaldehyde is a highly toxic and volatile compound, which has many mutagenic and carcinogenic effects both in cell culture and animal studies.[3] It has been shown to cause point mutations in the hypoxanthine-guanine phosphoribosyl transferase locus in human lymphocytes.[52] Furthermore, it may induce sister chromatid exchanges and gross chromosomal aberrations.[53,54] Acetaldehyde may also interfere with the DNA repair by inhibiting O^6-methylguanine transferase, an enzyme that is important for the repair of adducts caused by alkylating agents.[55] The covalent binding to DNA and the formation of stable adducts is one mechanism by which acetaldehyde could trigger the occurrence of replication errors in oncogenes or tumor suppressor genes.[56] Stable DNA adducts of acetaldehyde have been shown in different organs of alcohol-fed rodents and in leukocytes of alcoholics.[57]

In all different cell systems used in studies on the carcinogenic actions of acetaldehyde, a strong dose dependency with regard to acetaldehyde concentration has been observed. The induced damages occur after acetaldehyde treatment with acetaldehyde concentrations ranging from 40 to 1000 μM and incubation times from 1 to 90 h. These acetaldehyde concentrations are equal to those found after alcohol administration *in vivo* in human saliva and as well in the colonic contents of experimental animals.[58,8]

Folate is a crucial methyl group donor for many transmethylation reactions in the human body. Diminished folate leads to hypomethylation of the DNA that has been observed in experimental cancer models and in human cancer. The decreased levels of folic acid in alcoholics may be partly due to acetaldehyde, since it is able to catabolize folate via cleavage at the C^9–C^{10} bond.[59] It has been found that alcohol treatment for two weeks decreases colonic mucosal folate levels by 48% in rats.[60] This could be prevented with ciprofloxacin that also prevented the ethanol-induced increase in intracolonic acetaldehyde concentration.[60]

Long-term administration of acetaldehyde in drinking water to rats causes hyperplastic and hyperproliferating changes in the tongue, epiglottis, and the forestomach.[61] An acetaldehyde inhalation experiment in rats showed an increased incidence of carcinomas in the nasal mucosa.[62] Another inhalation study with hamsters resulted in enhanced numbers of laryngeal carcinomas.[63] *In vitro* studies with the human adenocarcinoma cell line CACO-2 show that acetaldehyde decreases some brush border enzyme activities and alters certain cell properties including an increase in the proliferation rate and disturbed cell differentiation.[64,65] These results suggest more aggressive and invasive tumor behavior *in vivo*.

According to the International Agency for Research on Cancer there is sufficient evidence to identify acetaldehyde as a carcinogen in animals.[3] Most recent epidemiological, genetic and biochemical studies strongly support the view that acetaldehyde produced either by microbes representing normal gut flora or by salivary glands is a local carcinogen also in humans.[9–11]

22.3.2.2 Microbial Acetaldehyde Production in the Saliva

There is an array of microbial alcohol dehydrogenases (ADH). Under anaerobic conditions ADH-containing microbes are capable of producing energy from glucose through alcoholic fermentation. The reaction runs as follows:

Alcoholic fermentation

$$\text{ADH}$$
$$\text{Glucose} \rightarrow \text{Acetaldehyde} \leftrightarrow \text{Ethanol}$$

Under aerobic or microaerobic conditions the last ADH-mediated reaction is reversed with acetaldehyde as an end-product.[66] An example of this type of reversed reaction is acetaldehyde production *in vitro* by human mouth- and bronchopulmonary washings.[67] *In vivo*, microbial acetaldehyde production from ethanol has been reported to occur in the oropharynx of healthy subjects,[68] and in the intestinal contents of rats with a jejunal blind-loop.[69]

Marked amounts of acetaldehyde can be detected in the saliva of healthy volunteers after ingestion of a moderate dose of ethanol (0.5 g/kg body weight) (Figure 22.1).[58] This is 10 to 20 times more than systemic blood acetaldehyde levels after even considerably higher doses of alcohol. Salivary acetaldehyde levels show remarkable interindividual variation and are clearly reduced after a 3-d use of an antiseptic mouthwash (Figure 22.1).[58] This emphasizes the role of oral microflora in the production of salivary acetaldehyde.

After a moderate dose of alcohol acetaldehyde levels in saliva range between 18 and 143 μM and are achieved within 40 min after alcohol ingestion.[58] These are acetaldehyde levels that are known to be able to cause mutagenic effects. *In vitro* results show that microbial acetaldehyde production in saliva is strongly associated with the ethanol concentration and is pH-dependent.[58]

As stated earlier in this chapter, smoking, heavy drinking, and poor dental status are well-known risk factors of the upper digestive tract cancers, as well as also the strongest factors increasing salivary acetaldehyde production.[70,71] Smoking shows a positive linear correlation between salivary acetaldehyde levels and cigarette use.[70] It can be estimated that a smoker with a daily consumption of approximately 20 cigarettes has a 50 to 60% increased salivary acetaldehyde production. This implies that even after moderate alcohol intake smokers produce markedly higher concentrations of carcinogenic acetaldehyde in the oral cavity than nonsmokers.

Regarding the microbiological mechanisms, an increase in yeast infections, e.g., *Candida albicans*, has been demonstrated among smokers.[72] This in accordance with findings of an increased incidence and also higher loads of yeasts among high acetaldehyde producers.[72] In general, a microbial "switch" with a significant increase

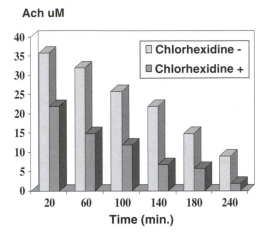

Ach uM

FIGURE 22.1 Acetaldehyde (Ach) in human saliva after a moderate dose of ethanol (0.5 g/kg body weight): effect of chlorhexidine (0.2%) mouth rinsing (twice daily for 60 sec). (Adapted from Homann, N. et al., High acetaldehyde levels in saliva after ethanol consumption: Methodological aspects and pathogenetic implications, *Carcinogenesis*, 18, 1739, 1997.)

in the production of Gram-positive vs. Gram-negative bacteria has been described in smokers.[73] In accordance with this observation almost all aerobic Gram-positive bacteria are significantly increased in "high" acetaldehyde-producing salivas, whereas the Gram-negative aerobic bacteria are not associated with high acetaldehyde production.[70] Thus, there is in general a good link between microbial observations that some species are associated with higher acetaldehyde production and the well-known effect of smoking on the oral microflora.

Regarding alcohol consumption, only heavy drinking (>40 g/d) seems to be associated with increased acetaldehyde production in saliva.[70] However, when an increase is observed it is dose-dependent and increases salivary acetaldehyde levels by about 50%. As compared to smoking, microbial changes in the oral microflora of alcoholics have been less intensively described.[74] Since high salivary acetaldehyde production is observed only among heavy drinkers, induction of microbial enzymes might be an explanation for this finding.

It can be concluded that smoking and alcohol together increase the salivary acetaldehyde production by about 100% as compared to nonsmokers and moderate drinkers.[70] Therefore the main risk factors for upper digestive tract cancer both independently and jointly increase the salivary microbial acetaldehyde production.

Poor oral hygiene is a risk factor for oral cavity cancer and leads to bacterial overgrowth, periodontitis, and caries. In a study with 132 volunteers, poor oral hygiene showed an approximately twofold increase in salivary acetaldehyde production and this was confirmed after adjustment for smoking, alcohol consumption, age and gender.[71] Studies on human saliva producing either very high or low acetaldehyde levels from ethanol show that mainly aerobic bacteria and yeasts are associated with an increased acetaldehyde production.[71,75,76] High acetaldehyde-producing salivas have been shown to express stronger yeast colonization than the low acetaldehyde-producing salivas.[75] Among yeast carriers, the density of yeasts is higher in high acetaldehyde producers than in low producers. Moreover, *Candida albicans* strains isolated from the high acetaldehyde-producing salivas form significantly higher acetaldehyde levels from ethanol than *Candida albicans* strains from low acetaldehyde-producing salivas.[75]

22.3.2.3 Microbial Acetaldehyde Formation in the Stomach

Achlorhydric atrophic gastritis is a well-known premalignant condition of gastric cancer.[77] Many theories of the pathogenetic mechanisms behind increased gastric cancer risk in patients with atrophic gastritis have been published, and still there is no final explanation. Enhanced local microbial production of endogenous ethanol and endogenous acetaldehyde could be one explaining factor for increased gastric cancer risk among patients with achlorhydric atrophic gastritis.

Due to its acidity, the normal human stomach is free of microbes. However, microbes may survive with a pH over 4.0 and bacterial proliferation can be expected when the pH rises over 5.0.[78] Bacterial overgrowth in achlorhydric stomach leads to the formation of minor concentrations of endogenous ethanol and acetaldehyde after glucose infusion in man.[79] After ethanol infusion the mean intragastric acetaldehyde level of the atrophic gastritis patients increases within an hour to 6.5-fold as compared to the healthy controls.[79]

22.3.2.4 Microbial Acetaldehyde Formation in the Large Intestine

In 1990s it was demonstrated in rats that after an acute dose of ethanol, acetaldehyde levels higher than in the liver or in the blood are found in colonic mucosa.[80] Since in that study mucosal acetaldehyde levels were significantly lower in germ-free than in normal animals, mucosal acetaldehyde was suggested to be generated at least in part through bacterial ethanol oxidation. Later studies have proved that this assumption was correct.

The reversed microbial ADH reaction produces striking amounts of acetaldehyde when human colonic contents are incubated *in vitro* at 37°C with increasing ethanol concentrations.[81] This reaction is active already at comparatively low (10 to 100 mg%) ethanol concentrations known to exist in the colon during and after normal drinking.[8] Moreover, acetaldehyde formation catalyzed by microbial ADHs takes place at a pH normally found in the colon and is rapidly reduced with lowering of the pH.[81]

Not only microbes but also colonic mucosal cells express ADH and ALDH enzymes, but in much lower activities than the liver.[82,83] It has been estimated that the ALDH activity of colonic mucosa could be sufficient for the removal of the acetaldehyde produced by colonic mucosal ADH during ethanol oxidation. It may, however, be insufficient for the removal of the acetaldehyde produced by intracolonic bacteria.[83]

Antibiotics can be used to examine the role of bacterial flora in the regulation of intracolonic acetaldehyde concentration. The reduction of aerobic gastrointestinal flora with ciprofloxacin decreases the total ethanol elimination rate by about 10% both in rats and man.[84,85] This associates with a significant decrease in the mean ADH activity of the fecal samples, in almost total abolishment of the formation of endogenous ethanol in the colon, and in a remarkable reduction of the intracolonic acetaldehyde production from ethanol.[84,86]

22.3.2.5   Human "Knockout" Model for Long-Term Acetaldehyde Exposure

As mentioned earlier many recent epidemiological studies have shown that the risk of ethanol-associated digestive tract cancers is remarkably increased in Asian subjects with partially inactive ALDH2 enzyme.[27,28] In the initial epidemiological studies the carcinogenic action of acetaldehyde was related to the elevation of blood acetaldehyde among ALDH2-deficient subjects.[87] However, by this means it is not possible to explain why cancer risk is not increased among ALDH2-deficient subjects in organs such as liver and kidneys.[27]

Another possibility is that after alcohol drinking, acetaldehyde levels are increased locally, for instance, in the saliva. Indeed, after ingestion of a moderate dose of alcohol (0.5 g/kg body weight), ALDH2-deficient Asians have two to three times higher acetaldehyde levels in their saliva than those with the normal enzyme throughout the whole observation period of 240 min (Figure 22.2).[88] Cannulation of the duct of the parotid glands showed that the additional salivary acetaldehyde was produced in the ALDH2-deficient subjects by the salivary glands.[88] Obviously, ALDH2-deficient parotid glands were not able to detoxify acetaldehyde derived from ethanol by their own ADH. Furthermore, ALDH2-deficient individuals had nine times higher acetaldehyde levels in their saliva than in their blood.[88] This indicates that the origin for additional salivary acetaldehyde in ALDH2-deficiency can be located to the parotid gland and not to the blood.

The ADH of somatic cells is inhibited effectively by 4-methylpyrazole, but that of microbes is hardly affected. In line with this fact, 4-methylpyrazole decreased significantly salivary acetaldehyde concentration after alcohol drinking in ALDH2-deficient subjects but not at all in those with the normal ALDH2 enzyme.[89] This indicates that in general the major source of salivary acetaldehyde after alcohol drinking is the ADH-containing microbes representing normal oral flora.[89]

ALDH2-deficient Asian heavy drinkers form an exceptional human knockout model for long-term acetaldehyde exposure. Whenever they drink, they are exposed for hours afterwards to abnormally high levels of salivary acetaldehyde (Figure 22.2) and this is associated with a remarkably increased risk of digestive tract cancers (Table 22.5). In the light of the epidemiological data discussed before, the Asian human knockout model for deficient acetaldehyde oxidation proves that acetaldehyde produced from ethanol by oral microbes or salivary glands is a local and topical carcinogen in man. Since 30 to 50% of Asians do have a deficient ALDH2 enzyme, it can be estimated that the combination of the ALDH2-deficiency gene and heavy drinking exposes about 15 to 30 million people to the preventable cancer risk that exists only among Asian populations.

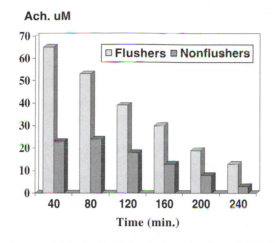

Ach. uM

Time (min.)

FIGURE 22.2 *In vivo* acetaldehyde (Ach) levels in oral saliva of ALDH2-deficient Asians (flushers) and of those with the normal ALDH2 enzyme (nonflushers) after a moderate dose of alcohol (0.5 g/kg body weight). (Adapted from Väkeväinen, S. et al., High salivary acetaldehyde after a moderate dose of alcohol in ALDH2-deficient subjects: Strong evidence for the local carcinogenic action of acetaldehyde, *Alcohol. Clin. Exp. Res.*, 24, 873, 2000.)

22.4 FUTURE PREVENTIVE STRATEGIES

Based on genetic, epidemiological, and biochemical evidence, it can be concluded that acetaldehyde derived from ethanol oxidation by microbes representing normal gut flora is a local and topical carcinogen in the digestive tract of not only the Asians but of all human beings. With regard to cancer prevention all mechanisms that may have an effect on the regulation of acetaldehyde concentration either in the saliva or intestinal contents are of crucial importance (Table 22.6). The message for prevention is that one should take care to maintain good oral hygiene and avoid smoking, heavy drinking, and drinking to intoxication. Future clinical studies are warranted to examine the possible role of topically administered acetaldehyde binding L-cysteine in cancer prevention.[90] Other topics of interest are to screen of possible microbes producing particularly effectively acetaldehyde from ethanol among cancer patients and to establish the role of nutritional factors, and pre- and probiotics in the regulation of acetaldehyde concentration in the saliva, gastric juice, and contents of the large intestine.

22.5 SUMMARY

Excessive alcohol consumption and heavy smoking are the main risk factors of upper digestive tract cancers. Cancer risk is dose-dependent and alcohol and smoking have synergistic effects. Alcohol is not carcinogenic. However, its first metabolite — acetaldehyde — has been shown to be a local carcinogen both in experimental animals and in man. Microbes representing normal human gut flora are able to produce acetaldehyde from ethanol. After alcohol drinking this results in high local

TABLE 22.6
Factors Having an Effect on the Concentration of Carcinogenic Acetaldehyde in Saliva, Gastric Juice, or in the Contents of Large Intestine

Factor	Effect on Acetaldehyde Concentration/Mechanism
Increasing alcohol concentration	Highly significant positive correlation between ethanol and acetaldehyde concentration in saliva (r = 0.95) and in the large intestine.[58,8]
Smoking	Salivary acetaldehyde production from ethanol increases, and this is associated with an increase in the number and quality of microbes producing acetaldehyde.[70]
Heavy drinking	Salivary acetaldehyde production from ethanol increases probably due to the induction of microbial enzymes.[70]
Poor oral hygiene	Salivary acetaldehyde production from ethanol increases and this is associated with an increase in the number and quality of microbes producing acetaldehyde.[71]
ALDH2-deficiency	Salivary acetaldehyde concentration after alcohol drinking increases *in vivo* since, in addition to microbes, parotid glands also produce acetaldehyde from alcohol.[88]
Rinsing of mouth with antiseptic chlorhexidine	Salivary acetaldehyde production from ethanol decreases due to the decrease in the number of oral microbes.[58]
L-cysteine tablet	Salivary acetaldehyde concentration after alcohol drinking decreases *in vivo* since L-cysteine binds acetaldehyde to a nonreactive derivative.[90]
Ciprofloxacin	Intracolonic acetaldehyde concentration after alcohol administration decreases *in vivo* and this is associated with a decrease of aerobic ADH-containing flora.[84–86]
Metronidazole	Intracolonic acetaldehyde concentration after alcohol administration increases *in vivo* and this is associated with an increase of aerobic ADH-containing flora.[86,91]
Disulfiram	Intracolonic acetaldehyde concentration after alcohol administration increases *in vivo* since colonic mucosal ALDH activity decreases.[92]
Drugs inhibiting gastric acid secretion	Acetaldehyde increases after alcohol drinking in the gastric juice and this is associated with the bacterial colonization of the stomach.[93]
Atrophic gastritis	Acetaldehyde increases in the gastric juice after alcohol drinking and this is associated with the bacterial colonization of the stomach.[79]

Data from Salaspuro, M., Microbial metabolism of ethanol and acetaldehyde and clinical consequences, *Addiction Biol.*, 2, 35, 1997; Homann, N., Alcohol and upper gastrointestinal tract cancer: the role of local acetaldehyde production, *Addiction Biol.*, 6, 309, 2001; Salaspuro, M., Acetaldehyde, microbes and cancer of the digestive tract, *Crit. Rev. Clin. Lab. Sci.*, 40, 183, 2003.

acetaldehyde concentrations in the saliva and contents of the large intestine. Most importantly, those environmental and hereditary factors that are associated with increased risk of digestive tract cancers are also factors that increase the local concentrations of carcinogenic acetaldehyde in human saliva. These include, for instance, smoking, heavy drinking, poor oral hygiene, and a hereditary deficiency of the acetaldehyde-metabolizing enzyme, aldehyde dehydrogenase (ALDH2). Due to this genetic deficiency to detoxify acetaldehyde, Asian heavy drinkers form an exceptional human knockout model for long-term acetaldehyde exposure. The risk of alcohol-related digestive tract cancers is particularly high among this population. The combined evidence derived from the epidemiological and biochemical studies strongly suggests that acetaldehyde produced locally in the digestive tract by microbes representing normal gut flora is a local and topical carcinogen. This opens a new microbiological approach to the pathogenesis of digestive tract cancer and may have an influence on future preventive strategies.

With regard to cancer prevention all mechanisms which have an effect on salivary or intracolonic acetaldehyde concentration are of importance. The message for prevention is that one should take care of good oral hygiene and avoid smoking, heavy drinking, and drinking to intoxication.

References

1. Doll, R. et al., Alcoholic beverages and cancers of the digestive tract and larynx, in *Health Issues Related to Alcohol Consumption*, 2nd ed., Macdonald, I., Ed., Bodmin, MPG Books, Cornwall, U.K., 1999, Appendix 1.
2. IARC. *Alcohol Drinking*, IARC monographs on the evaluation of the carcinogenic risk to humans, Lyon, WHO International Agency for Research on Cancer, Lyon, France, 1988, 44.
3. IARC. Acetaldehyde, in *Re-Evaluation of Some Organic Chemicals, Hydrazine and Hydrogen Peroxide*, IARC monographs on the evaluation of the carcinogenic risk to humans, WHO International Agency for Research on Cancer, Lyon, France 1999, 71, Part 2, p. 319.
4. Seitz, H.K. and Simanowski, U.A. Alcohol and carcinogenesis, *Annu. Rev. Nutr.*, 8, 99, 1988.
5. Seitz, H.K., Pöschl, G., and Simanowski, U.A., Alcohol and cancer, in *Galanter*, M. (Ed.), *Recent Developments in Alcoholism*, Plenum Press, New York, 1998, 14, p. 67.
6. Halsted, C.H., Robles, S.A., and Mezey, E., Distribution of ethanol in the human gastrointestinal tract, *Am. J. Clin. Nutr.*, 26, 831, 1973.
7. Jones, A.W., Distribution of ethanol between saliva and blood in man, *Clin. Exp. Pharmacol. Physiol.*, 6, 53, 1979.
8. Jokelainen, K. et al., High intracolonic acetaldehyde values produced by a bacterio-colonic pathway for ethanol oxidation in piglets, *Gut*, 39, 100, 1996.
9. Salaspuro, M., Microbial metabolism of ethanol and acetaldehyde and clinical consequences, *Addiction Biol.*, 2, 35, 1997.
10. Homann, N., Alcohol and upper gastrointestinal tract cancer: the role of local acetaldehyde production, *Addiction Biol.*, 6, 309, 2001.
11. Salaspuro, M., Acetaldehyde, microbes and cancer of the digestive tract, *Crit. Rev. Clin. Lab. Sci.* 40, 183, 2003.
12. Lamu, L., Etude de statistique clinique de 131 cas de cancer de l'oesophage et du cardia, *Arch. Malad. Appar. Diges. Malad. Nutr.*, 4, 451, 1910.
13. La Vecchia, C. et al., Epidemiology and prevention of oral cancer, *Oral Oncol.*, 33, 302, 1997.

14. Boffeta, P. and Garfinkel, L., Alcohol drinking and mortality among men enrolled in an American Cancer Society prospective study, *Epidemiology*, 1, 342, 1990.
15. Ng, S.K.C., Kabat, G.C., and Wynder, E.L., Oral cavity cancer in non-users of tobacco, *J. Nat. Cancer Inst.*, 85, 743, 1993.
16. Tavani, A. et al., Risk factors for oesophageal cancer in lifelong nonsmokers, *Cancer Epid. Biomark. Prev.*, 3, 387, 1994.
17. Tuyns, A.G., Oesophageal cancer in non-smoking drinkers and in non-drinking smokers, *Int. J. Cancer*, 32, 443, 1983.
18. Rothman, K. and Keller R., The effect of joint exposure of alcohol and tobacco on risk of cancer of the mouth and pharynx, *J. Chron. Dis.*, 25, 711, 1972.
19. Tuyns, A.J., Pequignot, G., and Jensen, O.M., Les cancers de l'oesophage an Ille-et-Villaine en fonction des niveaux de consommation d'alcool et de tabac, Des risques qui se multiplient, *Bull. Cancer*, 64, 45, 1977.
20. Castellasagué, X. et al., Independent and joint effects of tobacco smoking and alcohol drinking on the risk of esophageal cancer in men and women, *Int. J. Cancer*, 82, 657, 1999.
21. Lands, W.E.M., A review of alcohol clearance in humans, *Alcohol*, 15, 147, 1998.
22. Crabb, D.W. et al., Genotypes for aldehyde dehydrogenase deficiency and alcohol sensitivity. The inactive ALDH2*2 allele is dominant, *J. Clin. Invest.*, 83, 314, 1989.
23. Goedde, H.W. et al., Distribution of ADH2 and ALDH2 genotypes in different populations, *Hum. Gen.*, 88, 344, 1992.
24. Harada, S., Agarwal, D.P., and Goedde, H.W., Aldehyde dehydrogenase deficiency as cause of facial flushing reaction to alcohol in Japanese, *Lancet*, 2, 982, 1981.
25. Peng, G.S. et al., Involvement of acetaldehyde for full protection against alcoholism by homozygosity of the variant allele of mitochondrial aldehyde dehydrogenase gene in Asians, *Pharmacogenetics*, 9, 463, 1999.
26. Chen, C.C. et al., Interaction between the functional polymorphism of the alcohol-metabolism genes in protection against alcoholism, *Am. J. Hum. Gen.*, 65, 795, 1999.
27. Yokoyama, A. et al., Alcohol-related cancers and aldehyde dehydrogenase-2 in Japanese alcoholics, *Carcinogenesis*, 19, 1383, 1998.
28. Murata, M. et al., Genotype difference of aldehyde dehydrogenase 2 gene in alcohol drinkers influences the incidence of Japanese colorectal cancer patients, *Jpn. J. Cancer Res.*, 90, 711, 1999.
29. Bosron, W.F. and Li, T.K., Genetic polymorphism of human liver alcohol and aldehyde dehydrogenases, and their relationship to alcohol metabolism and alcoholism, *Hepatology*, 6, 502, 1986.
30. Coutelle, C. et al., Laryngeal and oropharyngeal cancer, and alcohol dehydrogenase 3 and glutathione S-transferase M1 polymorphism, *Hum. Gen.*, 99, 319, 1997.
31. Harty, L.C. et al., Alcohol dehydrogenase 3 genotype and risk of oral cavity and pharyngeal cancers, *J. Nat. Cancer Inst.* 89, 1698, 1997.
32. Bouchardy, C. et al., Role of alcohol dehydrogenase 3 and cytochrome P-4502E1 genotypes in susceptibility to cancers of the upper aerodigestive tract, *Int. J. Cancer*, 87, 734, 2000.
33. Olshan, A.F. et al., Risk of head and neck cancer and the alcohol dehydrogenase 3 genotype, *Carcinogenesis*, 22, 57, 2001.
34. Benhamou, E. et al., Incidence des cancers en France 1978–1982. INSERM, Paris, 1990.
35. Launoy, G. et al., Oesophageal cancer in France: potential importance of hot alcoholic drinks, *Int. J. Cancer*, 71, 917, 1997.

36. Wynder, E.L. et al., Environmental factors in cancer of upper alimentary tract: Swedish study with special reference to Plummer-Vinson (Paterson-Kelly) syndrome, *Cancer*, 10, 470, 1957.

37. Day, N.E., Some aspects of the epidemiology of esophageal cancer, *Cancer Res.*, 35, 3304, 1975.

38. Franceschi, S. and La Vecchia, C., Alcohol and the risk of cancers of the stomach and rectum, *Digest. Dis.*, 12, 276, 1994.

39. Kato, I., Tominaga, S., and Matsumoto, K., A prospective study of stomach cancer among a rural Japanese population: a 6-year survey, *Jpn. J. Cancer Res.*, 83, 568, 1992.

40. Kune, G.A. and Vitetta, L., Alcohol consumption and the etiology of colorectal cancer: a review of the scientific evidence from 1957 to 1991. *Nutr. Cancer*, 18, 97, 1992.

41. Longnecker, M.P. et al., A meta-analysis of alcoholic beverage consumption in relation to risk of colorectal cancer, *Cancer Causes Contrib.*, 1, 59, 1990.

42. Scheppach, W. et al., WHO Consensus statement on the role of nutrition in colorectal cancer, *Eur. J. Cancer Prev.*, 8, 57, 1999.

43. Hiriyama, T., Association between alcohol consumption and cancer of the sigmoid colon: observations from a Japanese cohort study, *Lancet*, ii, 725, 1989.

44. Winn, D.M. et al., Mouthwash use and oral conditions in the risk of oral and pharyngeal cancer, *Cancer Res.*, 51, 3044, 1991.

45. Salo, J.A., Ethanol-induced mucosal injury in rabbit oesophagus, *Scand. J. Gastroenterol.*, 18, 713, 1983.

46. Cohen, S.M. and Ellwein, L.B., Cell proliferation in carcinogenesis, *Science*, 249, 1007, 1990.

47. Blot, W.J., Alcohol and cancer, *Cancer Res. (Suppl.)*, 52, 2119, 1992.

48. Maier, H. et al., The effect of chronic ethanol consumption on salivary gland morphology and function in the rat, *Alcohol. Clin. Exp. Res.*, 10, 425, 1986.

49. Kaufman, S.E. and Kaye, M.D., Induction of gastrooesophageal reflux by alcohol. *Gut*, 18, 336–338, 1978.

50. Seitz, H.K., Alcohol effects on drug-nutrient interaction, *Drug Nutr. Interact.*, 4, 143, 1985.

51. Lieber, C.S., Microsomal ethanol oxidizing system (MEOS): the first 30 years (1968–1998) — a review, *Alcohol. Clin. Exp. Res.*, 23, 991, 1999.

52. He, S.M. and Lambert, B., Acetaldehyde-induced mutation at the hprt locus in human lymphocytes *in vitro*, *Environ. Mol. Mutagen,*. 16, 57, 1990.

53. Helander, A. and Lindahl-Kiessling, K., Increased frequency of acetaldehyde-induced sister chromatid exchanges in human lymphocytes treated with an aldehyde dehydrogenase inhibitor, *Mut. Res.,* 264, 103, 1991.

54. Obe, G., Jonas, R., and Schmidt, S., Metabolism of ethanol *in vitro* produces a compound which induces sister chromatid exchanges in human peripheral lymphocytes *in vitro*: acetaldehyde not ethanol is mutagenic, *Mut. Res.,* 174, 47, 1986.

55. Espina, N. et al., *In vitro* and *in vivo* inhibitory effect of ethanol and acetaldehyde on O^6-methylguanine transferase, *Carcinogenesis,* 9, 761, 1988.

56. Fang, J.L. and Vaca, C.E., Development of a 32P-postlabelling method for the analysis of adducts arising through the reaction of acetaldehyde with 2´-deoxyguanosine-3_-monophosphate and DNA, *Carcinogenesis*, 16, 2177, 1995.

57. Fang, J.L. and Vaca, C.E., Detection of DNA adducts of acetaldehyde in peripheral white blood cells of alcohol abusers, *Carcinogenesis*, 18, 627, 1997.

58. Homann, N. et al., High acetaldehyde levels in saliva after ethanol consumption: methodological aspects and pathogenetic implications, *Carcinogenesis*, 18, 1739, 1997.

59. Shaw, S. et al., Cleavage of folates during ethanol metabolism, *Biochem. J.*, 257, 277, 1989.

60. Homann, N., Tillonen, J., and Salapuro, M., Microbially produced acetaldehyde may increase the risk of colon cancer via folate deficiency, *Int. J. Cancer,* 86, 169, 2000.

61. Homann, N. et al., Effects of acetaldehyde on cell regeneration and differentiation of the upper gastrointestinal tract mucosa, *J. Nat. Cancer Inst.,* 89, 1692, 1997.

62. Woutersen, R.A. et al., Inhalation toxicity of acetaldehyde in rats. III. Carcinogenicity study, *Toxicology*, 41, 213, 1986.

63. Feron, V.J., Kruysse, A., and Woutersen, R.A., Respiratory tract tumours in hamsters exposed to acetaldehyde vapor alone or simultaneously to benzo(a)pyrene or dieth-ylnitrosamine, *Eur. J. Cancer. Clin. Oncol.*, 18, 13, 1982.

64. Koivisto, T. and Salaspuro, M., Effects of acetaldehyde on brush border enzyme activities in human colon adenocarcinoma cell line Caco-2, *Alcohol. Clin. Exp. Res.,* 21, 1599, 1997.

65. Koivisto, T. and Salaspuro, M., Acetaldehyde alters proliferation, differentiation and adhesion properties of human colon adenocarcinoma cell line Caco-2, *Carcinogenesis*, 19, 2031, 1998.

66. Salaspuro, V. et al., Ethanol oxidation and acetaldehyde production *in vitro* by human intestinal strains of *Escherichia coli* under aerobic, microaerobic and anaerobic conditions, *Scand. J. Gastroenterol.*, 34, 967, 1999.

67. Miyakawa, H. et al., Oxidation of ethanol to acetaldehyde by bronchopulmonary washings: role of bacteria, *Alcohol. Clin. Exp. Res.,* 10, 517, 1986.

68. Pikkarainen, P.H. et al., Contribution of oropharynx microflora and of lung microsomes to acetaldehyde in expired air after alcohol ingestion, *J. Lab. Clin. Med.,* 97, 631, 1981.

69. Baraona, E. et al., Role of intestinal bacterial overgrowth in ethanol production and metabolism in rats, *Gastroenterology*, 90, 103, 1986.

70. Homann, N. et al., Increased salivary acetaldehyde levels in heavy drinkers and smokers: a microbiological approach to oral cavity cancer, *Carcinogenesis,* 22, 663, 2000.

71. Homann, N. et al., Poor dental status increases the acetaldehyde production from ethanol in saliva: a possible link to the higher risk of oral cancer among alcohol-consumers, *Oral Oncol.*, 37, 153, 2001.

72. Holmstrup, P. and Besserman, M. Clinical, therapeutic and pathogenetic aspects of chronic oral multifocal candiasis, *Oral Surg. Oral Med. Oral Path.*, 56, 388, 1983.

73. Colman, G. et al., Cigarette smoking and the microbial flora of the mouth, *Aust. Dent. J.*, 21, 111, 1976.

74. Harris, C.K. et al., Oral health in alcohol misusers, *Comm. Dent. Health,* 13, 199, 1996.

75. Tillonen, J. et al., Role of yeasts in the salivary acetaldehyde production from ethanol among risk groups for ethanol-associated oral cavity cancer, *Alcohol. Clin. Exp. Res.,* 23, 1409, 1999.

76. Muto, M. et al., Acetaldehyde production by non-pathogenic *Neisseria* in human oral microflora: Implications for carcinogenesis in upper aerodigestive tract, *Int. J. Cancer,* 88, 342, 2000.

77. Morson, B.C. et al., Precancerous conditions and epithelial dysplasia in the stomach, *J. Clin. Pathol.*, 33, 711, 1980.

78. Stockbruegger, R.W. et al., Pernicious anaemia, intragastric bacterial overgrowth and possible consequences, *Scand. J. Gastroenterol.*, 19, 355, 1984.
79. Väkeväinen, S. et al., Ethanol-derived microbial production of carcinogenic acetaldehyde in achlorhydric atrophic gastritis, *Scand. J. Gastroenterol.*, 37, 648, 2002.
80. Seitz, H.K. et al., Possible role of acetaldehyde in ethanol-related rectal cocarcinogenesis in the rat, *Gastroenterology*, 98, 406, 1990.
81. Jokelainen, K. et al., *In vitro* acetaldehyde formation by human colonic bacteria, *Gut*, 35, 1271, 1994.
82. Yin, S.J. et al., Genetic polymorphism and activities of human colon alcohol and aldehyde dehydrogenases: no gender and age differences, *Alcohol. Clin. Exp. Res.*, 18, 1256, 1994.
83. Koivisto, T. and Salaspuro, M., Aldehyde dehydrogenases of rat colon: comparison with other tissues of the alimentary tract and the liver, *Alcohol. Clin. Exp. Res.*, 20, 551, 1996.
84. Jokelainen, K. et al., Inhibition of bacteriocolonic pathway for ethanol oxidation by ciprofloxacin in rats, *Life Sci.*, 61, 1755, 1997.
85. Tillonen, J. et al., Ciprofloxacin decreases the rate of ethanol elimination in humans, *Gut*, 44, 347, 1999.
86. Visapää, J.-P. et al., Inhibition of intracolonic acetaldehyde production and alcoholic fermentation in rats by ciprofloxacin, *Alcohol. Clin. Exp. Res.*, 22, 1161, 1998.
87. Yokoyama, A. et al., Multiple primary esophageal and concurrent upper aerodigestive tract cancer and aldehyde dehydrogenase-2 genotype of Japanese alcoholics, *Cancer*, 77, 1986, 1996.
88. Väkeväinen, S. et al., High salivary acetaldehyde after a moderate dose of alcohol in ALDH2-deficient subjects: strong evidence for the local carcinogenic action of acetaldehyde, *Alcohol. Clin. Exp. Res.*, 24, 873, 2000.
89. Väkeväinen, S. et al., 4-Methylpyrazole decreases salivary acetaldehyde levels in ALDH2-deficient subjects but not in subjects with normal ALDH2, *Alcohol. Clin. Exp. Res.*, 25, 829, 2001.
90. Salaspuro, V. et al., Removal of acetaldehyde from saliva by a slow-release buccal tablet of L-cysteine, *Int. J. Cancer*, 97, 361, 2002.
91. Tillonen, J. et al., Metronidazole increases intracolonic but not peripheral blood acetaldehyde in chronic ethanol-treated rats, *Alcohol Clin. Exp. Res.*, 24, 570, 2000.
92. Visapää, J.-P., Tillonen, J., and Salaspuro, M., Microbes and mucosa in the regulation of intracolonic acetaldehyde concentration during ethanol challenge, *Alcohol*, 37, 322, 2002.
93. Väkeväinen, S. et al., Hypochlorhydria induced by a proton pump inhibitor leads to intragastric microbial production of acetaldehyde from ethanol, *Aliment. Pharmacol. Ther.*, 14, 1511, 2000.

23 Mineral/Electrolyte-Related Diseases Induced by Alcohol

Ragnar Rylander

CONTENTS

23.1 INTRODUCTION

The normal functioning of the body is highly dependent on optimal concentrations of a variety of agents that have different chemical characteristics and take part in various cellular and other reactions. Examples of such groups of agents are antioxidants, vitamins, and trace metals. One group of agents of particular interest in connection with alcohol intake is composed of three important minerals acting as electrolytes. Potassium, magnesium, and calcium are of critical importance for the normal functioning of the body and a deficiency in either or all of them may lead to the development of symptoms and severe disease. They are influenced by alcohol in two ways: first, the intake of these minerals is often low among those consuming alcohol due to a deficient diet and, second, alcohol by itself influences the regulatory mechanisms for these minerals.

This chapter will initially give a brief description of the physiology of the three minerals, followed by information on how alcohol influences their homeostasis. Finally, it describes the different clinical diseases attributable to a deficiency of potassium, magnesium, and calcium. Some considerations on the public health impact will close the chapter.

23.2 THE ROLE OF MINERALS/ELECTROLYTES

A large number of minerals is known to be necessary for the body and its functions. In this context, we will focus on three of these in which a considerable increase in our knowledge has taken place during the last decades and in which the information is now so complete that it is well motivated from an ethical point of view to perform intervention trials in population groups which are deficient. Potassium, magnesium, and calcium, each by itself or in collaboration with one another, play pivotal roles in many of the basic functions of the body.

23.2.1 POTASSIUM

Potassium is mainly present intracellularly with 97% of the body burden in the cell cytosol. It is a regulator of cell function, particularly conductance in nerves, heart muscle, and skeletal muscle, and blood vessel smooth muscle. The intake is mainly through vegetables, bananas, fruit juices, and nuts.

The intracellular level is controlled by a complex regulatory mechanism involving aldosterone, angiotensin, insulin, and hormones. The excretion is proportional to the flow in the distal nephron, and persons with a high intake of fluid are thus at risk for depletion. Data suggest that the potassium balance is closely related to magnesium. In experimentally induced hypomagnesemia, there was a concomitant loss of potassium, and the effect of magnesium supplementation in deficient patients is improved if potassium is administered simultaneously.

Potassium deficiency causes tiredness, muscular weakness, and disturbances of the cardiac rhythm. Chronic acidosis, in contrast to acute, increases potassium loss by inhibiting proximal tubular sodium chloride and water reabsorption. The composition of modern food favors the development of acidosis. During prolonged exercise, potassium is released from skeletal muscle into the extracellular fluid and this condition may lead to cardiac arrhythmia and sudden death.

23.2.2 MAGNESIUM

In the body, about 99% of the magnesium is present intracellularly with half the amount in bone and high proportions in skeletal muscle and the heart. The proportion of free ionized magnesium is very low and serum levels are thus poor indicators of the body burden.

Magnesium is a cofactor in all enzymes involved in the phosphate transfer reactions that utilize ATP and other nucleotide triphosphates as substrates. It is involved in the regulation of cellular permeability through regulation of channel activity and neuromuscular excitability.

The major intake is through leafy green vegetables, whole grain cereals, beans, nuts, and shellfish. Intake through drinking water is physiologically important even if this contributes relatively little to the total intake.

The principal regulator of magnesium homeostasis is the kidney.[1] Reabsorption takes place in the nephron through transepithelial transport where magnesium-depleted cells provide the intrinsic control of the transport.[2] The transport is also partly regulated by magnesium/calcium sensors in the epithelial cells, and it has been shown that vitamin D plays a role in the regulation of the uptake.[3] Diuretics such as spironolactone and furosemide may influence the reabsorption.[4]

Magnesium deficiency will increase the risk for muscle-related pathological effects through the decreased reaction threshold and lead to cardiac muscle arrhythmia, tremor, ataxia, and nystagmus. There is also a risk for hypocalcemia. Low magnesium levels increase the reactivity of arteries to vasoconstrictor agents, attenuate responses to vasodilators, promote vasoconstriction, and increase peripheral resistance.[5]

23.2.3 CALCIUM

Calcium is the most common mineral in the body and comprises 1 to 2% of the body weight. More than 99% is present in the skeleton. Calcium is important for cell function, particularly signal transmission in the cell interior. Blood coagulation, blood vessel wall muscular tension, and skeletal muscle contraction are the most important physiological functions determined by calcium. The initial discoveries that calcium is required for muscular contractility were followed by research data showing its role in cell division, cellular motility, hormone secretion, neural activity, apoptosis, and many others.

Intake of calcium is via milk and other dairy products. Leafy green vegetables, particularly cabbage, are other important sources of calcium in food. Intake through drinking water is also of importance.

Calcium levels in the extracellular space are, in contrast to potassium and magnesium, 1000- to 10,000-fold higher, and the gradient across the cell wall is maintained by the aid of calcium pumps on the cell surface membrane. Calcium excretion is regulated through Na^+/K^+-ATPase activity in the proximal tubular cells and a decrease in this activity will lead to an increased excretion of calcium. A major part of the normal calcium secretion is through feces and the regulatory mechanisms of the gastrointestinal tract are thus important for calcium homeostasis. Bone calcium is regulated by parathyroid hormone activity. This hormone regulates plasma calcium levels through bone resorption, activating vitamin D that increases intestinal absorption and increases renal absorption.

Lack of calcium causes increased muscle and nerve excitability, and may cause muscular cramps and, in severe cases, tetanus. Hypercalciuria may also stimulate the production of parathyroid hormone, which would work to increase serum calcium levels, but also increases the blood pressure.

23.3 CLINICAL DISEASE RELATED TO POTASSIUM, MAGNESIUM, AND CALCIUM DEFICIENCY

23.3.1 THE CONCEPT OF SYNERGISM

The relation between a deficiency in potassium, magnesium, and calcium and clinical disease has also been evaluated in a number of clinical and epidemiological studies. Although these have often focused on one of the agents, it is becoming increasingly clear that the agents work in conjunction with one another and that no causality for a single agent is likely to be present. It has already been illustrated how the secretion of magnesium is followed by an increased secretion of potassium and, in cases where a pathological relation has been related to one agent, this is, in reality, present in a complex mixture of several compounds. It is thus not possible to draw conclusions regarding causality. Likewise, a number of intervention experiments have been reported with a small, if any, effect on the clinical parameter when one single agent such as magnesium is used. The effect is more often significant if a mixture of agents is given — for instance, a diet rich in fruit and vegetables.

In addition to the factors discussed, it has also been shown that the acid-base balance is important for the homeostasis of the minerals discussed. Due to a decreased ability to excrete acid and in combination with an increased, nutritional acid load, an increased general loss of minerals from the skeleton occurs with increasing age.[6] In view of the above, the effects of alcohol on potassium, magnesium, and calcium need to be considered jointly.

23.3.2 CARDIOVASCULAR DISEASE

There is abundant information that a deficiency in potassium, magnesium, or calcium is related to an increased risk for cardiovascular disease. The mechanisms behind cardiovascular disease comprise alterations in the blood vessel wall induced by blood vessel wall pathology, and muscular contractility related to blood pressure, and decreased muscle reaction threshold, related to arrhythmia. Increased blood pressure is a major risk factor for coronary heart disease, stroke, and kidney failure. An abnormal regulation of muscular tone and reaction threshold could thus be a pathophysiological phenomenon, contributing to the risk. The previously presented information on the cellular effects of deficiencies in potassium, magnesium, and calcium supports a hypothesis that these changes are important risk factors for cardiovascular and muscular disease.

Several studies have evaluated the importance of potassium, magnesium, and calcium for cardiovascular disease on a public health level. A number of ecological and cohort studies has been performed in different populations. In this context, reference will only be made to some of these studies as examples of the plethora of such studies available in the literature.

In a study from the U.S., data from a national health and nutrition study were used to assess the relation between potassium and cardiovascular disease in a population sample of 9805 persons.[7] Dietary potassium intake was determined using questionnaires over the period 1971 to 1992. The risk for stroke was significantly

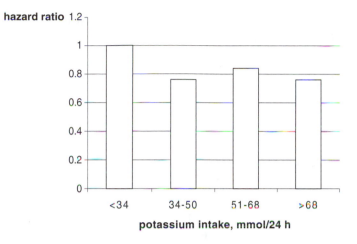

FIGURE 23.1 Risk for stroke in relation to intake of potassium in diet. (Modified from Bazzano, L.A. et al. Dietary potassium intake and risk of stroke in U.S. men and women. NHANES I Epidemiologic Follow-Up Study. *Stroke* 32, 1473–1480, 2001.)

and negatively related to the potassium intake although a dose–response relationship could not be found (Figure 23.1).

It has long been known that mortality from ischemic heart disease (IHD) is lower in areas with a higher hardness of the drinking water.[8,9] Many of the studies showed a relation between cardiovascular deaths and the drinking water level of either magnesium or calcium or both. In a case-control study from the south of Sweden, an inverse relation was found between magnesium in drinking water and death from acute myocardial infarction, and for females, also, between calcium and death.[10] Similar findings were reported in a previous study from the same area[11] (Figure 23.2) and in studies from Taiwan.[12,13] In a study using a U.S. population register, serum magnesium was inversely related to morbidity from ischemic heart disease.[14]

Although these and other studies on drinking water and cardiovascular disease have found relationships with magnesium, the real life exposure involves other minerals as well. In studies on the amount of minerals in different diets, a protective effect from diets rich in vegetables and fruit has been found. These dietary items also contain high amounts of several minerals.[15,16]

The relation between calcium and blood pressure is the subject of several studies and a meta-analysis has been published.[17] In this, 25 studies were analyzed and it was concluded that intake of calcium-rich food or calcium provided some evidence for an association but there was a severe lack of prospective studies.

A number of intervention studies have been performed to assess the effect of minerals for markers of cardiovascular disease. A meta-analysis of 33 studies on potassium intervention concluded that there might be a beneficial effect on blood pressure.[18] Several of the studies reviewed were, however, were dietary intervention studies, where the real intervention comprised several minerals and other agents.

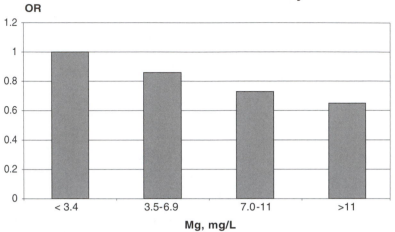

FIGURE 23.2 Relation between risk to die in myocardial infarction and drinking-water magnesium levels. (Modified from Rubenowitz, E., Axelsson, G., and Rylander, R., Magnesium and calcium in drinking water and death from acute myocardial infarction in women. *Epidemiology* 10, 31–36, 1999.)

Regarding single minerals, several studies have been reported where hypertensive persons were treated orally with nutritional doses of magnesium; a review has recently been published.[19] It was concluded that there was a suggestion of a dose-dependent reduction in blood pressure from the magnesium intervention but that the relationship had to be confirmed in larger studies, using higher doses of magnesium. The present information was not considered sufficient for clinical and treatment purposes. Patki et al.[20] found no effect of magnesium supplementation but a decrease in blood pressure after treatment with potassium. Two studies reported a very small effect of calcium supplementation.[21,22]

It has recently been shown in a group of 30 alcoholics that they had increased levels of vascular cell adhesion molecules, suggesting the presence of an inflammation.[23] This study is of particular interest as there is increasing insight that cardiovascular disease has a strong inflammatory component in its pathology.

23.3.3 OSTEOPOROSIS

Osteoporosis and the related fractures are a major health problem in Western countries. It has been estimated that the lifetime risk of a fracture exceeds 40% for women and 13% for men.[24] The osteoblastic activity in the bone is reduced, leading to a decreased rate of bone osteoid deposition. The disease is usually not related to a deficiency in calcium intake but to other underlying pathological conditions such as lack of estrogen secretion, vitamin C, and exercise. Some data suggest, however, that mineral intake may be important. An intervention trial with magnesium in osteoporotic women resulted in slower bone loss and fewer fractures.[25] An evaluation of the Framingham heart study in the U.S. based on 5209 males and females demonstrated an association between magnesium intake and bone mineral density in one hip site and the arm.[26] The general loss of minerals from the skeleton including calcium and magnesium due to the reduced ability to excrete acid among the elderly has been demonstrated.[6]

23.3.4 MIGRAINE AND TENSION HEADACHES

Migraine is a widespread suffering in different populations and causes a considerable use of drugs against pain. The underlying pathology has strong vascular and muscular components resulting in vasospasm. This may lead to ischemic exhaustion of smooth muscle contraction with loss of vascular tone. A similar pathology probably lies behind ordinary tension headaches.

Results from one intervention study demonstrated a decrease in duration and intensity of the attacks after supplementation with oral magnesium for 12 weeks.[27] Epidemiological studies on the intake of magnesium in food or water and the risk for migraine or intervention studies controlling for the supply in water or in food in relation to risk have not been performed. In one study with magnesium-rich water supplementation to migraine patients, an increase in intracellular magnesium was found after 2 weeks.[28]

23.4 EFFECTS OF ALCOHOL CONSUMPTION IN CLINICAL STUDIES

The effects of alcohol consumption on potassium, magnesium, and calcium have been studied in animal models and among alcoholic subjects. As stated previously, it is evident from these results that an increased secretion of one mineral is often accompanied by deficiencies in the others and often via the same mechanisms.[29]

The earliest studies on magnesium deficiency among consumers of alcohol were reported in 1936 and 1938.[30,31] Since then, numerous studies have demonstrated that intake of alcohol results in a deficit in potassium, magnesium, and calcium, and that the situation normalizes when alcohol intake ceases.[32] As an example in a study on 127 alcoholic patients, hypomagnesemia was the most common electrolyte disturbance.[33] These patients often had acid-base and electrolytic disturbances such as hypokalemia, hypocalcaemia, and respiratory alkalosis. Serum magnesium levels were correlated with potassium excretion.

As serum magnesium levels are a poor predictor of the body burden, several investigators have used a magnesium-loading test. In a study on 16 alcoholics with normal renal function, the test persons excreted less magnesium in the urine than a control group during 24 h after an intravenous administration of magnesium.[34] After a diet supplementation with magnesium-rich food, the excretion increased, suggesting an increased body burden of magnesium. In a study on regular consumers of alcohol who were not chronic alcoholics, an oral loading test with magnesium was performed.[35] After the loading test, the urinary excretion of magnesium and calcium was higher among persons consuming alcohol and was dose related to the amount consumed (Figure 23.3).

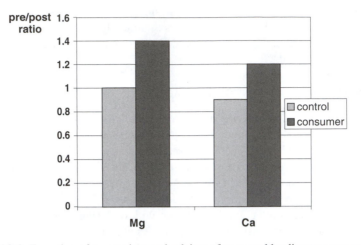

FIGURE 23.3 Excretion of magnesium and calcium after an oral loading test among controls and consumers of alcohol. (Modified from Rylander, R. et al. Moderate alcohol consumption and urinary excretion of magnesium and calcium. *Scand. J. Clin. Lab. Invest.* 61, 401–406, 2001.)

The reason for the increased secretion of these minerals after consumption of alcohol is probably a dysfunction of the renal tubuli.[36] This study investigated renal tubular function among 61 patients with chronic alcoholism and 42 control subjects with no or only minor consumption of alcohol. Among the alcoholics, there were significant decreases of maximal reabsorptive ability for glucose and increases in the fractional excretion of β_2-microglobulin in 38% of the patients. Other abnormalities were aminoaciduria and defects in tubular acidification. Glomerular filtration rates were not different between alcoholics and controls. After 4 weeks of abstinence, the pathological findings decreased.

There is also evidence that consumption of alcohol causes a deficiency in potassium and calcium. In a study on 127 alcoholics, serum potassium levels were found to be significantly lower than in a control group.[37] These patients also had hypomagnesemia and the authors suggested that this caused an opening of the potassium channels in the loop of Henle, increasing the excretion of potassium. In a study on 43 alcohol-intoxicated persons, serum calcium levels as well as magnesium levels were related to serum alcohol concentrations.[38]

A syndrome with coarse tremor of the hands and tongue, athetoid movements of the extremities, and convulsions has been described among a variety of conditions with severe magnesium deficiency.[39] It is also known that alcoholics suffer from muscular weakness, sometimes referred to as alcoholic myopathy.[4,40,41] This myopathy is independent from malnutrition and liver disease as well as from peripheral neuropathy. Apart from decreased muscle strength, there is also an increased blood level of muscle enzymes, reflecting the action of alcohol and its metabolite acetaldehyde on muscle protein synthesis.

Alcohol consumption interferes with the normal balance of minerals required for normal bone density. In addition, there are other factors possibly also related to alcohol consumption such as impaired parathyroid hormone secretion and reductions in vitamin D serum levels. Alcohol consumption thus probably increases the risk for osteoporosis.

23.5 PUBLIC HEALTH IMPLICATIONS

Changes in the way of life and the environment often have consequences that alter the risks for disease in the population. This is particularly clear concerning the intake of different nutrients in the daily diet. The supply of vital nutrients in food and water consumed in modern society is often inadequate. This problem is accentuated among the elderly, who often have an inadequate intake of nutrients, due to low food consumption in general or due to economical limitations regarding food purchase. A consensus statement from a group of European scientists reported that inadequate nutrition contributes to a loss of function and the development and progression of disease, and that adequate nutrition is not achieved by all groups of the elderly.[42]

From an ecological point of view, the inherent risk for disease due to changes in dietary habits in modern life is exemplified by an analysis of the intake of different nutrients in an evolutionary perspective. There are important differences in diet between Neolithic man and modern humans, based on evidence from archaeology and paleontology.[43] According to this study, the intake of fibers by modern humans is lower and the intake of fat higher than that of Neolithic man. Both these dietary items are highly related to risk for disease. Regarding minerals, the study reported that the intake of sodium for modern humans is higher whereas the intake of potassium, calcium, and magnesium is lower than for Neolithic man. Thus the ecological changes in intake of nutrients brought about by civilization and urbanization comprise deficiencies in the natural nutrition that may constitute a risk for negative health effects. Another example is the source of drinking water. Most of the supply of drinking water in ancient times was from wells, which often had a high content of different minerals. With urbanization and the increasing consumption of water, surface water is nowadays the most important source, meaning that the population consumes water with very low levels of minerals.

The third critical change in the way of life of particular interest in this context is the consumption of distilled alcohol. This was introduced around the turn of the first millennium and became particularly widespread among the populations in the temperate regions of the northern hemisphere. In ancient civilizations such as those of the South American Indians, wine was known but only used in connection with religious ceremonies, chiefly by the priests. The introduction of "social drinking," a habit that is also spreading into the young age groups, is thus a new phase of our adaptation to a lifestyle that implies severe risks for health effects.

The previous review of diseases related to a suboptimal content of potassium, magnesium, and calcium in the body has demonstrated that the health effects are extensive. From a public health point of view, it is thus highly relevant to perform prevention programs directed against factors that cause these deficiencies.

Regarding alcohol, most of the studies on potassium, magnesium, and calcium have been performed on persons with a high intake. From a research point of view, this is relevant as the effects are most pronounced at the upper end of the dose scale.

It must be remembered, though, that alcohol acts as a poison and that poisons exhibit dose–response relationships. It is thus conceivable that the same effects as studied among the extreme consumers will be present, albeit less severe, also among persons consuming less alcohol. Evidence for such dose–response relationships has been published[35,38] and implies that society is dealing with a potential health problem that is more widespread than that revealed by investigations on alcoholics only.

For prevention purposes, apart from the limitation of alcohol consumption, which is an obvious conclusion, there should also be further research and preventive efforts concerning the role of dietary intakes, including drinking water, and possibly the intervention with tablets and/or waters rich in minerals. In this context, it is of value to identify groups at risk, which would be those with a low intake of the minerals as well as those with a high intake of alcohol, affecting the homeostasis of the compounds.

References

1. Quamme, G.A. and de Rouffignac, C. Epithelial magnesium transport and regulation by the kidney. *Front. Biosci.* 5, D694–D711, 2000.
2. Stegman, W. and Quamme, G.A. Determination of epithelial magnesium transport with stable isotopes. *J. Pharmacol. Toxicol. Methods* 43, 177–182, 2000.
3. Ritchie, G. et al. 1,25(OH)$_2$D$_3$ stimulates Mg^{2+} uptake into MDCT cells: modulation by extracellular Ca $^{2+}$ and Mg^{2+}. *Am. J. Physiol. Renal. Physiol.* 280, F868–F878, 2001.
4. Aagaard, N.K. et al. Muscle strength, NA-K-pumps, magnesium and potassium in patients with alcoholic liver cirrhosis — relation to spironolactone. *J. Intern. Med.* 252, 56–63, 2002.
5. Touyz, R.M. et al. Effects of low dietary magnesium intake on development of hypertension in stroke-prone spontaneously hypertensive rats: role of reactive oxygen species. *J. Hypertens.* 20, 2221–2232, 2002.
6. Frassetto, L. et al. Diet, evolution and aging. *Eur. J. Nutr.* 40, 200–213, 2001.
7. Bazzano, L.A. et al. Dietary potassium intake and risk of stroke in US men and women. NHANES I Epidemiologic Follow-Up Study. *Stroke* 32, 1473–1480, 2001.
8. Rylander, R. Environmental magnesium deficiency as a cardiovascular risk factor. *J. Cardiovasc. Risk* 3, 4–10, 1996.
9. Marx, A. and Neutra, R.R. Magnesium in drinking water and ischaemic heart disease. *Epidemiol. Rev.* 19, 258–272, 1997.
10. Rubenowitz, E., Axelsson, G., and Rylander, R. Magnesium and calcium in drinking water and death from acute myocardial infarction in women. *Epidemiology* 10, 31–36, 1999.
11. Rubenowitz, E., Axelsson, G., and Rylander, R. Magnesium in drinking water and death from acute myocardial infarction. *Am. J. Epidemiol.* 143, 456–462, 1996.
12. Yang, C.Y. and Chiu, H.F. Calcium and magnesium in drinking water and the risk of death from hypertension. *Am. J. Hypertens.* 12, 894–899, 1999.
13. Young, D.B, Lin, H., and McCabe, R.D. Potassium's cardiovascular protective mechanisms. *Am. J. Physiol.* 268, R825–R837, 1995.
14. Ford, E.S. Serum magnesium and ischaemic heart disease: findings from a national sample of US adults. *Int. J. Epidemiol.* 28, 645–651, 1999.

15. McCarron, D.A. and Reusser, M.E. Are low intakes of calcium and potassium important causes of cardiovascular disease? *Am. J. Hypertens.* 14, 206S–212S, 2001.

16. Fang, J., Madhavan, S., and Alderman, M.H. Dietary potassium intake and stroke mortality. *Stroke* 31, 1532–1537, 2000.

17. Cutler, J.A. and Brittain, E., Calcium and blood pressure. An epidemiologic perspective. *Am. J. Hypertens.* 3, 137S–146S, 1990.

18. Whelton, P.K. et al. Effects of oral potassium on blood pressure. Meta-analysis of randomized controlled clinical trials. *JAMA* 277, 1624–1632, 1997.

19. Jee, S.H. et al. The effect of magnesium supplementation on blood pressure: a meta-analysis of randomized clinical trials. *Am. J. Hypertens.* 15, 691–696, 2002.

20. Patki, P.S. et al. Efficacy of potassium and magnesium in essential hypertension: a double blind, placebo controlled, crossover study. *BMJ* 301, 521–523, 1990.

21. Bucher, H.C. et al. Effects of dietary calcium supplementation on blood pressure. a meta-analysis of randomized controlled trials. *JAMA* 275, 1016–1022, 1996.

22. Cappucio, F.P., Siani, A., and Strazzullo, P. Oral calcium supplementation and blood pressure: an overview of randomized trials. *J. Hypertens.* 7, 941–946, 1989.

23. Sacanella, E. et al. Chronic alcohol consumption increases serum levels of circulating endothelial cell/leukocyte adhesion molecules E-selectin and ICAM-1. *Alcohol Alcohol.* 34, 678–684, 1999.

24. Kanis, J. WHO study group. Assessment of fracture risk and its applications to screening for postmenopausal osteoporosis: synopsis of a WHO report. *Osteoporosis Int.* 4, 368–381, 1994.

25. Stendig-Lindberg, G., Tepper, R., and Leichter, I. Trabecular bone density in a two-year controlled trial of per oral magnesium in osteoporosis. *Magnes. Res.* 6, 155–163, 1993.

26. Tucker, K.L. et al. Potassium, magnesium, and fruit and vegetable intakes are associated with greater bone mineral density in elderly men and women. *Am. J. Clin. Nutr.* 69, 727–736, 1999.

27. Peikert, A., Wilimzig, C., and Köhne-Volland, R. Prophylaxis of migraine with oral magnesium: results from a prospective, multi-center, placebo-controlled and double-bland randomised study. *Cephalagia* 16, 257–263, 1996.

28. Thomas, J. et al. Free and total magnesium in lymphocytes of migraine patients — effect of magnesium-rich mineral water intake. *Clin. Chim. Acta* 295, 63–75, 2000.

29. Elisaf, M. et al. Hypokalaemia in alcoholic patients. *Drug Alcohol Rev.* 21, 73–76, 2002.

30. Cline, W.B. and Coleman, J.B. The treatment of delirium tremens. *JAMA* 107, 404, 1936.

31. Nicholson, W.M. and Taylor, H.M. The effect of alcohol on water and electrolyte balance in man. *J. Clin. Invest.* 17, 279–283, 1938.

32. Shane, S.R. and Flink, E.B. Magnesium deficiency in alcohol addiction and withdrawal. *Magnes. Trace Elem.* 92, 10: 263–268, 1991.

33. Elisaf, M., Merkouropoulos, M., and Tsianos, E.V. Pathogenetic mechanisms of hypomagnesemia in alcoholic patients. *J. Trace Elem. Med. Biol.* 9, 210–214, 1995.

34. Bohmer, T. and Mathiesen, B. Magnesium deficiency in chronic alcoholic patients by an intravenous loading test. *Scand. J. Clin. Lab. Invest.* 42, 633–636, 1982.

35. Rylander, R. et al. Moderate alcohol consumption and urinary excretion of magnesium and calcium. *Scand. J. Clin. Lab. Invest.* 61, 401–406, 2001.

36. De Marchi, S. et al. Renal tubular dysfunction in chronic alcohol abuse — effects of abstinence. *N. Engl. J. Med.* 329, 1927–1934, 1993.

37. Elisaf, M. et al. Hypokalaemia in alcoholic patients. *Drug Alcohol Rev.* 21, 73–76, 2002.
38. Petroianu, A. et al. Acute effects of alcohol ingestion on the human serum concentrations of calcium and magnesium. *J. Int. Med. Res.* 19, 410–413, 1991.
39. McCollister, R.J., Flink, E.B., and Lewis M. Urinary excretion of magnesium in man following ingestion of ethanol. *Am. J. Clin. Nutr.* 12, 415–420, 1963.
40. Preedy, V.R. et al. Alcoholic skeletal muscle myopathy: definitions, features, contribution of neuropathy, impact and diagnosis. *Eur. J. Neurol.* 8, 677–687, 2001.
41. Sacanella, E. et al. Chronic alcoholic myopathy: diagnostic clues and relationship with other ethanol-related diseases. *Occup. J. Med.* 88, 811–817, 1995.
42. Bates, C.J. et al. Nutrition and aging: a consensus statement. *J. Nutr. Health Ageing* 6, 103–116, 2002.
43. Eaton, S.B., Konner, M., and Shostak, M. Stone ages in the fast lane: chronic degenerative diseases in evolutionary perspective. *Am. J. Med.* 84, 739–749, 1988.

Index

A

acetaldehyde, 399
  carcinogen, 400
  microbial acetaldehyde formation in the
      large intestine, 403
  saliva, 401
  stomach, 403
  translational control, 131
alcohol abuse, 80
  alcohol and body fat, 371
  BMI, 370
  malnutrition, survival, 10
  mortality, 90
  nondrinkers, 372
  weight gain adiposity, 368
  weight gain, 372
alcohol consumption, pattern of, 92–93
  beverage, 92, 398
  high-risk groups, 94
  mechanisms, 93
alcoholic beverage cardiovascular disease,
    22
  chlorogenic acid, 32
  homocysteine, 31
alcoholic muscle disease, 275
alcoholic pancreatitis, 8
alcohol intake in dietary surveys, 206
  Belgian Interuniversity Research on
      Nutrition and Health, 212
  consumption worldwide, 202
  HANES I, 208
  serum gamma-glutamyltransferase, 207
  total energy intake, 214
alcohol levels metabolism of nutrients, 46
alcohol metabolism, 173, 192
  ADH and ALDH polymorphisms, 193
  alcohol dehydrogenase, 174, 188
  alcohol metabolizing enzymes, 188
aldehyde dehydrogenases, 178, 190

nomenclature, 189
alcohol pro-oxidant, 29
ALDH2 activity,180
  ALDH2 deficiency, 395
angiotensin-converting enzyme gene
      polymorphism, 133
animal models of alcohol, 270
  cerebrovascular spasms, 346
  Kupffer cells, 345
  pair-feeding, 270
  red and white wine, 350
  vitamin E, 345, 347
antioxidants lipid peroxidation, 51
apoptosis, 275, 317
  apoptosis, alcohol-induced, 132
  cell death, 157
  transactivation, 318
  unregulated cell proliferation, 318
arachidonic acid, 249
  arachidonate supplement in alcoholics,
    256
  arachidonic acid supplement, 251
  fatty acid, 250
  liver phospholipids, 253
  liver tissue, 254–255
  liver triglyceride, 252
  prostanoid, 255
  serum alanine aminotransferase, 252
arrhythmias, 117
  alcohol intoxication, 118
  arterial fibrillation, 119
atherogenesis, 109
atherosclerosis, 108

B

betaine, 61
beverage, 106
blood lipids CHD, 324
  blood lipids, 325

425